Head and Neck Oncology

Cancer Treatment and Research

WILLIAM L MCGUIRE, *series editor*

Livingston RB (ed): Lung Cancer 1. 1981. ISBN 90-247-2394-9.
Bennett Humphrey G, Dehner LP, Grindey GB, Acton RT (eds): Pediatric Oncology 1. 1981.
ISBN 90-247-2408-2.
DeCosse JJ, Sherlock P (eds): Gastrointestinal Cancer 1. 1981. ISBN 90-247-2461-9.
Bennett JM (ed): Lymphomas 1, including Hodgkin's Disease. 1981. ISBN 90-247-2479-1.
Bloomfield CD (ed): Adult Leukemias 1. 1982. ISBN 90-247-2478-3.
Paulson DF (ed): Genitourinary Cancer 1. 1982. ISBN 90-247-2480-5.
Muggia FM (ed): Cancer Chemotherapy 1. ISBN 90-247-2713-8.
Bennett Humphrey G, Grindey GB (eds): Pancreatic Tumors in Children. 1982. ISBN 90-247-2702-2.
Costanzi JJ (ed): Malignant Melanoma 1. 1983. ISBN 90-247-2706-5.
Griffiths CT, Fuller AF (eds): Gynecologic Oncology. 1983. ISBN 0-89838-555-5.
Greco AF (ed): Biology and Management of Lung Cancer. 1983. ISBN 0-89838-554-7.
Walker MD (ed): Oncology of the Nervous System. 1983. ISBN 0-89838-567-9.
Higby DJ (ed): Supportive Care in Cancer Therapy. 1983. ISBN 0-89838-569-5.
Herberman RB (ed): Basic and Clinical Tumor Immunology. 1983. ISBN 0-89838-579-2.
Baker LH (ed): Soft Tissue Sarcomas. 1983. ISBN 0-89838-584-9.
Bennett JM (ed): Controversies in the Management of Lymphomas. 1983. ISBN 0-89838-586-5.
Bennett Humphrey G, Grindey GB (eds): Adrenal and Endocrine Tumors in Children. 1983.
ISBN 0-89838-590-3.
DeCosse JJ, Sherlock P (eds): Clinical Management of Gastrointestinal Cancer. 1984.
ISBN 0-89838-601-2.
Catalona WJ, Ratliff TL (eds): Urologic Oncology. 1984. ISBN 0-89838-628-4.
Santen RJ, Manni A (eds): Diagnosis and Management of Endocrine-related Tumors. 1984.
ISBN 0-89838-636-5.
Costanzi JJ (ed): Clinical Management of Malignant Melanoma. 1984.
ISBN 0-89838-656-X.
Wolf GT (ed): Head and Neck Oncology. 1984. ISBN 0-89838-657-8.

Head and Neck Oncology

edited by

GREGORY T. WOLF
Department of Otolaryngology
Head and Neck Surgery Division
University of Michigan
Ann Arbor, Michigan, USA

RC 280
H4
H388
1984

1984 **MARTINUS NIJHOFF PUBLISHERS**
a member of the KLUWER ACADEMIC PUBLISHERS GROUP
BOSTON / DORDRECHT / LANCASTER

Distributors

for the United States and Canada: Kluwer Academic Publishers, 190 Old Derby Street, Hingham, MA 02043, USA

for the UK and Ireland: Kluwer Academic Publishers, MTP Press Limited, Falcon House, Queen Square, Lancaster LA1 1RN, England

for all other countries: Kluwer Academic Publishers Group, Distribution Center, P.O. Box 322, 3300 AH Dordrecht, The Netherlands

Library of Congress Cataloging in Publication Data

```
Main entry under title:

Head and neck oncology.

   (Cancer treatment and research)
   Includes index.
   1. Head--Cancer--Treatment.  2. Neck--Cancer--
Treatment.  I. Wolf, Gregory T.  II. Series.  [DNLM:
1. Head and Neck Neoplasms--therapy.  W1 CA693 / WE 707
H4319]
RC280.H4H388  1984      616.99'49106      84-6129
ISBN 0-89838-657-8
```

ISBN 0-89838-657-8 (this volume)

Contents

Part III – Advances in chemotherapy and immunotherapy

Cancer Treatment and Research

Foreword

Where do you begin to look for a recent, authoritative article on the diagnosis or management of a particular malignancy? The few general oncology textbooks are generally out of date. Single papers in specialized journals are informative but seldom comprehensive; these are more often preliminary reports on a very limited number of patients. Certain general journals frequently publish good in-depth reviews of cancer topics, and published symposium lectures are often the best overviews available. Unfortunately, these reviews and supplements appear sporadically, and the reader can never be sure when a topic of special interest will be covered.

Cancer Treatment and Research is a series of authoritative volumes which aim to meet this need. It is an attempt to establish a critical mass of oncology literature covering virtually all oncology topics, revised frequently to keep the coverage up to date, easily available on a single library shelf or by a single personal subscription.

We have approached the problem in the following fashion. First, by dividing the oncology literature into specific subdivisions such as lung cancer, genitourinary cancer, pediatric oncology, etc. Second, by asking eminent authorities in each of these areas to edit a volume on the specific topic on an annual or biannual basis. Each topic and tumor type is covered in a volume appearing frequently and predictably, discussing current diagnosis, staging, markers, all forms of treatment modalities, basic biology, and more.

In Cancer Treatment and Research, we have an outstanding group of editors, each having made a major commitment to bring to this new series the very best literature in his or her field. Martinus Nijhoff Publishers has made an equally major committment to the rapid publication high quality books, and worldwide distribution.

Where can you go to find quickly a recent authoritative article on any major oncology problem? We hope that Cancer Treatment and Research provides an answer.

WILLIAM L. MCGUIRE
Series Editor

Preface

The effectiveness of conventional surgery or radiation therapy in curing patients with squamous carcinoma of the head and neck is well established. Single modality treatment strategies employing surgery or radiation therapy for small, locally confined tumors have resulted in 5-year survival rates of 70–90%. In patients with extensive primary tumors or regional metastases, however, the 5-year survival rates range from 0–60%. Combinations of surgery and radiation in patients with advanced tumors have not significantly improved the generally poor overall survival rates achieved with surgery alone. This has been attributed to failures in the control or prevention of distant metastases despite occasional reductions in local recurrence rates and prolongation of disease-free interval.

These grim statistics combined with the severe functional and cosmetic disabilities associated with treatment have stimulated clinical and basic science research efforts directed at refining established treatment methods and exploring innovative treatment strategies for patients with advanced head and neck cancer. Although those activities have principally involved conventional treatment modalities of surgery and radiation therapy, considerable recent interest has been evident in defining the role of adjuvant chemotherapeutic and immunotherapeutic approaches. The objectives of these research efforts have been to decrease the functional and cosmetic disability associated with head and neck cancer therapy, improve rehabilitation and increase survival rates. Progress in rehabilitation has been evident while little improvement has been demonstrated thus far in survival statistics. The current volume reviews areas of head and neck oncology where progress is evident and areas where new approaches hold promise for significantly improving treatment results. Recent experiences with the management of regional metastases, soft tissue reconstruction, vocal rehabilitation and tumors of the paranasal sinuses and skull base are described in detail. Advances in radiation therapy with the use of newer particles, radiation sensitizers and hyperthermia are described. Finally, the current status of adjuvant chemotherapy and immunotherapy is reviewed. It is hoped that the broad scope of this volume will provide an overview of advances in treatment and research that will be useful across the multiple disciplines involved in the care of patients with head and neck cancer. Exchange of information and intellectual cross-fertilization among the various disciplines will undoubtedly enhance the development of future research efforts and ultimately translate into clinical benefit for patients with head and neck cancer.

GREGORY T. WOLF

List of contributors

Shan R. Baker, M.D., F.A.C.S.
Department of Otolaryngology – Head and
   Neck Surgery
University of Michigan Medical Center
Ann Arbor, Michigan, USA

Pierre Bataini, M.D.
Department of Radiotherapy
Institut Curie
Paris, France

Jürgen Bier, M.D.
Department for Dental, Oral, Maxillofacial
   and Plastic Surgery of the Face –
   Head & Neck Oncology
Rhenish – Westphalian Technical Universi-
   ty
Aachen, Federal Republic of Germany

Eric D. Blom, M.D.
Head and Neck Surgery Associates
Indianapolis, Indiana, USA

Giulio Cantù, M.D.
Oncologia Clinica C
Istituto Nazionale Tumori
Milan, Italy

Fausto Chiesa, M.D.
Oncologia Clinica C
Istituto Nazionale Tumori
Milan, Italy

C. Norman Coleman, M.D.
Division of Radiation Therapy and Medi-
   cal Oncology
Stanford University School of Medicine
Stanford, Michigan, USA

Aurora Costa, M.D.
Oncoologia Sperimentale C
Istituto Nazionale Tumori
Milan, Italy

J.B. Dubois, M.D.
Department of Radiotherapy
Centre Paul Lamarque
Montpellier, France

Mario R. Eisenberger, M.D.
Cancer Therapy Evaluation Program
Division of Cancer Treatment
National Cancer Institute
Bethesda, Maryland 20205, USA

Nemetallah A. Ghossein, M.D.
Director of Radiotherapy
Albert Einstein College of Medicine
Bronx, New York, USA

Malcolm D. Graham, M.D.
Department of Otolaryngology – Head and
   Neck Surgery
University of Michigan Medical Center
Ann Arbor, Michigan, USA

Thomas W. Griffin, M.D.
Department of Radiation Oncology
University of Washington School of Medicine
Seattle, Washington, USA

Ronald C. Hamaker, M.D., F.A.C.S.
Head and Neck Surgery Associates
Indianapolis, Indiana, USA

Waun Ki Hong, M.D.
Medical Oncology Section
Boston Veterans Administration Medical Center
Boston, Massachusetts, USA

Daniel F. Hoth, M.D.
Cancer Therapy Evaluation Program
Division of Cancer Treatment
National Cancer Institute
Bethesda, Maryland, USA

Charlotte Jacobs, M.D.
Department of Medicine/Oncology
Stanford University Medical Center
Stanford, California, USA

Michael E. Johns, M.D.
Department of Otolaryngology –
Head and Neck Surgery,
Johns Hopkins Hospital,
Baltimore, Maryland, USA

Mary Johnson, Ph.D.
Division of Biometrics
Food and Drug Administration
Washington, D.C., USA

Michael J. Kaplan, M.D.
University of Virginia Medical Center
Charlottesville, Virginia, USA

John L. Kemink, M.D.
Department of Otolaryngology – Head and Neck Surgery
University of Michigan Medical Center
Ann Arbor, Michigan, USA

Stephen J. Kleinschuster, Ph.D.
College of Live Sciences and Agriculture
Agriculture Experimental Station
University of New Hampshire
Durham, New Hampshire, USA

Padmakar P. Lele, M.D., D.Phil.
Harvard M.I.T. Health Sciences Program
Massachusetts Institute of Technology
Cambridge, Massachusetts, USA

Robert Makuch, Ph.D.
Biostatistics and Data Management Section
Division of Cancer Treatment
National Cancer Institute
Washington, D.C., USA

Franco Mattavelli, M.D.
Oncologia Clinica C
Istituto Nazionale Tumori
Milan, Italy

Peter E. Maxim, Ph.D.
Senior Scientist
CooperBiomedical, Inc.
Malvern, Pennsylvania, USA

Roberto Molinari, M.D.
Head and Neck Oncology Department
Istituto Nazionale Tumori
Milan, Italy

Juan G. Posada, M.D.
Cancer Therapy Evaluation Program
Division of Cancer Treatment
National Cancer Institute
Bethesda, Maryland, USA

James D. Popkin, M.D.
Medical Oncology Section
Boston Veterans Administration Medical Center
Clinical Assistant Professor of Otolaryngology
Boston University School of Medicine
Boston, Massachusetts, USA

Joost Ruitenberg, Ph.D.
National Institute of Public Health
Bilthoven, the Netherlands

David E. Schuller, M.D.
Department of Otolaryngology
Ohio State University
Columbus, Ohio, USA

Stanley M. Shapshay, M.D.
Department of Otolaryngology
Lahey Medical Center
Boston, Massachusetts, USA

Rosella Silvestrini, M.D.
Oncologia Sperimentale C
Istituto Nazionale Tumori
Milan, Italy

Mark I. Singer, M.D., F.A.C.S.
Head and Neck Surgery Associates
Indianapolis, Indiana, USA

James Y. Suen, M.D.
Department of Otolaryngology and Maxil-
    lofacial Surgery
University   of   Arkansas   for   Medical
    Sciences
Little Rock, Arkansas, USA

Robert W. Veltri, Ph.D.
Director of Research and Development

CooperBiomedical, Inc.
Malvern, Pennsylvania, USA

Fabio Volterrani, M.D.
Istituto di Scienze Radiologiche
University of Milan
Milan, Italy

Todd H. Wasserman, M.D.
Department of Radiology
Mallinckrodt Institute of Radiology
Washington University School of Medi-
    cine
St. Louis, Missouri, USA

Stephen Wetmore, M.D.
Department of Otolaryngology and Maxil-
    lofacial Surgery
University   of   Arkansas   for   Medical
    Sciences
Little Rock, Arkansas, USA

Richard Wheeler, M.D.
University of Alabama at Birmingham
Comprehensive Cancer Center
Birmingham, Alabama, USA

Gregory T. Wolf, M.D.
Department of Otolaryngology – Head and
    Neck Surgery
University of Michigan Medical Center
Ann Arbor, Michigan, USA

1. Clinical management of regional metastases

STEPHEN J. WETMORE and JAMES Y. SUEN

Introduction

The presence of metastatic disease in the neck is a major factor in determining survival of patients with malignant neoplasms of the head and neck
and is at least as important, if not more so, as the size of the primary
lesion.

Incidence

The incidence of cervical metastases in patients with head and neck cancer
varies depending on primary site, from as low as 1% for T_1 glottic cancers [1] to as high as 80% for nasopharyngeal cancer [2]. Malignancies arising in the nasopharynx, oropharynx, or hypopharynx have a high metastatic
rate, ranging from 50% to 80%. The high incidence of cervical metastases in
these sites results from a combination of factors, including the rich lymphatic supply to the pharynx and the difficulty of examining these areas, which
often causes delayed diagnosis and, consequently, advanced disease at time
of diagnosis.

In previously untreated patients, the pattern of metastatic spread to the
neck is very predictable. Nasopharyngeal carcinomas usually spread initially
to the non-palpable retropharyngeal nodes and then to the nodes of the
jugulodigastric-upper posterior cervical triangle areas (Fig. 1). From there,
metastases proceed along the deep jugular chain in the anterior cervical
triangle or along the spinal accessory chain in the posterior cervical triangle.
Oropharyngeal cancers usually metastasize to the jugulodigastric nodes and
then inferiorly along the deep jugular chain [3]. Anterior oral cavity lesions
usually spread to submental or submandibular sites. Laryngeal and hypopharyngeal carcinomas metastasize to the upper or midjugular nodes.

Bilateral cervical metastases occur more frequently with large primary

Gregory T. Wolf (ed), Head and Neck Oncology.
© *1984 Martinus Nijhoff Publishers, Boston. ISBN 0-89838-657-8. Printed in The Netherlands.*

2

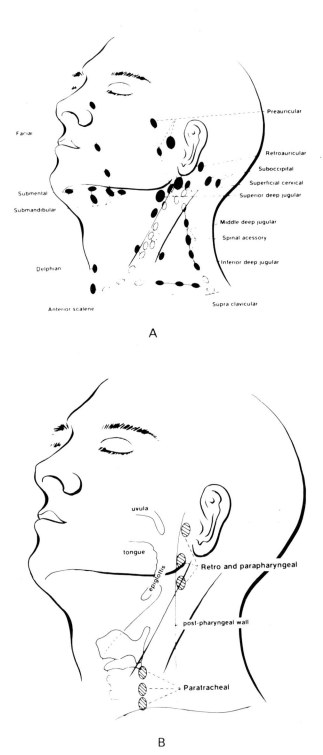

Figure 1. Cervical lymph nodes.

tumors or tumors that are close to the midline of the neck. The highest incidence of bilateral metastases (40%) is seen with nasopharyngeal carcinomas [2]. However, while it is unusual to see cervical metastases skip nodes in previously untreated patients, the usual pattern of metastases may be altered following surgery or radiotherapy.

Evaluation

Palpation is the primary method of evaluating the neck for metastatic disease. Many studies [4–7] have confirmed the inaccuracies of palpation, with the incidence of clinical false negatives ranging from 20% to 56%. Even when diagnosing the node on palpation as clinically positive for involvement, frequently the extent of disease is inaccurately estimated.

Computerized tomography (C.T. scanning) that is used primarily to determine the extent of disease in areas such as the pterygopalatine a fossa, infratemporal fossa, and parapharyngeal space that are difficult to assess by direct visualization or palpation, may also be useful to diagnose cervical node metastases and to assess the resectability of large neck masses [8]. C.T. scanning appears to be more accurate than palpation in diagnosing occult neck nodes [9].

When the primary site of a malignancy has been identified, it is biopsied and the palpable neck nodes are assumed to represent metastases. When the primary malignancy is not identified or when recurrent disease in the neck is suspected, a needle biopsy may be considered. Although the role of the needle biopsy is still somewhat controversial, needle biopsies are being used with increasing frequency. The classic large bore needle biopsy provides a core of tissue for histologic examination but has the disadvantages of possible seeding of the needle tract with tumor and of missing a small node. The fine needle biopsy [10, 11] provides an aspirate for cytological examination but may be more difficult for the pathologist to interpret. Essentially no tumor seeding has been reported with fine needle biopsy. An additional drawback to either large or fine needle biopsies is that lymphoma is usually difficult for most pathologists to diagnose with this method.

For years it has been taught that suspicious neck nodes should not be biopsied prior to a thorough diagnostic evaluation. Although it seems logical that open biopsy of a node increases not only the risk of local seeding but also morbidity due to the surgical wound, until recently there was no information in the literature to validate this notion. In 1978, McGuirt and McCabe [12] reported a study of 715 radical neck dissections, in which 64 (8.9%) of the patients had undergone cervical node biopsy prior to definitive treatment. They found that wound necrosis, local neck recurrence, and distant metastases occurred significantly more frequently in those patients

4

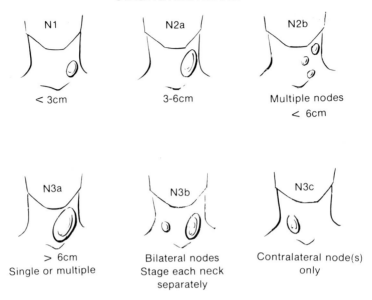

Figure 2. Cervical node classification system.

who had undergone prior biopsy than in the remainder of patients who had no biopsy or who had had biopsy only at the time of definitive treatment.

Staging

The American Joint Committee for Cancer Staging and End Results Reporting [13] provides the most commonly used classification system (Fig. 2) for describing cervical metastases:

N_X Nodes cannot be assessed.

N_0 No clinically positive nodes.

N_1 Single clinically positive homolateral node, 3 cm or less in diameter.

N_2 Single clinically positive homolateral node, more than 3 cm but no more than 6 cm in diameter, or multiple clinically positive homolateral nodes, none more than 6 cm in diameter.

N_{2a} Single clinically positive homolateral node, more than 3 cm but no more than 6 cm in diameter.

N_{2b} Multiple clinically positive homolateral nodes, none more than 6 cm in diameter.

N_3 Massive homolateral node(s), bilateral node(s), or contralateral node(s).

    N_{3a} Homolateral clinically positive node(s), at least one greater than 6 cm in diameter.

    N_{3b} Bilateral clinically positive nodes (in this situation, each side of the neck should be staged separately; that is N_{3b}: right, N_{2a}; left, N, for example).

    N_{3c} Only contralateral clinically positive node(s).

The TNM classification system relies primarily on the *size* of neck nodes to determine prognosis. Two recent reports, however, suggested that the size of the largest node in a neck dissection specimen was not a critical factor in survival [14, 15]. Sessions [14], in a study of 791 patients with laryngeal and hypopharyngeal primaries, showed no correlation between size of the largest node and prognosis, with the exception of patients with pyriform sinus lesions having large nodes. A problem in interpreting this study is that node measurements were made from the pathological specimens rather than from the clinical evaluation, since a neck node measuring 8 cm clinically may be composed of several 3 cm nodes pathologically. Schuller *et al.* [25] demonstrated no difference in 5-year survival rates among patients with various sizes of ipsilateral nodes except in Stage III and IV carcinomas of the larynx, in which large nodes adversely affected survival. This retrospective clinical study only included patients who underwent RND and therefore excluded patients who presented with massive unresectable nodes. A report by Shah and Tollefsen [7] concurs with the generally accepted belief that prognosis worsens as the 'N' status progresses from N_0 to N_3.

The presence of multiple positive nodes usually implies a poorer prognosis, according to the TNM classification system, but the current literature does not completely substantiate this hypothesis. Sessions [14] reported no correlation between survival and number of positive nodes for glottic and supraglottic primaries but did report decreased survival in pyriform sinus primaries with more than one positive node. Schuller *et al.* [15] reported no difference in survival between patients who had one positive node versus those who had multiple ipsilateral positive nodes.

The anatomical level of lymph node metastases does seem to influence prognosis. Spiro *et al.* [16] analyzed the level of node involvement in 580 patients with metastases from oral cavity or oropharyngeal primaries and reported that the prognosis was directly related to the level of node involvement. No 5-year survivors were reported in the 15 patients who manifested supraclavicular nodes. Schuller [15] demonstrated a significantly worse 5-year survival in patients with posterior triangle disease compared to all other nodal sites. He also reported no survivors among 12 patients with non-contiguous node involvement, compared with a 25% (47/187) 5-year survival in patients with contiguous nodal site involvement. Multiple level involvement is an adverse factor in survival compared with single level involvement.

Clinically negative neck

General comments

The appropriate treatment of the clinically negative neck in head and neck cancer patients continues to be controversial, with several questions unresolved. When, if ever, should an elective neck dissection (END) be performed? Should the node dissection be a standard radical neck dissection (RND) or is a modification adequate? Is radiotherapy or surgery the preferred treatment? Is the prognosis any worse if treatment of the neck is delayed until a node becomes palpable?

Elective dissection for the clinically negative neck

The main argument in favor of END is the recognized inaccuracy of palpation in determining the presence of metastatic neck disease. Sako et al. [5] reported a 28% incidence of histologically positive nodes in 123 patients who underwent elective neck dissection for a variety of head and neck primary sites. For cancers of the tonsil, oral tongue, and base of tongue, the occult metastatic rate was 36%, 38%, and 55% respectively. Likewise, Southwick et al. [4] reported a 40% metastasis rate in clinically negative necks in patients with intraoral cancer.

Other points in favor of END include the following: (1) When the surgeon must enter the neck to remove the primary and the risk of metastasis is over 25%, it seems logical to also remove the nodes most likely to be involved in metastatic disease; (2) neck dissections result in relatively low morbidity and mortality; (3) it is often difficult to detect clinically positive nodes early on routine follow-up; (4) the modified neck dissection (MND) procedure provides a means of removing nodes with minimal functional or cosmetic deformity; and (5) END may be used as a staging procedure to determine if postoperative radiotherapy is necessary and to help predict prognosis.

The primary arguments against END are the following: (1) several studies indicate that the cure rate may not be significantly worse if one waits for occult nodes to become clinically positive [7, 17–20]; (2) routine END results in a number of unnecessary procedures; and (3) radiotherapy, though expensive, time consuming, and also possibly unnecessary, may be as effective as neck dissection for the eradication of occult lymph node metastases.

A number of studies [4, 6, 7, 17–26] have examined the issue of END. Skolnick *et al.* [26] divided their surgically treated patients into two groups. The first group had surgical treatment of the primary only; the neck was not treated. This group showed a 13% (17/132) recurrence rate in the neck and all but two of the cases had recurrence of the primary. The second surgical group, which taken on a whole had a higher 'T' status than the first group, underwent resection of the primary plus radical neck dissection (RND) and this group exhibited a 21% (49/228) recurrence rate in the neck. Although 20/49 patients whose primary tumors were controlled had neck recurrences, only five of the recurrences were in the ipsilateral RND treated neck, resulting in a 2.5% (5/199) neck recurrence rate when the primary tumor was controlled. This study showed a low incidence of neck recurrence for untreated as well as surgically treated patients when the primary remains controlled. Ogura *et al.*, [6] using a probability model, estimated that if occult nodes were allowed to become palpable prior to treatment, the 3-year survival rate would decrease 4% for patients with supraglottic carcinomas and 11% for patients with pyriform sinus carcinomas. They felt, therefore, that END was probably warranted. On the other hand, Shah and Tollefson [7] computed only a 5% improvement in 5-year survival rate for patients having supraglottic laryngeal tumors with occult nodes compared with those patients who had clinically palpable nodes and concluded that routine END was not indicated for patients with supraglottic carcinomas.

Elective radiotherapy for the clinically negative neck

The main advantages of radiotherapy as treatment in the clinically negative neck are the apparent decreased incidence of cervical recurrences and the ease of administering radiotherapy to the neck when the primary lesion is being irradiated. The disadvantages of radiotherapy are: (1) a large number of patients may undergo unnecessary treatment; (2) morbidity and mortality are increased if subsequent surgical therapy is needed; (3) a large field of radiotherapy may be difficult for the patient to tolerate in terms of mucositis, pain, and weight loss; (4) long term side effects such as dryness of the mouth and pharynx, as well as fibrosis of the neck tissues, usually occur; and (5) radiation fibrosis increases the difficulty of diagnosing recurrent disease, especially in the patient with a thick neck.

Elective radiotherapy has been proposed as an alternative to END. Recent reports [27–29] show a 13% to 19% recurrence rate in the neck after elective radiotherapy which improved to 1% to 4% after excluding patients who had also developed recurrences in the primary site. The majority of the metastases in all three of these studies occurred in patients who had recurrence at the primary site. It is impossible to determine whether the clinical metastases were due to inability of radiotherapy to eradicate microscopic disease in the neck as well as gross disease in the primary site, or due to re-seeding from the uncontrolled primary site.

Fletcher [30] reported the results of radiotherapy versus no radiotherapy in the contralateral N_0 neck of a large number of patients with head and neck cancer, most of whom had clinically positive nodes on the ipsilateral neck. Only 3% (6/187) of patients receiving radiotherapy developed subsequent contralateral metastases compared with a fairly high incidence, 24% (46/187), without neck irradiation.

Goffinet et al. [31] reported that 40% (7/18) of patients with oral cavity carcinomas treated only with radium implants developed neck metastases, compared with none in 34 patients in whom the neck as well as the oral cavity were irradiated.

Treatment recommendations

We have formulated our philosophy of treatment for the clinically negative neck to encompass recent advances in surgical technique and radiotherapy and yet individualize treatment according to the patient. In general, if the chance of occult metastases is felt to be greater than 25%, the neck should be treated. If the primary tumor is being treated with radiotherapy, then the fields should be expanded to treat the neck(s) to 5000 rads.

If the primary is being treated with surgery alone, an elective modified neck dissection is recommended. With a midline lesion, such as in the tongue base, epiglottis, or anterior floor of mouth, we feel a bilateral MND is warranted. Since it is rare in previously untreated patients for neck metastases to skip groups of nodes, the primary node groups (first and second echelon) are the most important to remove. The MND may vary in extent: For cancers of the anterior floor of mouth, a bilateral supraomohyoid dissection should be adequate. In cancers that first metastasize to the jugular chain, the posterior cervical triangle does not necessarily have to be resected completely. Should clinically or pathologically positive nodes be identified during the MND, the operation can be converted to a RND.

In advanced cases when the primary tumor is to be treated with surgery and postoperative radiotherapy and the neck is clinically negative, we recommend that if the neck is exposed in order to approach the primary cancer, a MND be performed. If the neck is found pathologically to be positive, it is included in the field of irradiation. An alternative to END is to resect only the primary cancer and the irradiate both the primary site and the neck.

Clinically positive neck

The treatment of neck metastases is usually done in conjunction with treatment of the primary tumor unless the primary is unknown, previously treated, or not in the head and neck.

Surgery

In the surgical assessment of the patient with metastatic neck disease, the ultimate question is whether the disease is resectable. If either the primary neoplasm or the cervical nodes are deemed unresectable, or if there are distant metastases, the patient is usually treated palliatively with radiotherapy and/or chemotherapy.

There are several factors to be considered in determining resectability. Nodal fixation represents extracapsular spread to contiguous structures but does not imply unresectability if the structure to which the nodal mass is attached can be resected and reconstructed with acceptable functional results. Although nodes fixed to the carotid artery are frequently resectable by dissecting the tumor in a subadventitial plane off the internal or common carotid arteries, it is nevertheless associated with a very poor (7% 5-year survival) prognosis [32].

Johnson *et al.* [33] examined the incidence of extracapsular spread of tumor in lymph nodes with respect to nodal size and patient survival. They found extracapsular spread in 65% of N_1 necks and 75% of N_{2-3} necks. The 3-year survival in those patients with positive nodes but without extranodal spread was 52%, which was similar to the 62% 3-year survival in those patients with histologically negative necks; however, in those patients with extracapsular spread of tumor the 3-year survival dropped to 28%. Other factors adversely affecting resectability are the presence of Horner's syndrome, vagus nerve paralysis, and phrenic nerve paralysis. The presence of any of these signs indicates extensive neck involvement with tumor that is usually unresectable.

Neck dissection

The standard surgical treatment for neck metastases is the radical neck dissection as described by Crile in 1906 [34]. This procecure consists of a unilateral cervical node dissection plus removal of the submandibular gland, tail of the parotid gland, sternocleidomastoid muscle, internal jugular vein, and the spinal accessory nerve. The most significant factor in long term morbidity from this procedure is the removal of the spinal accessory nerve with resultant shoulder discomfort and disability. To decrease this morbid-

10

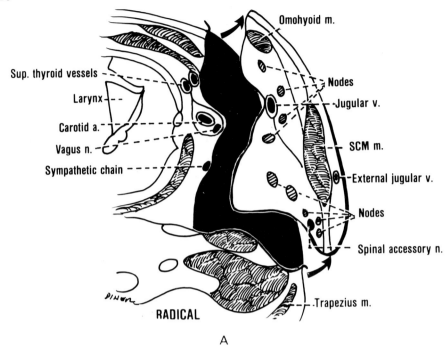

Sup. thyroid vessels

Larynx

Carotid a.

Vagus n.

Sympathetic chain

Omohyoid m.

Nodes

Jugular v.

SCM m.

External jugular v.

Nodes

Spinal accessory n.

Trapezius m.

RADICAL

A

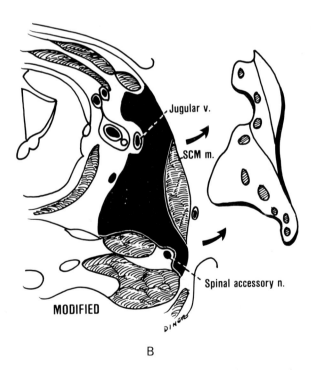

Jugular v.

SCM m.

Spinal accessory n.

MODIFIED

B

Figure 3. (a) Radical neck dissection; (b) modified neck dissection.

ity some surgeons try to preserve the spinal accessory nerve in selected cases of RND. This is done when the clinically positive nodes do not involve the spinal accessory nerve anywhere in its course or when the neck is clinically negative.

Some surgeons go a step further and advocate modification of the radical neck dissection so that only the lymphatic structures are removed. This procedure, known as the modified or functional neck dissection, was described and popularized by Bocca in 1967 [35], although it was originally described by O. Suarez earlier in this century. The MND is more variable in the extent of dissection than is the well-standardized RND. This factor is both a strength and a weakness of this technique. The lack of standardization makes comparison of statistics more difficult but, on the other hand, allows the surgeon to tailor the operation to the patient. Proponents of the MND do not suggest that it be used in place of RND except in selected situations. From an oncologic viewpoint, the lymph nodes are removed with the same fascial envelope in a MND as in a RND (Fig. 3) with the exception that this envelope is opened to dissect the spinal accessory nerve. The carotid sheath is opened in a MND as in a RND except that instead of sacrificing the internal jugular vein, it is skeletonized using sharp dissection. In addition, the sternocleidomastoid muscle is usually saved in a MND.

The contents of the submandibular and submental triangle may or may not be removed, depending upon the primary site. The extent of dissection posteriorly in the posterior cervical triangle and inferiorly in the supraclavicular triangle may vary depending on the primary tumor site and the philosophy of the surgeon.

Roy and Beahrs [36] selectively preserved the spinal accessory nerve during RND in about one-half of a series of 250 patients. When examining the subgroup of patients with histologically positive necks, they reported a 36% recurrence rate in the neck when the nerve was sacrificed compared with a 17% recurrence rate when the nerve was preserved. This study suggests that in selected patients, saving the spinal accessory nerve does not adversely affect the recurrence rate.

Jesse et al. [37] described a study of three types of neck dissection: (1) RND for patients with advanced neck disease; (2) RND with sparing of the spinal accessory nerve in patients with tumor involvement of the sternocleidomastoid muscle or suspected posterior triangle disease but without tumor involvement of the spinal accessory nerve; and (3) MND for those patients with less disease in the neck than the preceding groups. Postoperative radiotherapy was used if the neck was histologically N_2 or if the primary tumor was large. Excluded from this study were patients who died within 18 months and had no neck recurrence. Recurrence rates in the neck were 16% with RND (18/115), 13% with RND and sparing of the XI nerve (3/24), and 11% (18/171) with MND.

Lingeman *et al.* [38] reported on 347 RNDs and 98 MNDs performed over a ten-year period. Sixty-nine percent of the RND patients and 59% of the MND patients also received pre- or post-operative radiotherapy. Of the 113 N_0 patients undergoing RND, 17 (14%) had local recurrence in the neck compared with no recurrence in 70 patients undergoing MND. All 17 of the N_0 RND group with neck recurrence also had recurrent primary disease present. The recurrence rates in the neck for N_{1-2} disease were identical between RND and MND patients.

Bocca [39, 40] reported comparable 5-year survival rates of patients with laryngeal carcinoma treated with RND compared with MND, both for N_0 necks and for N_{1-2} necks. Radiotherapy was not employed.

All of the above reports were retrospective studies of selected patients who underwent RND with nerve sparing or MND. The technique for MND varied from surgeon to surgeon and frequently from case to case, depending upon tumor factors. In addition, a varying percentage of patients received radiotherapy. While these reports indicate that MND is as effective as RND in treating clinically negative necks as well as some N_1 and N_2 necks, prospective randomized studies are needed to confirm these observations.

We suggest the following guidelines for RND and MND based on published reports and on our own extensive experience with both types of neck dissections [41]:

Radical neck dissection

Indications
1. Clinically positive resectable cervical node(s) associated with a resectable primary.
2. Resectable nodes involving two or more levels of the neck.
3. Clinically positive nodes when surgery is the only treatment planned.
4. Cervical metastases appearing after the primary has been controlled with surgery, radiation, or combined therapy.
5. Recurrent or persistent positive nodes after radiotherapy to the neck.
6. Fixed neck mass that becomes mobile following radiotherapy or chemotherapy.
7. High risk of occult positive nodes (elective neck dissection) if the surgeon does not accept modifications of neck dissections or is inexperienced in doing MND.

Contraindications
1. Uncontrolled cancer of the primary site.
2. Evidence of distant metastasis.
3. Fixed nodes unchanged by radiotherapy or chemotherapy.

Advantages
1. Straightforward, well described, and well known procedure.
2. Low likelihood of leaving nodal disease behind.

Disadvantages
1. Trapezius muscle dysfunction with shoulder drop resulting in pain and limitation of motion.

2. Mild to moderate neck deformity.
3. Occasional occurrence of painful neuromas.
4. Prolonged facial and/or cerebral edema if bilateral simultaneous RND performed.

Modified neck dissection

Indications
1. Elective neck dissection when there is a 25% or greater risk of occult positive nodes.
2. N_1 neck when surgery is to be followed by radiotherapy, e.g., in $T_3-T_4N_1M_0$ neoplasms of oral cavity, oral pharynx, or hypopharynx.
3. Papillary or follicular carcinoma of the thyroid with neck metastases.
4. For the lesser involved side when bilateral neck dissection is indicated; postoperative radiotherapy should be used in this situation.

Contraindications
1. Clinically positive nodes when surgery is the only treatment modality to be used.
2. Clinically positive nodes after radiotherapy to the neck.
3. Clinically positive nodes after previous modified or regional neck dissection.
4. Melanoma with clinically positive nodes.
5. Inexperienced surgeon.

Advantages
1. Low incidence of shoulder drop and shoulder disability.
2. Low morbidity and mortality when performed on one side during bilateral neck dissection.
3. Protection for the carotid artery.
4. Useful as a staging procedure in the N_0 neck to determine both the need for postoperative radiotherapy and the ultimate prognosis.
5. Avoidance of cosmetic deformity produced by RND.
6. Avoidance of major sensory deficit and painful neuroma if the cervical plexus is preserved.
7. Preservation of head and neck venous drainage.
8. Possibility for conversion to a radical neck dissection if multiple clinically positive nodes are noted during surgery.

Disadvantages
1. Possible omission of occult positive nodes in the neck specimen if a limited MND is performed.
2. Increased risk of cutting into positive nodes and seeding neck.
3. Increased risk of hematoma under the sternocleidmastoid muscle.
4. Increased difficulty and operative time over that of a radical neck dissection if a full MND is performed.
5. Increased difficulty in performing a secondary RND if neck disease recurs.

Radiotherapy

Although the preceding discussion has implied that the first major decision on treating neck metastases is the determination of resectability, there are some tumors, such as nasopharyngeal carcinomas that are best treated with radiotherapy even if the neck metastases are deemed clinically resectable.

Furthermore, some radiotherapists feel that radiotherapy can effectively be used as the primary therapy for metastatic neck disease. Schneider *et al.* [42] reported 94 cases of N_1 neck disease treated over a period of 20 years in which they show a 19% rate of recurrence in the neck when the primary was controlled. They concluded that control of a single non-fixed metastatic cervical node with 6500 rads is excellent; however, if nodes are greater than 3 cm or are multiple, external radiotherapy alone cannot be relied upon for control and a neck dissection should follow.

Wizenberg [43] reported an 8% neck failure rate when the primary was controlled, and a 26% failure rate of the neck and primary site in a series of 113 patients treated with 7000 to 7500 rads to the neck. Excluded from this study were 128 patients, 68 of whom had advanced local disease or poor general health. The 5-year survival rate was only 28% for Stage III patients and 19% for Stage IV patients. Fayos and Lamp [44] reported only a 24% absolute 5-year survival in 66 patients with N_1 necks treated with radiotherapy, despite neck dissection in 23 of these patients for recurrent disease. These three studies show that high dose radiotherapy may be effective in the treatment of N_1 neck disease but the overall survival rate of these patients does not appear to be as high as with surgical therapy.

Combined therapy

In an effort to improve local and regional control of head and neck cancer and improve survival, many physicians have advocated combining surgery and radiotherapy for those patients who have a relatively poor prognosis when either form of therapy is used alone.

Three prospective randomized studies have examined the effects of low dose preoperative radiotherapy. E.W. Strong [45] reported that 2000 rads given preoperatively significantly decreased the incidence of neck recurrence compared with unirradiated controls but did not improve the 3-year survival rate. Lawrence *et al.* [46] reported no beneficial effects of 1400 rads. M.S. Strong *et al.* [47] reported that 2000 rads reduced neither the recurrence rate in the neck nor survival but did adversely affect the incidence of distant metastases. In addition to providing conflicting results, these studies used a lower dose of radiotherapy than most physicians currently advocate.

No prospective randomized studies of moderate dose preoperative radiotherapy versis surgery alone are available but several studies comparing preoperative with postoperative radiotherapy have been reported. Vandenbruck *et al.* [48] reported that patients with pyriform sinus and aryepiglottic fold carcinomas had a 5-year survival rate of 20% with 5500 rads of preoperative radiotherapy versus 56% with 5500 rads postoperatively. However, results for control of neck metastases were not separately described.

A number of retrospective studies have looked at surgery versus combined therapy for treatment of neck metastases. In patients with nodal involvement ranging from N_0 to N_2, Byers [49] reported a 20% neck recurrence rate for RND alone versus a 15% neck recurrence rate for RND plus radiotherapy. De Santo et al. [50] reported a 37% recurrence rate for patients with N_2 necks treated with RND alone compared with a 54% recurrence rate with preoperative radiotherapy of 4000 rads or more followed by RND. Lee and Krause [51] looked at survival rates rather than recurrence rates when examining their patients who underwent either surgery or combined therapy of a clinically positive neck. They reported identical 60% 5-year determinant survival rates for surgery and combined therapy groups after deleting patients who developed local recurrences. The above studies do not support the proposition that combined therapy is better than surgery alone.

Jesse and Fletcher [52] reported the recurrence rates in the neck for surgically treated patients as 14% for N_1, 26% for N_2, and 34% for N_3 compared with recurrence rates for a combined treatment group of 2% for N_1, 11% for N_2, and 25% for N_3. This data was based on 311 patients who survived 24 months with the primary lesion controlled.

This brief review of retrospective studies of combined therapy provides conflicting results. At our institution, RND alone or MND plus postoperative radiotherapy is used for the N_1 neck and RND plus radiotherapy for N_2 and N_3 disease. The size and location of the primary are also factors in recommending combined therapy.

Chemotherapy

Although many papers discuss the response rate of head and neck tumors to chemotherapy, few papers discuss the chemotherapeutic effect on nodal metastases. In a preliminary report of a multi-institutional study of preoperative cis-platinum and bleomycin, Baker et al. [53]showed nodal response rates of 70% for N_1, 66% for N_2, and 29% for N_3 necks. The response rates strongly correlated with response of the primary site.

Neck metastases from unknown primary

The incidence of neck metastases from an unknown primary is low, since in most instances the primary lesion is found after a careful search. Search for a head and neck primary should include endoscopy under anesthesia with selected random biopsies of the nasopharynx, tonsils, base of tongue, and any suspicious areas. If the node is located in the upper two-thirds of the neck, a head and neck primary should be suspected although lymphoma may also present in the upper neck. If the node is located in the supraclavicular triangle, the most likely site for the primary tumor is below the clavicles, such as the breast, lung, stomach or gonads.

If the neck mass is resectable and a careful search does not identify the primary, an excisional biopsy should be performed unless one suspects a carotid body tumor. In that case a contrast enhanced CT scan or an arteriogram should be obtained. When frozen section of the neck mass shows squamous cell carcinoma a radical neck dissection is usually performed. An alternate treatment is a MND followed by full course radiotherapy to the upper aerodigestive tract in hopes of also treating the unknown primary. A diagnosis of adenocarcinoma usually contraindicates neck dissection due to the poor prognosis, unless a salivary gland or thyroid neoplasm is suspected. The diagnosis of lymphoma requires further studies to assess the stage of disease.

All reports agree that the prognosis for patients presenting with supraclavicular nodes [54–58] or with adenocarcinoma [55, 56, 58] is poor. For patients with squamous cell carcinoma, however, the 3-year survival rates range from 40% to 53% [55, 58] and the 5-year survival ranges from 25% to 54% [54–56].

Reports [55, 56] from two large series of patients indicate that if the primary is aggressive enough to ultimately manifest itself the prognosis is worse than if it were to remain occult. Jesse et al. [55] reported a 58% 3-year survival rate if the primary remained occult versus a 31% 3-year survival if a primary above the clavicles was eventually found. Likewise, Coker et al. [56] reported a 5-year survival of 60% if the primary remained occult versus 30% if it were found. However, Barrie et al. [54] and Leipzig et al. [58] reported no difference in survival whether the primary remained occult or was eventually discovered. Furthermore, Dickson and Vargas [57] reported an 18% 5-year survival rate for patients with occult primaries versus 25% if the primary were found. The main difference between this report and the preceding reports was that Dickson and Vargas treated their patients primarily with radiotherapy while the other authors either used surgery or surgery plus radiotherapy.

When looking more closely at treatment results of surgery versus radiotherapy, it is difficult to arrive at valid conclusions because all previous reports have been retrospective evaluations and selection criteria were usually not well established. Jesse et al. [55] in the largest series, reported a 3-year absolute survival rate of 57% (59/104), 48% (25/52), and 47% (13/28) for surgery, radiotherapy and combined therapy respectively, but the radiotherapy group had the largest percentage of N_3 necks.

Treatment recommendations

A reasonable plan of therapy for neck disease from an unknown primary would be a RND for the N_1 neck, and surgery plus radiotherapy for the N_2 and the resectable N_3 neck. For the patient who presents after ungoing excisional node biopsy, full course radiotherapy may be an alternative to RND. Patients with adenocarcinoma or metastases to supraclavicular nodes should receive radiotherapy and/or chemotherapy because of their poor prognosis.

Palliative therapy to the neck

In patients with far-advanced local or regional disease or with distant metastases, therapy is usually palliative rather than curative. In borderline cases when the chance of cure is small, the patient and his family should be informed of the risks and complications of potentially curative versus palliative treatment and encouraged to choose the treatment. When the chance of cure is minimal, palliative therapy should be instituted to try to alleviate the patient's symptoms and perhaps also to give the patient a glimmer of hope.

Surgical therapy for palliation is rarely indicated, with the exception of procedures such as tracheotomy for airway obstruction, ligation of vessels for severe hemorrhage or for impending carotid artery rupture, and feeding esophagostomy for severe malnutrition.

Radiotherapy is frequently used for palliation. Some radiotherapists may recommend a full course of therapy in the hope that an occasional patient will actually be cured. Other radiotherapists will administer a moderate dose in a short time span in order to minimize treatment time and prolong the patient's time at home.

Chemotherapy is gaining a larger role in palliation. It is frequently used after surgery and radiotherapy for treating persistent or recurrent disease. Since response rates for chemotherapy are usually higher if it is administered prior to other treatment, a rational approach would be to try a course of chemotherapy prior to palliative radiotherapy. Protocols using concomitant chemotherapy and radiotherapy have been used but for the most part have not achieved encouraging results.

Most chemotherapy studies have not looked at cervical metastases alone but have focused on different primary sites. Methotrexate and cis-platinum are the most active agents, with response rates of 25% to 40%. Many multi-drug protocols have been espoused with varying response rates, but even with responses to multi-drug regimens, when they occur, they usually last only for a few months. More data on chemotherapy are found in Chapters 12–15.

Other types of therapy such as cryotherapy and hyperthermia have been advocated. Cryotherapy is not indicated for cervical metastases. Hyperthermia is dealt with in Chapter 11.

Non-squamous head and neck cancers

Melanoma metastatic to cervical nodes

Approximately 20% of melanomas arise in the head and neck [59]. Since metastatic neck nodes adversely affect survival [60, 61], the presence of resectable clinically positive nodes is considered an indication for a RND, assuming the patient has a primary melanoma that is also resectable and no distant metastases. Depending upon the location of the primary melanoma, an extended neck dissection may be indicated that includes nodes not normally removed with a RND, such as suboccipital nodes or parotid nodes. Frequently the platysma located between the primary and the nodal disease is removed in hopes of catching 'in-transit' metastases.

The treatment of the clinically negative neck in the patient with a primary melanoma in the head and neck region is controversial. Some retrospective studies indicate that the rate of occult metastases found at elective neck dissection ranges from 11% to 19% [60, 62, 63], compared with the later occurrence of metastatic nodes in patients with untreated necks, that ranges from 23% to 30% [60, 62]. The difference between these two groups of figures probably represents micrometastases that were present but not detectable in the patient undergoing neck dissection. Since patients with histologically detectable metastases, whether clinically occult or clinically evident, have a similarly poor prognosis, the overall survival figures [60, 62] of 70% to 77% for patients undergoing elective neck dissection versus 49% to 61% for patients observed until metastasis occurred probably represent the control of patients with micrometastases.

To more precisely determine which patients might benefit from elective neck dissection, the Clark classification of levels of invasion and the Breslow technique [65, 66] for measuring thickness of the primary melanoma have been used to correlate the degree of invasion of the primary with the likelihood of metastatic disease. Storm *et al.* [61] report that only 10% of patients with Clark Level II (papillary dermis involvement) had histologically involved nodes, compared with 33% to 43% nodal involvement with Levels III, IV, and V tumors. Hansen and McCarten [67], in a study of 154 cases, one-third of which were in the head and neck, report that patients with lesions less than 1.5 mm in thickness were virtually all long term survivors regardless of type of treatment, whereas those patients with lesions greater than 1.5 mm had a definitely lower survival rate that was significantly ($p < 0.01$) improved with elective neck dissection.

Treatment recommendations

We suggest RND, or extended RND when indicated, for patients with resectable, clinically positive neck nodes from a primary melanoma in the head and neck. For the patient with a clinically negative neck we recommend END if the primary melanoma extends into Clark levels III, IV, or V, or if the primary measures greater than 1.5 mm in thickness. We would probably use an MND but convert it to a RND if positive nodes were found at surgery.

Thyroid carcinoma metastatic to the neck

The treatment of neck nodes in patients with thyroid carcinoma depends on the histologic type of carcinoma and the presence of clinically or surgically positive nodes. The frequency of nodal metastases from papillary carcinoma ranges from 21% to 82% [68–70]. A MND is indicated for treating papillary carcinoma with clinically palpable metastatic nodes. Marchetta *et al.* [71] reported no recurrence in the operated neck of 30 patients followed for up to 10 years, despite widespread cervical involvement. The incidence of positive nodes ranged from 79% to 87% in the mid-jugular, lower jugular, and visceral compartments to 16% in the upper jugular region, 13% in the spinal accessory area, and 11% in the submandibular triangle.

Treatment of the neck in patients with papillary carcinoma who do not have clinically positive nodes is controversial. Attie *et al.* [69] performed elective MND in 115 of 212 patients with papillary carcinoma and found that 69% had histologic evidence of metastases. The 97 patients, who for various reasons did not undergo MND, did undergo paratracheal node dissections with positive findings in 23%. Other surgeons such as Crile and Hawk [72] do not perform elective neck dissection unless cervical nodes are grossly involved at the time of exploration.

Follicular carcinoma has a lower incidence of cervical metastases than does papillary carcinoma, although it exhibits a higher distant metastatic rate [68]. Woolner *et al.* [68] reported a 10% cervical metastatic rate in follicular carcinoma patients who demonstrated moderate or marked capsular invasion of the thyroid gland compared with a 1% metastatic rate in patients with slight or no capsular invasion. Tollefsen *et al.* [73] reported a 25% incidence of clinically positive nodes. For follicular carcinoma of the thyroid most surgeons would perform a MND for clinically positive nodes or for histologically confirmed occult nodes.

Medullary carcinoma comprises only 5% to 10% of thyroid malignancies [74–76]. Most tumors arise spontaneously, but about 10% of patients manifest an inherited form of the disease. Serum calcitonin levels obtained after infusion of calcium are helpful in screening family members of patients suspected of having the hereditary type of medullary carcinoma [77]. The incidence of neck nodes is similar (50%) in both the spontaneous and inherited forms [76], although the presence of bilateral thyroid lobe involvement is higher and the age of presentation is earlier in the inherited from.

The occurrence of metastatic nodes adversely affects survival; Chong *et al.* [76] report an 86% 10-year survival when nodes are uninvolved, compared with 46% survival when nodes are involved. The same authors report a recurrence rate of 62% after MND compared with a recurrence rate of 44% after RND.

A combination of surgery plus radiotherapy has not been proven to be beneficial although external radiotherapy may be helpful for palliation [75, 77]. Radioiodine is not used for treatment because medullary carcinoma cells do not take up iodine.

Undifferentiated or anaplastic carcinoma occurs mainly in the sixth and seventh decades of life [68] and constitutes 5% to 15% [68, 78] of all thyroid malignancies. Anaplastic carcinoma grows rapidly and presents with fixation to adjacent neck structures, enlarged cervical nodes, and frequently, distant metastases. The one-year survival is 10% to 23% [68, 74]. Due to the aggressive nature of the disease, neck dissection is usually not feasible. A recent report [79] in which surgery, radiotherapy, and chemotherapy with Actinomycin D were combined has encouraging results but these have not been confirmed by other investigators [70].

Treatment recommendations

We recommend subtotal or total thyroidectomy for papillary, follicular, and medullary carcinoma. For papillary carcinoma, if clinically positive nodes are present a MND is done, including dissection of the tracheoesophageal nodes. If the neck is clinically negative, the tracheoesophageal and inferior jugular nodes are examined. If frozen section of suspicious nodes reveals metastatic disease, MND is done including a tracheoesophageal dissection. Bilateral MND is done if nodes are present bilaterally. RND may be indicated for extensive nodal disease.

Follicular carcinoma is approached in the same fashion as papillary carcinoma.

Medullary carcinoma with clinically positive nodes is treated with MND or RND depending on the extent of metastasis. If nodes are clinically negative MND may be considered because of the high incidence of metastasis in this disease. As with other types of thyroid carcinoma, a tracheoesophageal node dissection should be included in the neck dissection when clinically positive nodes are present. If surgery is performed for undifferentiated or anaplastic carcinoma with neck metastases, RND is usually done with resection of the primary. Frequently this neoplasm is so advanced at the time of presentation that definitive surgery is not performed. Tracheotomy may be necessary to avoid asphyxiation from tracheal invasion.

Salivary gland neoplasms metastatic to the neck

Approximately 80% of all salivary gland neoplasms arise in the parotid gland, 5% to 10% arise in the submandibular gland, and 10% to 15% in the minor salivary glands and in the sublingual gland [80, 84]. Conley and Baker [81] report the incidence of malignant neoplasms in a series of 1,280 salivary gland neoplasms as follows: parotid gland 20% to 30%, submandibular gland 30% to 50%, sublingual gland 80% to 90%, and minor salivary glands, 40% to 65%.

Most series [80, 81] show that mucoepidermoid carcinoma is the most common malignant salivary gland neoplasm. Mucoepidermoid carcinomas are usually divided into two categories: a low grade, relatively benign type, or a high grade, aggressively malignant type. Spiro *et al.* [82] in a study of parotid malignancies report no neck metastases from the low grade type but a 44% incidence of metastases with intermediate and high grade types (Table 1). The only other histologic types of salivary gland malignancies with relatively high metastatic rates were epidermoid carcinoma and adenocarcinoma. Other malignancies such as adenoid cystic carcinoma, acinous cell carcinoma, and malignant mixed tumors had a relatively low cervical metastatic rate [82–85].

Spiro *et al.* [87] report a 37% incidence of cervical metastases from malignant submandibular gland tumors. As seen in Table 2, the occult meta-

Table 1. Cervical lymph node metastases secondary to parotid malignancies (from Spiro *et al.* [82])

Lesion	Patients	Percent with positive nodes
Mucoepidermoid carcinoma, low grade	56	0
Mucoepidermoid carcinoma, intermediate and high grade	89	44
Malignant mixed tumor	53	21
Acinous cell carcinoma	33	18
Adenocarcinoma	28	36
Adenoid cystic carcinoma	20	10
Epidermoid carcinoma	10	70
Total	288	26

Table 2. Cervical lymph node metastases secondary to submandibular gland malignancies (from Spiro et al. [86])

Lesion	Patients	Percent with positive nodes
Adenoid cystic carcinoma	42	21
Malignant mixed tumor	23	22
Mucoepidermoid carcinoma, intermediate and high grade	19	58
Epidermoid carcinoma	15	60
Adenocarcinoma	14	50
Mucoepidermoid carcinoma, low grade	4	—
Anaplastic/unclassified carcinoma	3	100
Acinous cell carcinoma	1	—
Total	121	37

static rate is high for anaplastic, epidermoid, intermediate and high grade mucoepidermoid, and adenocarcinomas. They selected approximately half of their patients for elective RND and found positive nodes in 42%.

Conley [81] reports a 31% incidence of neck metastases for malignant minor salivary gland tumors.

Treatment recommendations

From reviewing the literature and from our own experience, we suggest a RND for any clinically positive nodes associated with salivary gland malignancies from any site, assuming that both the primary and the cervical metastases are resectable. For high grade mucoepidermoid, epidermoid, anaplastic and adenocarcinoma, an elective neck dissection, either a MND ·or RND, is probably worthwhile. An alternative to an elective neck dissection would be a regional node dissection to remove the first echelon nodes draining the primary; if any of these nodes are positive on frozen section, a complete MND or RND would be performed.

Postoperative radiotherapy is usually employed if histological examination shows multiple metastatic nodes or if the tumor is a particularly aggressive one such as anaplastic or high grade mucoepidermoid.

Chemotherapy may play a role in the more aggressive lesions and in recurrent or unresectable neck disease [87].

Acknowledgement

Figures 1, 2, and 3 reproduced with permission of Churchill Livingstone, Inc., from Suen and Myers, (eds.), Cancer of the head and neck, 1981.

References

1. Till JE, Bruce WR, Elway A, Till MJ, Niederer V, Reid J, Hawkins NV, Rider WD: A preliminary analysis of end results for cancer of the larynx. Laryngoscope 85(2):259–275, 1975.
2. Chiang TC, Griem ML: Nasopharyngeal cancer. Surg Clin North Am 53(1):121–133, 1973.
3. Lindberg R: Distribution of cervical lymph node metastases from squamous cell carcinoma of the upper respiratory and digestive tracts. Cancer 29(6):1446–1449, 1972.
4. Southwick HW, Slaughter DP, Trevino ET: Elective neck dissection for intraoral cancer. Arch Surg 80:905–909, 1960.
5. Sako K, Pradier RN, Marchetta FC, Pickren JW: Fallibility of palpation in the diagnosis of metastases to cervical nodes. Surg Gynecol Obstet 118(5):989–990, 1964.
6. Ogura JH, Biller HF, Wette R: Elective neck dissection for pharyngeal and laryngeal cancers: An evaluation. Ann Otol Rhinol Laryngol 80:646–653, 1971.
7. Shah JP, Tollefsen HR: Epidermoid carcinoma of the supraglottic larynx. Am J Surg 128:494–499, 1974.
8. Mancuso AA, Maceri D, Rice D, Hanafee W: CT of cervical lymph node cancer. AJR 136(2):381–385, 1981.
9. Friedman M, Shelton V, Mafee M, Bellity P, Grybauskas V, Skolnik E: Metastatic neck disease: Evaluation by computerized tomography. Read in part before the American Society for Head and Neck Surgery, Palm Springs, California, March 13, 1983.
10. Young JEM, Archibald ST, Shier KJ: Needle aspiration cytologic biopsy in head and neck masses. Am J Surg 142:484–489, 1981.
11. Frable MAS, Frable WJ: Fine-needle aspiration biopsy revisited. Laryngoscope 92(12):1414–1418, 1982.
12. McGuirt WF, McCabe BF: Significance of node biopsy before definitive treatment of cervical metastatic carcinoma. Laryngoscope 88(4):594–597, 1978.
13. Beahrs OH, Carr DT, Rubin P: Manual for staging of cancer 1978, American Joint Committee for Cancer Staging and End-results Reporting. Chicago, 1978.
14. Sessions DG: Surgical pathology of cancer of the larynx and hypopharynx. Laryngoscope 86(6):814–839, 1976.
15. Schuller DE, McGuirt WF, McCabe BF, Young D: The prognostic significance of metastatic cervical lymph nodes. Laryngoscope 90(4):557–570, 1980.
16. Spiro RH, Alfonso AE, Farr HW, Strong EW: Cervical node metastasis from epidermoid carcinoma of the oral cavity and oropharynx. Am J Surg 128:562–567, 1974.
17. Harrold CC: The case against unlimited prophylactic neck dissection. In: Conley J (ed) Cancer of the Head and Neck. Washington, D.C., Butterworths, 1970, pp 186–190.
18. Reed F, Miller WA: Elective neck dissection. Laryngoscope 80(8):1292–1304, 1970.
19. Stell PM: The management of cervical lymph nodes in head and neck cancer. Proc Roy Soc Med 68:83–85, 1975.
20. Mendenhall WM, Million RR, Cassisi NS: Elective neck irradiation in squamous cell carcinoma of the head and neck. Head Neck Surg 3(1):15–20, 1980.
21. Skolnik EM, Tenta LT, Tardy ME, Wineinger DM: Elective neck dissection in head and neck cancer. Arch Otolaryngol 87(5):471–476, 1968.
22. Kremen AJ: The case for elective (prophylatic) neck dissection. In: Conley J (ed) Cancer of the Head and Neck. Washington D.C., Butterworths, 1970, pp 183–185.
23. Spiro RH, Strong EW: Epidermoid carcinoma of the oral cavity and oropharynx. Arch Surg 107(9):382–384, 1973.
24. Martis CS, Karakasis DT: Prophylactic neck dissection in oral carcinomas. Int J Oral Surg 3:293–296, 1974.

24

25. Nahum AM, Bone RC, Davidson TM: The case for elective prophylactic dissection. Trans Am Acad Ophthalmol Otolaryngol 82:603–612, 1976.
26. Skolnik EM, Katz AH, Mantravadi R, Becker SP, Stal S: Evolution of the clinically negative neck. Ann Otol Rhinol Laryngol 89(6):551–555, 1980.
27. Staley CJ, Herzon FS: Elective neck dissection in carcinoma of the larynx. Otolaryngol Clin North Am 3(3):543–554, 1970.
28. Rabuzzi DD, Chung CT, Sagerman RH: Prophylactic neck irradiation. Arch Otolaryngol 106(8):454–455, 1980.
29. Mantravadi R, Katz A, Haas R, Liebner EJ, Sabato D, Skolnik E, Applebaum EL: Radiation therapy for subclinical carcinoma in cervical lymph nodes. Arch Otolaryngol 108(2):108–111, 1982.
30. Fletcher GH: Elective irradiation of subclinical disease in cancers of the head and neck. Cancer 29(6):1450–1454, 1972.
31. Goffinet DR, Gilbert EH, Weller SA, Bagshaw MA: Irradiation of clinically uninvolved cervical lymph nodes. Canadian J Otolaryngol 4(5):927–933, 1975.
32. Kennedy JT, Krause CH, Loevy S: The importance of tumor attachment to the carotid artery. Arch Otolaryngol 103(2):70–73, 1977.
33. Johnson JT, Barnes EL, Myers, EN, Schramm VL, Borochovitz D, Sigler BA: The extracapsular spread of tumors in cervical node metastasis. Arch Otolaryngol 107:725–729, 1981.
34. Crile, G: Excision of cancer of the head and neck. J Am Med 47:1780–1786, 1906.
35. Bocca E, Pignataro O: A conservation technique in radical neck dissection. Ann Otol Rhinol Laryngol 76:975–987, 1967.
36. Roy PH, Beahrs OH: Spinal accessory nerve in radical neck dissection. Am J Surg 118:800–804, 1969.
37. Jesse RH, Ballantyne AJ, Larson D: Radical or modified neck dissection: a therapeutic dilemma. Am J Surg 136:516–519, 1978.
38. Lingeman RE, Stephens R, Helmus C, Ulm J: Neck Dissection: Radical or conservative. Ann Otol Rhinol Laryngol 86:737–744, 1977.
39. Bocca E: Critical analysis of the techniques and value of neck dissection. Nuovo Arch Ital di Otol 4(2):151–158, 1976.
40. Bocca E, Pignataro O, Sasaki CT: Functional neck dissection. Arch Otolaryngol 106:524–527, 1980.
41. Suen JY, Wetmore SJ: Cancer of the neck. In Suen JY, Myers EN (eds): Cancer of the Head and Neck. New York, Churchill Livingstone, 1981, pp 185–211.
42. Schneider JJ, Fletcher GH, Barkley HT: Control by irradiation alone of nonfixed clinically positive lymph nodes from squamous cell carcinoma of the oral cavity, oropharynx, supraglottic larynx, and hypopharynx. AJR 123:42–48, 1975.
43. Wizenberg MJ, Bloedorn FG, Weiner S, Gracia J: Treatment of lymph node metastases in head and neck cancer. A radiotherapeutic approach. Cancer 29(6):1455–1462, 1972.
44. Fayos JV, Lampe I: The therapeutic problem of metastatic neck adenopathy. AJR 114:65–75, 1972.
45. Strong EW: Preoperative radiation and radical neck dissection. Surg Clin North Am 49(2):271–276, 1969.
46. Lawrence W, Terz JJ, Rogers C, King RE, Wolf JS, King ER: Preoperative irradiation for head and neck cancer: a retrospective study. Cancer 33:318–323, 1974.
47. Strong MS, Vaughan CW, Kayne HL, Aral IM, Ucmakli A, Feldman M, Healy GB: A randomized trial of preoperative radiotherapy in cancer of the oropharynx and hypopharynx. Am J Surg 136:494–500, 1978.
48. Vandenbrouck C, Sancho H, LeFur R, Richard JM, Cachin Y: Results of a randomized clinical trial of preoperative irradiation versus postoperative in treatment of tumors of the hypopharynx. Cancer 39:1445–1449, 1977.

49. Byers RM: Symposium: Adjuvant cancer therapy of head and neck tumors. The use of postoperative irradiation – its goals and 1978 attainments. Laryngoscope 89:567–572, 1979.

50. DeSanto LW, Holt JJ, Beahrs OH, O'Fallon WM: Neck dissection: Is it worthwhile? Laryngoscope 92(5):502–509, 1982.

51. Lee JG, Krause J: Radical neck dissection: elective, therapeutic, and secondary. Arch Otolaryngol 101(11):656–659, 1975.

52. Jesse RH, Fletcher GH: Treatment of the neck in patients with squamous cell carcinoma of the head and neck. Cancer (Suppl) 39:868–872, 1977.

53. Baker SR, Makuch RW, Wolf GT: Preoperative cisplatin and bleomycin therapy in head and neck squamous carcinoma. Arch Otolaryngol 107:683–689, 1981.

54. Barrie JR, Knapper WH, Strong EW: Cervical nodal metastases of unknown origin. Am J Surg 120:466–470, 1970.

55. Jesse RH, Perez CA, Fletcher GH: Cervical lymph node metastasis: unknown primary cancer. Cancer 31:854–859, 1973.

56. Coker DD, Casterline PF, Chambers RG, Jaques DA: Metastases to lymph nodes of the head and neck from an unknown primary site. Am J Surg 134:517–522, 1977.

57. Dickson R, Vargas DR: Occult primary of the head and neck. J Otol 8:427–434, 1979.

58. Leipzig B, Winter ML, Hokanson JA: Cervical nodal metastases of unknown origin. Laryngoscope 91:593–598, 1981.

59. Harris TJ, Hinckley DM: Melanoma of the head and neck in Queensland. Head Neck Surg 5:197–203, 1983.

60. Ballantyne AJ: Malignant melanoma of the skin of the head and neck. An analysis of 405 cases. Am J Surg 120(10):425–431, 1970.

61. Storm FK III, Eilber FR, Morton DL, Clark WH Jr: Malignant melanoma of the head and neck. Head Neck Surg 1:123–128, 1978.

62. Simon JN: Malignant melanoma of the head and neck. Am J Surg 116(10):494–498, 1968.

63. Harris MN, Roses DF, Culliford AT, Gumport SL: Melanoma of the head and neck. Ann Surg 182(1):86–91, 1975.

64. Clark WH Jr, From L, Bernardino EA, Mihm MC: The histogenesis and biologic behavior of primary human malignant melanomas of the skin. Ca Res 29:705–715, 1969.

65. Breslow A: Thickness, cross-sectional areas and depth of invasion in the prognosis of cutaneous melanoma. Ann Surg 172(5):902–908, 1970.

66. Breslow A: Tumor thickness, level of invasion and node dissection in stage I cutaneous melanoma. Ann Surg 182(5):572–575, 1975.

67. Hansen MG, McCarten AB: Tumor thickness and lymphocytic infiltration in malignant melanoma of the head and neck. Am J Surg 128:557–561, 1974.

68. Woolner LB, Beahrs OH, Black BM, McConahey WM, Keating FR: Classification and prognosis of thyroid carcinoma. A study of 885 cases observed in a thirty year period. Am J Surg 102:354–387, 1961.

69. Attie JN, Khafif RA, Steckler RM: Elective neck dissection in papillary carcinoma of the thyroid. Am J Surg 122:464–471, 1971.

70. Bumsted RM: Thyroid disease: A guide for the head and neck surgeon. Ann Otol Rhinol Laryngol 89 (Suppl 72):3–16, 1980.

71. Marchetta FC, Sako K, Matsuura H: Modified neck dissection for carcinoma of the thyroid gland. Am J Surg 120:452–455, 1970.

72. Crile G Jr, Hawk WA: Carcinomas of the thyroid. Cleve Clin Q 38:97–104, 1971.

73. Tollefsen HR, Shab JP, Huvos AG: Follicular carcinoma of the thyroid. Am J Surg 126:523–528, 1973.

74. Fletcher JR: Medullary (solid) carcinoma of the thyroid gland: a review of 249 cases. Arch Surg 100:257–262, 1970.

75. Hill CS Jr, Ibanez ML, Samaan NA, et al.: Medullary (solid) carcinoma of the thyroid gland. Medicine 52(2):141–171, 1973.
76. Chong GC, Beahrs OH, Sizemore GW, Woolner LH: Medullary carcinoma of the thyroid gland. Cancer 35:695–704, 1975.
77. Baylin SB: Medullary carcinoma of the thyroid gland: Use of biochemical parameters in detection and surgical management of the tumor. Surg Clin N Am 54:309–323, 1974.
78. Maddox WA, Knott HW, Dowling EA: Carcinoma of the thyroid: review of fifteen years' experience. Am Surg 37(11):653–660, 1971.
79. Rogers JD, Lindberg RD, Hill CS Jr, Gehan E: Spindle and giant cell carcinoma of the thyroid: A different therapeutic approach. Cancer 34:1328–1332, 1974.
80. Eneroth CM: Salivary gland tumors in the parotid gland, submandibular gland, and the palate region. Cancer 27:1415–1418, 1971.
81. Conley J, Baker DC: Cancer of the salivary glands. In Suen JY, Myers EN (eds): Cancer of the Head and Neck. New York, Churchill Livingstone, 1981, pp 524–556.
82. Spiro RH, Huvos AG, Strong EW: Cancer of the parotid gland. A clinicopathologic study of 288 primary cases. Am J Surg 130:452–459, 1975.
83. Eneroth CM, Jakobson PA, Blanck C: Acinic cell carcinoma of the parotid gland. Cancer 19:1761–1772, 1966.
84. Spiro RH, Huvos AG, Strong EW: Adenoid cystic carcinoma of salivary origin. Am J Surg 128:512–520, 1974.
85. Spiro RH, Huvos AG, Strong EW: Acinic cell carcinoma of salivary origin. A clinicopathologic study of 67 cases. Cancer 41:924–935, 1978.
86. Spiro RH, Hajdu ST, Strong EW: Tumors of the submaxillary gland. Am J Surg 132:463–468, 1976.
87. Suen JY, Johns MF: Chemotherapy for salivary gland cancer. Laryngoscope 92(3):235–239, 1982.

2. Advances in the management of paranasal sinus tumors

MICHAEL E. JOHNS and MICHAEL J. KAPLAN

Introduction

Cancer of the paranasal sinuses is rare, but because of a historically dismal prognosis and morbidity, these tumors deserve great attention. Advances necessary to improve the management of these tumors include: earlier diagnosis, better local control, and the development of new and better therapeutic modalities. Unfortunately, the natural history of the more common malignant tumors in this anatomic area confound these goals. Diagnosis is frequently delayed because early symptoms are lacking, misleading or ignored. When symptoms do occur, they frequently mimic benign disease such as allergy or a 'persistent cold'. Although locally advanced, cervical or distant metastatic spread is present at the time of diagnosis in only 5–15% of cases. Thus, local control is a realistic goal. Limiting factors, however, include extension of tumor to vital structures at the cribriform plate, pterygomaxillary space, orbital apex, sphenoid, and nasopharynx. The major challenge to the head and neck surgeon is to improve the chances of cure and yet provide functional and cosmetic reconstruction. This chapter will review the current status and recent advances in the recognition and delineation of disease extent, surgical techniques used to achieve local control and rehabilitation, and investigational therapy.

Anatomy

To understand the problems in managing paranasal sinus tumors a thorough detailed knowledge of the complex regional anatomy and routes of tumor spread is imperative [1]. Areas relevant to this discussion are highlighted with reference to excellent illustrations that may be found in many previously published sources [2, 3].

The maxillary sinuses are the largest of the paranasal sinuses, averaging 3.5–4.0 cm in height, 2.5 cm transversely, and 3 cm anteroposteriorly [2].

Gregory T. Wolf (ed), Head and Neck Oncology.
© *1984 Martinus Nijhoff Publishers, Boston. ISBN 0-89838-657-8. Printed in The Netherlands.*

Tumor can erode through the thin walls of the sinus in any direction, particularly medially through the natural ostium or through thin bone to penetrate the lateral wall of the nose. Anterolaterally, tumor erosion results in involvement of the cheek and malar bone. Posteriorly, tumor can penetrate into the pterygomaxillary and infratemporal spaces. Superiorly, the thin floor of the orbit separates the orbital periosteum from the antrum, and the maxilloethmoid plate separates ethmoid from antrum. Inferiorly, the hard palate and dental roots may be invaded. Approximately 80% of tumors of the paranasal sinuses appear to originate in the maxillary sinuses [5–10].

The ethmoid sinuses are the origin of most other paranasal tumors not presenting in the antrum. Only 1% of paranasal sinus malignancies originate in the frontal or sphenoid sinuses.

The ethmoid sinus consists of a variable number of air cells that lie between the medial wall of the orbit and the upper lateral wall of the nose. Like the antrum, they develop embryologically in the second trimester from mucosal invaginations that are lined by respiratory pseudostratified ciliated columnar epithelium, and reach full development in adolescence. The attachment of the middle turbinate roughly divides the ethmoid cells into two groups: an anterior group that drains into the middle meatus and a posterior group that drains into the superior meatus. The general shape of the ethmoid labyrinth is a truncated pyramid: wider posteriorly (1.5 cm) than anteriorly (0.5–1.0 cm), and wider superiorly than inferiorly. The anteroposterior dimension is 4–5 cm and the height 2–2.5 cm.

Local tumor spread can occur most easily through the lateral wall of the ethmoid complex (the lamina papyracea), to invade the medial orbital periosteum. Inferolaterally, erosion of the maxilloethmoid plate allows extension to or from the antrum. Tumor may extend medially into the nasal cavity and posteriorly into the sphenoid sinus or nasopharynx. Anteriorly, the ethmoid cells extend to the lacrimal bone and tumors arising in the ethmoid may therefore erode into the soft tissues beneath the medial canthus of the eye. The superior limit of the ethmoid complex is the fovea ethmoidalis lateral to the ethmoid attachment of the middle turbinate, and the cribriform plate medial to the middle turbinate. These structures lie at or just superior to the horizontal plane of the medial and lateral canthi. The right and left cribriform plate are separated only by the narrow perpendicular plate of the ethmoid bone and more anteriorly by the thicker crista galli. Extension of tumor superiorly may involve both cribriform plates, the anterior cranial fossa dura, olfactory bulb, and frontal lobe of the brain.

The lymphatic drainage of the antroethmoidal complex is limited, and forms from two capillary networks: the respiratory network and the olfactory network. The lymphatic system of the maxillary and much of the ethmoid sinuses connects with that of the nose. It drains posteriorly toward the nasopharyngeal and lateral retropharyngeal nodes, and from there to the subdigastric and internal jugular nodes. The olfactory mucosa is drained by lymphatics running perineurally posteriorly to the lateral pharyngeal nodes in the parapharyngeal space, and from there the internal jugular nodes [10, 11].

The most important mechanism of tumor spread in paranasal sinus malignancies is by direct extension through thin bony margins. Despite the usually advanced local disease at the time of presentation, only 10–15% of antroethmoid squamous cell carcinoma presents with cervical metastases [4, 6, 7, 12]. Thus, metastases do not usually occur until tumor extends beyond the limited lymphatic capillary networks of the paranasal sinuses to areas rich in lymphatic drainage.

Classification

A classification system fulfills its purpose if it produces a clinically useful means of communication and provides a sound basis for therapeutic planning and the evaluation of therapeutic efficacy. Although there have been many staging schemes proposed for cancer of the paranasal sinuses, no classification system has found general acceptance. Two logical, well-reasoned classifications for maxillary sinus cancer are reproduced here [13, 14]. The American Joint Committee on Cancer, 1978, proposed a modification of Sisson's 1963 staging system that recognized that inferiorly located tumors had a better prognosis than superiorly located ones (Table 1). Harrison's 1978 proposal for staging is perhaps in some ways superior for therapeutic planning because the T class correlates better with the extent of surgical resection necessary to extirpate the tumor (Table 2). Evolving philosophies of treatment, including recent enthusiasm for extended craniofacial resection, have changed the implications of some of the critical parameters in evaluation, such as anterior cranial fossa involvement. Intrinsic technological difficulties in evaluating extent of disease have also hampered efforts to achieve a uniform staging system.

Table 1. American joint committee on cancer staging system for maxillary sinus tumors [13]

Primary tumor

TX Tumor cannot be assessed by rules

T1 Tumor confined to antral mucosa of the infrastructure (below Ohngren's line, which is a theoretical plane between the medial canthus of the eye and the angle of the mandible), with no bone erosion or destruction

T2 Tumor confined to suprastructure mucosa without bone destruction or infrastructure tumor with bony destruction of only medial or inferior walls

T3 Tumor invasion of cheek, orbit, anterior ethmoids, or pterygoid muscle

T4 Massive tumor with invasion of cribriform plate or base of skull, posterior ethmoid, sphenoid, nasopharynx, or pterygoid plate

Table 1. (continued)

Cervical nodes

NX   Cannot be assessed
N0   No clinically positive nodes
N1   Single clinicaly positive homolateral node <3 cm in diameter
N2a Single homolateral node 3–6 cm in diameter
N2b Multiple homolateral nodes, none >6 cm
N3a >6 cm homolateral node(s)
N3b Bilateral nodes (stage each side separately)
N3c Contralateral node(s) only

Stage

I   = $T_1N_0M_0$
II   = $T_2N_0M_0$
III = $T_3N_0M_0$, $T_{1-3}N_1M_0$
IV   = $T_4N_{0-1}M_0$, any N_{2-3}, any M_1

Table 2. Staging system for maxillary sinus tumors, (based on Harrison [14])

Primary tumor

T1   Confined to antral mucosa with no bony erosion
T2   Bony erosion but no evidence of involvement of facial skin, orbit, pterygopalatine fossa, or
     ethmoids
T3   Involvement of orbit, ethmoid, or facial skin
T4   Involvement of nasopharynx, sphenoid sinus, cribriform plate, or pterygopalatine fossa

The previous anatomical review of local pathways of tumor spread high-lights several critical points that are key in evaluating (or classifying) a paranasal sinus malignancy [15]. Maxillary and ethmoid sinus tumors can be discussed as one entity, antroethmoidal cancer, because it is so exceedingly rare for the frontal sinus or sphenoid sinus to be the primary site of disease. The antroethmoidal complex is most vulnerable to tumor spread where the bony confines are thinnest. These sites include lamina papyracea, orbital floor, and cribriform plate. The greatest morbidity occurs when extension involves functionally critical structures, such as the orbit, palate, or facial skin; or functionally critical structures that are unresectable, such as selected areas of the skull base.

Adequate diagrams of the tumor, particularly at the time of presentation, greatly facilitate subsequent therapeutic planning. Comparisons to initial diagrams may allow earlier recognition of recurrence. This requires synthesis of information gleaned from polytomography and CT scanning as well as from direct observation and biopsy. Though complex, a multilevel diagram similar to that published by Petruson [16] appears to be the minimum necessary to adequately picture and follow tumor involvement at the critical margin sites: cribriform plate and anterior cranial fossa, medial and inferior orbital periosteum, intraorbital contents, orbital apex, pterygomaxillary space, nose, nasopharynx, sphenoid sinus, and skin.

Pathology

Although the number of different histologic types of malignant tumors that have been reported in the paranasal sinuses is large (Table 3), squamous cell carcinoma is the predominant cancer, accounting for 80-85% of cases [3, 7, 9, 17]. As such, it has been the basis for most of the accrued knowledge regarding the biological behavior and therapeutic response of paranasal sinus tumors. Adenoid cystic carcinoma and adenocarcinoma account for about 5-10% of cases. Extranodal lymphomas [18-20], soft tissue sarcomas [8, 21], melanomas [22], and metastases [23, 24] (e.g., of renal, lung, or breast origin) comprise most of the other types of malignant tumors.

Esthesioneuroblastomas are infrequent tumors of neural crest origin [25, 28]. Because of the potential for histologic confusion due to the undifferentiated nature of these tumors, an adequate biopsy and competent

Table 3. Paranasal sinus malignancies*

---

1. Squamous cell carcinoma
2. Adenocarcinoma
3. Adenoid cystic carcinoma
4. Soft tissue sarcoma:
   Fibrosarcoma
   Osteogenic sarcoma
   Rhabdomyosarcoma
   Chondrosarcoma
   Leiomyosarcoma
   Vascular (e.g. hemangiopericytoma)
   Other (e.g. liposarcoma)
5. Extranodal lymphoma
6. Melanoma
7. Esthesioneuroblastoma
8. Metastases:
   Renal
   Lung
   Breast
   Other
9. Extramedullary plasmacytoma
10. Small cell carcinoma (neuroendocrine carcinoma)
11. Other (e.g. mucoepidermoid)

---

* This list does not include nonmalignant lesions such as juvenile angiofibroma, fibrous dysplasia, giant cell reparative granuloma, and certain fungal infections which may radiologically and clinically behave in a locally destructive manner.

interpretation is an especially critical step in planning therapy [30, 31]. Electron microscopy, special stains (including trichrome, reticulin, and possibly immunoperoxidase stains), and touch preps when lymphoma is a consideration, may be necessary if the typical pathological features of squamous cell carcinoma are not apparent.

Epidemiology

A clue to the etiology of paransal sinus malignancies is found in their epidemiology [32]. Animal studies and epidemiological studies in Europe, North American, and Japan, strongly suggest that nickel exposure from nickel refineries (nickel subsulfide and nickel carbonyl), and possibly from other industries using nickel, is a potent paranasal (and respiratory) carcinogen, increasing the risk of squamous cell carcinoma 800 times [32]. In Europe, Australia, and the United States, wood dust, which slows mucociliary transport, has been implicated as a carcinogen in nasoethmoid adenocarcinoma [32–34]. An increase in the incidence of adenocarcinoma has been found among furniture and other woodworkers and among shoe workers [35, 36]. Thorium dioxide, previously used in radiology, radium used in painting watch dials, mustard gas, isopropyl oil, and several other chemicals have been suspected to be potential carcinogens as well [31]. It is uncertain whether tobacco use is epidemiologically related to paranasal sinus cancer.

Signs and symptoms

Squamous cell carcinoma is most common in males, and may occur at any age but is more common between ages 50 and 70. Several series suggest that a prior history of chronic sinusitis may often be obtained. Because upper respiratory tract infections are so common, the criteria for the diagnosis of 'chronic' sinusitis has varied, and because in retrospect these may be early symptoms of tumor, it is unlikely that the history of prior sinusitis is clinically useful.

Although epidemiological and laboratory studies have identified likely risk factors, these risk factors are quite unusual in the presenting history of most patients. An additional difficulty for the early diagnosis of malignancy is the fact that early growth of sinus cancer is symptomatically silent. There is an average six-month delay, and often longer, between onset of symptoms and diagnosis of malignancy [6, 37, 38].

Nasal bleeding, nasal obstruction, and pain referred to the frontonasal areas or along the alveolar nerve to the gingiva are among the most common symptoms. For maxillary sinus tumors involving the infrastructure of the sinus, dental pain, loosened maxillary teeth, or a change in the fit of a maxillary denture are symptoms that may first be seen by a dentist.

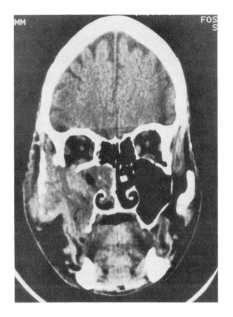
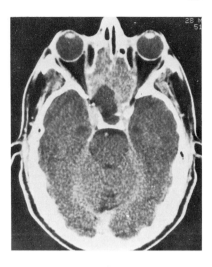

Figure 1A. Coronal CT through plane of sphenoid and posterior orbit (note rectus muscles and optic nerve). Destructive soft tissue mass (a T_4N_0 antral squamous cell carcinoma) erodes antral medial, inferior and lateral walls, floor of orbit, and extends into nasal cavity, soft tissue of cheek, and zygomatic arch. Tumor in orbit abuts the inferior rectus muscle.

Figure 1B. Axial CT with contrast through plane of eye (note lens, muscle cone, and optic nerves). Tumor (an esthesioneuroblastoma) occupies both ethmoid sinuses eroding the medial wall of both orbits, and extends posteriorly beyond the orbital apices into the sphenoid. The enhancing cavernous sinus on the left is well demarcated. The lucent area is probable necrotic tissue within tumor.

Signs and symptoms of more advanced disease are related to the invasion of adjacent structures. Proptosis, diplopia, infraorbital hypesthesia, and an inner canthal mass suggest orbital invasion. Trismus is an ominous sign of pterygoid muscle involvement. Posterior extension may also cause a middle ear effusion and a nasopharynx mass may be visible on indirect exam. Anterior extension can cause erythema, swelling, and paresthesias of the cheek. Inferior extension may cause a submucosal gingivobuccal sulcus mass, or eventually an oroantral fistula. Sinusitis may occur secondary to blockage of natural ostia; a headache may also occur secondary to increased intracranial pressure from penetration into the anterior cranial fossa. Only about 10–15% of cases present with cervical metastases.

Advances in diagnosis

X-Ray computed tomography

Although severe limitations remain, technological advances in radiological

34

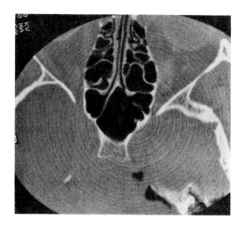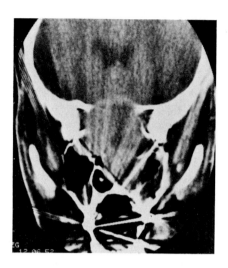

Figure 1C. Axial CT of normal ethmoid sinus for comparison, obtained at a similar level, but using 1.5 mm slices and a bone-enhancing computer algorithm. The narrowness of the ethmoid sinus medial to the middle turbinate is demonstrated well.

Figure 1D. Coronal CT with contrast at plane of orbital apex demonstrating invasion of tumor into anterior cranial fossa. (Same patient as Fig. 1B.)

imaging have made accurate delineation of tumor extent less difficult [39, 40]. The hallmark of malignancy in pluridirectional tomography and CT scanning is bone destruction (Fig. 1). Expansile lesions demonstrating periosteal new bone deposition appear radiologically as an expanded rim of bone. This appearance is more commonly associated with benign disease, although a slow-growing malignancy may also have this appearance. Minor salivary gland tumors, esthesioneuroblastoma, lymphomas, and some soft tissue sarcomas may all cause some bone remodeling. Aggressive bone destruction with no remodeling or reshaping is seen in 80% of patients presenting with squamous cell carcinoma in the paranasal sinuses [41–43]. These radiological changes are often difficult to see on plain films [44, 45]. They may be visible by tomography before the more obvious physical signs of malignancy appear. Because these tumors remain symptomatically silent throughout the early period of time when they are potentially most curable, a high index of suspicion and early use of computed or pluridirectional tomography is perhaps the most important advance necessary to improve the overall management and chance of cure of paranasal sinus tumors.

Imaging by X-ray computed axial tomography (CT), like pluridirectional tomography, is limited by the physical principles on which it is based: the presence of sufficiently different electron absorption coefficients of tumor and surrounding tissue. Computed tomography is excellent in differentiating high density bone from low density air or soft tissue. In the antrum, a soft tissue density may represent inflammatory tissue from sinusitis, blocked sinus secretions from sinusitis or tumor, or may represent malignant tissue. Air-fluid levels, although helpful in that they demonstrate fluid rather than solid tissue, may be the result of a blocked ostium from either inflammatory or malignant disease. Although CT scans differentiate tissue densities only 4% different from water [46], this is insufficient to distinguish the nearly identical electron absorption of malignant tissue and chronic inflammatory tissue. Contrast enhancement partially overcomes the problem by increasing the tissue density of some tumors that are highly vascular. This has proved particularly helpful in the delineation of juvenile angiofibromas. The detection by CT of intracranial extension at the cribriform plate in esthesioneuroblastoma and adenoid cystic carcinoma is not currently sufficiently sensitive to predict the absence of tumor. Contrast enhancement may at times accurately demonstrate malignant tissue superior to the cribriform, but the failure to demonstrate cribriform penetration does not necessarily mean the absence of pathology. A problem of CT scanning peculiar to the paranasal sinuses especially at the palate and skull base can be the presence of too much tissue density between air and bone [46]. The presence of metallic densities, as in tooth fillings, can also present technical artifacts.

Advances in the technology of CT scanning have overcome certain technical problems. Scanners such as the General Electric 8800 and 9800 have higher resolution because of increased sampling of electron absorption coefficients in decreased time. Thinner planes (slices), edge enhancement, and enhanced gray scales also have extended diagnostic capabilities. However, the determination of bone destruction often remains uncertain at precisely the areas it is most critical in judging resectability. Computed image reformation, such as the reconstruction of coronal views at the cribriform plate when actual coronal scanning is not possible or is unsafe, have aided diagnosis. Despite this improved technology, the extent of tumor is still underestimated in about 30% of cases [48].

Nuclear magnetic resonance (NMR)

An exciting complementary diagnostic tool for the future, though costly at present, is medical imaging by nuclear magnetic resonance (NMR) [49, 50]. Introduced for medical application in the early 1970's [51, 52], NMR, without requiring x-irradiation, exploits the intrinsic spin and specific resonant frequency possessed by all atomic nuclei. In the presence of a strong uniform magnetic field and a second specific oscillating magnetic field, nuclei emit very weak but detectable signals (10^{-12} that of an x-ray in conventional CT) as they change quantized energy levels. The study of the hydrogen nucleus (a proton) is best suited for diagnostic application because it is so abundant (in H_2O) in the body, and because of certain other physical characteristics of the proton [53–55].

Unlike x-ray tomography where only electron density is measurable, NMR can measure three parameters: the proton density and two relaxation times, T_1 and T_2. The proton density in NMR is analogous to the electron density in conventional x-ray tomography: the fundamental difference of course is that one maps protons in soft tissue and the other unrelated electrons, and these densities do not change in a parallel manner. The relaxation times T_1 and T_2 are rate constants characterizing the return to equilibrium after the second magnetic field is turned off. T_1 and T_2 may be changed by changing the strength of the magnetic fields and the method of detection. Thus, with increased experience, it should be possible to empirically adjust the strength of the magnetic fields and the method of detection in order to increase the resolution of whichever variable (proton density, T_1, or T_2) offers the most useful information in a particular clinical setting. Three dimensional reconstruction is performed by rotating field gradients in a manner similar to reconstructing the sweeps of conventional computed tomography.

In tumors of the paranasal sinuses, the major clinical problem is earlier detection. Currently, X-ray computed tomography is the most sensitive method of detecting a tumor before ominous physical signs are present. Even the astute physician, suspicious of a malignancy before it can be seen by rhinoscopy, has a problem: is he to perform a Caldwell-Luc on every patient whose symptoms persist? If he waits until CT demonstrates bone destruction, the tumor is usually already advanced. He may perform an antral exploration in all cases of unilateral antral opacification [56, 57], but even this has not affected the epidemiological fact that antroethmoidal cancer is not recognized early. If on the other hand there is not yet architectural bony changes by CT or pluridirectional tomography, it is difficult to strongly suspect malignancy.

It was first shown experimentally in 1971 that the relaxation times of malignant tissue are generally longer than in their normal tissue of origin [51]. Numerous reports have confirmed and expanded these observations, including reports of epithelial malignancies, numerous cell lines, and sera in patients with known tumors [50].

It is possible that NMR will be able to distinguish with modest sensitivity, chemical differences (the state of the water perhaps) between benign and malignant tissue before the tumor changes the anatomic shape of an afflicted organ. If so, it will then be used to complement the superior spatial resolution of CT. Importantly, since NMR uses no ionizing irradiation, it may be possible to use NMR as an early *screening* procedure for *any* patient with known risk factors or when early nonspecific symptoms of paranasal disease are present.

NMR imaging is a promising technique that is on the verge of practical application [58, 59]. Because it measures different variables than CT, it will become a complementary diagnostic tool. A major application in the management of paranasal sinus tumors may be the exploitation of differential relaxation times in order to reliably detect malignancy before bone destruction occurs. Harrison stated in 1976 that 'there is little hope of any worthwhile improvement except to ensure that those who are potentially curable are cured' [60]. NMR holds the promise of increasing the percentage of patients who are 'potentially curable'.

Advances in treatment

Current therapy

Since the first maxillectomy was performed in 1826 by Lizars, the philosophy of treatment of paranasal sinus cancer has evolved through stages. In 1933, Ohngren advocated partial surgical extirpation followed by radiation [61]. Radical surgery in the postwar era (1945–1955) produced cure rates no higher than 25–35%. Orthovoltage radiation alone generally resulted in even lower cure rates (10–30%). Subsequently, numerous reports have discussed various approaches using combinations of surgery and radiation. The initial failure to improve the 25–35% cure rates by combination approaches led to a reappraisal of the indications for orbital exenteration in the hopes of at least causing less morbidity. Various chemotherapy protocols were (and continue to be) actively investigated. Two themes however appear to be consistent: early detection of disease is rare and advanced disease responds poorly. That early diagnosis, as discussed in the previous section, would be a key to improved management is reinforced by a literature review demonstrating that the few cases that are truly found early respond with cure rates of 42–91% [6, 12, 37, 62].

Because antroethmoidal cancer is rare, series reported in the literature are of necessity retrospective. Paranasal cancers are usually included with tumors of the nasal cavity, and too often combine tumors of differing histologies in reporting treatment results. Because no staging system is universally accepted and because the degree of documentation varies, evaluation and comparison of treatment results from different centers is extremely difficult. Our current approaches rely on principles drawn from our own experience and on the reason and judgment of experienced clinicians like Harrison, Sisson, and Fitz-Hugh, who have observed and participated in the changes in treatment strategies over the past two decades.

Although not universally acknowledged, combined radiation and surgical approaches appear to have had the most success in treating antroethmoidal cancer [5, 9, 37, 63, 66]. Whether irradiation should be preoperative [6, 9, 12, 67] or postoperative [5, 48, 65, 68] has not been resolved. Though far from compelling, the results of these studies suggest preoperative radiation is perhaps superior.

Several questions are raised by the poor prognosis of advanced antroethmoidal cancer. Is there a subpopulation of patients considered still resectable in whom, in an effort to decrease the morbidity of maxillectomy and orbital exenteration, less radical surgery can be performed without decreasing the already low chance of cure? Selected series over the past 20 years suggest that when the orbital periosteum is uninvolved by tumor, the orbital contents may often be preserved [2, 38, 64, 69–71]. Reconstruction of the orbital floor is unnecessary when the orbital periosteum has been preserved.

Advances in surgery

A more hopeful question is: can recent advances in anterior skull base surgery improve the overall survival of patients with antroethmoidal cancers?

Between 1954 and 1963 [72–74], techniques for the combined craniofacial resection of ethmoidal tumors were first described. This raised the possibility of en bloc resection of those tumors that extend to the cribriform, ethmoidal roof, superior orbit, and dura or intracranial contents of the anterior cranial fossa. Several surgical objectives are met by this general approach. Most importantly, complete removal of the tumor is possible. In order to achieve this, the best procedure in theory is one providing the maximum necessary exposure for adequate evaluation and unrestricted surgical excision. Full repair of dural tears and cerebrospinal fluid leaks must be possible. Perioperative complications must be kept low.

Although different surgeons have discussed variations [71, 75–77], the technique outlined below (supraorbital approach with pericranial flap closure [77, 78] represents a basic approach that allows maximal anterior cranial fossa and supraorbital exposure, minimal brain retraction, and excellent protection against CSF leaks and meningitis.

General intubation anesthesia is achieved. Because of the length of the operative procedure, the patient is monitored by central venous and peripheral arterial lines. Continuous temperature monitoring is achieved with an esophageal thermometer. Urine output is monitored via bladder catherization. End-tidal CO_2 is also constantly monitored via a Beckman End-Tidal CO_2 monitor. The operative procedure is performed in cooperation with a neurosurgeon who is responsible for obtaining exposure from the intracranial route.

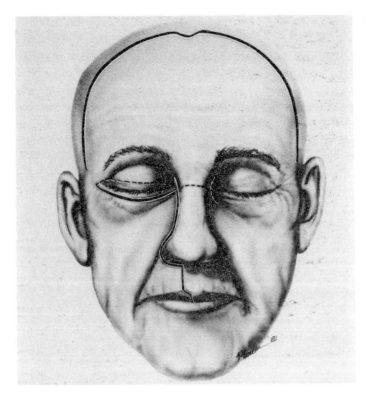

Figure 2. A bicoronal scalp flap is used to expose the skull for craniotomy. The facial incisions utilize an external ethmoidectomy, lateral rhinotomy, or Weber-Ferguson incision with modifications (dotted lines) depending on the extent of disease and of surgical exposure necessary.

In order to facilitate retraction of the frontal lobes for exposure of the floor of the anterior fossa, CSF is removed by a subarachnoid drain placed percutaneously into the lumbar subarachnoid space. After placement of these catheters, the patient is placed in the supine position with the head in slight extension so that the floor of the anterior fossa is perpendicular to the

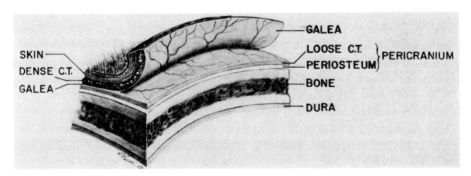

Figure 3. The scalp is composed of two discrete layers. The pericranium and the overlying loose connective tissue beneath the galea aponeurotica.

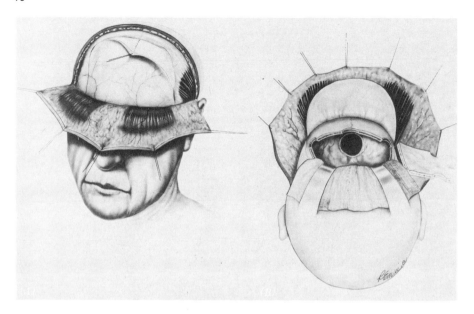

Figures 2, 3 and 4 are republished with permission from Johns et al., Laryngoscope 91:952–958, 1981.

Figure 4A. The pericranial flap is raised using electrocautery, reflected downward over the scalp flap, and covered with moist sponges. The blood supply is based inferiorly on the supraorbital and supratrochlear arteries and laterally on the supratemporal arteries. (B). The anterior cranial fossa defect which is to be covered with pericranial flap is seen. The bone flap is seen attached to skull by temporalis fascia and muscle.

horizontal. The hair is then shaven, standard betadine prepping completed, a bicoronal skin flap is outlined (Fig. 2), and the skin to be incised infiltrated with 1/2% lidocaine and 1:100,000 epinephrine. The bicoronal flap is reflected anteriorly to just beyond the superior orbital ridge. Pericranium is included in this flap (Fig. 3). At the superior orbital ridge, the periorbita is continuous with the pericranium. Separating the periorbita-pericranium from the orbital roof without lacerations prevents subsequent herniation of orbital fat into the field.* Burr holes are then created to facilitate the creation of a bone flap. One burr hole is made just posterior to the frontal process of the zygoma. A second paramidline burr hole is placed at the nasal process of the frontal bone on the side uninvolved by tumor. (As this second burr hole usually passes through the frontal sinus, it will be necessary to

---

* If no exposure of the orbital roof is required, then the bicoronal flap need be reflected only as far as the brow line. In this case the pericranium initially may be left attached to frontal bone in a manner identical to the bicoronal approach in a osteoplastic frontal procedure [2, 79]. The pericranial flap in this case must be developed at this time (Fig. 4A). The subsequent bone flap may then be created extending 4 cm to either side of the midline, with a height of 4 cm, and with the craniotomy defect beginning 4 cm above the brow line (Fig. 4B).

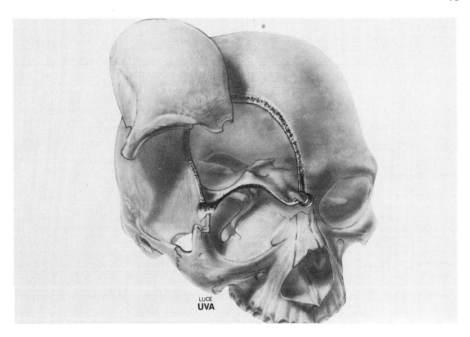

LUCE
UVA

Figure 5 is republished with permission from Janer et al., Neurosurgery 11:537–542, 1982.

Figure 5. Exposure of anterior skull base and superior orbital roof achieved by supratemporal approach. Although usually remaining attached by temporalis muscle or fascia, the bone flap may be removed as in this diagram.

remove mucosa and inner cortical lining of frontal sinus that is within the bone flap.)

Protecting the periorbita with a brain spatula, a gigli saw is used to connect the burr holes. The superior part of the bone flap is created with a craniotome after separating dura from inner bone table. The bone flap, which may be left attached laterally to the superficial temporalis facia and muscle, includes superior orbital rim and anterior orbital roof to provide maximum exposure of and access to both ethmoid complexes and the orbital contents (Fig. 5). If necessary, sufficient orbital roof may be removed to obtain exposure to within 2 cm of the anterior communicating artery complex. Dura is reflected from the recessed cribriform area and the olfactory nerves are individually cut. Where dura invaginates into bony crevices, clips are applied across the neck of these invaginations and the dura cut. The earlier placement of the lumbar subarachnoid drain to remove CSF allows exposure of the full extent of cribriform plate with minimal retraction of frontal lobe. Using frozen sections for guidance, as much involved dura as necessary is sacrificed. Any dural tears are repaired by primary closure or by using temporalis fascia or a pericranial flap. The craniotome is now used to make the superior bony cuts of the en bloc tumor resection. These bone cuts separate the cribriform plate and any other areas involved by tumor from remaining uninvolved orbital roof, frontal sinus, and cranial floor bilaterally.

At this point, exposure having been obtained from above, the head and neck surgeon commences the en bloc resection from the facial approach. To separate the sterile intracranial operative field from the facial operative field, that may be contaminated by nasal bacteria, a two layer antibiotic soaked gauze and towel (a Cushing's veil) is used. This veil is seated along the plane of the eyebrows and can therefore be reflected superiorly or inferiorly to exclude one or the other operative field.

Modifications of the Weber-Ferguson incision are used depending on tumor extent. An extension across the roof of the nose allows the entire external nose to be rotated out of the operative field. Inclusion of the orbital contents can be easily added if orbital periosteum is found to be involved by tumor (Fig. 2). If the tumor does not involve the maxilla or is limited to the upper inner quadrant of the maxillary sinus and the floor is free, the hard palate can be preserved. If the floor of the maxilla is involved, a maxillectomy will be necessary. The extent of the surgical procedure is increased or reduced based on tumor extent. Once the tumor is freed from all bony, muscular, and neural attachments with acceptable margins, the specimen is removed from below and contains as a minimum the entire ethmoid block including lamina papyracea, the middle, and superior turbinates on both sides.

Following en bloc resection, a pericranial flap reconstruction helps prevent cerebrospinal fluid rhinorrhea and, along with a skin graft placed inferior to the flap, reduces the chance of meningitis from nasal bacterial contamination. It also serves as a sling to help support the frontal lobes (Fig.6) [77]. If the pericranial flap has not yet been made, the pericranium may easily be separated from the bicoronal skin flap by first using 1/2% lidocaine with 1:100,000 epinephrine in the loose connective tissue to hydrodissect the galea from the periosteum. The pericranial flap is then dissected and sutured to the deepest parts of exposed dura on the anterior cranial fossa floor, creating a water-tight closure. The skin graft is placed thransethmoidally, sutured in place, and secured with packing brought out transnasally. Because the pericranium is vascularized, survival of the exposed skin graft is highly likely. Some surgeons have, in addition, recommended placement of a free split rib graft just superior to the skin graft to provide more solid support for the frontal lobe [80, 81]. We have not found this to be necessary. The bone flap is then replaced and stabilized with multiple stainless steel wires. Galea and skin incisions are then closed in standard fashion.

The patient is carefully monitored in the ICU for 48 hours including the use of an intracranial pressure screw [82]. In most cases, by the second post-

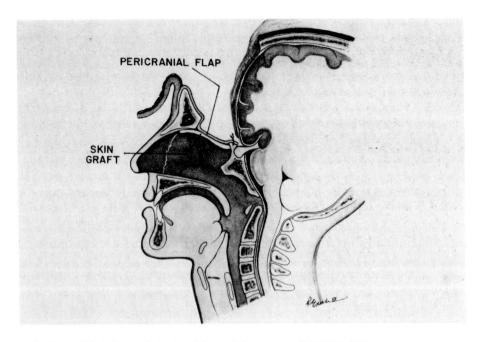

PERICRANIAL FLAP

SKIN GRAFT

Figure 6 is republished with permission from Johns et al., Laryngoscope 91:952–958, 1981.

Figure 6. The pericranial flap is brought into the craniotomy site and sutured in multiple locations to the deepest part of the exposed dura on the anterior cranial floor. A split thickness skin graft or dermal graft is placed against the nasal surface of the pericranial flap.

operative day, all monitoring lines are removed and the patient is discharged from the ICU for routine postoperative care. Sinus packing is removed on the fifth postoperative day, facial sutures are removed on the seventh postoperative day and the patient is discharged home on the 10th to 14th postoperative day, barring complications.

In deciding whether a combined craniofacial resection is necessary to achieve en bloc resection, it should be recalled that the cribriform is an area where radiological evaluation is imprecise. Understaging is common. In our experience with esthesioneuroblastoma, several patients undergoing craniofacial resection have had intracranial involvement that was not demonstrated by CT scan.

Improved survival rates without increased morbidity have been consistently seen using a combination of radiation and craniofacial surgery. Ketcham in 1973 reported a 53% determinant 5-year survival rate among 48 patients, including those with prior treatment [71]. Smaller series have realized similar success [83, 84]. This approach has been applied to patients with esthesioneuroblastoma [76, 77], juvenile angiofibroma [84–86], and other tumors [76] with good results and little or no cosmetic deformity.

Terz has extended the principle of craniofacial resection to include resection of the middle cranial fossa in cases of maxillary sinus carcinoma because tumor so often invades the pterygoid fossa [87, 88].

After raising a forehead flap on the side of the tumor to expose the frontal bone and temporal fossa, an anterior cranial dissection is completed in a manner similar to that described earlier. The head is then turned to explore the middle cranial fossa via an extradural subtemporal craniectomy. The middle meningeal artery is divided. The dura is elevated in order to transect the second and third divisions of the trigeminal nerve. An air drill is then used to connect the foramen spinosum, foramen ovale, and foramen rotundum. The bony incision is then extended posterolaterally and anterolateriall to complete the bony cuts in the middle cranial fossa floor. Posterolaterally the bone cut is extended anterior to the petrous ridge and through the temporomandibular joint. Anterolaterally, the bone cut curves from the foramen rotundum, through the sphenoid bone, and through the superior orbital fissure, and an orbital exenteration is included in the maxillectomy. These bony cuts in the middle cranial fossa demark the superior limits of the infratemporal space. The maxilla, pterygoid plate, mandibular ramus superiorly to temporomandibular joint, pterygoid muscles, nasal bone, and orbital contents may then be removed en bloc with the anterior cranial fossa contents previously dissected. If necessary, involved parts of the nasopharynx and oropharynx could be included.

Terz has reconstructed the defect using the forehead flap created at the beginning of the procedure. It is sutured to the remaining anterior and middle cranial fossa floors. The anterior bony plate is wired in place and an occipitofrontal skin flap rotated over it. Alternatively, the bicoronal – Weber Ferguson approach with a pericranial flap might be used to close the defect in a more cosmetically acceptable manner. The palate is usually reconstructed with an obturator (made from a cast of the hard palate preoperatively) wired to remaining teeth. Other skin flaps or prosthodontic approaches are possible for an edentulous patient.

Using this extended anterior-middle cranial fossa approach, Terz reported a 72% 3-year survival among 22 patients with squamous cell carcinoma when the sphenoid sinus and nasopharynx were initially histologically negative [88].

There appears to be little question that craniofacial resection, using the combined skills of a neurosurgical and a head and neck surgical team, is safe, and has extended the limits of surgical excision, while still allowing satisfactory reconstruction.

Investigational therapy

Improved survival rates of 50–70% are achievable only in a selected subpopulation of patients where the addition of craniofacial surgery permits en bloc resection. Although local recurrence ramains by far the predominant cause of failure in squamous cell carcinoma of the paranasal sinuses, cervical and distant metastases are not uncommon. Approximately 35% of patients with antral cancer develop neck nodes at some time [8, 89, 90]. Distant metastases have appeared even in the absence of local recurrence after craniofacial resection.

Because of these problems, there is much current interest in the use of chemotherapeutic drugs in conjunction with other treatment modalities. Various protocols for advanced squamous cell carcinoma of the head and neck using combinations of cis-platinum, bleomycin, methotrexate, vincristince, and 5-fluorouracil, have often produced dramatic cytoreduction. Complete response rates however remain very low and as of yet, there has been no demonstrated increase in patient survival.

In maxillary sinus cancer, several small series of patients treated with intraarterial regional chemotherapy in conjunction with surgery and radiation have been reported. A variety of chemotherapeutic agents including 5-fluorouracil [91], bleomycin and methotrexate [92], and cis-platinum [93], have been utilized with inconclusive results. A review of thirteen cases of esthesioneuroblastoma suggest that this tumor may be responsive to a combination of vincristine and cyclophosphamide [94].

The use of chemotherapy in the treatment of epithelial tumors of the paranasal sinuses remains an experimental approach to be studied in rigorously controlled clinical protocols. Investigation of new chemotherapeutic drugs may offer more promise in the future.

Advances in radiation therapy: radiosensitizers

The fact that hypoxic cells demonstrate increased radioresistance was reported in the English literature fifty years ago [95]. The reasons for this observation have been extensively investigated in hope of discovering methods to sensitize hypoxic cells to irradiation [96]. The inhibition of sublethal cellular repair by Actinomycin D [97], hyperthermia [98], and in hypoxic cells by the depletion of intracellular thiols has been extensively studied [99, 100]. Cis-platinum, better known because of its direct chemotherapeutic action in head and neck squamous cell carcinoma, is also a potential radiosensitizer [101, 102]. Electron affinic compounds such as the nitro compounds and metabolically unstable nitroxyl free radicals act as oxygen mimetics, thereby sensitizing hypoxic cells.

The clinical application of radiosensitizers is in a developmental stage. Phase II and III studies with misonidazole, a nitro compound, have been carried out with many different tumors, including head and neck squamous cell carcinoma [103, 104]. Early studies demonstrate modest response rates, no improved control, and a high incidence (15–20%) of peripheral neuro-pathy using the drug. More effective nitro compound sensitizers that are less neurotoxic than misonidazole and some non-nitro compounds are being actively investigated. Borrowing from the experience with multiple drugs used in chemotherapy, it may be possible to enhance the effects of radio-sensitizers by combining compounds that act by different mechanisms thereby enhancing efficacy and reducing overall toxicity.

Advances in radiation therapy: heavy particles

As an alternative to X-ray and gamma rays, the medical application of heavy charged particles has been suggested. They offer several theoretical potential advantages: (1) a decreased oxygen enhancement ratio (OER); (2) altered dose distribution; and 3) altered primary biological effect. The most important advantage of heavy particles is that, like chemical radiosensitiz-ers, they reduce the radioresistant effect of hypoxia in tumors. The radior-esistance of hypoxic cells is less for neutrons, heavy ions, and pi-mesons than for X-rays [105, 106]. This lower oxygen enhancement ratio (OER) offers a modest therapeutic advantage in the hypoxic conditions common to many tumors.

Secondly, unlike the physical dose distribution of X-rays, gamma rays and neutrons, all of which reduce exponentially with depth, the dose distri-bution of charged heavy ions is such that the most radiation damage occurs at a calculable depth from the surface, the Bragg peak, where the particles stop. Thus, localized, densely ionizing high radiation dose can be delivered to a deep seated tumor while significantly sparing surrounding normal tis-sue. This principle has thus far found its widest clinical use in proton ther-apy of choroidal melanoma [106].

The Bragg peak can be spread over several centimeters with ridge filters in order to treat a larger field. Particles of higher atomic number such as carbon, neon, and argon are more effective in reducing the OER but also have reduced depth-dose effectiveness [105, 106]. For the relatively shallow depth required for the treatment of paranasal sinus tumors, argon is perhaps the most appropriate element in this regard [108].

The third theoretical advantage of charged particles relates to the *in vivo* radiobiological effect of the radiation [105, 106, 108]. It is thought that the slowness and inaccuracy of repairing double-stranded DNA breaks is an important cause of cellular lethality. One effect of heavy ions is that they cause many more double-stranded breaks than do X-rays. X-rays cause more rapidly repairable single-stranded breaks. Inaccurate repair of double-stranded breaks during S phase (DNA synthesis) of the cell cycle also makes the DNA less resistant to high LET radiation than to X-rays. This decreases the variation in tumor radiosensitivity caused by that proportion of cells in this less radiosensitive phase of the cell cycle.

The question that needs to be addressed is whether these costly new treatments increase radiocurability. Neutrons have been shown to hold an advantage over photons in one study of head and neck carcinoma [109, 110], but not in several other studies [111–113]. Phase I trials of heavy ion therapy are underway for head and neck cancers. An increase in late complications has been seen by some investigators using neutrons with low dose per fraction. Despite initial disappointment, more data must be acquired before reliable clinical conclusions can be reached.

The future

Major advances in therapy will no doubt come about in large part as a result of the application of increased basic understanding of the molecular biology of cancer and the immune system. Intense studies of gene mappings, monoclonal antibodies, and the role of oncogenes have made initial advances in the diagnosis of leukemia. The implications of these studies suggest far reaching therapeutic manipulations. Study of keratin differentiation among squamous cells is promising. Improved tissue culture methods for squamous cell carcinomas and other tumors should allow development of *in vitro* biological models and may have a role in chemotherapeutic sensitivity studies. Continued support of research at the molecular level is the foundation for our hopes of understanding both normal intracellular control mechanisms and abnormal ones, which we call cancer.

Summary

Cancer of the paranasal sinuses represents a major challenge in diagnosis and treatment. These antroethmoidal malignancies are insidious in onset, and extend early to vital adjacent structures, producing disability in comfort, function, and self image.

A major goal necessary to improve the overall pessimistic outlook associated with these cancers is certainly early diagnosis. This goal has been elusive. Nuclear magnetic resonance imaging is likely to be a safe screening measure that may be able to distinguish tumor from inflammatory disease before the presence of bone destruction. For these reasons, NMR imaging is likely to hold great promise for the early recognition of sinus malignancy.

The major therapeutic advance in the management of paranasal tumors in the past decade has been the demonstrated success of craniofacial resections of the anterior skull base. Unfortunately for too many patients, tumor has

48

already extended beyond the limits of en bloc resection at time the of diagnosis. Although it is likely that earlier recognition could increase the proportion of patients in whom potentially curative en bloc resection is feasible, there will no doubt remain a substantial group for whom the prognosis will remain poor. Advances in molecular biology and immunobiology, along with continued basic clinical research of investigational therapies, such as new chemotherapeutic drugs, radiosensitizers, high energy particle radiation, and immunotherapy, may provide the information necessary to open new horizons in the treatment of these malignancies.

References

1. Gray H: In: Warwick R, Williams PL (eds) Gray's Anatomy, 35th edn. London, Longman, 1973.
2. Montgomery WW: Surgery of the Upper Respiratory System, 2nd edn. Philadelphia, Lea and Febiger, 1979.
3. Boone MLM, Harle TS, Higholt HW: Paranasal sinuses and nasal cavity. In: Fletcher GH, Jing B-S (eds) The Head and Neck. Chicago, Year Book Medical Publishers, Inc, 1968, pp 235–313.
4. Lederman M: Tumors of the upper jaw. Natural history and treatment. J Laryngol Otol 84:369–401, 1970.
5. Lewis JS, Castro EB: Cancer of the nasal cavity on paranasal sinuses. J Laryngol Otol 86:255–262, 1972.
6. Jackson RT, Fitz-Hugh GS, Constable WC: Malignant neoplasms of the nasal cavities and paranasal sinuses: (A retrospective study). Laryngoscope 87:726–736, 1977.
7. Robins PE, Powell, DJ, Stansbie JM: Review: Carcinoma of the nasal cavity and paranasal sinuses: Incidence and presentation of different histological types. Clin Otolaryngol 4:431–456, 1979.
8. Batsakis, JG: Tumors of the Head and Neck: Clinical and Pathological Consideration, 2nd edn. Baltimore, Williams and Wilkins, 1979.
9. Sisson GA, Becker SP: Cancer of the nasal cavity and paranasal sinuses. In: Suen JY, Myers EN (eds) Cancer of the Head and Neck. New York, Churchill Livingston, 1981, pp 242–279.
10. Haagensen CD, Feimd CR, Herter FP, Slanetz CA Jr., Weinberg JA: The Lymphatics in Cancer. Philadelphia, W.B. Saunders, 1972.
11. Bleehen NM: Ethmoid sinus cancer. JAMA 219:346–347, 1972.
12. Cheng VST, Wang CC: Carcinoma of the paranasal sinuses. A study of sixty-six cases. Cancer 40:3038–3041, 1977.
13. Staging of cancer of head and neck sites and of melanomas, 1980. Chicago, American Joint Committee on Cancer, 1980.
14. Harrison DFN: Critical look at the classification of maxillary sinus carcinomata. Ann Otol Rhinol Laryngol, 87:3–9, 1978.
15. Harrison DFN: A critical evaluation of present day attitudes to the treatment of antro-ethmoidal cancer. J Otolaryngol 11:148–150, 1982.
16. Petruson B: A form to show extension of tumors in the nose and sinus. Arch Otolaryngol 108:460–461, 1982.
17. Batsakis JG, Rice DH, Solomon AR: The pathology of head and neck tumors: Squamous and mucous gland carcinomas of the nasal cavity, paranasal sinuses, and larynx, part 6.

Head Neck Surg 2:497–508, 1980.

18. Fu YS, Perzin KH: Nonepithelial tumors of the nasal cavity, paranasal sinuses and naso-pharynx. A clinicopathological study. X. Malignant lymphomas. Cancer 43:611–621, 1979.

19. Gottlieb TH, Meriwether WD: Lymphosarcoma of paranasal sinuses. Arch Otol 93:199–202, 1971.

20. Wang CC: Primary malignant lymphoma of the oral cavity and paranasal sinuses. Radiology 100:151–153, 1971.

21. Goepfert H, Lindberg RD, Sinkovics JG, Ayala AG: Soft tissue sarcoma of the head and neck after puberty. Treatment by surgery on postoperative radiation therapy. Arch Otolaryngol 103:365–368, 1977.

22. Lund V: Malignant melanoma of the nasal cavity and paranasal sinuses. J Laryngol Otol 96:347–355, 1982.

23. Nahum AM, Bailey BJ: Malignant tumors metastatic to the nose and paranasal sinuses: Case report and review of the literature. Laryngoscope 73:942–953, 1963.

24. Bernstein JM, Montgomery WW, Balogh K: Metastatic tumors to the maxilla, nose, and paranasal sinus. Laryngoscope, 76:621–650, 1966.

25. Chaudhry AP, Haar JG, Koul A, Nickerson PA: Olfactory neuroblastoma (esthesioneuro-blastoma). A light and ultrastructural study of two cases. Cancer 44:564–579, 1979.

26. Elkon D, Hightower SI, Lim ML, Cantrell RW, Constable WC. Esthesioneuroblastoma. Cancer 44:1987–1094, 1979.

27. Trojanowski JQ, Lee V, Pillsbury N, Lee S: Neuronal origin of human esthesioneuroblas-toma demonstrated with anti-neurofilament monoclonal antibodies. N Engl J Med 307:159–161, 1982.

28. Gown AM: Neuronal origin of human esthesioneuroblastoma. Letter to the editor. N Engl J Med 307:1457, 1982.

29. Silva E, Batsakis JG: Neuronal origin of human esthesioneuroblastoma. Letter to the editor. N Engl J Med 307:1457–1458, 1982.

30. Cantrell RW, Ghorayeb BV, Fitz-Hugh GS: Esthesioneuroblastoma: Diagnosis and treatment. Ann Otol Rhinol Laryngol 86:760–765, 1977.

31. Oberman HA, Rice DH: Olfactory neuroblastomas. A clinicopathologic study. Cancer 38:2494–2502, 1976.

32. Roush GC: Epidemiology of cancer of the nose and paranasal sinuses: Current concepts. Head Neck Surg 2:3–33, 1979.

33. Acheson ED, Cowdell RH, Hadfield E, Macbeth RG: Nasal cancer in woodworkers in the furniture industry. Br Med J 2:587–596, 1968.

34. Engzell U: Occupational etiology and nasal cancer. An internordic project. Acta Otolaryngol (Suppl) 360:126–128, 1979.

35. Acheson ED, Cowdell RH, Jolles B: Nasal cancer in the Northhampton boot and shoe industry. Br Med J 1:385–393, 1975.

36. Acheson ED: Nasal cancer in the furniture and boot and shoe manufacturing industries. Prev Med 5:295–315, 1976.

37. Schechter GL, Ogura JH: Maxillary sinus malignancy. Laryngoscope 82:796–806, 1972.

38. Weymuller EA, Reardon EJ, Nash D: A comparison of treatment modalities in carcinoma of the maxillary antrum. Arch Otolaryngol 106:625–629, 1980.

39. Mancuso AA, Hanafee WN: Paranasal sinuses – normal anatomy, methodology, and pathology. In: Computed Tomography of the Head and Neck. Baltimore, Williams and Wilkins, 1982, pp 203–243.

40. Schindler E, Reck R: Value and limits of computer-assisted tomography. Head Neck Surg 2:287–292, 1980.

41. Som PM, Shugar JMA: The significance of bone expansion associated with the diagnosis of malignant tumors of paranasal sinuses. Radiology 136:97–100, 1980.

50

42. Dubois PJ, Schultz JC, Perrin RL, Dastur KJ: Tomography in expansile lesions of the nasal and paranasal sinuses. Radiology 125:149–158, 1977.
43. Som PM: The role of CT in the diagnosis of carcinoma of the paranasal sinuses and nasopharynx. J Otolaryngol 11:340–348, 1982.
44. De St Jeor, Konradh, Hanafee WN: Tomography of paranasal sinus disease undetected by routine views. Appl Radio 9:73–80, 1980.
45. Jeans WD, Gilani S, Bullimore J: The effect of CT scanning on staging of tumors of the paranasal sinuses. Clin Radiol 33:173–179, 1982.
46. Thomsen J, Gyldensted C, Lester J: Computer tomography of cerebellopontine angle lesions. Arch Otolaryngol 103:65–69, 1977.
47. Jing BS, Goepfert H, Close LG: Computerized tomography of paranasal sinus neoplasms. Laryngoscope 88:1485–1503, 1978.
48. Robin PE, Powell DJ: Diagnostic errors in cancers of the nasal cavity and paranasal sinuses. The essential role of surgery. Arch Otolaryngol 107:138–140, 1981.
49. Kaufman L, Crooks LE, Margulis A: Nuclear Magnetic Resonance Imaging in Medicine. New York, Igaku-Shoin, 1981.
50. Partain CL, James AE Jr, Rollo FD, Price RR: Nuclear Magnetic Resonance (NMR) Imaging. Philadelphia, WB Saunders Company, 1983.
51. Damadian R: Tumor detection by nuclear magnetic resonance. Science 171:1151–1153, 1971.
52. Lauterbur PC: Image formation by induced local interactions: example employing nuclear magnetic resonance. Nature 242:190–191, 1973.
53. Pykett IL, Newhouse JH, Buonanno FS, et al.: Nuclear magnetic resonance Principle of nuclear magnetic resonance imaging. Radiology 143:157–168, 1982.
54. James AE Jr, Partain CL, Holland GN, et al.: Nuclear magnetic resonance imaging: The current state. AJR 138:201–210, 1981.
55. Hounsfield GN: Computed medical imaging. Nobel lecture, December 8, 1979. J Comput Assist Tomogr 4:665–674, 1980.
56. Eichel BS: The medical and surgical approach in management of the unilateral opacified antrum. Laryngoscope 87:737–750, 1977.
57. Eichel BS: Criteria for selection of patients undergoing paranasal sinus surgery. Candidate's thesis to the American Laryngological, Rhinological and Otological Society, Inc., 1976.
58. Marx JL: NMR opens a new window into the body. The uses of nuclear magnetic resonance for medical diagnosis hovers on the brink of practical applications. Science 210:302–305, 1980.
59. Bydder GM, Steiner RE, Young IR, et al.: Clinical NMR imaging of the brain: 140 cases. AJR 139:215–236, 1982.
60. Harrison DFN: Problem in surgical management of neoplasms arising in the paranasal sinuses. J laryngol Otol 90:69–74, 1976.
61. Ohngren LG: Malignant tumors of the maxillo-ethmoidal region: A clinical study with special reference to the treatment with electrocautery and irradiation. ACTA Otolaryngol (Suppl) 19:1–476, 1933.
62. Ellingwood KE, Million RR: Cancer of the nasal cavity and ethmoid/sphenoid sinuses. Cancer 43:1517–1526, 1979.
63. Robin PE, Powell DJ: Treatment of carcinoma of the nasal cavity and paranasal sinuses. Clin Otolaryngol 6:401–414, 1981.
64. Som ML: Surgical management of carcinoma of the maxilla. Arch Otolaryngol 99:270–273, 1974.
65. Jesse RH, Goepfert H, Lindberg RD: Carcinoma of the sinuses: A review of treatment. In: Chambers RG, Jansen de Limpeus AMP, Jaques DA, Routledge RT (eds) Cancer of the Head and Neck. Amsterdam, Excerpta Medica; New York, American Elsevier Publ Co, 1975, pp 153–159.

66. Sisson GA: Symposium. III. Treatment of malignancies of paranasal sinuses: Discussion and summary. Laryngoscope 80:945–953, 1970.

67. Yu-Hua H, Gui-Yi T, Yu-Qin Q, et al.: Comparison of pre- and postoperative radiation in the combined treatment of carcinoma of maxillary sinus. Lat J Radiation Oncol Biol Phys 8:1045–1049, 1982.

68. Ahmad K, Cordoba RB, Fayos JV: Squamous cell carcinoma of the maxillary sinus. Arch Otolaryngol 107:48–51, 1981.

69. Larson DL, Christ JE, Jesse RH: Preservation of the orbital contents in cancer of the maxillary sinus. Arch Otolaryngol 108:370–372, 1982.

70. Adkins WY Jr: Maxillectomy with preservation of orbital function. Surg Forum 27:548–550, 1976.

71. Ketcham AS, Chretien PB, Van Buren TM, Hoye RC, Beazley RM, Herdt JR: The ethmoid sinuses: A re-evaluation of surgical resection. Am J Surg 126:469–476, 1973.

72. Smith RR, Klopp CT, Williams JM: Surgical treatment of cancer of the frontal sinus and adjacent areas. Cancer 7:991–994, 1954.

73. Malecki J: New trends in frontal sinus surgery. Acta Otolaryngol 50:137–140, 1959.

74. Ketcham AS, Wilkins RH, Van Buren JM, Smith RR: A combined intracranial facial approach to the paranasal sinuses. Am J Surg 106:698–703, 1963.

75. Shah JP, Galicich JH: Craniofacial resection for malignant tumors of ethmoid and anterior skull base. Arch Otolaryngol 103:514–517, 1977.

76. Schramm VL, Myers EN, Maroon JC: Anterior skull base surgery for benign and malignant disease. Laryngoscope 89:1077–1091, 1979.

77. Johns ME, Winn HR, McLean WC, Cantrell RW: Pericranial flap for the closure of defects of craniofacial resections. Laryngoscope 91:952–958, 1981.

78. Jane JA, Park TS, Pobereskin LH, Winn HR, Butler AB: The supraorbital approach: Technical note. Neurosurgery 11:537–542, 1982.

79. Bridger GP, Shaheen OH: Radical surgery for ethmoid cancer. J Laryngol Otol 82:817–824, 1968.

80. Sisson GA, Bytell DE, Becker SP, Ruge D: Carcinoma of the paranasal sinuses and cranial-facial resection. J Laryngol Otol 90:59–68, 1976.

81. Schuller D: Personal communication.

82. Winn HR, Dacey RG, Jane JA: Intracranial subarachnoid pressure recording: Experience with 650 patients. Surg Neurol 8:41–47, 1977.

83. Bridger GP: Radical surgery for ethmoid cancer. Arch Otolaryngol 106:630–634, 1980.

84. Terz JJ, Young HF, Lawrence W Jr: Combined craniofacial resection for locally advanced carcinoma of the head and neck. II. Carcinoma of the paranasal sinuses. Am J Surg 140:618–624, 1980.

85. Jafek BW, Nahum AM, Butler RM: Surgical treatment of juvenile nasopharyngeal angiofibroma. Laryngoscope 83:707–720, 1973.

86. Krekorian EA, Katu RH: Surgical management of nasopharyngeal angiofibroma with intracranial extension. Laryngoscope 87:154–164, 1977.

87. Standefer J, Holt GR, Brown WE, Gates GA: Combined intracranial and extracranial excision of nasopharyngeal angiofibroma. Laryngoscope. in press.

88. Terz JJ, Alksne JF, Lawrence W Jr: Craniofacial resection for tumors invading the pterygoid fossa. Am J Surg 118:732–740, 1969.

89. Windeyer BW: Malignant tumors of the upper jaw. Br J Radiol 16:362–366, 1943.

90. Larsson LG, Mortensson G: Maxillary antial cancers. JAMA, 219:342–345, 1972.

91. Goepfert H, Jesse RH, Lindberg RD: Arterial indusions and radiation therapy in the treatment of advanced cancer of the nasal cavity and paranasal sinuses. Am J Surg 126:464–468, 1973.

92. Moseley HS, Thomas LR, Sverts EC, Stevens KR, Ireland KM: Advanced squamous cell carcinoma of the maxillary sinus. Results of combined regional infusion chemotherapy,

radiation therapy and surgery. Am J Surg 141:522–525, 1981.

93. Arbit E, Sundareson N, Galicich JH, Shab J: Craniofacial resection following chemotherapy. Surg Neurol 13:395–399, 1980.

94. Wade PM, Smith RE, Johns ME: Response of esthesioneuroblastoma to chemotherapy. Report of five cases and review of the literature. Arch Otolaryngol, in press.

95. Crabtree HG, Cramer W: The action of radium on cancer cells. II. Some factors determining the susceptibility of cancer cells to radium. Proc R Soc Lond (Biol) 113:238–250, 1933.

96. Stratford IJ: Mechanisms of hypoxic cell radiosensitization and the development of new sensitizers. Int J Radiat Oncology Biol Phys 8:391–398, 1982.

97. Piro AJ, Taylor CC, Bell JA: Interaction between radiation and drug damage in mammalian cells. II. The effect of Actinomycin D on the repair of sub-lethal damage in plateau phase cells. Cancer 37:2697–2702, 1976.

98. Ben-Hur E, Elkind MM, Bronk BV: Thermally enhanced radio-response of cultured Chinese hamster cells: Inhibition of repair of sublethal damage and enhancement of lethal damage. Radiat Res 58:38–51, 1974.

99. Bump EA, Brown JM: The use of drugs which deplete intracellular glutathione as radiosensitizers of hypoxic tumor cells *in vivo*. Int J Radiat Oncol Biol Phys 8:439–442, 1982.

100. Varnes ME, Biaglow JE, Koch CJ, Hall EJ: Depletion of non-protein thiols of hypoxic cells by misonidazole and metronidazole. In: Brady LW (ed) Radiation Sensitizers. New York, Masson, 1980, pp 121–124.

101. Douple EB, Richmond RC: Platinum complexes as radiosensitizers of hypoxic mammalian cells. Br J Cancer 37 (Suppl III):98–102, 1978.

102. Stratford IJ, Williamson C, Adams GE: Combination studies with misonidazole and a cis-platinum complex: Cytotoxicity and radiosensitization *in vitro*. Br J Cancer 41:517–523, 1980.

103. Fazekas JT: The value of adjuvant misonidazole in the definitive irradiation of advanced head and neck squamous cancer. An RTOG pilot study (#78–02). Int J Radiat Oncol Biol Phys 5 (Suppl 2):186–187, 1979.

104. Sealy R, Williams A, Cridland S, Stratford M, Minchinton A, Hallet C: A report on misonidazole in a randomized trial in locally advanced head and neck cancer. Int J Radiat Oncol Biol Phys 8:339–342, 1982.

105. Hall ET: Radiobiology for the Radiologist. Hagerstown, Maryland, Harper and Row, 1978.

106. Hall EJ: The particles compared. Int J Radiat Oncol Biol Phys 8:2137–2140, 1982.

107. Gragoudas ES, Goitein M, Koehler A, *et al.*: Proton irradiation of choroidal melanomas. Arch Ophthalmol 96:1583–1591, 1978.

108. Tobias CA, Blakely EA, Alpen EK, *et al.*: Molecular and cellular radiobiology of heavy ions. Int J Radiat Oncol Biol Phys 8:2109–2120, 1982.

109. Catterall M, Sutherland I, Bewley DK: First results of a randomized clinical trial of fast neutrons compared with X or gamma rays in treatment of advanced tumors of the head and neck. Br Med J 2:653–656, 1975.

110. Catterall M, Bewley DK: Fast Neutrons in the Treatment of cancer. London, Academic Press; New York, Grune and Stratton, 1979.

111. Duncan W, Arnott SJ, Orr JA, Kerr GR: The Edinburgh experience of fast neutron therapy. Int J Radiat Oncol Biol Phys 8:2155–2157, 1982.

112. Cohen L: Absence of a demonstrable gain factor for neutron beam therapy of epidermoid carcinoma of the head and neck. Int J Radiat Oncol Biol Phys 8:2173–2176, 1982.

113. Griffin TW, Laramore GE, Hussey DH, Hendrickson FR, Rodriquez-Antunez A: Fast neutron beam radiation therapy in the United States. Int J Radiat Oncol Biol Phys 8:2165–2168.

3. Advances in the diagnosis and management of neoplasms of the skull base

JOHN L. KEMINK and MALCOLM D. GRAHAM

Both benign and malignant lesions involving the skull base occur in one of the most inaccessible areas of the body. Furthermore, surgical resections in this area have been limited by the critical structures located at the skull base and the severity of complications risked with surgery in this area. While neurosurgeons, head and neck oncologic surgeons, and otologists all have their own approach to the skull base, it was not until fifteen years ago that a systematic interdisciplinary surgical approach to the skull base emerged. Essential to the development of these approaches were recent technical advances in preoperative diagnostic evaluation and surgical equipment. Accurate determination of tumor extent through advances in polytomography and computerized axial tomogram scanning has enabled careful patient selection and surgical planning. The surgical endeavor has been made more efficient by the use of the operating microscope and the air drill with constant water suction irrigation.

Surgical approaches to the skull base are difficult and the risks of neurological deficits are significant. The spinal cord, the arteries and veins supplying the brain and intracranial structures, and virtually all cranial nerves exit the skull base. Neurological deficits that may result from disease or surgery of the skull base can affect all the senses. Thus the challenges are obvious. With present techniques, the risks of serious disability and death in the removal of benign lesions of the skull base have been minimized and now these surgical approaches are being extended collaboratively to the removal of malignant neoplasms involving the skull base while preserving maximum cosmetic appearance and neurologic function. In this chapter, the evaluation of patients with primarily benign tumors of the skull base and the selection of surgical approaches to the lesions are described in detail since the application of recently developed skull base surgical techniques represents a new frontier in the management of malignant neoplasms involving the base of the skull.

Gregory T. Wolf (ed), Head and Neck Oncology.
© *1984 Martinus Nijhoff Publishers, Boston. ISBN 0-89838-657-8. Printed in The Netherlands.*

Acoustic neuroma

Presentation

The signs and symptoms of a cerebellopontine angle tumor were well described in the classic monograph by Cushing [1]. Althought the acoustic neuroma is most commonly a lesion of the vestibular portion of the 8th cranial nerve, it is usually the function of the auditory portion of the 8th nerve that is initially affected. The sensorineural hearing loss associated with acoustic neuroma is most often of gradual onset, but can occur as a sudden or stepped loss. The sensorineural hearing loss is retrocochlear and characterized by reduced discrimination and auditory fatigue. The vestibular symptoms generally are absent or subtle. Mild dysequilibrium is common, but on occasion, vertigo characterized by pulsion or rotary symptoms is noted. As the tumor enlarges the symptoms progress to include facial and hypopharyngeal hypesthesia (5th and 9th cranial nerves), vocal cord paresis (10th cranial nerve), and facial weakness (7th cranial nerve). Cerebellar symptoms, papilledema, and blindness are late effects of the intracranial mass of acoustic tumors [2].

Evaluation

Diagnosis of acoustic tumors requires a high degree of suspicion. Complete evaluation of the patient with asymmetric hearing loss is indicated. The diagnosis of an acoustic neuroma may be difficult due to other concomitant otologic conditions, including chronic suppurative otitis media, otosclerosis, Meniere's disease, or the symptoms of tinnitus and fullness. Physical examination in all but the largest tumors may be normal except for the hearing loss. However, evaluation of the cranial nerves may reveal a decreased corneal reflex or hypesthesia of the posterior external auditory canal (Hittselberger's sign). Facial nerve symptoms are infrequent. Large acoustic tumors may begin to produce facial hypesthesia from trigeminal nerve involvement. Currently, it is increasingly uncommon to see patients with advanced neurological deficits at the time of initial diagnosis. However, despite an increasing awareness of acoustic tumors, extension into the posterior cranial fossa at time of diagnosis is common.

The audiometric evaluation includes a pure-tone audiogram with speech discrimination and auditory brain stem response testing. Asymmetric or unilateral hearing loss is most frequent, and poor discrimination increases the suspicion for acoustic tumor. Although special audiometrics including tone decay, stapedial reflex decay, small increment sensitivity index, and Bekesy audiometry may be helpful in diagnosis, they have generally been replaced by auditory brain stem response (ABR) testing [3–6]. Auditory brain stem response testing produces a characteristic wave form thought to be representative of the progression of nerve potentials in the acoustic nerve and brain stem. The wave forms are generated by repetitive clicks or tone pips which are time-locked and computer averaged. Increased interwave latencies are produced by tumor pressure on the cochlear nerve, resulting in conduction time delays and desynchronization of nerve impulses. The ABR appears to be highly accurate for the diagnosis of acoustic neuroma, and can be helpful in the evaluation of primary brain stem abnormalities including demyelinating diseases, stroke, and brain stem tumors.

Evaluation of the vestibular portion of the 8th cranial nerve is most reliably accomplished with electronystagmography. Linthicum and Churchill reported reduced vestibular responses in 40% of small acoustic neuromas, in 84% of medium sized acoustic neuromas, and in 91% of large tumors [7]. A reduced vestibular response is found in approximately 80% of all patients with acoustic neuromas.

Radiologic evaluation begins with standard petrous pyramid X-rays. This series of films should consist of multiple views of the internal auditory canal including Stenvers, Towns, transorbital, and base views. Careful examination of the internal auditory canal in all views is necessary, since an enlarged canal will not necessarily be identifiable in all views. Care must be taken to compare the internal auditory canal diameter at identical points between the vestibule laterally and the posterior lip of the porous acousticus medially. Normal fluting of the porous medial to the internal auditory canal may be inappropriately interpreted as internal auditory canal enlargement. Petrous pyramid polytomograms are helpful in evaluating the internal auditory canal when petrous pyramid pneumatization obscures the canal [8]. Crabtree and Gardner [9] have found only a small improvement in assessment of the internal auditory canal with polytomograms, and do not recommend their use as a routine screening examination (Fig. 1).

Computer axial tomography (CAT) can be used to evaluate the presence and extent of tumors in the posterior cranial fossa. The majority of scans

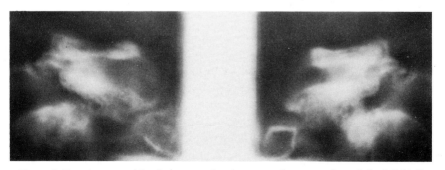

Figure 1. Petrous pyramid polytomography demonstrating expansion of the left IAC.

56

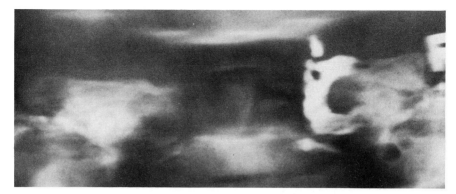

Figure 2. Pantopaque IAC meatography demonstrating a medium sized acoustic neuroma protruding into the posterior fossa.

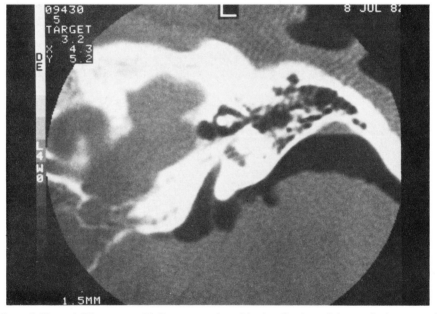

Figure 3. Normal CO_2-contrast IAC meatography with visualization of the vestibular nerves in the IAC.

used in the evaluation of the cerebellopontine angle are performed with contrast administration since acoustic neuromas will not enhance without its administration. The newer generation CAT scans have been able to diagnose progressively smaller tumors. Advances in CAT scanner technology are on the verge of allowing the evaluation of the presence of tumor in the internal auditory canal without contrast. Since CAT cannot yet reliably evaluate the contents of the internal auditory canal without contrast, and will occasionally miss a small posterior fossa lesion, a patient with suspected tumor may require a posterior fossa myelogram. Air or contrast myelogra-

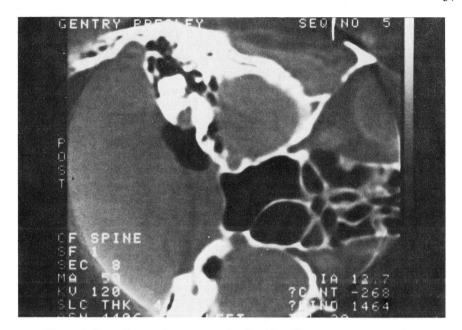

Figure 4. A small acoustic neuroma visualized by CO_2-contrast meatography.

phy with the use of the newer generation CAT scanners should provide a definitive evaluation [10] (Figs. 2–4). The use of air (CO_2) contrast has recently become popular and is effective in the evaluation of the cerebello-pontine angle [11]. With the further development of the high resolution computer axial scanner, the nerves of the internal auditory canal can be imaged and invasive myelography may become unnecessary.

Surgical approach

There are several surgical approaches to acoustic tumor removal. Decision regarding surgical route is determined by tumor size, hearing and vestibular status, and surgeon familiarity. The most common routes are suboccipital, translabyrinthine, retrolabyrinthine, and middle cranial fossa.

In the lateral suboccipital route, the posterior fossa is exposed through a craniotomy. The usual anterior limit to the craniotomy is the sigmoid sinus, the superior limit is the transverse sinus, and inferiorly bone may be removed to open the foramen magnum. The approach is versatile and gives adequate exposure for removal of both medium and large tumors. The facial nerve may be difficult to identify on the deep side of the tumor. Theoretically, hearing may be preserved.

The benefit of the translabyrinthine approach is the positive identification of the facial nerve. House [12] and Glasscock and Hays [13] have reported preservation of facial nerve function in approximately 95% of all tumors. After wide mastoidectomy, labyrinthectomy, and skeletonization of the facial nerve, the internal auditory canal is opened and the facial nerve is identified and dissected free from tumor. The facial nerve usually passes on the anterior superior surface of the acoustic tumor and the nerve most frequently becomes attenuated over the mass. Careful identification and dissection of the nerve from lateral to medial as it stretches over the tumor is essential for its preservation. Occasionally the facial nerve will enter the tumor itself. The tumor is then removed from the brain stem, preserving vascular structures including the anterior inferior cerebellar artery. If necessary, the translabyrinthine approach can be extended anteriorly transcochlear. This will allow access to the anterior dome of the cerebellopontine angle, anterio-medial petrous pyramid, and the clivus.

With the retrolabyrinthine approach, the labyrinth is preserved and potentially hearing can be saved. Identification of the facial nerve is more difficult since the lateral internal auditory canal is not exposed [14]. Access to the cerebellopontine angle is posterior to the labyrinth, but anterior to the sigmoid sinus. The occipital cortical bone is removed and the sigmoid sinus is depressed posteriorly to allow adequate access.

The middle cranial fossa approach is indicated only for removal of small tumors in patients with serviceable hearing [6, 7, 15, 16]. The approach is extradural through a craniotomy in the temporal squamous bone. Dura is elevated from the middle cranial fossa floor; the internal auditory canal is unroofed, and the tumor is removed. Removal of larger tumors extending into the posterior fossa via this route is not recommended, since surgical exposure and vascular control are limited.

The choice of the surgical approach is not only determined by tumor size and hearing levels, but also by other patient factors. A small tumor in an elderly individual might be followed by serial computer axial scanning. A large lesion in such an individual might be decompressed and not totally removed, thereby potentially reducing surgical risks and postoperative morbidity [17]. Total removal of a large lesion in a young adult is indicated, and may be removed by either a combined or a two-stage approach [18]. The combined approach consists of both translabyrinthine and suboccipital procedure at one sitting. In two stages, the first approach is by translabyrinthine route to identify and preserve the facial nerve, and the second stage suboccipitally to remove the bulk of tumor extending toward the foramen magnum. There is an unusual group of patients with bilateral acoustic tumors. These are most likely an axial form of neurofibromatosis and may present without the stigmata of skin nodules or cafe-au-lait spots [19]. These patients frequently have a family history of acoustic tumors and present with other benign and sometimes malignant tumors including meningiomata, astrocytomas, ependymonas, and neuromatous involvement of the cranial, spinal, autonomic, and peripheral nerves [20]. Although preservation of hearing and facial function is imperative, it is a formidable task in these patients due to the apparent rapid tumor growth in young adults and tendency for these tumors to invade the facial nerve.

Prognosis

The present goals of acoustic tumor surgery are total tumor removal with preservation of facial nerve function, and hearing. The probability of attainment of these goals has improved considerably over recent decades. The first sign of advancement was the dramatic decrease in surgical mortality reported by Cushing [1] and Dandy [2]. The era of grading the acceptability of surgical results by the percentage of total removal and preservation of facial nerve function came with House's [12] ability to consistently preserve facial nerve function after total removal of acoustic neuromas in over 90% of cases. Presently preservation of hearing in those patients with serviceable hearing is being investigated.

Present day standards for tumor removal appear to be 80–90% total removal of tumor with a similar incidence of preservation of the facial nerve. Attempts at preservation of hearing have met with some success in smaller tumors. Removal of tumor extending into the cerebellopontine angle, with some exceptions, has resulted in loss of cochlear function.

Surgery for the removal of acoustic tumors is an excellent example of recent advances in skull base surgery. Whereas the original concern was for operative mortality, we are now in an era of treatment refinements aimed at limiting postoperative disabilities.

Glomus tumors of the temporal bone

The signs, symptoms, and classification of glomus tumors of the temporal bone were clearly described by Alford and Guilford in 1964 [21]. They divided glomus tumors into two categories based on their site of origin, the glomus tympanicum and glomus jugulare. Guild [22] described the cell of origin, the glomus body, noting the glomus bodies were found both in the dome of the jugular bulb and on the promontory of the middle ear associated with Jacobsen's nerve and the auricular branch of the vagus nerve. The clinical occurrence of this tumor was first reported by Rosenwasser [23] in 1945. The glomus tympanicum tumor arises from the glomus bodies on the promontory of the middle ear while the glomus jugulare arises in the dome of the jugular bulb.

Presentation

The glomus tympanicum most frequently presents with the insidious onset of pulsatile tinnitus and a conductive hearing loss, although they also may be discovered as an incidental finding on routine physical examination. The glomus jugulare arises within the well of the dome of the jugular bulb and commonly presents late after considerable growth and bony destruction. They also may present with pulsatile tinnitus and conductive hearing loss after expanding from the jugular bulb onto the mesotympanum. Glomus jugulare tumors may cause deficits in the function of the cranial nerves near the jugular bulb (cranial nerves IX–XII), facial nerve paresis due to tumor extension into the mastoid, or sensorineural hearing loss from bony erosion of the labyrinth [64]. Occasionally either a glomus tympanicum or jugulare tumor may erode the tympanic membrane and present as a bleeding mass in the external auditory canal. Glomus tumors in the head and neck may be multiple [25], with the most common example being an ipsilateral glomus tympanicum and carotid body tumor.

Evaluation

Accurate diagnosis and evaluation of the extent of a glomus tumor of the temporal bone requires appropriate physical examination and radiologic assessment. The physical examination infrequently differentiates between the glomus tympanicum and the glomus jugulare tumor. Only if all borders of the tumor are visible through the tympanic membrane can one assume it to be a glomus tympanicum. If all borders are not visible behind the tympanic membrane, the tumor may be either a large glomus tympanicum or the superior margin of a much larger glomus jugulare tumor that extends from the jugular bulb into the hypotympanum. If there are cranial nerve abnormalities associated with a lesion, it is most likely a glomus jugulare tumor.

Brown described a diagnostic test that demonstrated the pulsatile vascularity of this lesion [26]. With the use of the pneumatic otoscope, the tympanic membrane is depressed against the tumor to demonstrate the vascular pulsations. These pulsations may be recordable on a tympanogram.

Although physical examination and cranial nerve mapping is helpful in determining the existence and extent of tumor, radiographic techniques including polytomography, high resolution computer axial scanning, arteriography, and jugular venography are definitive. The radiologic workup must address jugular bulb involvement since determination of the tumor category and subsequent management is based on this knowledge. Petrous pyramid plain films may show jugular foramen erosion, but are not helpful in deli-

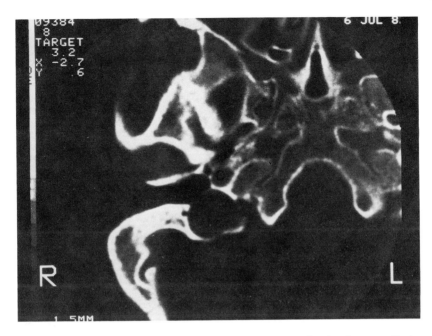

Figure 5. A jugular bulb dehiscent into the hypotympanum. JF – jugular foramen; C – internal carotid artery.

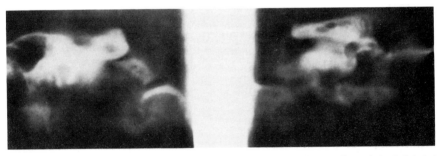

Figure 6. A-P polytomography of the temporal bone demonstrating erosion of the left inferior temporal bone.

neating tumor extent. One must be careful not to over-interpret the significance of assymmetry in the size of jugulare foramina. Most frequently the jugular foramina are asymmetric with the right side being larger (Fig. 5). Anterior-posterior and lateral petrous pyramid polytomography is generally most helpful (Fig. 6). The lateral projection best demonstrates erosion of the bony 'keel' between the carotid artery anteriorly and the jugular bulb posteriorly (Fig. 7). This erosion is highly suggestive of a glomus jugulare tumor. High resolution computer axial scanning and arteriography should provide an accurate estimation of tumor size and intracranial extension. The vascular blush obtained by arteriography is highly diagnostic of a glo-

62

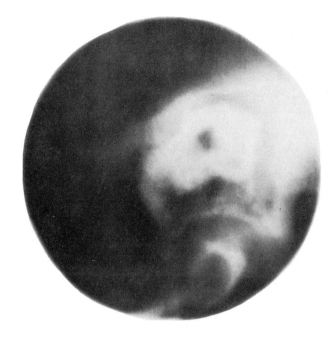

Figure 7. Lateral polytomography demonstrating erosion of the bony 'keel' between the internal carotid artery and the jugular bulb.

mus tumor (Fig. 8). Jugular venography is performed to evaluate the presence of tumor within the jugular bulb and extension intraluminally into the jugular vein. Care must be taken in positioning the patient to 'unfold' the jugular bulb so it is completely evaluated. On occasion, the venous phase of the arteriogram will have sufficient radiopaque contrast to provide this information. When the venous phase is inadequate or the jugular bulb is occluded, jugular venography is necessary to determine the inferior extent of tumor within the jugular vein (Fig. 9).

Surgical approach

Only small glomus tympanicum tumors whose borders are clearly visible through the tympanic membrane can be removed via the external auditory canal [27]. When removing this tumor it must be clearly differentiated from a dehiscent carotid artery. The presence of the promontory bone just deep to the lesion will make this clear. Injury to the carotid artery in its intratemporal portion is hazardous and may require carotid artery ligation for control.

In radiologically proven glomus tympanicum tumors whose borders are not entirely visible through the tympanic membrane, the extended facial recess approach is recommended [27]. Occasionally the facial recess will be

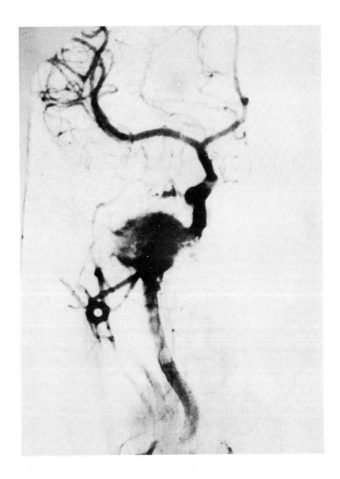

Figure 8. Carotid arteriography demonstrating a medium sized glomus jugulare tumor.

narrow requiring removal of all or part of the bony posterior external auditory canal.

The removal of glomus jugulare tumors is a major surgical task [27–30]. It requires identification in the neck of the cranial nerves of the jugular foramen, transposition of the facial nerve, and removal of all the bone lateral to the tumor and jugular bulb. A wide mastoidectomy is performed. The facial nerve is identified from the cochleariform process into the parotid gland and is usually transposed anteriorly. Others have reported the preservation of the bony facial canal [31]. Bone is removed lateral to the jugular bulb. The sigmoid sinus is opened and packed off, and the jugular vein is divided and ligated in the neck. The jugular vein is then elevated superiorly up to the jugular bulb, taking care to visualize and preserve the cranial nerves on its anterio-medial surface. The tumor mass is then dissected working the tumor margin in a circumferential fashion. As the tumor bleeds it is packed off with Surgicel and a new area is dissected. Anteriorly, care must be taken

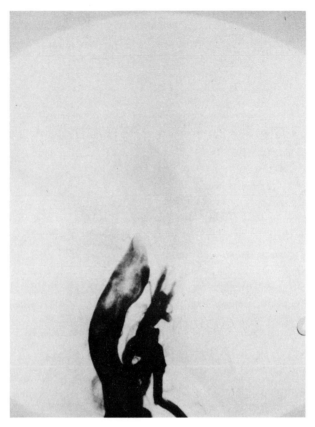

Figure 9. Jugular venogram demonstrating extension of a glomus jugulare tumor down the jugular vein into the neck.

to avoid injury to the carotid artery. Identification of the carotid artery remote from the tumor may be helpful in the development of this plane, but conservative resection is indicated in this area unless carotid artery ligation or reconstruction is anticipated. Resection of posterior fossa dura, facial nerve, cochlea, and semicircular canals may be required in larger tumors. Dural defects when present are repaired and the surgical defect is packed with an abdominal fat graft. The external auditory canal is oversewn after removal of deep external auditory canal skin.

For large glomus jugulare tumors with intracranial extension, a combined neuro-otologic and neuro-surgical procedure may be required. Combined suboccipital, transtemporal approaches have been described by Hilding and Greenberg [32] and Kinney [33].

While radiation therapy is not the treatment of choice for surgically resectable glomus tumors of the temoral bone, tumor reductions following radiation therapy have been recorded [34, 35]. Glomus tumors have been shown to have non-uniform responses, and tumor sterilization by radiation therapy is infrequent [36]. Radiation therapy is useful for management of recurrences and unresectable lesions. Some support has been advanced for combined surgical and radiation therapy approaches [37].

Prognosis

Glomus tumors are slow growing, benign tumors and complete removal indicates an excellent prognosis. Present surgical methods are designed to minimize cranial nerve deficits. Identification in the neck of the cranial nerves at the jugular bulb generally allows preservation of these nerves and their function. Mobilization and transposition of the facial nerve from the cochleariform process to the parotid gland is frequently associated with immediate postoperative paresis and subsequent complete recovery. Those patients who lose the function of cranial nerves VII, IX, X, XI and XII have significant morbidity both immediately and long term. In those patients who lose these functions acutely, a tracheotomy should be considered for postoperative airway protection.

Facial nerve neuroma

Neuromas may involve the facial nerve along its intracranial, intratemporal, or extratemporal course. This discussion will focus on the diagnosis and treatment of intratemporal and intracranial neuromas of the facial nerve.

Presentation

Altmann [38] in 1935 presented the first comprehensive description of a facial nerve neuroma, and felt that the symptomatology of facial nerve neuroma was sufficiently pathognomic that they could be diagnosed clinically. The earliest reported cases were diagnosed late, usually presenting with longstanding facial paralysis and obstruction of the external auditory canal with tumor. More recently there has been an increased awareness of this clinical entity, and improved neurotologic diagnostic methods have resulted in earlier diagnosis.

Facial paralysis has been the most common presenting sign in a number of series [39–42]. However, other authors have reported patients with no evidence of facial dysfunction [42, 43]. Classically, there is a history of slowly progressive facial paralysis, although sudden onset of paralysis and a fluctuating paresis may occur. Bailey and Graham [43] reported a case of facial nerve neuroma with a history of sudden onset of facial paralysis followed by partial recovery and some associated mass motion. May and Hardin [44] noted that a progressive facial paralysis over a period greater than 3 weeks suggested tumor etiology. They also noted that in approximately one-third of their series of 20 patients with ipsilateral recurrent facial palsy, there was a neoplastic etiology. Fisch and Ruttner [45] and Pulec [46] reported a sudden onset of facial paralysis, while facial twitching or hemispasm have also been noted as symptoms suggesting tumor involvement of the facial nerve [42, 47].

Hearing loss is the second most common presenting symptom [48]. Conductive hearing loss may occur with middle ear involvement due to tumor expansion and pressure on or disruption of the ossicular chain. In these cases a gray-white polypod mass frequently is present behind the posterior superior tympanic membrane, or may fill the middle ear, erode tympanic membrane, and obstruct the external auditory canal. Sensorineural hearing loss may result from erosion into the labyrinth or tumor compression on the cochlear nerve. Otalgia and vertigo may be presenting symptoms, but are unusual, and chorda tympani involvement can precipitate loss of taste.

Facial neuroma involving the internal auditory canal may present with an initial onset of sensorineural hearing loss in a similar way to the acoustic neuroma. Tumor enlargement may subsequently cause facial paralysis and intracranial symptoms.

Evaluation

An intratemporal facial nerve neuroma generally extends along the course of the facial nerve for a greater distance than clinically or radiographically anticipated. The neuroma visualized in the middle ear may extend intracranially into the internal auditory canal and cerebello-pontine angle, or extratemporally into the parotid gland. Preoperative radiologic assessment addresses this potential spread.

Topographic testing of facial nerve function including tearing, stapedial reflex, taste, and salivation may be helpful, but is not definitive in the evaluation of the extent of facial nerve neuroma [40]. Definitive assessment of fallopian canal enlargement may be made with petrous pyramid polytomography. High resolution computer axial scanning may demonstrate a cerebello-pontine angle tumor or dilatation of the fallopian or internal auditory canals (Fig. 10). Special attention should be paid to the area of the geniculate ganglion, as Fisch and Ruttner [45] have reported that a variety of tumors including facial neuroma occur in this area. Extension into the posterior fossa or the internal auditory canal may be evaluated with air-contrast or pantopaque myelography.

An intracranial facial nerve neuroma may present with many of the find-

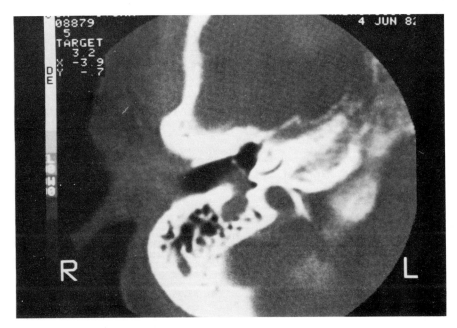

Figure 10. CAT Scan of a facial nerve neuroma demonstrating fallopian canal erosion with tumor extension into the mesotympanum.

ings of, and be clinically indistinguishable from, an acoustic neuroma. Pure tone audiometry may show sensorineural hearing loss, and auditory brain stem response testing may show latency delay. Electronystagmography may show reduced vestibular response. Thus, differentiation of an acoustic from facial nerve neuroma may not be possible prior to surgical exposure.

Despite thorough investigation, false negatives may occur. Jackson *et al.* [42] recommended surgical exploration of all progressive facial palsies that occur over an extended period of time, or show no return of tone or function after six months. Conley and Janecka [41] reported involvement of the facial nerve in the deep lobe of the parotid gland, and recommended parotid exploration if another etiology could not be identified.

Surgical approach

The treatment goals of facial nerve neuroma surgery are complete removal of the tumor with preservation of hearing and restoration of facial nerve function. A surgical approach to the facial nerve is the sole treatment and may require exposure of the nerve in the parotid, mastoid, intralabyrinthine, and internal auditory canal segments. Although radiologic evaluation may demonstrate an area of fallopian canal expansion, the histologic extent of tumor is usually beyond these dimensions. Exposure of the nerve for a distance beyond the radiologic abnormality must be anticipated. A comprehensive account of contemporary transtemporal techniques for surgical exposure of the facial nerve has been provided by Graham [49]. Most commonly, the transmastoid and middle fossa approaches are adequate for exposure of neuromas of the intracanallicular or intralabyrinthine facial nerve segments. In those patients with nonserviceable hearing, a translabyrinthine exposure of the facial nerve and internal auditory canal may be indicated.

Rarely, a small tumor may be resected with preservation of the nerve trunk [40]. Surgical removal and cable grafting of the nerve with frozen section histologic control is necessary in most cases. The nerve graft is usually placed in the fallopian canal and its ends are approximated and stabilized with packing. Approximation of the cable graft to the facial nerve stump in the internal auditory canal is difficult. When the involved segment of nerve is limited to less than 1 cm, a facial nerve transposition and primary anastomosis can be performed. If primary anastomosis or cable grafting fail, hypoglossal anastomosis may be necessary.

Recently we have elected to decompress the facial nerve neuroma in several patients with normal facial nerve function. We do not know if this will delay the progression of facial nerve paresis. Resection and grafting of the nerve would then be performed when facial nerve weakness progresses and before significant atrophy of the facial musculature occurs. This approach may be particularly useful in the elderly patient.

Prognosis

Resection and grafting of the facial nerve usually results in adequate facial nerve function. Although mild asymmetry of facial nerve function and synkinesis may result, facial resting tone and protective function (i.e., mouth, eye) are generally adequate. Restoration of facial motion will occur between 6–18 months after grafting depending on the location of the repair. Anastomosis in the internal auditory canal is difficult and may lead to poor results. When graftable facial nerve stumps are present, the results are generally better with grafting than with all other static reconstructions or dynamic reinnervations of the face, including fascial slings, temporal muscle flaps, and cranial nerve XII-VII anstomoses.

In the immediate postoperative period, attention should be given to protection of the eye. Although postoperatively there is considerable variability in eye closure, all patients are asked to wear eye protection. Some patients will have good eye closure despite facial nerve paralysis, and require only occasional use of artificial tears. Others will have considerable difficulty, and will need an extensive medical regime of artificial tears, lubricants, moisture chambers, and eyelid support with taping techniques. Occasionally a tarsorrhaphy is required despite anticipated facial nerve recovery.

Congenital cholesteatoma

Congenital cholesteatoma of the temporal bone may be divided into four anatomical groups. These are the congenital cholesteatomas of the middle ear, perigeniculate area, petrous apex, and cerebellopontine angle. These cholesteatomas arise from epithelial rests and should be distinguished from acquired cholesteatoma, and from congenital external auditory canal cholesteatoma associated with group I abnormalities in congenital atresia of the external auditory canal.

Presentation

The clinical presentation of congenital cholesteatoma varies depending upon cholesteatoma location. Cholesteatoma of each area, (the middle ear/mastoid, perigeniculate area, petrous apex, and cerebello-pontine angle) may have a distinctive presentation. Middle ear congenital cholesteatomas were originally reported by House [50] in 1953 and have been reviewed recently by House and Sheehy [51] and Curtis [52]. Conductive hearing loss and a bulging whitish mass behind an intact tympanic membrane are common findings in middle-ear/mastoid congenital cholesteatomas [53]. Fifty percent of cases will present with recurrent otitis media and may fistulize through the tympanic membrane. Differentiation of congenital middle ear cholesteatoma from acquired cholesteatoma may be difficult. They may also be discovered incidentally at the time of myringotomy in the pediatric-aged population. Congenital cholesteatoma of the mastoid may present with postauricular pain and/or swelling, and on occasion facial paralysis [50].

Perigeniculate and petrous apex cholesteatomas usually present with insidious or rapidly progressive facial nerve paralysis [54, 55]. Sensorineural hearing loss from labyrinthine or internal auditory canal erosion is common, but a conductive hearing loss may also result from cholesteatoma extension into the middle ear or blockage of the eustachian tube. Facial twitching may occur in the presence of congenital cholesteatoma as well as with facial nerve neuromas. Vestibular dysfunction may complete the symptom complex. On occasion the cholesteatoma may erode into the middle or posterior fossa and expand markedly before producing symptoms. Preservation of hearing despite extensive destruction of the labyrinth has been reported [56, 57].

Congenital cholesteatomas of the cerebello-pontine angle account for six

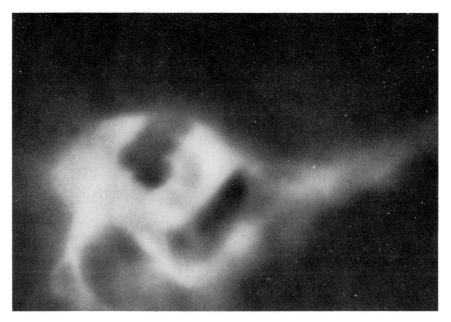

Figure 11. Lateral polytomography of a congenital cholesteatoma superior to the IAC.

to seven percent of lesions in this area [55]. They may present in a manner identical to an acoustic neuroma or on occasion may produce trigeminal neuralgia [58]. Their frequent occurence in the younger adult age group with symptoms of facial nerve twitching or paresis may help differentiate them from an acoustic neuroma.

Evaluation

Congenital cholesteatoma of the temporal bone may have sensorineural or conductive hearing loss with or without facial nerve paralysis, depending on the area of involvement. Plain films of the temporal bone may demonstrate large cholesteatomas of the temporal bone, with a truncated medial aspect of the petrous pyramid being typical of petrous apex congenital cholesteatomas. Polytomographic techniques may not identify cholesteatoma in the middle ear, but will be helpful in evaluating the bony erosion of perigeniculate or petrous pyramid cholesteatomas (Fig. 11). More recently, high resolution CAT scanning may identify these bony defects as well as soft tissue extension. Congenital cholesteatomas appear cystic and will not enhance with imaging techniques. Air or contrast myelography may be required in the evaluation of the posterior fossa. Posterior fossa cholesteatoma will classically show a scalloped border.

Surgical approach

Surgical management of congenital cholesteatoma requires either complete removal of the cholesteatoma matrix or permanent exteriorization. The isolated middle ear cholesteatoma may be removed transtympanically. The surgeon must be prepared to detach the tympanic membrane from the malleus and to follow the cholesteatoma into the protympanum and expose the attic, antrum, or middle fossa to remove cholesteatoma. Care must be taken with removal of cholesteatoma adjacent to the facial nerve since this nerve is often dehiscent. Routine middle ear reconstructive techniques may be used if ossicles are eroded or removed, or the tympanic membrane is sacrificed.

Removal of congenital cholesteatomas of the perigeniculate area or petrous apex areas may be accomplished by the transmastoid or middle cranial fossa approach, or by a combination of both procedures. Frequently, cholesteatoma must be dissected from the facial nerve, and occasionally the intralabyrinthine portion of the nerve must be mobilized to completely remove a perigeniculate cholesteatoma. This may require sectioning of the greater superficial petrosal nerve and transposition of the facial nerve posteriorly. The cholesteatoma may also insinuate itself between dura and the middle fossa floor, and may extend for a considerable distance along the middle cranial fossa floor. Petrous apex cholesteatoma may act similarly and erode the bony labyrinth or the internal auditory canal. Only careful and often tedious dissection will prevent injury to these structures. Cholesteatoma of the petrous apex may be exteriorized into the mastoid cavity or the sphenoid sinus, however, frequent cleansing of debris from the cholesteatoma cavity is required to prevent inspissation and subsequent infection [59]. Removal of cholesteatoma debris from the sphenoid sinus is particularly difficult, as the surgical fistula tract has a propensity for stenosis leading to inspissation of debris.

Surgical removal of congenital cholestatomas from the cerebellopontine angle may be accomplished utilizing surgical approaches similar to those utilized in acoustic tumor surgery [59, 60]. Spillage or retention of cholesteatomatous debris intradurally may result in an intense aseptic meningitis.

Prognosis

Complete removal of cholesteatoma matrix will prevent recurrence. Olivecrona reported six cases of cerebellopontine angle cholesteatomas in which matrix was left, that failed to demonstrate recurrences during a ten year follow-up [58]. Longstanding facial nerve paralysis from congenital cholesteatoma has a poor prognosis for recovery. Recently the authors have treated a patient with a perigeniculate congenital cholesteatoma who developed rapidly progressive facial nerve paralysis in the immediate preoperative period. She subsequently had good delayed facial nerve recovery with mild weakness and synkinesis.

Carcinoma of the external auditory canal and middle ear

A wide variety of malignant tumors may involve the external auditory canal, middle ear, and mastoid. Squamous cell carcinoma is the most frequent histologic type in both the external auditory canal and middle ear [61]. Although the high incidence of squamous cell carcinoma of the mastoid is well documented in radium-dial painters, the inciting cause in the majority of external auditory canal and middle ear cancers in unknown [62]. While ultraviolet light is considered to be a causative factor in squamous cell carcinoma of the pinna, chronic eczematoid external and chronic suppurative otitis have been proposed as a causative factor in squamous cell carcinoma of the external auditory canal and middle ear [63, 64]. Adenoid cystic carcinoma and a wide variety of other carcinomas including basal cell carcinoma, melanoma, mucoepidermoid carcinoma, and ceruminous gland adenocarcinoma have been reported in this location [61, 65].

Presentation

A majority of patients with external auditory canal carcinomas present with otorrhea, bleeding, pain and decreased hearing. Frequently these symptoms occur in an ear with previous otologic disease including chronic suppurative otitis media and chronic dermatoses. Although many authors have emphasized the importance of pain as a symptom in carcinoma, it is not a consistent finding. However, pain is frequently an early symptom with adenoid cystic carcinoma. Sensorineural hearing loss, vertigo, or facial nerve paralysis may be present in advanced cases regardless of history.

Characteristically, an external auditory canal carcinoma appears as a poorly defined polypoid mass or plaque with friability, fissuring, bleeding, and a build up of epithelial debris. Nodular and ulcerative presentations have also been observed.

In carcinoma of the mastoid, early diagnosis is difficult due to concealment of the tumor. With growth and destruction of bone, headache and pain may occur. The carcinoma may become apparent as it erodes into the external auditory canal or through the mastoid cortex into the skin. Cranial nerve deficits will occur as the tumor destroys the skull base. Cervical metastases may occur early, but distant metastases usually occur late in the course of disease. Death from local extension is the rule.

Evaluation

Biopsy of the lesion will frequently provide the histologic diagnosis. Usual varieties of both benign and malignant tumors in this are may require special histologic or electron microscopic study for diagnosis. Tumor extent and surgical resectability are determined by cranial nerve involvement and radiologic evaluation including petrous pyramid polytomography and high resolution CAT scanning.

Surgical approach

Isolated carcinomas of the external auditory canal that do not extend into the middle ear may be managed by mastoidectomy and sleeve resection of the external auditory canal. Lateral temporal bone resection provides preservation of the facial nerve with minimal cosmetic and functional disability [66]. In these cases superficial parotidectomy and mandibular condylectomy or resection of the middle cranial fossa floor above the external auditory canal may be indicated. Postoperative radiation therapy may also be considered.

With carcinomas extending into the middle ear or mastoid, more extensive surgical procedures with greater cosmetic and functional disabilities may be necessary. In 1951 Ward, Loch, and Lawrence [67] and Campbell, Volk, and Burkland [68] applied the concept of en bloc temporal bone dissection for carcinomas involving the middle ear. This procedure involves subtotal resection of the temporal bone lateral to the carotid artery. Further modifications in technique were described by Parsons and Lewis [69], Conley and Novack [66], Arena [70], and Gacek and Goodman [71] and reviewed by Neeley and Forrester [72]. Recently, Fisch and Pillsbury presented an infratemporal fossa approach to lesions of the temporal bone and base of skull [73]. They reviewed their experience using this approach to the petrous pyramid, clivus, parasellar, and parasphenoid areas in fifty-one patients. Hilding [74] and Graham and Associates [75] have reported three patients with total temporal bone resection after planned ligation of the internal carotid artery (Fig. 12). It is not known if these more extensive surgical resections improve long term prognosis. Postoperative radiation therapy should be strongly considered in any extensive lesion.

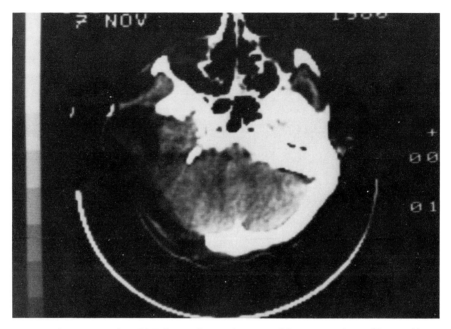

Figure 12. A postoperative CAT Scan of a total temporal bone resection with carotid artery ligation for squamous cell carcinoma of the middle ear.

Prognosis

Although no current staging system for temporal bone malignancies exist, patients with localized tumors that require only lateral temporal bone resection appear to have a better prognosis. Crabtree and Associates [76] reported favorable survival rates with 'en bloc dissection of the external auditiory canal'. Other authors have reported similar findings. Radiotherapy was used in a minority of these cases. Radiotherapy alone is felt to result in unacceptably high local recurrence rates.

Combined treatment is the therapy of choice in most advanced lesions. Despite aggressive surgery and tumoricidal doses of radiation, survival statistics are dismal [64, 77]. Patients considered for surgical resection should be carefully chosen. Debulking of tumor followed by radiation therapy has had some support, but beneficial results have not been adequately documented. In procedures requiring sacrifice of the facial nerve, immediate grafting should be considered. Temporary tracheostomy should be performed in the older age group or patients suspected of having vagus nerve injury. Cosmetic reconstruction and carotid artery protection are provided with local or regional flaps.

Encephalocele and CSF leaks of the temporal bone

Post surgical and postinfectious encephalocele through the tegmen tympani and tegmen mastoideum are well recognized complications in otology [78–81]. Temporal lobe herniation into the mastoid cavity is secondary to loss of both bone and dural support. Subsequent management must deal with cerebrospinal fluid (CSF) leak, herniation of brain into the mastoid cavity, and skin and cholesteatoma matrix in the middle ear and mastoid. Less frequently recognized is a spontaneous congenital encephalocele associated with cerebrospinal fluid otorrhea or rhinorrhea [80–88]. Encephalocele and/or cerebrospinal fluid leak may also be secondary to temporal bone fracture or rarely tumor.

Presentation

Presentation of postsurgical encephalocele may occur early or late in the postoperative course. Early occurrences are generally associated with maceration of exposed brain and CSF leak. Late occurrences are associated with pulsatile, progressive prolapse of skin-covered brain into the mastoid cavity. Subsequently, desquamated skin may accumulate behind the prolapsed brain and infection may ensue.

Spontaneous congenital encephalocele has been recognized more recently. This entity may present as serous otitis media, cerebrospinal fluid rhinorrhea, or cerebrospinal fluid otorrhea through a tympanic membrane perforation. The history frequently includes prior myringotomy and pressure equalizing tube placement that resulted in chronic otorrhea, subsequently recognized as cerebrospinal fluid. Profuse rhinorrhea with bending over may also be a presenting finding.

Temporal bone encephalocele and CSF leak may also present after blunt or penetrating temporal bone trauma. Other syndromes, including the giant apical air cell syndrome, may present with transtemporal CSF leak [89].

Evaluation

Physical examination has generally been most helpful in the evaluation of a postsurgical encephalocele. The size and extent of the prolapse may be visualized in the mastoid cavity. Sensorineural hearing levels and facial nerve function are usually normal unless previously surgically injured. With intact canal wall procedures, a postsurgical encephalocele may be hidden and present with signs and symptoms similar to a spontaneous congenital encephalocele.

With spontaneous congenital encephaloceles, serous otitis media and CSF rhinorrhea are the most common presentations. On occasion prolapsed brain may present as a mass behind the tympanic membrane. CSF rhinorrhea frequently requires further evaluation including sinus films, RISA scan, and CSF contrast studies. In the experience of some authors, petrous pyramid polytomography and computer axial scanning have not been helpful in locating the small and often multiple defects in the bony tegmen and dura that are typical of this entity [90]. Others have found these tests useful [81, 87]. Surgical exploration of the tegmen is indicated in the presence of documented middle ear CSF even in the face of negative radiologic evaluation. Although meningitis has not occurred in our experience with six cases, it has occurred in others [82, 91].

Following traumatic temporal bone injury, complete assessment of the patient's physical and neurologic status including cranio-facial injuries and cranial nerve deficits is required. In these cases, radiologic evaluation is most helpful for determining the priorities of surgical intervention. Surgery for traumatic encephalocele and CSF leak should await neurologic stabilization. Meningitis is a common sequelae of unrepaired traumatic CSF leaks.

Surgical approach

Temporal bone encephaloceles and CSF leaks may be surgically approached either transmastoid or through the middle cranial fossa intradurally or extradurally. While the transmastoid repair of the defect is frequently successful, repair through the middle cranial fossa provides greater visualization. Techniques for repair of the tegmen defect via transmastoid approach have included both placement of reconstructive material (i.e. fascia, cartilage, or prosthetics) from the mastoid intracranially and obliteration of the mastoid with flaps or free tissue [80, 81, 87, 88, 91, 92]. A middle cranial fossa approach for repair provides greater visualization and can be either extra or intradural. A variety of closure techniques including primary dural repair and fascia, bone, cartillage, or synthetic supports have been used [82, 93–96].

Bony defects of postsurgical encephaloceles are frequently large. Repair can be either transmastoid or via the middle cranial fossa. The transmastoid approach offers limited access to the dural defect. Repair is accomplished by 'tucking' the fascia and supporting materials (bone, cartillage, or synthetics) along the floor of the middle fossa to occlude the defect. Obliteration of the mastoid and/or middle ear may be performed simultaneously to secure the repair. Intradural or extradural repair via the middle cranial fossa approach is accomplished by wide overlaping of the dural edges with fascia and supporting materials. The authors prefer an extradural middle cranial fossa reconstruction using a fascia-bone-fascia sandwich [96]. The bone used is a portion of the craniotomy flap from the temporal bone squama and the fascia is temporalis fascia. With all approaches, care must be taken not to entrap skin in the repair.

The bony and dural defects in spontaneous congenital encaphaloceles are routinely small and multiple [92]. Frequently an encephalocele is present in the anterior epitympanium where visualization may be inadequate and surgical repair via a transmastoid approach is difficult without ossicular disruption. Although the authors routinely explore these cases transmastoid to define the defect, repair is accomplished through the middle fossa. The bony defects are usually small and do not require repair. The dural defects can be sealed by wide coverage of the middle cranial fossa floor with a temporalis fascia graft.

Great care must be exercised in the exploration of traumatic injuries of the temporal bone. Simple fractures of the temporal bone do not require surgical repair, however, such is not the case with fractures associated with immediate facial nerve paralysis, encephalocele, or a persistent CSF leak. In all cases surgical exploration should await neurological stabilization.

In traumatic temporal bone fractures associated with encephalocele or persistent CSF leak, the middle fossa approach provides wide exposure of the middle cranial fossa floor with clear identification of the pathology. Wide dural repairs and extensive bony reconstruction can be performed with minimal risk. In our experience, and intradural repair has not been necessary. Transmastoid exposure may risk hearing or facial nerve function when surgical orientation is difficult due to severe comminution of bone.

Chordoma

Cranial chordomas are dysontogenic neoplasms that arise in residual embryonic notochord [97]. These neoplasms are of concern to the skull base surgeon because they arise in the clivus and progressively destroy the base of the skull. Frequently they extend ventrally into the nasopharynx, nose or sinuses and cause nasal obstruction [98]. Headache, loss of vision, and cranial nerve deficits with involvement of the abducens, trigeminal, facial, and acoustic nerves are common presenting complaints [99]. Central nervous system symptoms can be the result of intracranial extension. Submental vertex radiographs, polytomography, and high resolution axial scanning will help delineate tumor extend and base of skull destruction (Fig. 13). Because of the relative inaccessibility of the tumor site, surgical exposure and tumor removal is difficult. Surgical debulking of the tumor followed by high dose radiation therapy is the treatment of choice, and may afford good palliative

78

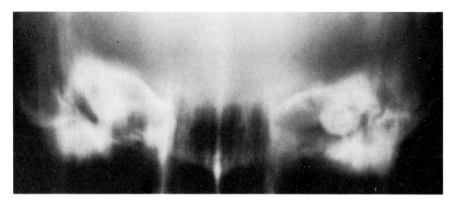

Figure 13. Polytomography demonstrating extensive involvement of the right petrous apex with chordoma.

results [97]. The overall prognosis is poor since residual disease is left. Due to the difficult accessibility, surgical control of chordomas is a unique challenge to the skull base surgeon and lends itself to creative surgical approaches.

Summary

To successfully remove even benign lesions of the skull base, it is apparent that new concepts and techniques must be considered and utilized. Mobilization and rerouting of cranial nerves, resection of mandible and zygoma for access, carotid artery resection or bypass, en bloc resection of the temporal bone and carotid artery, staging of procedures, debulking tumor, exteriorization of cholesteatoma of the petrous apex and posterior fossa, and fat obliteration of bone and dural defects to prevent cerebrospinal fluid leakage are all examples of new concepts of skull base surgery. These concepts are being applied increasingly to the management of malignant tumors involving the temporal bone, pterygomaxillary space, nasopharynx and sphenoid bone. Further technical advances are envisioned that should allow more effective surgical treatment approaches for tumors in this most difficult anatomic area. Together with the advent of effective adjuvant chemotherapy and immunotherapy, surgery for skull base malignancies should play a major role in improving the dismal prognosis associated with these tumors.

References

1. Cushing H: Tumors of the Nervus Acosticus and the Syndrome of the Cerebellopontine Angle. W.B. Saunders CO, Philadelphia, 1917.
2. Bucy PC: Tumors of the cerebellopontine angle. Arch Otolaryngol, 73:29–36, 1961.

3. Eggermont JJ, Don M, Brackmann DE: Electrocochleography and auditory brain stem electric responses in patients with cerebellopontine angle tumors.

4. Clemis JC, McGee T: Brain stem electric response audiometry in the differential diagnosis of acoustic tumors. Laryngoscope 89:31-42, 1979.

5. Selters WA: Acoustic tumor detection with brain stem electric response audiometry. Arch Otolaryngol 103:181-187, 1977.

6. Glasscock ME, Jackson CG, Josey AF, et al.: Brain stem evoked response audiometry in a clinical practice. Laryngoscope 89:1021-1035, 1979.

7. Linthicum FH Jr, Churchill D: Vestibular test results in acoustic tumor cases. Arch Otolaryngol 88:56-59, 1968.

8. Glasscock ME, III, Overfield RE, Miller GW: Polytomograph in an otologic practice. Southern Medical Journal 69:1433-1437, 1976.

9. Crabtree and Gardner: Radiographic findings in cerebellopontine angle tumors. In: House, Luette (eds) Acoustic Tumor, Vol I: Diagnosis. University Park Press, PP 241-251.

10. Scanlan RL: Positive contrast medium (Iophendylate) in diagnosis of acoustic neuroma. Arch Otolarngol 89.

11. Kricheff II, Pinto RS, Bergeron RT, Cohen N: Air-CT Cisernography and canalography for small acoustic neuromas. AJNR 1:57-63, 1980.

12. House WF: Acoustic Neuroma. Arch Otolaryngol (Mongraph II) 88:575-715, 1968.

13. Glasscock ME, III, Hayes JW: The translabyrinthine removal of acoustic and other cerebellopontine angle tumors. Arch Otolaryngol 82:415-427, 1973.

14. Domb GH, Chole RA: Anatomical studies of the posterior petrous apex with regard to hearing preservation in acoustic neuroma removal. Laryngoscope 90:1769-1776, 1980.

15. House FW: Middle cranial fossa approach to the petrous pyramid. Arch Otolaryngol 78:460-46, 1963.

16. Glasscock ME, III, Hays JW, Miller GW, et al.: Preservation of hearing in tumors of the internal auditory canal and cerebellopontine angle. Laryngoscope 88:43-55, 1978.

17. House WF: Partial tumor removal and recurrence in acoustic tumor surgery. Arch Otolaryngol 88éé-654, 1968.

18. Glasscock ME, III, Hays JW, Jackson CG, et al.: A one-stage combined approach for the management of large cerebellopontine angle tumors. Laryngoscope 88:1563-1575, 1978.

19. Linthicum FH jr, Brackmann DE: Bilateral acoustic tumors. Arch Otolaryngol 106:729-733, 1980.

20. Hittselberger WE, Hughes RL: Bilateral acoustic tumors and neurofibromatosis. Arch Otolaryngol 88:152-163, 1968.

21. Alford BR, Guilford FR: A Comprehensive study of tumors of the glomus jugulare. Laryngoscope 765-787, Jan 1962.

22. Guild SR: The glomus jugulare, a nonchromaffin paraganglion, in man. Ann Otol 62:1045-1071, 1953.

23. Rosenwasser H: Cartoid body tumor of the middle ear and mastoid. Arch Otolaryngol 4:64-67, 1945.

24. Spector GJ, Gado M, Ciralsky R, et al.: Neurologic implications of glomus tumors in the head and neck. Laryngoscope, 1387-1395, 1974.

25. Spector GJ, Ciralsky R, Maisel FH, et al.: Multiple glomus tumors in the head and neck, Laryngoscope 1066-1075, 1974.

26. Brown LA: Glomus jugulare tumor of the middle ear. Laryngoscope 63:281-292, 1953.

27. House WF, Glasscock ME, III: Glomus tympanicum tumors. Arch Otolaryngol 87:550-554, 1968.

28. Shapiro MJ, Irvington NJ, Neues DK: Technique for removal of glomus jugulare tumors. Arch of Otolaryngol 79:219-224, 1964.

29. Fisch U, Pillsbury HC: Intratemporal fossa approach to lesions in the temporal bone and base of the skull. Arch of Otolaryngol 105:99-107, 1979.

30. Glasscock ME, III, Harris PF, Newsome G: Glomus tumors: diagnosis and treatment. Laryngoscope 84:2006-2032, 1974.
31. Mischke RE, Balkany TJ: Skull base approach to glomus jugulare. Laryngoscope 90:89-93, 1980.
32. Hilding DA, Greenberg A: Surgery for large glomus jugulare tumor. Arch Otolaryngol 93:227-231, 1971.
33. Kinney SE: Glomus jugulare tumors with intracranial extension. Amer J of Otology 1:67-71, 1979.
34. Brackmann DE, House WE, Tery R, et al.: Glomus jugulare tumors: effect of irradiation. Tr Am Acad Ophth & Otol 76:1423-1431, 1972.
35. Silverstone SM: Radiation therapy of glomus jugulare tumors. Arch Otolaryngol 97:43-48, 1973.
36. Spector GJ, Maisel RH, Ogura JH: Glomus jugulare tumors, II: a cliniopathologic analysis of the effects of radiotherapy. Ann Otol 83:26-32, 1974.
37. Gardner G, Cocke EW, Robertson JT, et al.: Combined approach surgery for removal of glomus jugulare tumors. Laryngoscope 87:665-688, 1977.
38. ALTMANN F: Uber neurogene tumoren des abstcigcndcn facialistcilcs. Monatsschr f Ohrenh 69:1032, Sept 1935.
39. Neely JG, Alfordo BR: Facial nerve neuromas. Arch Otolaryngol 100:298-301, 1974.
40. Pulec JL: Facial nerve neuroma. laryngoscope 82:1160-1176, 1972.
41. Conley J, Janecka I: Schwann cell tumors of the facial nerve. Laryngoscope 84:958-962, 1974.
42. Jackson CG, Glasscock ME, Hughes G, Sismanis A: Facial paralysis of neoplastic origin: diagnosis and management. Laryngoscope 90:1581-1595, 1980.
43. Bailey CM, Graham MD: Intratemporal facial nerve neuroma: a discussion of five previously unpublished cases. J of Laryn & Otolog 97(1):65-72, Jan 1983.
44. May M, Hardin WB: Facial palsy: interpretation of neurologic findings. Trans Am Acad Ophthalmol Otolaryngol 84:710-722, 1977.
45. Fisch U, Ruttner J: Pathology of intratemporal tumors involving the facial nerve. In: Fisch U (ed) Facial Nerve Surgery. Kugler Publ, BV, Amstelveen, The Netherlands and Aesculapius Publ Co, Birmingham, AL, 448-456, 1977.
46. Pulec JL: Facial nerve tumors. Ann Otol 78:962-982, 1969.
47. Cawthorne T: Intratemporal facial palsy. Arch Otolaryngol 90:789-799, 1969.
48. Horn KL, Crumley RL, Schindler RA: Facial neurilemmomas. Laryngoscope 91:1326-1331, 1981.
49. Graham MD: Surgical exposure of the facial nerve: contemporary transtemporal tecniques. Am J Otol 1:137-146, 1980.
50. House HP: An Apparent primary cholesteatoma: case report. Laryngoscope 63:712-713, 1953.
51. House JW, Sheehy JL: Cholesteatoma with intact tympanic membrane. Laryngoscope 90:70-76, 1980.
52. Curtis AW: Congenital middle ear cholesteatoma: two unusual cases and a review of the literature. Laryngoscope 89:1159-1165, 1979.
53. Peron DL, Schuknecht HF: Congenital cholesteatoma with other anomalies. Arch Otolaryngol 101:498-505, 1975.
54. Fisch U: Congenital cholesteatoma. Clin Otolaryngol 3:369-376, 1978.
55. Nager GT: Epidermoid involving the temporal bone: clinical, radiological and pathological aspects. Laryngoscope 85:1-21, 1975.
56. Bumsted R, Dolan K, Sade J, McCabe BF: Preservation of cochlear function after extensive labyrinthine destruction. Ann Otol 86:131-137, 1977.
57. Thomsen J, Barfoed C, Fleckenstein P: Congenital cholesteatoma. J Laryngol and Otol 94:263-268, 1980.

58. Olivecrona H: Cholesteatomas of the cerebellopontine angle. Acta Psychiat Et Neurol 24:639–643, 1944.
59. Gacek RR: Evaluation and management of primary petrous apex cholesteatoma. Otolaryn Head and Neck Surg 88:519–523, 1980.
60. Housse WF, Doyle JB: Early diagnosis and removal of primary cholesteatoma causing pressure to the VIIIth nerve. Laryngoscope 00:1053–1063, 1962.
61. Batsakis JG: Epidermal carcinomas of the integument of the nose and ear. In: Tumors of the Head and Neck, 2nd edn. Williams & Wilkins Co, pp 420–430, 1979.
62. Beal DD, Lindsay JR, Ward PH: Radiation-induced carcinoma of the mastoid. Arch Otolaryngol 81:9, 1965.
63. Graham MD: personal communication.
64. Johns ME, headington JT: Squamous cell carcinoma of the external auditory canal. Arch of Otolaryngol 10:45–49, 1974.
65. Pulec JL: Glandular tumors of he external auditory canal. Laryngoscope 87:161–1612, 1977.
66. Conley JJ, Novack AJ: The surgical treatment of malignant tumors of the ear and temporal bone: Part I. Arch Otolaryngol 71:635–652, 1960.
67. Ward GE, Loch WE, Lawrence W, Jr: Radical operation for carcinoma of the external auditory canal and middle ear. Am J Surg 82:169–178, 1951.
68. Campbell E, Volk BM, Burkland CW: Total resection of temporal bone for malignancy of the middle ear. Ann Surg 134:397–404, 1951.
69. Parsons H, Lewis JS: Subtotal resection of the temporal bone for cancer of the ear. Cancer 7:995–1001, 1954.
70. Arena S: Tumor surgery of the temporal bone. Laryngoscope 84:645–670, 1974.
71. Gacek RR, Goodman M: Management of malignancy of the temporal bone. Laryngoscope 87:1622–1634, 1977.
72. Neely JG, Forrester M: Anatomic considerations of the medial cuts in the subtotal temporal bone resection. Otolaryngol Head Neck Surg 90:641–645, 1982.
73. Fisch U, Pillsburg HC: Infratemporal fossa approach to lesions in the temporal bone and base of the skull. Arch Otolaryngol 105:99–107, 1979.
74. Hilding DA, Selker R: Total resection of the temporal bone for carcinoma. Arch Otolaryngol 89:98–107, 1969.
75. Graham MD, Kemink JL, Sataloff RT, et al.: Total en bloc resection of the temporal bone and carotid artery for malignant tumors of the ear and temporal bone, in preparation.
76. Crabtree JA, Britton BH, Pierce MK: Carcinoma of the external auditory canal. Laryngoscope 86:405–415, 1976.
77. Lewis JS: Squamous carcinoma of the ear. Arch Otolaryngol 97:41–42, 1973.
78. Baron SH: Herniation of the brain into the mastoid cavity. Arch Otolaryngol 90:779–785.
79. Paparella MM, Meyerhoff WL, Oliviera CA: Mastoiditis and brain hernia (mastoiditis Cerebri). Laryngoscope 88:1097–1106, 1978.
80. Glasscock ME, Dickins JRE, Jackson CG, et al.: Surgical management of brain tissue herniation into the middle ear and mostoid. Laryngoscope 89:1743–1754, 1979.
81. Kamerer DB, Caparosa RJ: Temporal bone encephalocele: diagnosis and treatment. Laryngoscope 92:878–882, 1982.
82. Schurr PH: Endaural cerebral hernia. Br J Surg 17:414–417, 1960.
83. Dysart BR: Spontaneous cerebrospinal otorrhea: Report of a case with successful surgical repair. Trans Am Laryngol Rhinol Soc 62:381, 1959.
84. Mealy J Jr: Chronic cerebrospinal fluid otorrhea: report of a case associated with chronic infection of the ear. Neurology 11:996–998, 1961.
85. Blatt IM: Surgical repair for cerebrospinal otorrhca due to middle ear and mastoid disease: report of six cases. Laryngoscope 73:446–460, 1963.

86. Koch H: Meningocele of the temporal bone. Acta Otolaryngol (Stockh) 38:59–62, 1950.

87. Jahrsdoerfer RA, Richtsmeier WJ, Cantrell RW: Spontaneous CSF otorrhea. Arch Otolaryngol 107:257–261, 1981.

88. Neely JG, Neblett CR, Rose JE: Diagnosis and treatment of spontaneous cerebrospinal fluid otorrhea. Laryngoscope 92:609–612, 1982.

89. Kraus EM, McCabe BF: The giant apical air cell syndrome. Ann Oto Rhinol Laryngol 91:237–239, 1982.

90. Graham MD: personal communication.

91. Briant TDR, Bird R: Extracranial repair of cerebrospinal fluid fistula. J of Otolaryngol 11:191–197, 1982.

92. Jahn AF: Endaural Brain hernia: repair using conchal cartilage. J of Otolaryngol 10:471–475, 1981.

93. Hall GM, Pulec JL, Hallberg OE: Persistent cerebrospinal fluid otorrhea. Arch Otolaryngol 86:43–47, 1967.

94. Fernandez-Blasini N, Longo R: Surgical correction of dural herniation into the mastoid cavity. Laryngoscope 88:1841–1846, 1977.

95. Spetzler RF, Wilson CB: Management of recurrent CSF rhinorrhea of the middle and posterior fossa, J Neurosurgery 49:393–397, 1978.

96. Graham MD: Surgical management of dural and temporal lobe herniation into the radical mastoid cavity. Laryngoscope 92:329–331, 1982.

97. Batsakis JG: Soft tissue tumors of the head and neck: unusual forms. In: Tumors of the Head and Neck,, 2nd edn, pp 350–368, 1979.

98. Batsakis JG, Kittleson AC: Chordomas; otorhinolaryngologic presentation and diagnosis. Arch Otolaryngol 78:168–175, 1963.

99. Dahlin DC, MacCarty CS: Chordoma: a study of fifty-nine cases. Cancer 5:1170–1178, 1952.

4. Surgical restoration of the voice after laryngectomy

MARK I. SINGER, ERIC D. BLOM and RONALD C. HAMAKER

1. Introduction

In 1974, the Centennial Conference on Laryngeal Cancer was held at Toronto, Canada, commemorating the 100 years of progress since Billroth's first laryngectomy. The Congress assembled from throughout the world all of the disciplines interested in carcinoma of the larynx to engage in formal debate and informal discussions to further the state of knowledge and to try to understand differences in rationale and practice. Douglas Bryce stated in the first Conacher Memorial Lecture 'the Centennial Conference, because of the stature of its faculty, has a great challenge to be a source of information – and to develop an unequalled bank of information which can be widely disseminated across the world' [1]. He went on to say that 'it is the necessity to conserve the faculty of human communication by speech that complicates our considerations of the proper primary treatment of patients with this disease'. It was the hope that out of the conference would come a 'great leap forward' to stimulate new efforts in the treatment of cancer of the larynx.

The history of the development of laryngectomy is marked in the latter part of the 19th Century by intense controversy over the propriety of biopsy and safety of the treatment methods. Holinger noted that 'loss of voice was regarded by many as more terrible than loss of limb or sight, or of life itself' [2]. Although even Hayes Martin considered extrinsic laryngeal carcinoma hopeless; Gluck, Soerensen, and in the United States, Solis-Cohen reported successful total laryngectomy operations. The statistics improved in the early 20th Century, although the controversy between conservative versus radical surgery continued and was heightened by the introduction of radiation therapy. The divergence of ideas regarding treatment continues to this day.

With the historic report 'The First Laryngectomy Performed on Humans. As Carried Out By Theodore Billroth, and the Utilization of Artificial

Gregory T. Wolf (ed), Head and Neck Oncology.
© *1984 Martinus Nijhoff Publishers, Boston. ISBN 0-89838-657-8. Printed in The Netherlands*

Larynx', voice restoration by a prosthetic device was introduced [3]. Since the Second World War, a number of secondary methods for voice restoration have been reported using tracheopharyngeal shunts and sometimes ingenious valved devices and cannulas. They have been described by Briani, Conley, Asai, Komorn, Taub, Shedd, Weinberg, Sisson, McConnel, Traissac, and Mozolewski, and have been reported in detail elsewhere [4–12]. These methods have been complicated by shunt stenosis, breakdown, leakage, and death in a few cases. In some instances, voice production has been good, but the methods used were not readily available to many patients.

This chapter will not review the secondary methods for voice restoration, in that they are primarily of historical note only, but will focus on primary vocal restorative procedures that accompany laryngectomy. At the Centennial Congress in Canada, investigators from around the world assembled and presented their successful methods. Ten years have elapsed and with it, a depth of perspective on results has developed that permits a selective review of the status of these procedures. Finally, a personal technique is reviewed as a suggested answer to the historical problems and as a stimulus to future improvements. The 100 years since Billroth have been dedicated to the improved control of laryngeal cancer, and to the achievement after therapy of a better quality of life. This review will seek to answer how well that has been done.

2. Selected contemporary review

In Kobe, Japan, Asai developed the principles of secondary and primary 'laryngoplasty' as a surgical procedure for vocal rehabilitation after laryngectomy. He recognized that only 'a limited number of laryngectomees' acquired satisfactory communication by esophageal speech or the artificial larynx. He felt that 'simulation of the movements of the glottis is impracticable' and voice could be achieved by constructing a communication between the trachea and pharyngeal cavity [13].

These efforts were refined to the development of a primary 'laryngoplasty' immediately following laryngectomy. It was recognized that total laryngectomy should not be limited or compromised by the phonatory reconstruction; the main contraindication being subglottic extension of greater than 1 cm from the inferior margin of the true vocal cords. Also, patients with limited pulmonary reserve should be excluded. The procedure was introduced in 1974, and by 1982 had been performed in 21 patients.

The laryngectomy is traditionally wide field, removing the hyoid bone and transecting the trachea below the cricoid cartilage. The residual mucous membrane of the anterior pharyngeal wall is preserved intact and reflected inferiorly to join the first treacheal ring. The flap is sutured circumferential-

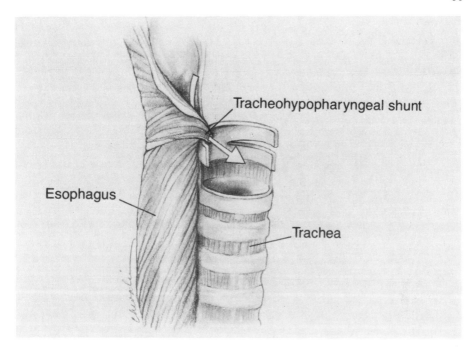

Tracheohypopharyngeal shunt

Esophagus

Trachea

Reprinted by permission of the *Laryngoscope*, Vol. 93.

Figure 1. Asai's tracheopharyngeal shunt primarily constructed at laryngectomy.

ly to the trachea and the lateral margins then approximated to form a mucosa lined tube (Fig. 1). A strut from the superior cornua of the thyroid cartilage is introduced between the pharyngeal flap and the esophageal mucous membrane to maintain the length of the mucosal tube, and a rubber catheter is used as a stent for this tube for a period of three weeks.

Voice production is accomplished by occluding the tracheostoma to divert air into the pharynx. With continued practice, the patient is reported to develop good conversational ability. Of the series of 21 patients, 15 were successful with voice production. Six patients developed either stenosis or secondary infection with subsequent breakdown of the shunt. Nine of the patients had no problems, while three had some aspiration, two experienced 'constant cough' controlled by compressing the anterior neck during swallowing, and one had severe, chronic aspiration of liquids.

Intelligibility of speech as assessed by volunteers listening to random word lists ranged from 53–83%. The resultant speech quality was generally 'rougher' than normal speech. Comments regarding radiation therapy or adjunctive treatments are not available nor is followup with reference to recurrence rates.

Another one-stage primary technique for voice rehabilitation was proposed by the Japanese investigator, Amatsu of Kobe, Japan [14]. The indi-

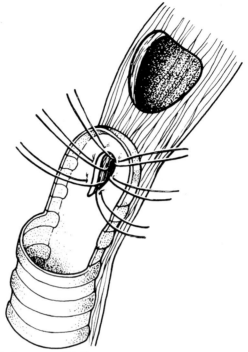

Reprinted by permission of the *Laryngoscope*, Vol. 93.

Figure 2. Side to side tracheoesophageal fistula with preservation of membranous trachea (after Amatsu).

cations for selection were similar to Asai's. Although previously irradiated cases were accepted, higher pressures were necessary for speech production.

The larynx is usually removed at the first tracheal ring, and a tracheostoma is established at the third or fourth ring. The membranous trachea is preserved after resection of the anterior wall forming an inferiorly-based flap usually measuring 2×4 cm. A side-to-side tracheoesophageal anastomosis is constructed at the superior aspect of the tracheal flap (Fig. 2). The tracheoesohageal shunt is created by tubing the tracheal flap over a stent catheter, and the hypopharynx is closed in the customary fashion (Fig. 3).

Speech is permitted after two weeks by digital occlusion of the tracheostoma, and effortless phonation develops with daily practice. The shunt develops increased resilience with repeated insufflations during daily conversation. Sound is produced by the vibrating effect of expired air on the walls of the esophagus.

During the period from 1976 to 1978, 30 patients underwent the procedure. Although 28 patients initially developed useful speech ability, only 23 patients had conversational ability that was durable. One patient had spasmodic speech, and one had a closure procedure because of inability to use the shunt. Two developed wound infections with shunt dehiscence, three

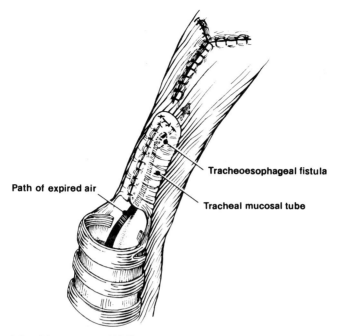

Path of expired air

Tracheoesophageal fistula

Tracheal mucosal tube

Reprinted by permission of the *Laryngoscope*, Vol. 93.

Figure 3. Tubed membranous trachea completing tracheoesophageal shunt (after Amatsu).

had spontaneous shunt closures, and one could not produce speech despite a patent shunt.

Aspiration was present to varying degrees in nine patients. Control of this problem was usually accomplished by digital pressure on the shunt. Nine patients had received preoperative radiation, and of these, six developed 'good speech'. Data regarding long term tumor control was not provided, but is not expected to be significantly different from that associated with conventional laryngectomy.

The Italian laryngologist, Staffieri, proposed another method for primary tracheopharyngeal shunt formation which was reported between 1969–1977 [15]. The method was attempted subsequently by a number of other investigators. The technique is analogous to the Japanese procedures reviewed above. The trachea is transected similarly at the first ring, and the hypopharynx is separated from the membranous trachea. The phonatory shunt or 'neoglottis fonatoria' is delicately created by exteriorization of the pharyngeal mucosa separate from the submucosal connective tissue and muscular layers (Fig. 4). This is sutured to the anterior surface of the hypopharynx and is then fixed to the postero-superior trachea, completing the shunt.

Indications for Staffieri's procedure include: Endolaryngeal lesions which require total laryngectomy with or without radical neck dissection. Contra-

88

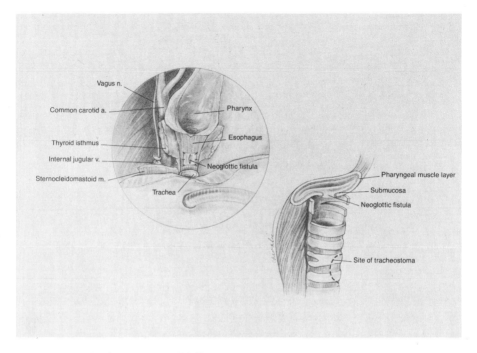

Reprinted by permission of the *Laryngoscope*, Vol. 93.

Figure 4. Tracheoesophageal fistula ('Neoglottis fonateria') by Staffieri's technique.

indicated are T3 lesions with posterior extension encroaching upon the anterior wall of the esophagus, or T4 lesions with soft tissue extension. Ideal requirements of the phonatory shunt are closure during passage of food and saliva and ease of opening during phonation by the 'thrust' of expiratory air with a closed tracheostoma.

Staffieri reported a series of 97 patients personally treated between 1970–1977. Six deaths were attributed to medical complications, leaving 91 evaluable patients. Results in eighty-four cases (92.3%) were judged satisfactory, while 21 (23%) required surgical revision of the shunt which was not properly functioning; and four required 'completion' laryngectomy. Five patients (5.4%) achieved a satisfactory voice result following revision, while the others did not.

It is stated that the neoglottic speech as described by Staffieri is natural and easily produced. Fluency exceeds esophageal speakers without fatigue, and vocal quality that is more natural regarding intensity and timbre. The author does not give incidence figures for 'primary incontinence' of the neoglottis but suggests that this occurence is best managed by early shunt revision (one month). Primary stenosis may also occur because of edema and esophageal wall scarring, and this also requires early revision by retrograde tracheal dilatation. Late incontinence may occur at months or years postoperatively and includes liquid and solid food aspiration. It is suggested that this is related to atrophy of the walls of the shunt and successful revision is usually possible. There were 29 revisions reported in 21 patients with good results in 17 cases.

In a review of the 'pseudoglottis procedure' from Northwestern University, 26 cases were performed by the method of Staffieri for tumors classified as T3 or T4. 13 of these were also N1 [16]. Of greatest significance was the occurrence of six early recurrences of which four were reportedly at the primary site. This left 18 evaluable cases from the standpoint of voice and swallowing function. Nine patients experienced serious aspiration, four required revision surgery of the pseudoglottis, and four were converted or underwent completion laryngectomy. Shunt stenosis was identified in one patient. The overall success rate relative to voice production was 65% of cases.

Leipzig from the University of Texas reported that of 50 patients undergoing the Staffieri neoglottic reconstruction, nine had recurrent disease over a $3\frac{1}{2}$ year period [17]. There were three recurrences at the stoma, three regional metastases, and three distant metastases. 'Significant' aspiration was experienced in 20 patients (40%), requiring shunt revision in 14 cases with one-half requiring closure to control aspiration. Speech function was reported to be satisfactory in only 50% of patients.

Radiation experience was also reported. Twenty-seven patients had received some form of this adjunctive therapy, of which 13 developed voice; however, 14 required revision surgery to control a major complication, usually aspiration.

At Emory University, McConnel and Teichgraeber reported experience with Staffieri neoglottic reconstruction in patients followed as long as five years [18]. All 13 patients obtained speech from two weeks to three months postoperatively. Five patients required shunt dilatation, and one required revision for stenosis. Seven patients had 'troublesome' aspiration and required revision which was successful in four cases. One patient died of neck and distal metastases. There were six cases of pneumonia, and three required closure of the neoglottis.

The radiation experience in this series is unique. No patients who experienced radiation failure were selected for neoglottic reconstruction. In cases selected for radiation therapy postoperatively, the neoglottis was shielded with a dose of 5000 rads given to the primary and neck, and 1000 rads to the neoglottic shunt.

The authors concluded that the major complication rate abruptly increased after three years, dimming earlier successful reports of the technique. From their experience, it was stated: 'primary neoglottis reconstruction is a questionable alternative to total laryngectomy and esophageal speech for rehabilitation'.

2.1. Interpretive summary

As experience was gained with conservation laryngeal surgical techniques, it became evident that partial laryngectomy was feasible, and that voice could be preserved with a normal airway, and swallowing function maintained with little disruption. The major importance of adequate tumor resection and tolerance to therapeutic radiation was accepted and represents unquestionably one of the single greatest advances in therapy of laryngeal carcinoma.

As the structure of the larynx is progressively resected by either the thyrotomy approach of the vertical laryngectomy or the pharyngotomy approach of the horizontal laryngectomy, the ability to preserve a satisfactory functional larynx decreases for the critical aspects of deglutition and airway maintenance. Either the sphincter activity during swallowing is significantly impaired or the glottic and subglottic airway are narrowed to the extent that decannulation is not possible.

It is generally accepted on oncologic grounds that carcinomas extending across the ventricle (transglottic carcinoma) are not 'amenable' to conservation procedures. Transglottic carcinomas invade the supraglottic lymphatic compartment and are not effectively dealt with by the vertical procedure. On the other hand, when supraglottic carcinoma invades the ventricle, it will commonly spread to involve the paraglottic space, and horizontal resection is no longer a safe approach.

It occurred to a number of investigators that 'near total' resections of the larynx were possible with functional preservation of the structure, although some increase in complications would be encountered. The Italian surgeon, Serafini, demonstrated in animals as early as 1963, a 'simplified organ' that was apparently adequate after laryngectomy [19]. Initially the trachea was elevated to the level of the hyoid bone, and a tracheopharyngeal anastomosis was established just inferior to the stump of the suprahyoid epiglottis. The results of this technique were satisfactory in dogs, and the application to humans is reviewed.

3. Subtotal laryngectomy with airway preservation

Serafini's experience began in 1970; and by 1975, 40 patients had undergone his procedure [20]. The technique preserves the hyoid and suprahyoid epiglottic structure with attachments maintaining the vallecula. The perichondrium is reflected from the thyroid cartilage and preserved, while the larynx is resected at the first tracheal ring. The trachea is mobilized from the anterior esophageal wall for advancement to the tongue base. The lower edge of the pharyngostoma is sutured to the posterior edge of the tracheostoma. Anteriorly the tracheopharyngeal anstomosis is completed with the inferior raw edge of the preserved epiglottis. The hyoid bone is used to support the anastomosis, and the suture line is buttressed with the cricopharyngeus muscle.

It was stated that the trachea could be elevated 4 cm with this maneuver, and was maintained in this position affer complete healing. In an initial report of 25 selected cases, Serafini reported one local recurrence and two metastases. Phonation developed in all cases and compared favorably to conventional esophageal voice. Normal resumption of alimentation was rapid, but 'liquids presented some difficulty for a few weeks'. Significantly, 15 patients tolerated occlusion of the tracheostoma for normal respiration.

In a further review of this technique reported in 1976, Serafini's results of 35 patients revealed that successful speech occurred in 100% of patients, with 30% experiencing normal inspiration through the 'neolarynx' [21]. Four patients suffered bronchopneumonia secondary to aspiration while four others had prolonged difficulty swallowing liquids. Local recurrences occurred in eight cases, and were treated by completion laryngectomy, radical neck dissection, and radiotherapy. Twelve cases developed cervical lymph node disease over a three year period. Overall survival was 25 of 35 patients (71.5%). The causes of death were related to local recurrence in four cases, recurrent neck disease in two cases, distant metastases in one case, and intercurrent disease in three cases.

A larger international experience using the technique of Serafini has been reported that represented 122 cases submitted by 14 laryngologists from Italy, Spain, Austria, Japan, and France. A postoperative mortality occurred in seven cases (4%). Five cases had tracheal necrosis, 11 had aspiration pneumonia, and 11 (9%) had early local recurrence [21]. Excluding the deaths and early recurrences, 106 evaluable cases remained. Success, as measured by definitive decannulation, satisfactory speech and swallowing, was reported in no more than 16 cases (15%). Partial success, as characterized by satisfactory speech and swallowing, but inability to decannulate was noted in 60 cases (57%). Complete failure representing inability to decannulate, severe deglutition problems with or without speech was reported in 30 cases (28%).

Because of the considerable problems noted above, a functional laryngectomy was described in France during 1970 to 1975 that varied the resection by preservation of more of the larynx. The historical basis for this technique is traced to Foeder (1899) who suggested preservation of the cricoid ring, and arytenoid [22]. LaBayle proposed in 1971, a cricohyoidopexy [23]. The limits of resection were excision of the epiglottis with the pre-epiglottic space, excision of the ventricular bands, the vocal cords and the thyroid cartilage in continuity with the superior part of the cricoid ring and one arytenoid. The cricoid was advanced and supported by the hyoid bone, and apposition of the remaining arytenoid to the tongue base served to close the neolarynx and protect the lower respiratory tract. Results in 48 cases revealed definitive decannulation in 89% (43 patients) with satisfactory swallowing and phonation. Five cases could not be decannulated and had severe disturbance of deglutition. Piquet, also in France, improved on the functional results for glottic carcinomas by conservation of the entire cricoid ring and both arytenoids with preservation of 3/4 of the epiglottis [24]. This increased the functional success rate to 94% of patients. Local recurrence was encountered in 2 of 23 patients (9%) and required completion laryngectomy. One patient died of 'laryngeal edema'.

The Japanese investigators, Iwai and Koike, reported a primary technique in 1973, called a 'laryngoplasty type III' [25]. Preservation of the cricoid lamina and posterior thyroid alae was found essential for minimizing aspiration. This surgical procecure was a variation of narrow field laryngectomy, in which the larynx was reconstructed by fracturing and rotating the superior cornua medially and suturing them together to simulate the arytenoid eminence. Inferiorly based hypopharyngeal mucosal flaps were developed and rotated to resurface the neolarynx. The thyroid alar remnants were closed on themselves and elevated to the hyoid bone.

The resultant laryngoplasty was used in 19 cases, and five developed pharyngeal fistulae. No recurrences were detected, and aspiration occurred with inspiration or during swallowing in most of the patients but was generally felt to be tolerable. The voice was described as hoarse, but of a better quality than conventional esophageal voice. A number of patients were able to tolerate airway decannulation. The authors concluded that this was an effective procedure to 'preserve vocal function without sacrificing the curability of surgery for the extended laryngeal malignancy'.

4. Arytenoid mucosal shunts

Another approach was proposed by the Polish investigator, Mozolewski [26]. He recognized that the aim of phonatory surgery is the creation of a voicing system that functions with expiratory air flows under appropriate pressures to the pharynx. It was his feeling that concomitant preservation of respiratory function with a physiologic airway was yet experimental. In consideration of this, a method was developed and used since 1970, to rehabilitate speech and also protect the lower airway.

Three variations of 'autoplastic' vocal shunts were used. The arytenoid mucosal shunt was the most commonly described procedure representing a case experience of 60 patients. In the most favorable situation, one mucosa covered arytenoid and cricoid cartilage can be preserved. The shunt is formed from an inferiorly pedicled mucosal flap of the hypopharynx, that is tubed and sutured to the laryngeal mucosa overlying the arytenoid.

The results of this procedure are summarized as follows: Thirty-five of 60 had 'good' speech and 12 had average speech as defined by phonatory pressures not exceeding 35 cm H_2O. Thirteen patients were considered failures or lacking speech, which was the result of a closed shunt. The fundamental problem of shunt continence for food or saliva was demonstrated with a series of radiographic examinations. Twenty-one of the 60 cases were completely continent, and 16 were 'practically' tight, i.e., continent of saliva but minimal leakage of liquids was present. In 20 patients, there was little protection of the airway.

Successful treatment was analyzed in the following manner. Including an additional 20 supracrioid and supratracheal shunts, local recurrence was detected in 3 of 81 cases. Parastomal recurrence occurred in 9 of 81 cases and perioperative mortality in 5% of the cases.

4.1. Interpretive summary

It has been stated by Pearson that total laryngectomy is 'not truly necessary to obtain adequate margins' [27]. Further, he relates that 'historically, total laryngectomy was as much a response to the needs of respiration and deglutition as the needs of oncology. Currently, attempts to preserve the principle of total laryngectomy tend to be rationalized as oncologic'. The historical record reports Billroth's landmark achievement of total laryngectomy as a cancer treatment for therapeutic failure by the lesser procedure of thyrotomy. Separation of the 'airway' and 'foodway' was, in fact, accomplished by a diverting pharyngostomy. The scientific foundations for conservation surgery were provided by Pressman's 'compartmentalization' of the laryngeal lymphatic drainage routes, and Ogura's major study of the surgical pathology of laryngeal cancer [28, 29]. T3 cancers of the larynx are generally not 'amenable' to accepted conservation techniques on oncologic or physiologic grounds.

Pearson's contention that 'techniques that build their reconstructive strategy on anything less than a total laryngectomy have never attracted much support in North America' is an accurate reflection of the situation [27]. He feels that our understanding of the laryngoplastic techniques as described by Mozolewski, Iwai, or LaBayle, has been minimal. The review presented above is a contemporary 10-year assessment of the results of methods that represent variations in techniques with the common feature of attempts to preserve cricoid, arytenoid, and other parts of the endolarynx for the formation of useful phonatory shunts.

The critical aspect of the analysis is tumor control. Although only historical controls are available, the most disconcerting finding is the rate of midline or primary tumor recurrences reported by Staffieri, Serafini, Mozolewski, and LaBayle that exceeds the incidence after wide field laryngectomy. The data regarding radiation experience is important and must not be neglected; however, the data are not sufficient for reliable interpretation. By North American standards, radiation therapy would be used far more widely for T3 disease in combination with surgery than is used in Europe and is justified by improved disease control rates [30]. On the other hand, primary vocal rehabilitative procedures are not generally applicable when the patient has had preoperative radiation therapy because of well-documented failures and even mortality. Although postoperative radiation therapy is a standard modality in combined management of laryngeal carcinoma, the majority of laryngoplastic reconstructions have not received this therapeutic modality.

The common theme of aspiration that characterizes this literature review accounts for 25–50% of cases. However, the aspiration reported is generally tolerated with few cases of bronchopneumonia. A small but significant number of reconstructions must be converted to total laryngectomy (completions) to eventually manage this problem. The results of phonation are rarely reported in a scientific or quantitative manner but are generally stated to be of low pressure or 'good intelligibility'. Successful speakers are reported at rates of 65–100% which are assumed to exceed acquisition rates for conventional esophageal speech.

5. Extended hemilaryngectomy for subtotal laryngectomy

The reports of extended hemilaryngectomy and subtotal laryngectomy by Pearson *et al.* include 16 evaluable cases [31]. The operative technique involves resection of approximately one-half the cricoid ring with ipsilateral larynx and hyoid bone. The preserved endolaryngeal mucosa including arytenoid, vocalis muscle and portion of vocal cord is too narrow to tube for formation of a shunt, but adequately bridges the defect from the trachea to the pharynx. An inferiorly based hypopharyngeal flap is raised from the remaining mucosa and is rotated to augment the endolaryngeal bridge. This is subsequently tubed to form a shunt from the trachea to the pharynx (Fig. 5). The fistula walls are reportedly muscular and innervated by branches of the vagus nerve, while the recurrent laryngeal nerve contralateral to the cancer is preserved for arytenoid innervation.

Each of the 16 patients was reported to achieve a good 'fistula speech' with minimum of effort. Six of the patients experienced aspiration of varying degree without pulmonary complications, and none required revision or closure for this problem. Local recurrence was not detected, although

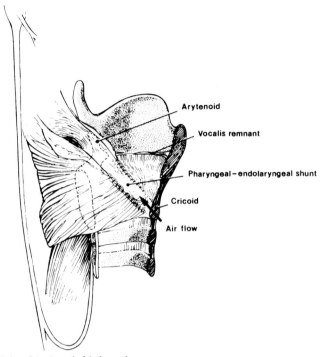

Reprinted by permission of the *Journal of Otolaryngology.*

Figure 5. Extended hemilaryngectomy (subtotal laryngectomy) variation of arytenoid mucosal shunt (after Pearson).

follow-up was admittedly short with eight patients under 15 months. One patient had received preoperative radiation therapy and four postoperative therapy. Twelve patients underwent radical neck dissection with five having histologically positive nodes, and two patients had recurrence in the *contralateral* neck.

5.1. Interpretive summary

Pearson concludes from his experience that this method may replace total laryngectomy as the optimum procedure for T3 laryngeal cancer. Also 'unless the results of radiation therapy for T3 laryngeal cancer are considerably improved, it should also supplant this modality completely' [31]. This remarkable statement is not substantiated by experience or time. The active sphincteric mechanism of this form of arytenoid mucosal shunt is not documented, and in theory the muscular attachments of the 'innervated' arytenoid are disrupted, rendering purposeful motion most unlikely. There is no clear evidence for an active phonetic function of the arytenoid shunt. Finally, it seems incumbent on the investigators that laryngeal whole section histopathology be used to evaluate the specimens and tumor behavior in preference to frozen section biopsies, that may be fraught with sampling errors. This is of particular importance in light of at least two cases of contralateral cervical metastases. Until these issues are addressed, this modified technique of arytenoid mucosal shunt must be viewed with the cautious skepticism reserved for the proponents of the other subtotal laryngectomies.

It is not surprising that laryngeal reconstructions using tissues continuously bathed in contaminated secretions, partially devitalized by the tumor resection, and commonly irradiated, are not capable of effectively simulating glottic and supraglottic functions. A vocal rehabilitative method is measured by its ability to meet a number of important criteria. There is no excuse for limitation of adequate cancer treatment with regard to either extent of surgical resection or use of conventional dose radiation therapy. Deglutition and handling of secretions must be physiologic and reacquired postoperatively with minimal delay. The patient should be free from dependence on complicated valves, tubes, and prostheses; while frequent endoscopy with dilatations and revisions ought not be required.

6. Tracheoesophageal puncture

Considerations for safety, conventional cancer treatment standards, and rapid uncomplicated return to near normal life without excessive costs are fundamental concerns of the voice restoration method of tracheoesophageal phonation employing a silicone valved prosthesis. In 1978, Singer and Blom proposed an uncomplicated surgical technique and simple silicone valve device that adequately answers many of the historical problems reviewed [32, 33].

An endoscopic method for voice restoration after esophageal speech failure using a silicone valve, Blom-Singer® voice prosthesis, is effective and reproducible with satisfactory success rates. By 1981, an accumulated experience of 129 patients was reported [34]. The criterion for success was based on fluency and intelligibility of the speakers. Acoustic, aerodynamic, and intelligibility studies of tracheoesophageal speakers were analyzed and reported in a number of publications [35–37]. In general the assessments often equaled or exceeded those of excellent esophageal speakers.

Postoperative problems have been insignificant and limited primarily to occasional extrusion of the prosthesis or minimal tracheitis. Although salivary contamination has been observed, no patients experienced aspiration pneumonia. Two patients of 129 developed intractable aspiration despite a functioning valve, and required a secondary closure procedure. Nine pa-

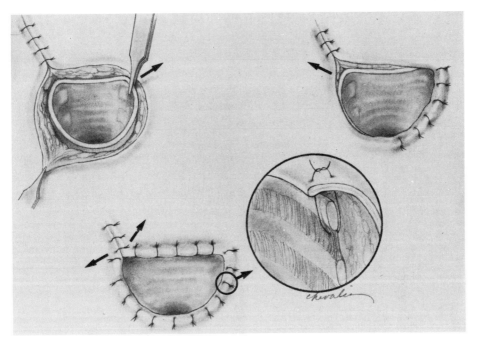

Figure 6. Tracheostoma construction by 'opening' the cartilaginous ring and fixing it to the inferior skin. Half-vertical mattress technique.

tients experienced some aspiration and responded to shunt cautery to enhance stenosis, effectively eliminating any leakage.

The success of this method of endoscopic voice restoration employing a prosthesis encouraged us to apply this to the rehabilitation at laryngectomy for early vocal function. A standard wide field total laryngectomy is performed with resection of a margin of the tongue base, hyoid bone with pre-epiglottic space contents, partial hypopharyngectomy, cricoid cartillage and post cricoid mucosa, 2–3 tracheal rings, strap muscles, ipsilateral thyroidectomy, and ipsilateral neck dissection when indicated. The trachea is beveled in order that the posterior wall is 5–7 mm superior to the anterior wall. The tracheal cartilage is sutured to the inferior skin flap using a half vertical mattress suture technique (Fig. 6). The tracheal ring is subsequently opened to a broad 'C' by traction from the inferio-lateral skin. This stabilizes the stoma by using the forces of wound contraction to maintain the patency.

The posterior or membranous trachea is supported laterally and care is exercised to avoid separating it from its attachments to the anterior esophagus. A point is selected for development of a tracheoesophageal shunt corresponding to 5 mm from the postero-superior margin or level with the anterior margin (Fig. 7). A curved hemostat is passed through the pharyngotomy defect to distend the membranous tracheal wall. A horizontal inci-

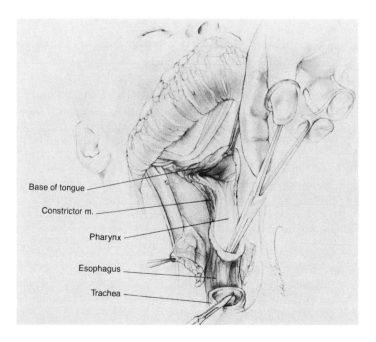

Figure 7. Primary tracheoesophageal puncture placement after laryngectomy.

sion is made through the tracheal and esophageal walls, allowing the tip of the hemostat to perforate and dilate the incision. This 'puncture' is stented by drawing a Foley catheter into the esophagus and inflating the balloon to prevent dislodgement (Fig. 8).

This maneuver will permit the formation of a horizontal side-to-side shunt of 9 mm in length. The shunt is truly esophageal at this level and inferior to the cricopharyngeal muscle and esophageal lip. It must be noted that a puncture of this type without mobilization of the esophageal mucosa and fixing it to the trachea is not permanent, but by definition is an esophagotomy. If the stent or valve (see below) is removed, the walls of the puncture will collapse, and the esophageal defect will usually heal. The tracheal defect behaves in a similar manner. For this reason, we refer to this as a 'puncture' rather than a 'fistula', and consider the procedure usually reversible without surgical intervention.

Although the tracheoesophageal shunt formed in this manner is short and horizontal, leakage of liquids or saliva will occur unless it is obturated or valved. The silicone valve successfully used in the secondary rehabilitative method of endoscopic voice restoration is also used in this primary setting. The valve is referred to as a voice prosthesis, but restores laryngeal function only as a sphincter, since the sound source is substituted by the apposition of vibrating pharyngoesophageal mucous membranes. The valve function is based on a 'slit design' permitting closure by the natural recoil of the mate-

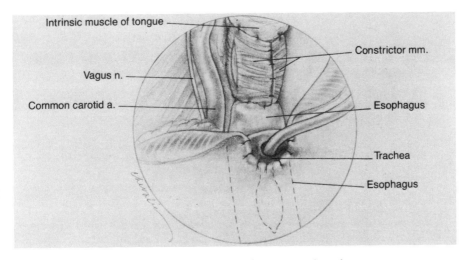

Figure 8. Balloon catheter stent of tracheoesophageal puncture.

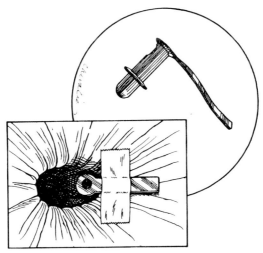

Figure 9. Silicone 'duckbill' voice prosthesis (Blom-Singer®).

rial. The Blom-Singer® voice prosthesis is 5.4 mm in diameter and has variable lengths (Fig. 9). At the esophgeal end, the slit valve opens under positive airway pressures, permitting flows of 50–100 cc. per second. The valve closes competently when air flow stops. We have descriptively termed this valve system a 'duckbill'.

The valve prosthesis occupies the tracheoesophageal puncture and usually maintains a horizontal or slightly antegrade inclination. It remains reliably closed during swallowing, maintaining a competent barrier to foods, liquids, or secretions. Although the axial length of the tracheoesophageal puncture is

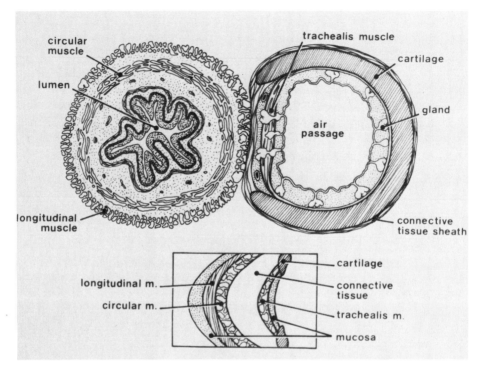

Figure 10. Arrangement of muscle and connective tissue layers of the tracheoesophageal 'common' wall.

not great, it is uncommon to have leakage around the valve or dilatation of the tissues over time or with continuous use. This is explained by two possible mechanisms. The esophagotomy and tracheotomy of each end of the tracheoesophageal puncture maintain a constant stenosing capacity or viewed differently, healing capability. This maintains a precise fit circumferentially about the cylindrical valve. Repetitive movement or piston effect of the valve will produce dilatation and must be avoided by proper technique for its use.

The second theory of tracheoesophageal puncture-valve continence concerns the anatomy of the tracheoesophageal wall at this level. Analysis of this region demostrates that the two parallel tubular structures are mucosa lined, with a sheet of smooth muscle deep to the tracheal mucosea that inserts on either side of the posterior cartilaginous rings known as the trachealis muscle (Fig. 10). This layer contributes tone to the membranous trachea. A layer of dense fascia occupies the space between the trachealis and anterior esophagus which progressively attenuates from the level of the cricoid to the thoracic esophagus. The anterior esophageal wall is composed of two layers of muscle, the outer longitudinal and the inner circular which are in continuity with the interior pharyngeal constrictor muscles. This region of the upper trachea and esophagus supports the silicone valve voice prosthesis without uncontrolled fistulization, leakage, or breakdown, and permits the simple horizontal shunt to function with little risk to the patient or to impose complicated technical demands on the clinicians.

The valve is comfortable and convenient to maintain at its superior tracheal location. Simple removal and cleansing after 2–3 days is the minimum requirement with easy replacement. The environment of the pharynx affects the silicone little, and a replacement is required after 3–4 months' continuous use.

Effective tracheoseophageal phonation occurs with pharyngoesophageal airflows of 100 cc per second a tracheal pressures ranging from 35–60 cm H_2O. Strain, tightness, or lack of fluency may occur if the resistance exceeds these measures. In consideration of this finding, esophageal distention may produce reflexive hypertonicity at the upper esophageal sphincter, and failure to relax may prevent phonation. This problem was reported to occur in 12% of unselected esophageal speech failures with complete failure of tracheoesophageal phonation, and up to 40% of patients with varying degrees of speech difficulty [34, 38].

The use of pharyngeal constrictor myotomy as a secondary method for speech salvage can be successfully added to the primary voice restoration technique. It is reasoned that this adds little hazard to the laryngectomy and optimizes the vocal tract for the higher airflows of tracheoesophageal puncture.

The operative field following conventional laryngectomy is suitable for a thorough, safe, and technically easy myotomy when the pharynx remains open (pharyngotomy). The mucosa is placed on tension with noncrushing clamps and is stretched over the operator's finger (Fig. 11). The posterior midline of the pharynx is identified at the level of the tongue base, and the muscular fibers of the middle pharyngeal constrictor are divided to permit entry of a curved hemostat which is used to complete a midline tunnel to the cervical esophagus. With the hemostat in place to maintain the midline orientation, the tented constrictor muscles are sharply incised vertically from the base of the tongue to the esophagus. The myotomy is then continued through the cricopharyngeus by stretching this muscle as well. This method requires little time and is advantageous for preservation of the vascularity of the remaining pharyngeal musculature and, in turn, the underlying mucosa.

The pharyngotomy is closed with an inverting suture technique to avoid tension at the base of the tongue. This may be accomplished by a 'T' shaped closure or a V-Y advancement. The second layer is established by burying the mucosal suture line, and a third layer is formed by reapproxi-

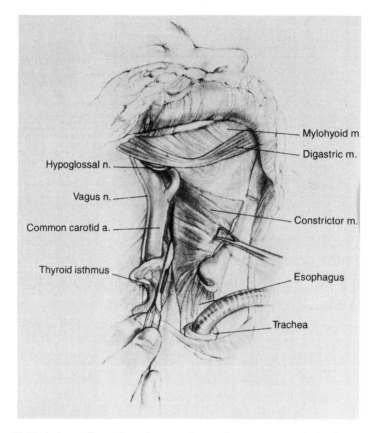

Figure 11. Technique of complete pharyngeal constrictor myotomy during laryngectomy.

mating the remaining constrictor musculature over the anterior midline as in a conventional closure method.

If no evidence of salivary fistula is detected, the nonradiated patients begin oral alimentation on the sixth or seventh postoperative day, and previously radiated patients on the tenth or eleventh day. The silicone voice prosthesis is inserted one to two days after the resumption of oral alimentation, and phonation may proceed immediately.

6.1. Results of primary vocal rehabilitation by tracheoesophageal puncture

Thirty patients who failed the criteria for conservation laryngectomy underwent total laryngectomy and primary voice reconstruction during a two-year period between 1980–1982. There were 23 males and seven females with ages ranging from 44 to 79 years. Nineteen of the group (63%) developed voice rapidly and maintained the silicone valve without dislodgement. Five of the patients had pectoralis major flaps, five were unplanned radiation patients, and seven received postoperative radiation therapy.

Nine patients were partially successful, in that voice was acquired, but five of these could not maintain the prosthesis during postoperative radiation therapy, and the tracheoesophageal puncture closed. Of the other four, speech was delayed three months in one, one lost the valve six weeks postoperatively, one had a pharyngeal reconstruction for stricture formation, and one developed incurable neck disease.

The complete failures were two. The mean age was older among failures (72 years versus 55 years). One developed a pharyngocutaneous fistula and one had a total pharyngeal reconstruction with a pectoralis major myocutaneous flap. There was no placement of the valve postoperatively, and speech was not evaluated. Both patients went on to complete courses of postoperative radiation therapy.

The time for satisfactory speech development for the 19 completely successful cases was two weeks for 10, four weeks for seven, six weeks for one (unplanned fistula), and four months for one patient. Five of the patients who lost the valve due to tracheoesophageal puncture closure were reopened endoscopically with successful voicing subsequently.

Some general observations can be made from this 30 patient experience. The method results in effective tracheoesophageal phonation, but long term use is limited by the inability of the newly laryngectomized patient to manage a tracheostoma and a prosthesis simultaneously. There were no problems of uncontrolled aspiration, no major delays in receiving adjunctive radiation therapy, but four (13%) fistulae were noted.

The patients were satisfied with the resultant communication status, but some did not comprehend the laryngectomized condition and were delayed in their necessary adjustments to it. A number expected secondary closure of the tracheostoma or an eventual return to normal speech with the tracheoesophageal puncture merely as an interim measure. If stomal stenosis developed, the addition of a tracheal cannula or vent tube further complicated the problem of managing a fresh stoma. Patients with a voice prosthesis in place who then received radiation therapy experienced increased tracheitis, bleeding, and eventual loss of prosthetic voice after four weeks of radiation.

6.2. Interpretive summary

The effective therapy of laryngeal carcinoma has a 100 year history characterized by many techniques proposed to preserve the ability to speak. The location of the neoplasm and its biological behavior necessarily direct the critical decisions regarding surgery and radiaiton therapy. The development of conservation laryngectomy procedures permits adequate tumor resection and voice preservation, however wider resection of the laryngeal sphincter mechanism allows uncontrolled aspiration and its consequences.

Alaryngeal patients may acquire voice from the efficient activation of the pharyngoesophageal mucous membranes by skilled air trapping or tracheal shunts. The valved silicone devices placed in a controlled tracheoesophageal puncture serve this purpose by providing needed airway protection and permitting voice production by the vibrating effect of expired pulmonary air on the pharyngoesophageal membranes. Deglutition remains physiologic with the valve functioning in the tracheoesophageal puncture.

The accepted surgical residua of total laryngectomy can be effectively used for the patient's rehabilitation with little alteration and no compromise of the principles of surgical oncology. The combination of modern valve technology, a simple horizontal tracheoesophageal shunt, and skilled patient instruction will allow nearly all laryngectomees intelligible and natural vocal rehabilitation.

Treatment decisions for laryngeal cancer can be made sympathetic to the patient's despair of an uncertain future with cancer and voicelessness. Restoration of voice is a goal sharing importance with that of effective therapy of laryngeal cancer. The diligent efforts described in the historical record reveal repeated refinements of earlier ideas and treatment methods, as well as a better understanding of the mechanisms of voice production. Improvements will appear in future reports based on an understanding of earlier methods and the ultimate goals of improved therapy of cancer and preservation of the sound producing continuity of the aerodigestive system.

References

1. Bryce DP: The Conacher memorial lecture: '100 years of effort'. Laryngoscope 85:241, 1975.
2. Holinger PH: A century of progress of laryngectomies in the northern hemisphere. Laryngoscope 85:322, 1975.
3. Gussenbauer C: Ueber die erste durch Th Billroth am Menschen ausgefuhrte Kehlkopf-Extirpation und die Anwendung eines kunstlichen Kokopfes. Arch Klin Chir 17:343–356, 1874.
4. Briani A: Riabilitazione fonetica di laringectomizzati a mezzo della corrente aerea espiratoria polmonare. Arch Ital Otol Rhinol Laryngol 63:469, 1952.
5. Conley JJ, DeAmesti F, Pierce JK: A new surgical technique for vocal rehabilitation of the laryngectomized patient. Ann Otol Rhinol Laryngol 67:655–664, 1958.
6. Asai R: Asai's new voice production method: a substitution for human speech. Paper presented at the Eighth International Congress of Otorhinolaryngology, Tokyo, 1965.
7. Komorn RM: Vocal rehabilitation in the laryngectomized patient with a tracheoesophageal shunt. Ann Otol Rhinol Laryngol 83:445–451, 1974.
8. Taub S, Shapiro RH: Vocal rehabilitation of laryngectomees: Preliminary report of a new technique. Am J Surg 124:87–90, 1972.

9. Shedd D, *et al.*: Further appraisal of reed fistula speech following pharyngolaryngectomy. Can J Otolaryngol 4:503, 1975.

10. Sisson GA, McConnell FMS, Logemann J: Voice rehabilitation after laryngectomy. Results with the use of hypopharyngeal prosthesis. Arch Otolaryngol 101:178–181, 1975.

11. Traissac L, Pardes P, Vazel P: A report on 99 cases of surgical speech rehabilitation, reconstructive techniques. In: Shedd DP, Weinberg B (eds) Surgical and Prosthetic Approaches to Speech Rehabilitation. Boston, GK Hall Medical publishers, 1980, p 199.

12. Mozolewski E, Zietek E, Jach K: Mucosal vocal shunt, Annales Academiae Medcae Stefinensis Supp 24(15):36, 1978.

13. Asai R, Minatogawa T, Kumoi T: Primary laryngoplasty immediately following total laryngectomy. Hyogo College of Medicine, Hyogo, Japan (in press).

14. Amatsu M: A one stage surgical technique for postlaryngectomy voice rehabilitation. Laryngoscope 90:1378–1386, 1980.

15. Staffieri M, Serafini I: La riabilitazione chirurgica della voce e della respirazione dopo laringectomia totale. 29th National Congress of the Associazione Otologi Ospedalieri Italiana. Bologna: Associazione Otologi Ospedalieri Italiana: 57–111, 1976.

16. Sisson GA, Bystell D, Becker SP: Total laryngectomy and reconstruction of the pseudoglottis: problems and complications. Laryngoscope 88:639–647, 1978.

17. Leipzig B, Griffiths CM, Shea JP: Neoglottic reconstruction following total laryngectomy: the Galveston experience. Ann Otol Rhinol Laryngol 89:204–208, 1980.

18. McConnel FMS, Teichgraeber J: Neoglottis reconstruction following total laryngectomy: the Emory experience. Otolaryngol Head and Neck Surg 90:569–575, 1982.

19. Arslan M: Techniques of laryngeal reconstruction. Laryngoscope 85:862, 1975.

20. Arslan M, Serafini I: Restoration of laryngeal functions after total laryngectomy. Report on the first 25 cases. Laryngoscope 82:1349, 1972.

21. Serafini I, Staffieri M: La riabilitazione chirurgica della voce e della respirazione dopo laringectomia totale. 29th National Congress of the Associazione Otologi Ospedalieri Italiana. Bologna: Associazione Otologi Ospedalieri Italiana, 1976.

22. Foeder O: Zur technik der laryng-extirpation, Arch fur Klin chirurgie, Ed 58, Heft 4, 802, 1899.

23. LaBayle J: Restorative total laryngectomy. In: Shedd DP, Weinberg B (eds) Surgical Prosthetic Approaches to Speech Rehabilitation. Boston, GK Hall Medical Publishers, 1980, pp 55–66.

24. Piquet JJ: Functional laryngectomy. In: Shedd DP, Weinberg B (eds) Surgical Prosthetic Approaches to Speech Rehabilitation. Boston, GK Hall Medical Publishers, 1980, pp 41–53.

25. Iwai H, Koike Y: Primary laryngoplasty. Laryngoscope 85:929, 1975.

26. Mozolewski E, Zietek E, Jach K: Mucosal vocal shunt. Annales Academiae Medcae Stefinensis Supp 24(15):9, 1978.

27. Pearson BW: Subtotal laryngectomy. Laryngoscope 91:1905, 1981.

28. Pressman JJ: Cancer of the larynx: Laryngoplasty to avoid laryngectomy. Arch Otolaryngol 59:355–412, 1954.

29. Ogura JH: Surgical pathology of cancer of the larynx. Laryngoscope 65:867–926, 1955.

30. Wang CC: Treatment of squamous cell carcinoma of the larynx by radiation. Radiologic Clinics of North America 16:209, 1978.

31. Pearson BW, Woods RD, Hartman DE: Extended hemilaryngectomy for T3 glottic carcinoma with preservation of speech and swallowing. Laryngoscope 90:1904, 1980.

32. Singer MI, Blom ED: Preliminary results with the tracheoesophageal fistula technique of Amatsu. In: Shedd DP, Weinberg B (eds) Surgical Prosthetic Approaches to Speech Rehabilitation. Boston, GK Hall Medical Publishers, 1980, p 3.

33. Singer MI, Blom ED: Tracteoesophageal puncture: A surgical prosthetic method for post laryngectomy speech restoration. Read before the third international symposium on plastic

and reconstructive surgery on the head and neck. New Orleans, 1979.

34. Singer MI, Blom ED, Hamaker RC: Further experience with voice restoration after total laryngectomy. Ann Otol Rhinol Laryngol 90:498–502, 1981.

35. Robbins J, *et al.*: An acoustic study of voice after tracheoesophageal puncture. Presented to the annual convention of the American Speech-Language-Hearing Association. Detroit, MI, 1980.

36. Weinberg B, *et al.*: Airway resistance during esophageal phonation. J Speech Hear Dis 47:194–199, 1982.

37. Dudley BL, *et al.*: An intelligibility study of tracheoesophageal puncture speakers and esophageal speakers. Presented tothe annual convention of the American Speech-Language-Hearing Association. Detroit, MI, 1980.

38. Singer MI, Blom ED: A selective myotomy for voice restoration after total laryngectomy. Arch Otolaryngol 107:670–673, 1981.

5. Myocutaneous flaps in reconstructive surgery of the head and neck

The physiologic basis and utilization of myocutaneous flaps is not new. The latissimus dorsi myocutaneous flap, for example, was first described by Tansini in 1896 [1]. But it was only until the late 1970s when the use of these flaps received widespread attention for the reconstruction of defects in the head and neck. The description of a new myocutaneous flap using the pectoralis major muscle was originally described by Krizek and Ariyan in 1977 [2] and soon thereafter followed by a description of the identical flap by Baek and Biller [3]. Since the description of this new flap, reports subsequently followed [4, 5] that described new flaps based on different muscles within or adjacent to the head and neck. Other reports [6, 7] have subsequently appeared describing modifications and expanded usage of some of these flaps.

One of the most important methods of flap classification relates to the description of the blood supply. This classification readily separates the regional skin flaps from the myocutaneous flaps. Regional skin flaps represent the transfer of skin and subcutaneous tissue that contains blood vessels that are either in a direct arterial or a random pattern orientation. The myocutaneous flaps involve the transfer of skin whose attachment to the underlying musculature is undisturbed because that underlying muscle contains the blood supply which is reaching the skin through muscular perforating arteries. Therefore, the blood supply to the skin of a myocutaneous flap enters perpendicular to the plane of the skin versus the blood supply of a regional skin flap which is parallel to the plane of the skin flap.

Another important difference between these two types of flaps involves the relative strength of the blood supply. In a regional skin flap, the blood supply to the skin at a point more distal from the base is less than the blood supply at a more proximal location. Therefore, the shorter the length of a regional skin flap, the greater its chance for survival. With a myocutaneous flap, in contrast, the blood supply to the overlying segment of skin to be

Gregory T. Wolf (ed), Head and Neck Oncology.
© *1984 Martinus Nijhoff Publishers, Boston. ISBN 0-89838-657-8. Printed in The Netherlands.*

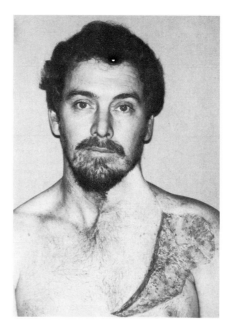

Figure 1. The thinness of the deltopectoral flap is the reason why the author prefers it for external neck resurfacing in a cancer patient.

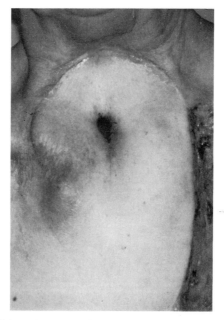

Figure 2. The thinness of the deltopectoral flap allows it to conform to concave cavities such as that created with resection of a tracheostomal recurrent cancer following mediastinal dissection.

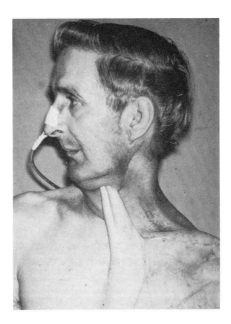

Figure 3. The deltopectoral flap, when used for pharyngeal reconstruction, results in an intentional pharyngocutaneous fistula as noted in this patient who has evidence of saliva draining through this fistula.

transferred is neither a function of its distance from the pedicle base of of the size of the skin island of the flap.

Although the myocutaneous flaps have resulted in a dramatic decrease in the frequency of usage of the regional skin flaps, they still have not made these flaps obsolete. There are still certain regional skin flaps, such as the deltopectoral flap, which are highly reliable, versatile, and are preferable to myocutaneous flaps for certain clinical situations. The thinness of the deltopectoral flap and its ability to be utilized in a one-stage procedure are two reasons whi it continues to preferred for external neck skin resurfacing (Fig. 1) rather than a myocutaneous flap which would be thicker because of the inclusion of the underlying muscle. Thin flaps provide easier examination of the cancer patient for the development of any recurrences or neck nodal metastases. The thinness of the deltopectoral flap makes it better suited to resurface certain defects, such as the large concavity created by resection of a tracheostomal recurrence with mediastinal dissection that involves removal of the manubrium and the proximal one-third of each clavicle (Fig. 2). The deltopectoral flap also provides an excellent mechanism of developing a functional pharyngocutaneous fistula in the patient whose clinical situation may be such that an intentional fistula is advisable (Fig. 3). However, any of the regional skin flaps result in a significant cosmetic insult and/or require multiple operations to complete the reconstruction and, therefore, have now been largely supplanted by the myocutaneous flaps.

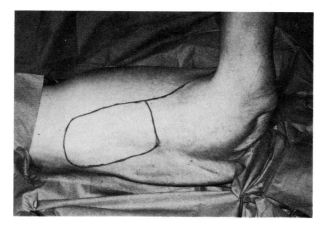

Figure 4. The latissimus dorsi myocutaneous flap has the capability of transferring a massive amount of tissue to reconstruct defects in the head and neck.

The head and neck surgical oncologist is now faced with performing major ablative procedures for advanced stage malignancies in patients who are part of combined therapy programs that oftentimes include not only radiation therapy but also chemotherapy. It is imperative that an effective reconstructive technique must not add an appreciable amount of operative time for these medically unstable, nutritionally deprived patients. Reconstructive techniques must be reliable with an excellent chance of success, and preferrably permits ablation and reconstruction in one operation so that subsequent planned treatment in a combined therapy program is not delayed.

Free flap reconstruction using microvascular techniques provides the identical capabilities for one-stage reconstruction as the myocutaneous flaps. However, the chances of successful transfer with free flaps does not yet approximate that of the myocutaneous flaps. Reports in the literature [7, 8] have documented an extraordinarily high chance of success with the myocutaneous flaps. One other major advantage over the free flaps centers on the relative technical ease of mycocutaneous flap transfer and the fact that no specialized equipment is required.

The myocutaneous flaps have been found to be versatile in terms of size and location of defects to be reconstructed. One can use the flap to transfer a small amount of tissue as with the temporalis myocutaneous flap or a massive amount of tissue with the latissimus dorsi flap (Fig. 4).

Although there are limitations to each of these flaps, there is no question that they represent a reliable and versatile technique that provides one-stage reconstructive capabilities without the need for specialized equipment or training and can be successfully used in a combined therapy setting for head and neck cancer patients.

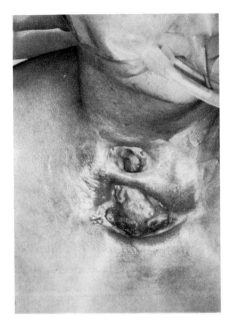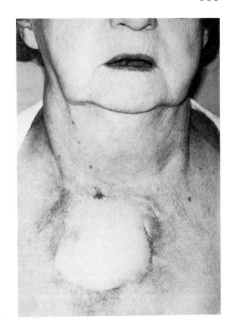

Figure 5. (a) Soft tissue defect resulting from sternal osteomyelitis and persistent tracheocutaneous fistula in an immunosuppressed patient. (b) One-stage reconstruction following debridement and then transfer using a pectoralis myocutaneous flap.

Pectoralis major flap

The pectoralis major myocutaneous flap is versatile, technically easy to use, and has a high degree of reliability. It represents one of the most commonly utilized flaps in the reconstruction of head and neck defects. It can be used for both internal reconstructions involving the oral cavity/pharynx or external resurfacing. It has the capability of transferring a small to large amount of tissue and can be used for reconstructing defects as high as the skull base and as low as the chest wall (Fig. 5).

The flap is initially designed so that the size of the skin island and its position over the pectoralis major muscle conform to the size and location of the defect. The position of the thoracoacromial artery is usually confirmed with the intraoperative use of the finger proble Doppler. In the majority of instances, the skin island is usually located over the inferomedial portion of the pectoralis major muscle. If one wants to decrease the thickness of the tissue in the area of the skin island, a portion of the skin island can be extended beyond the position of the pectoralis major muscle. Consequently, that portion of the skin island represents a random pattern flap with a more tenuous blood supply.

The skin island is then incised including the underlying subcutaneous tissue but the pectoralis major muscle is not disturbed. After the entire peri-

112

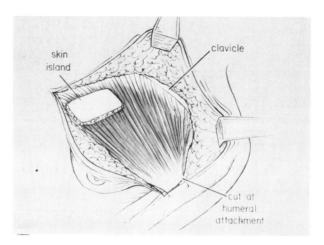

Figure 6. The pectoralis major muscle is exposed by elevating the skin and subcutaneous tissue away from it and making this chest flap continuous with the previously-undermined neck flaps.

meter of the skin island is cut, it is then secured to the underlying pectoralis major muscle with coated Vicryl sutures in an effort to protect the continuity of the musculocutaneous perforators in the area. A skin incision from the island is then made to the superior axiallary fold in an effort to preserve this upper chest wall skin for its use as a deltopectoral regional skin flap if needed at a later time. This superior chest wall skin in addition to the underlying subcutaneous tissue and pectoralis fascia is then undermined and elevated up to the clavicle where it is made continuous with the previously developed neck flaps (Fig. 6). At this point, the fibers of the pectoralis major muscle overlying a lower rib laterally are split and the muscle is mobilized away from the ribs at a horizontal plane on the level of the inferior end of the skin island. After the pectoralis major muscle is dissected away from the chest wall under the skin island, the inferior portion of the muscle is then incised around the skin island. The muscle incision is then incised both medially and laterally in an inferior to superior direction for a short distance. At this point, it is advisable to place another suture securing the skin island to the pectoralis major muscle and to tie this leaving it long enough to attach a hemostat as a means of retracting the flap. The pectoralis major is then bluntly dissected in an easily identifiable plane between it and the underlying pectoralis minor muscle up to the area where the clavipectoral fascia is identified at the superomedial corner of the pectoralis minor muscle. It is in this area that one will encounter the neurovascular pedicle to the flap.

The vein is usually readily seen and the thoracoacromial artery, which is a branch off the axillary artery and the main blood supply to this flap, is readily palpated. After the neurovascular pedicle has been identified, one

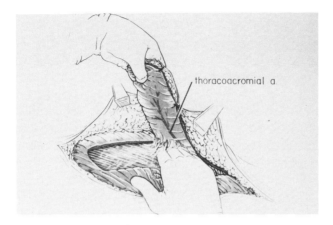

Figure 7. The flap can be elevated by incising the pectoralis muscle medially and laterally without danger of injury to the vascularity because it can be directly visualized throughout the procedure.

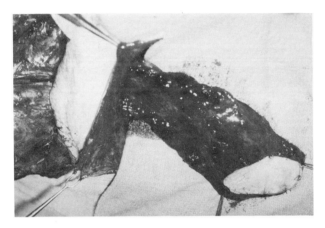

Figure 8. Appearance of pectoralis muscle flap following completion of the medial and lateral muscle incisions prior to its transfer under the chest wall skin into the area of the pharyngeal defect.

can then more safely incise the pectoralis muscle without danger of injury to the vascularity (Fig. 7). It is advisable for the medial muscular incision to be lateral to the sternocostal junction in an effort to avoid injuring the perforating branches of the internal mammary artery in the hopes of preserving that blood supply in case a deltopectoral flap is ever needed. The lateral muscle incision is carried out through the humeral origin of the muscle. It is at this level that multiple branches of the motor nerve to the pectoralis major muscle will be encountered and should be cut. The denervation of the muscle is important in eventually obtaining atrophy of the pectoralis major muscle. The medial and lateral incisions are then carried superiorly usually up to the level of the clavicle (Fig. 8). It is important to realize that the

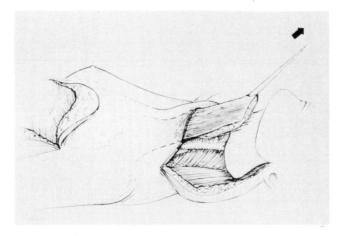

Figure 9. Pectoralis myocutaneous flap can be passed easily under skin of the chest wall and neck and advanced into the head and neck defect site.

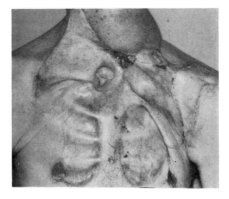

Figure 10. Skin grafts are necessary to resurface the flap donor sites in this thin patient who required the use of two large flaps for the neck skin resurfacing and tracheal reconstruction following mediastinal dissection with tracheal resection.

course of the thoracoacromial artery from the clavipectoral fascia oftentimes is in a lateral direction rather than in a straight course out to the distal portion of the muscle. Therefore, the lateral muscle incision needs to be performed carefully with continuous monitoring of the position of the artery. The muscle is incised to the level of the clavicle. The flap is then easily passed under the skin of the chest wall and neck and into the defect (Fig. 9).

The donor site of the flap can be enclosed primarily in the majority of instances after wide undermining. The only time in which that has not been feasible in the author's series has been when bilateral simultaneous pectoralis myocutaneous flaps had been utilized and then skin grafting was required (Fig. 10). Extra-large continuous pressure negative drainage tubes

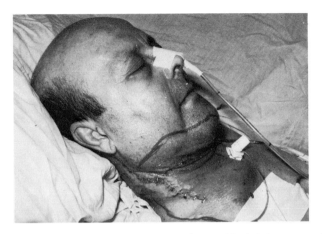

Figure 11. Because the flap pedicle is hidden under the neck skin, it is important that the nursing staff is aware of its location by outlining an area where there can be no contact with any pieces of equipment during the patient's postoperative care.

are laid across the chest wall of the donor site. It is important that upper position drains are sutured in position so that they do not inadventently come to lie in contact with the thoracoacromial artery which might conceivably compromise blood flow to the skin island.

When the flap is being used for internal reconstruction of the pharynx, the author has preferred to use a single layer closure with coated Vicryl sutures that oftentimes includes not only the skin but the underlying pectoralis muscle. Sufficient stitches are placed for a water tight closure, but not so many as to prevent neovascular ingrowth from the periphery. Following suturing of the skin island in the proper position, the pectoralis major muscle pedicle is then sutured to the underlying soft tussue of the neck in an effort to cover the carotid artery system. It is important that there be minimal tension on the muscular pedicle by the overlying neck skin. It is imperative that wide undermining of the neck flaps be undertaken so as to decrease that possibility. Multiple suction drainage tubes are placed as a means of hopefully preventing hematoma that can occur beceause of the cut muscle involved with this flap development.

An important feature of the postoperative care is to make the nursing staff aware of the location of the muscular pedicle so that they do not put any pressure in this area which might compromise blood flow. The area of the muscle pedicle is outlined on the patient with a marker as a means of identifying where there can be no contact by any pieces of equippent (Fig. 11).

This flap has been successfully used for a variety of reconstructive tasks. It actually can be transferred to a point as high as base of the skull. In addition to the usual reconstructive uses in the pharynx and oral cavity, it also can be utilized as part of a combined reconstructive technique with

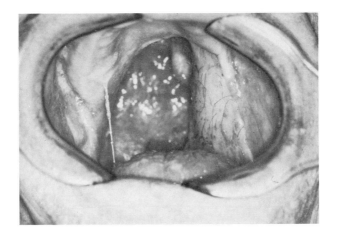

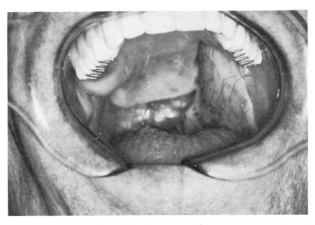

Figure 12. (a) Pharyngeal reconstruction with the pectoralis myocutaneous flap. (b) Palatal prosthesis in place directly abutting against the myocutaneous flap with no adverse effect on the flap.

prostheses (Fig. 12). It is strong enough to withstand the pressure of a prosthesis. The flap has been utilized successfully to reconstruct tongue base defects when combined with supraglottic laryngectomy (Fig. 13). These patients have been able to eat by mouth and talk in a normal fashion. The bulk of the flap seems to be especially beneficial for this particular reconstructive task. The only limitation for tongue base reconstruction in combination with supraglottic laryngectomy is when both hypoglossal nerves have been transected. In the one patient who had this situation, she was not able to successfully eat by mouth because of the adynamic tongue and the removed supraglottic larynx. The flap has even been used in combination with a prosthesis for tracheal reconstruction.

When the flap is transferred for either external facial and/or neck surfacing, certain technical points are important. The muscular pedicle of the flap

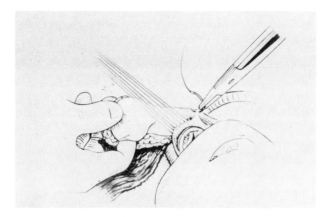

Figure 13. When the pectoralis myocutaneous flap is used for tongue base reconstruction following supraglottic laryngectomy, the skin island is sutured directly to the remaining perichondrium of the larynx, lateral pharyngeal wall, and the remaining tongue tissue.

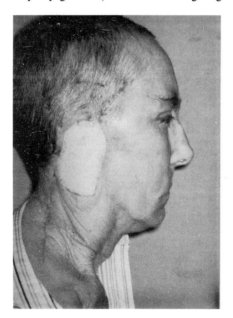

Figure 14. The use of the pectoralis myocutaneous flap for resurfacing temporal defects following temporal bone resection represents the most superior position that is possible in the majority of instances.

must rotate 180° for external defects. With this rotation, the tense bandlike motor nerve associated with the thoracoacromial artery and vein in the pedicle of the flap crosses the artery and cuts off blood flow with subsequent flap necrosis. Therefore, it is mandatory that the neurovascular pedicle be dissected and this nerve identified and cut to avoid this possibility. The superior limit of utilization for this flap of external defects is in the temporal area (Fig. 14).

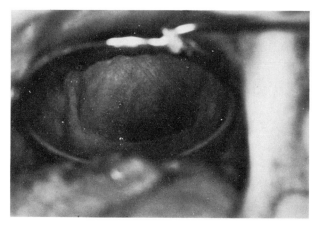

Figure 15. Appearance of the neocervical esophagus seen through a laryngeal mirror following reconstruction with the pectoralis myocutaneous flap.

Total cervical esophageal reconstruction remains a major challenge. The author's experience with the pectoralis major flap for this task has been variable. The current technique involves the use of a soft silastic esophageal tube used as a stenting device primarily at the time of reconstruction and kept in place for a protracted period of time. This technique seems to provided a reasonable chance for success (Fig. 15). However, the patients still have restrictions to the type of food capable of being swallowed. It is important to recognize that the alternatives to the use of this flap for cervical esophageal reconstruction such as jejunal transfer with microvascular technique, colon interposition or gastric pull-up all represent procedures with a substantial morbidity and even mortality. Whereas this particular technique with the pectoralis flap has not been uniformly successful, it seems to be reasonably well tolerated by the patients without the life-threatening complications associated with the other alternatives.

This flap has been found to be extremely versatile and highly reliable in the author's personal series now in excess of 100 pectoralis myocutaneous flaps for the reconstruction of major defects in the head and neck. There have been only two patients where there was total flap necrosis. The flaps have been utilized in a variety of clinical situations that have involved patients with poor nutrition and advanced age. The operative time required is actually less than that for the use of a deltopectoral flap because it is quicker to close the donor site.

The only drawback rests with the residual neck fullness that persists in a substantial number of patients [7]. Although this fullness actually provides a cosmetic benefit, it can make the examination of the neck for underlying recurrent or metastatic disease more difficult, especially if the neck has received postoperative radiation therapy (Fig. 16). But there is no question that the advantages of this flap far outweigh its drawbacks. It probably has

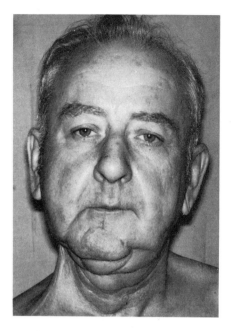

Figure 16. Two year postoperative appearance of patient's neck following the use of a pectoralis myocutaneous flap indicating the extent of persistent muscle bulk in spite of denervation of the muscle.

the greatest versatility of any of the myocutaneous flaps for head and neck reconstruction.

Trapezius flap

There are essentially two different types of trapezius myocutaneous flaps. The lower island trapezius flap is based on the transverse cervical vessels from the thyrocervical trunk as they course over the scalene muscles in the lower part of the neck to enter the trapezius muscle. It is possible to isolate a skin island with the underlying trapezius musculature attached to this vascular pedicle and then to subsequently transfer it into defects in the head and neck area. However, the position of these vessels in the neck makes them more vulnerable to possible metastatic involvement and inadvertent injury during the surgical treatment of neck nodal disease. The venous outflow of this flap has considerable variability and its adequacy is important to the maintenance of the flap viability. The arc of rotation for this flap is also limited by the vascular pedicle. The island trapezius myocutaneous flap is technically more demanding than the pectoralis with less versatility and therefore has not achieved the popularity of the pectoralis myocutaneous flap.

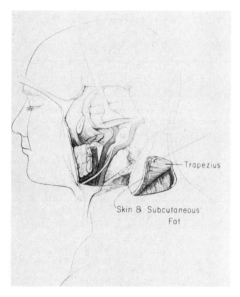

Figure 17. Superiorly based trapezius myocutaneous flap is an extension of the nape of neck regional skin flap but includes the underlying trapezius musculature.

In contrast, the superior trapezius myocutaneous flap is essentially an extension of the nape of neck regional skin flap. The design is identical except that the underlying trapezius musculature is included in its development (Fig. 17). This flap is technically easier to develop than the lower island trapezius flap and limitations of the vascular pedicle are not as stringent as with the former. It is utilized primarily for lateral neck and facial defects. There is somewhat of a drawback in that such a rotation invariably creates a substantial dog-ear which does not flatten out with time (Fig. 18). Therefore, it is necessary to undergo a second minor operation to excise the dog-ear which can be done under local anesthesia as an outpatient. Once again this flap's capabilities do not approximate that of the pectoralis major. But it is definitely a reliable and technically easy reconstructive technique for lateral neck or lateral facial reconstruction.

Sternocleidomastoid flap

This flap has been popularized by Ariyan [5]. The skin island overlying the sternocleidomastoid muscle derives its blood supply from the muscular perforators that traverse the sternocleidomastoid muscle and the platysma muscle enroute to the overlying neck skin. This vascular anatomy means that the sternocleidomastoid is not a myocutaneous flap in its strict definition. This flap can be utilized by either transecting the lower end or the

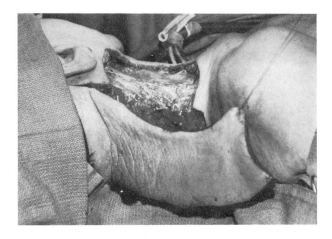

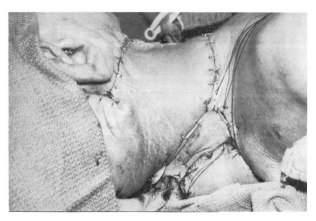

Figure 18. (a) This muscle flap can be quite long because of the improved vascularity, but (b) its 90° rotation for covering lateral neck or facial defects invariably creates a dog-ear deformity which requires a secondary procedure to excise.

upper end of the sternocleidomastoid muscle and then rotating the skin island into the defect. It is used primarily for smaller size intraoral defects. In order to use it in the cancer patient, it is mandatory that the surgical approach to clearing the neck nodal disease does not compromise the blood supply to the sternocleidomastoid muscle with the potential limitation of preserving a muscle that is routinely sacrificed in the traditional neck dissection.

It is not unusual for the skin component of these myocutaneous flaps to undergo necrosis with maintenance of the viability of the underlying muscle. The need for healing by migration of surrounding epithelium over this muscular bed adds another component of uncertainty to this flap. These limitations of restricted locations for reconstruction, potential injury to the muscle's vascularity during neck dissection, and the frequent loss of skin has

122

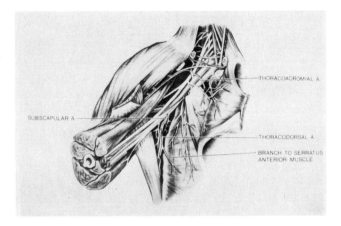

Figure 19. The main blood supply of the latissimus dorsi muscle is the thoracodorsal which is a branch from the subscapular artery coming from the axillary artery at a point distal to the take-off of the thoracoacromial artery.

resulted in this flap not being especially popular for anything other than rather small intraoral reconstructive tasks.

Latissimus dorsi flap

This is one of the oldest of the myocutaneous flaps and its use in head and neck reconstruction was pioneered by Quillen [9, 10]. There is no question that a flap utilizing the latissimus dorsi muscle is a reliable reconstructive technique. The latissimus dorsi muscle receives its blood supply from the thoracodorsal artery which again is another branch of the axiallary artery further distal than the thoracoacromial artery (Fig. 19). Occasionally this artery gives off a branch to the serratus anterior muscle. The artery does run on the undersurface of this large fan-shaped muscle that attaches on the lower thoracic and lumbar vertebrae and the iliac crest and comes to attach to the medial aspect of the humerus. Using this flap involves changing the patient to a lateral position following resection of the primary cancer in an effort to gain the exposure needed for development of the flap.

The technique is identical to the pectoralis major flap with respect to the skin island and securing it to the underlying muscle with stitches followed then by mobilization of the muscle into the head and neck defect area. The thoracodorsal artery is identified just lateral to the axialla and dissection is necessary through the axilla to gain mobility enough to permit utilization in the head and neck. The development of this flap is not technically difficult; however, it does require the head and neck surgeon to familiarize himself with axillary anatomy.

The latissimus dorsi flap has the advantage of providing the capabilities of transferring massive amounts of skin. The flap has the capabilities of being transferred to points more superiorly located than what is capable with the pectoralis myocutaneous flap. Its major disadvantage rests with the added operative time associated with the need for changing the patient's position. When a massive amount of skin is transferred, then primary closure is not feasible and skin grafting becomes necessary. Occasionally, problems can occur with healing of the skin graft in this particular flap donor site. There is no question that this flap represents a valuable tool for the reconstruction of large defects. However, the disadvantages associated with changing position preclude it from being a commonly utilized technique. Once again, the pectoralis major myocutaneous flap has the potential to reconstruct the overwhelming majority of defects without the disadvantages associated with the latissimus dorsi myocutaneous flap.

Karapandzic flap

The Karapandzic flap for lip defect reconstruction involves the principle that the obicularis oris muscle can be dissected away from its attachments to the surrounding mimetic muscles providing greater mobility while still being able to maintain the integrity of the neurovascular pedicles supplying this sphincteric muscle. It is utilized for the reconstruction of lip defects that cannot be closed primarily and is independent of the location of the defect. It provides the reconstructive potential of restoring not only form but also function.

The technique involves incising the skin in the nasolabial creases about the obicularis oris down to the defect (Fig. 20). Upper or lower lip defects can be reconstructed. This skin incision basically involves the total circumference of the mouth except for the area of the lip attached to the base of the nasal columella. It is important not to incise across this superior cupid's bow so that its midline position is maintained. After the skin incision is completed, the surgeon then begins to dissect and detach the fibers of the mimetic muscles from the obicularis oris while the arteries, veins, and nerve going to the obicularis oris are preserved (Fig. 21). Loupe magnification is a useful adjunct during this procedure. The flap can be developed under local anesthesia. After the mimetic muscles are totally separated and the obicularis oris is freed down to but not including the underlying oral mucosa, the lip defect is then closed by approximating the edges of the defect. The dramatic increase of tissue mobility with the separation of the obicularis oris from the mimetic muscles enables this closure to be completed without any tension. However, the mobilization of tissue changes the position of the oral commissures. It is at this point that the mimetic muscles are then reattached

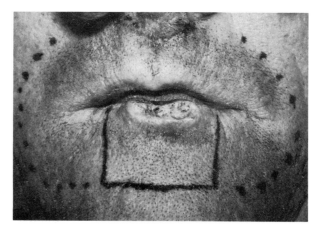

Figure 20. The Karapandzic flap involves a skin incision that follows the course of the nasolabial creases and the mental labial crease.

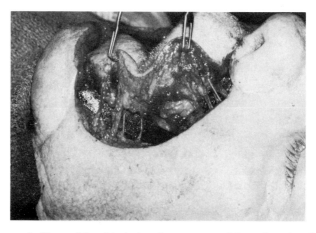

Figure 21. The muscle fibers of the obicularis oris are separated from the mimetic muscles with preservation of the multiple arteries, veins, nerves supplying this muscle.

to the new position of the oral commissures with absorbable sutures. These mimetic muscles define and establish the position and configuration of the oral commissures. The skin is approximated and the patient's aesthetic and functional reconstruction is completed (Fig. 22). There is no loss of movement of the reconstructed lips (Fig. 23).

It is possible to reconstruct large defects of the lips without the need for secondary oral commisuroplasties except in a relatively small number of patients who have had extensive portions of the lips reconstructed. The complications of this technique are minimal. It can be reliably and effectively utilized even in elderly patients because of the capabilities of performing the procedure under local anesthesia.

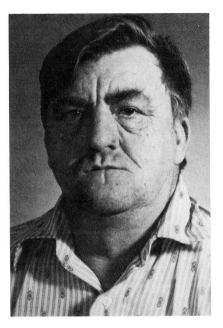

Figure 22. The flap provides the capability of restoring lip continuity and a satisfactory cosmetic result.

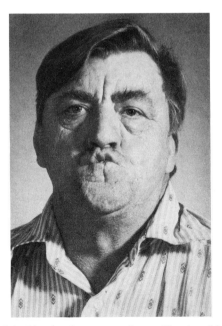

Figure 23. Preservation of the blood and nerve supply provides the added benefit of maintaining normal lip function.

126

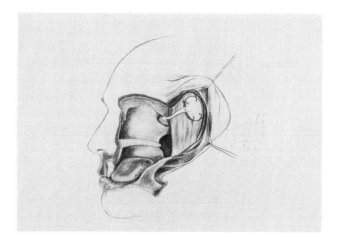

Figure 24. The temporalis myocutaneous flap involves utilization of lateral temporal skin attached to the underlying temporalis muscle and developing a muscular pedicle which is inferiorly based and corresponds to the origin of the blood supply to this muscle.

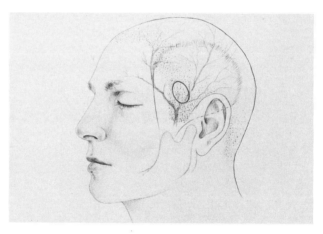

Figure 25. The flap can then be rotated to resurface skull base defects but only those defects which are located in lateral positions.

Temporalis flap

This flap has only recently been described [11] and provides the capabilities of resurfacing base of skull defects. It is developed by attaching a skin island to the underlying temporalis muscle (Fig. 24) and then releasing the muscle from the skull keeping it inferiorly pedicled, thus preserving the origin of its blood supply, and then rotating it into the position of the defect (Fig. 25). However, its use is limited to lateral skull base defects. It has the advantage of being developed in the hair-bearing skin and can be concealed without difficulty. The transfer of the muscle does result in some concavity in this area however the defect may be camouflaged with the adjustment of hair styling. Although this flap represents an example of the use of the principles of myocutaneous flaps to satisfy a particular reconstructive task, it certainly does not have the versatility of the previously mentioned flaps.

Extensions of myocutaneous flaps

As has been the case with the regional skin flaps, once the reliability of the myocutaneous flaps was demonstrated clinically, attempts were then begun to incorporate the transfer of bone for mandibular reconstruction. The pectoralis major myocutaneous flap has been used to transfer segments of rib to the mandible [12]. The sternocleidomastoid muscle flap has been used to transport a portion of the clavicle for the reconstruction of mandibular defects and the initial report was favorable [13]. However, the largest experience with such osteomyocutaneous flaps involves use of the trapezius muscle with the scapular spine as described by Panje [14]. It is important to realize that there is no extensive long-term experience yet with any of the techniques for the transfer of bone utilizing myocutaneous flaps. Therefore, it is premature to make any statements about their current value in mandibular reconstruction.

Other modifications have included the use of muscle flaps for the protection of underlying tissue such as following mediastinal dissection and for subcutaneous tissue augmentation. Once again, these reconstructive tasks take advantage of the rich vascularity of these muscles, especially the pectoralis major muscle. The objective of these muscle flaps is to enhance blood supply to an area that is relatively avascular and also for the augmentation of tissue or for the protection of nearby structures. Muscle flaps used in this manner are not a new technique.

Summary

This overview of the variety of myocutaneous flaps for the reconstruction of defects created by surgical ablation of head and neck malignancies documents their positive contribution to contemporary head and neck cancer surgery. The versatility and reliability of these flaps coupled with the technical ease of flap development resulted in their widespread use during the current era of combined therapy. Future experience with such flaps will undoubtedly help to define their value in the realm of bone transfer and in other areas.

128

References

1. Tansini I: Nuovo processo per l'amputazione della mammaella per cancro. La Riforma Medica 12:3–5, 1896.
2. Ariyan S, Krizek TJ: Reconstruction after resection of head and neck cancer. Read before the Clinical Congress of the American College of Surgeons, Dallas, October, 1977.
3. Baek S, Biller HF, Krespi YP, et al.: The pectoralis major myocutaneous island flap for reconstruction of the head and neck. Head and Neck Surg 1:293–300, 1979.
4. Panje WR: Myocutaneous trapezius flap. Head and Neck Surg 2:206–212, 1980.
5. Ariyan S: One stage reconstruction for defects of the mouth using a sternomastoid myocutaneous flap. Plast Reconstr Surg 63:618–625, 1979.
6. Schuller DE: Limitations of the pectoralis major myocutaneous flap in head and neck cancer reconstruction. Arch Otolaryngol 106:709–714, 1980.
7. Schuller DE: Pectoralis myocutaneous flap in head and neck cancer reconstruction. Arch Otolaryngol (in Press).
8. Baek SM, Lawson W, Biller HF: An analysis of 133 pectoralis major myocutaneous flaps. Plast Reconstr Surg 69:460–467, 1982.
9. Quillen CG, Shearing JH, Georgiade NG: Use of the latissimus dorsi myocutaneous island flap for reconstruction in the head and neck area. Plast Reconstr Surg 62:113–117, 1978.
10. Quillen CG: Latissimus dorsi myocutaneous flaps in head and neck cancer reconstruction. Plast Reconstr Surg 63:664–670, 1979.
11. Schuller DE, Goodman JH, Miller CA: Reconstruction of the skull base. Arch Otolaryngol (In Press).
12. Ariyan S, Cuono CB: Myocutaneous flaps for head and neck reconstruction. Head Neck Surg 2:321–345, 1980.
13. Barnes DR, Ossoff RH, Pecaro B, et al.: Immediate reconstruction of mandibular defects with a composite sternocleidomastoid musculoclavicular graft. Arch Otolaryngol 107:711–714, 1981.
14. Panje WR: Trapezius osteomyocutaneous is land flap for reconstruction of the anterior floor of the mouth and the mandible. Head Neck Surg 3:66–71, 1980.

6. Fast neutrons in the treatment of head and neck cancer

THOMAS W. GRIFFIN

Advances in the field of radiation oncology have, over the last two decades, resulted in a substantial improvement in the outlook for patients with carcinomas of the head and neck region. This improvement has been largely due to an increased understanding of the biology of the disease process and to the development of machines capable of optimizing radiation dose distributions. Nevertheless, there still remain a substantial number of patients in whom failure to control local disease contributes materially to their death. For the reasons outlined in the following paragraphs, particle beam radiation therapy might be expected to offer a therapeutic gain, as compared to conventional photon and electron beam therapy, in the management of these patients.

Currently, the following particle beams are being clinically tested: fast neutrons, protons, alpha particles, heavy ions (carbon, neon, argon), and negative pions. Fast neutrons are being investigated because they have radiobiological properties that are potentially superior to those of conventional X- and gamma rays. Protons and alpha particles are being studied because the dose distributions which may be achieved with these particles are superior, in many clinical situations, to those obtainable with photons or electrons. Heavy ions and pions have both a potential biological advantage and a dose distribution advantage.

1. Biological characteristics of particle beams

The biological effects of a radiation beam are dependent on the spatial distribution of the ionizing events produced in tissue. The rate at which charged particles deposit energy per unit distance is known as the linear energy transfer (LET), expressed in $Kev/\mu m$. Protons, electrons and photons are sparsely ionizing and are characterized by a low linear energy transfer.

Gregory T. Wolf (ed), Head and Neck Oncology.
© *1984 Martinus Nijhoff Publishers, Boston. ISBN 0-89838-657-8. Printed in The Netherlands.*

Fast neutrons, heavy ions and pions are densely ionizing and are referred to as high LET radiations.

In reviewing the possible causes of treatment failure in head and neck cancer with conventional radiation therapy, the major areas in which neutrons and other high LET radiations offer a potential biological advantage are:

1.1. Tumor cell hypoxia

Numerous studies in many biological systems have shown that hypoxic cells are significantly more resistant to the effects of X- and gamma irradiation than are well-oxygenated cells. While cells in most normal tissues are well oxygenated, most solid tumors are thought to have hypoxic regions which have outgrown their vascular supply. It has been postulated that these cells remain viable and provide a focus for local tumor recurrence [1].

The oxygen enhancement ratio (OER) is defined as the ratio of the dose of radiation required to produce a specified biological effect under anoxic conditions to the dose required to produce the same effect under well-oxygenated conditions. With photons, the OER for most mammalian cells is 2.5–3.0. With neutrons, heavy charged particles or pions, the OER is significantly smaller (1.4–1.7), and therefore, the protection conferred on tumor cells by hypoxia is diminished. Figure 1 illustrates survival for Chinese hamster ovary cells irradiated with ^{60}Co gamma rays or 50 MeV d→Be reaction. The OER for neutrons is 1.4, appreciably improved over the value of 2.4 for ^{60}Co gamma rays.

In practice, the clinical advantage of high LET radiation may be less than that suggested by this difference in OER. Not all tumor cells are severely hypoxic, and reoxygenation may occur during intervals between dose fractions, diminishing the influence of hypoxic cells on tumor recurrence.

1.2. Relative biological effectiveness

The relative biological effectiveness (RBE) of an ionizing radiation is the ratio of the dose of that radiation compared to the dose of a reference radiation required to produce a specific endpoint in a specific tissue.

Another potential area of therapeutic gain from high LET radiation exists when tumor cells are relatively radioresistant due to an increased capacity to accumulate sublethal radiation injury. This is reflected in a wide shoulder for the tumor cell survival curve. With neutrons and other high LET radiation, most cell killing results from single lethal events, leading to survival curves that are almost exponential in the range of clinical relevance (Fig. 2).

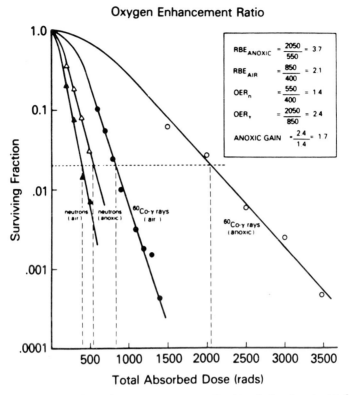

Figure 1. Survival curves for Chinese hamster ovary (CHO) cells irradiated with $^{60}Co_\gamma$ rays or 50 MeV$_{d\to Be}$ fast neutrons under aerated and anoxic conditions. At the survival level illustrated, the OER for neutrons is 1.4 compared to 2.4 for $^{60}Co_\gamma$ rays.

Tumors characterized by a large capacity to accumulate and repair sublethal radiation injury, such as some salivary gland tumors, should have a higher RBE for neutrons than normal tissue. It should be noted, however, that Howlett, Thomlinson and Alper have shown that RBE's of neutrons for different experimental tumors vary considerably and no general statement about which types of tumors are best treated with high LET radiation can be made at present [2].

1.3. Tumor cell kinetics

Because of the variation in radiosensitivity between cells in different stages of the cell cycle, redistribution between dose fractions results in an effective sensitization of proliferating cells that is not shared by nonproliferating normal cells. The latter are probably responsible for late radiation sequelae, which are the usual dose-limiting factors in radiation therapy. The cell-cycle-dependent variation of radiosensitivity is similar for neutrons and

132

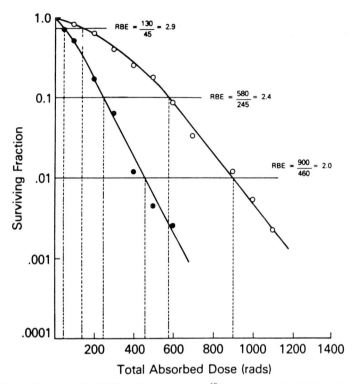

Figure 2. Survival curves for CHO cells exposed to $^{60}Co_{\gamma}$ rays or 50 MeV$_{d \rightarrow Be}$ fast neutrons illustrating the increase in RBE with decreasing dose per fraction. With fast neutron irradiation, most cell killing results from single-hit lethal events leading to survival curves with little or no shoulder.

gamma rays, but the magnitude of the difference is smaller for neutrons [3] (Fig. 3). Whether this property constitutes a therapeutic advantage for high LET radiation cannot be predicted. Tumors whose cells redistribute poorly, or whose spectrum is demonstrated by cells in resistant phases, would be more effectively treated with neutrons.

1.4. Repair of potentially lethal damage

The recovery from potentially lethal damage (PLD) occurs over a period of hours in cells irradiated *in vitro* when the postirradiation conditions are suboptimal for growth. Repair of PLD occurs following X- and gamma irradiation, but is less frequently observed following neutron irradiation [4] (Fig. 4). If, as has been suggested by Hall and Kraljevc, PLD repair after X- and gamma irradiation occurs in nutritionally-deprived tumor cells, but not

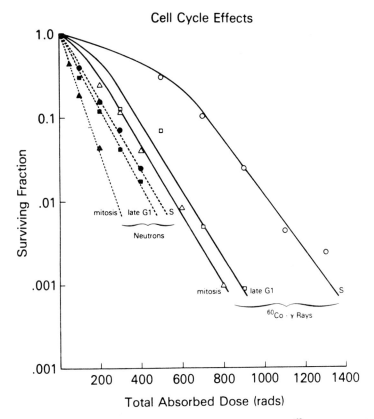

Figure 3. Survival curves for synchronized CHO cells irradiated with $^{60}Co_{\gamma}$ rays or 50 MeV$_{d\rightarrow Be}$ fast neutrons illustrating the variation in radiosensitivity with the position in the cell cycle. The cells were irradiated in three different positions in the cell cycle – mitosis, late G$_1$/early 5, and mid-to-late S phase. The cell-cycle-dependent variation in radiosensitivity is qualitatively similar for neutrons and γ rays, but the magnitude of the variation is reduced by a factor of 4 for neutrons.

in normal tissue cells, then the use of high LET beams would be therapeutically advantageous [5].

2. Physical characteristics of particle beams

Fast neutron beams can be generated for radiation therapy either by bombarding a target containing tritium (T) with accelerated deuterium (D) ions in a D-T generator or by bombarding a suitable target such as beryllium (Be) with protons (p) or deuterons (d) accelerated in a cyclotron or linear accelerator. The D-T generator produces a monoenergetic 14 MeV neutron beam whereas the proton-on-beryllium (p→Be) and deuteron-on-beryllium (d→Be) reactions produce neutron beams with a spectrum of energies.

134

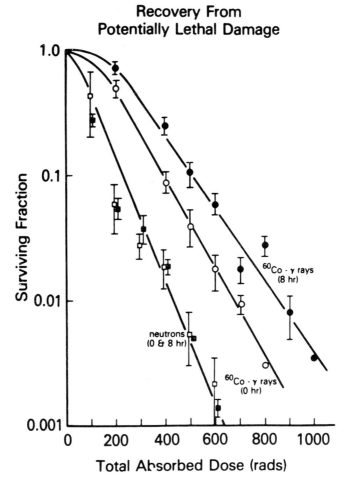

Figure 4. Potentially lethal damage (PLD): survival curves for plateau-phase CHO cells irradiated with $^{60}Co_\gamma$ rays (circles) or 50 MeV$_{d\to Be}$ fast neutrons (squares) and plated either immediately (open symbols) or 8 hours after irradiation (closed symbols). Repair of PLD occurs following irradiation with γ rays, but is not observed following neutron irradiation.

While protons, alpha particles, pions and heavy ions all have dose distribution advantages over conventional photons, neutrons do not. In fact, with the current limitation of physics-based machines with fixed horizontal treatment beams, the dose distributions achieved with neutrons are somewhat inferior to those achievable with modern megavoltage isocentric equipment. In 1984, new hospital-based neutron generators will begin operation at the University of Washington, UCLA, M.D. Anderson, and the University of Pennsylvania Hospitals. These new machines will allow dose distributions equivalent to modern 6 MeV linear accelerators.

3. Clinical studies

Fast neutron radiotherapy of head and neck cancer in the United States dates back to the 1940's when Stone and coworkers [6] used a neutron beam to treat patients having various advanced malignancies. Almost all of the long-term survivors had severe radiation sequelae in the normal tissue surrounding the tumor sites. This was initially interpreted as due to an increased relative biological effectiveness (RBE) for late effects as compared to acute effects and deterred further clinical investigation for approximately 20 years. In the 1950's, mammalian cell culture techniques were developed and it became apparent that the shapes of postirradiation cell survival curves were very different for high energy photons and fast neutrons. This meant that the clinically-used neutron fraction sizes corresponded to much higher RBE's than were extrapolated from the large-dose increment animal model studies prior to Stone's clinical work. Hence, nearly all of Stone's patients with serious radiation sequelae had inadvertently received extremely high radiation doses as reflected by calculated nominal standard doses (Ellis NSD formula) of 2000–3200 rets [7]. Clinical trials were first resumed at Hammersmith Hospital, London, England, in the 1960's. After several hundred patients with extensive cancers were treated, it was concluded that fast neutron radiotherapy was well tolerated and that many advanced malignancies responded amazingly well to fast neutron irradiation [8]. Based upon these very optimistic results, various centers throughout the world again began clinical trials with fast neutrons.

In the United States, patient treatments were started in 1972 at the M.D. Anderson Hospital, utilizing the Texas A & M University variable energy cyclotron (50 MeV d→Be reaction). Clinical trials were next instituted at the University of Washington utilizing a fixed energy cyclotron (22 MeV d→Be reaction) in 1973. Significant numbers of patients have also received neutron radiotherapy at the MANTA facility (35 MeV d→Be reaction) centered at George Washington University in Washington, D.C., at the GLANTA facility (25 MeV d→Be reaction) in Cleveland, Ohio, and at the Fermi Laboratory facility (66 MeV p→Be reaction) in Batavia, Illinois. Initially, Phase I clinical trials were carried out utilizing patients with advanced head and neck tumors who were felt to have less than a 10% five-year survival with conventional forms of treatment. This work yielded considerable information about the RBE's for different tissues and about the variation of the neutron RBE's from facility to facility. More recently, the majority of patients receiving fast neutron radiotherapy have been entered into randomized, prospective clinical trials designed to compare neutron irradiation with the best available photon control arm for a given tumor histology and site. Approximately 2500 patients have been treated in all, resulting in a fairly extensive patient data base.

The earliest clinically-significant results treating head and neck cancer with fast neutrons were reported from the Hammersmith Hospital, London, by Dr. Mary Catterall [9]. In a randomized trial of 133 patients with advanced cancers of the head and neck, neutron therapy showed a statistically significant superiority over photons for control of local-regional disease (Table 1). Neutrons were given in 12 fractions over 4 weeks to a total dose of 15.60 Gy_n. (Since Hammersmith investigators report only the neutron component of the beam and U.S. investigators report total radiation delivered, this is equivalent to 17 $Gy_{n\gamma}$.) Pilot studies using both neutrons alone and 'mixed beam' radiation therapy were started in the U.S. in 1972. Treatment with 'neutrons only' irradiated the primary tumor site and any region of clinically-involved cervical adenopathy to 17–22 $Gy_{n\gamma}$ according to one of the following three fractionation schemes: (a) 1.5 $Gy_{n\gamma}$ on Mondays and Fridays, (b) 1.0 $Gy_{n\gamma}$ on Mondays–Wednesdays–Fridays, or (c) 0.75 $Gy_{n\gamma}$ on Mondays–Tuesdays–Thursdays–Fridays. The term '$Gy_{n\gamma}$' refers to the *total* measured dose and includes the gamma ray contaminate produced by neutron-nucleii interactions (<10% at a depth of 10 cm). These three treatment schemes were 'normalized' to deliver 3.0 $Gy_{n\gamma}$ per week over seven weeks. The 'mixed beam' treatment consists of combined neutron and photon irradiation according to the following scheme: 0.6 $Gy_{n\gamma}$ on Mondays–Fridays and 1.8 Gy_γ on Tuesdays–Wednesdays–Thursdays. Assuming an RBE = 3, this corresponded to 9 Gy equivalent per week as did the 'neutrons only' form of treatment. The 'mixed beam' patients received between 65–70 Gy equivalent to the primary site and any region of clinically-involved cervical adenopathy. Table 2 summarizes the results from two U.S. pilot studies [10, 11], the Catterall trial [9], and studies accomplished by Drs. Batterman and Breuer in Amsterdam [12]. Patients in the Amsterdam trial received between 18 $Gy_{n\gamma}$ and 24 $Gy_{n\gamma}$ given in five fractions per week over four weeks. Although caution must be used when comparing results from different studies, there seems to be a trend favoring neutrons

Table 1. Results from the Hammersmith Hospital-MRC clinical trial of fast neutron therapy of head and neck cancer

All sites of head and neck region

Modality	Number of patients	Permanent local control	Complications	Survival at 2 years
Neutron	70	53 (76%) [+]	10/70 [*]	28 [**]
Photon	63	12 (19%)	2/63	15 [**]

[+] 53/70 > 12/63, $p < 0.001$.
[*] 10/70 > 2/63, $p < 0.05$.
[**] Actuarial percentages; difference is not significant.

Table 2. Two-year local control rates at the primary site and actuarial survival rates for patients with advanced head and neck cancers treated with fast neutron teletherapy

	Local control of primary (2-year actuarial)	Survival (2-year actuarial)
Hammersmith (Catterall *et al.*)		
Neutrons only (70 patients)	76%	28%
Amsterdam (Batterman and Breuer)		
Neutrons only (59 patients)	61%	17%
M.D. Anderson (Maor *et al.*)		
Neutrons only (48 patients)	43%	20%
Mixed beam (25 patients)	35%	25%
University of Washington (Laramore *et al.*)		
Neutrons only (62 patients)	20%	10%
Mixed beam (38 patients)	30%	40%

alone over mixed beam and a trend favoring 12 fractions in four weeks over a more prolonged fractionation scheme.

More recently, 199 evaluable patients with measurable cervical adenopathy were entered on a prospective, randomized RTOG study evaluating the use of fast neutrons in treatment of advanced, inoperable squamous cell carcinomas of the head and neck region. One hundred eleven patients were randomized to receive mixed beam radiation therapy, and 88 were randomized to the photon control treatment. The complete response rates were 86% for mixed beam vs 75% for photons for patients with class N_1 nodes, 62% for mixed beam vs 48% for photons for patients with class N_2 nodes, and 63% for mixed beam vs 53% for photons for patients with N_3 nodes. The percentages of patients remaining free of their adenopathy for two years were 78% for mixed beam vs 55% for photons for patients with N_1 nodes, 39% for both mixed beam and photons for patients with N_2 nodes and 24% for mixed beam vs 13% for photons for patients with N_3 nodes. The median disease-free status was 20.3 months for mixed-beam-treated patients and 6.4 months for photon-treated patients. The advantage for mixed beam irradiation as given in this study is statistically significant (Tables 3 and 4, Fig. 5) [15].

Studies using fast neutrons to treat salivary gland tumors have also been carried out in the United States and Europe. In a group of patients with advanced tumors, often recurrent after multiple prior operations, the local control rates varied between 72% and 94% [9, 12–14]. This control rate was felt by most of the investigators involved in the studies to be superior to that obtained with photon irradiated historical controls.

138

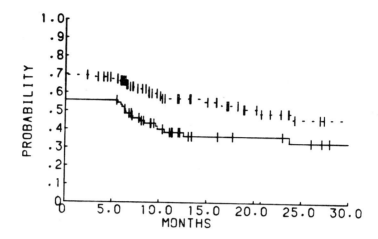

Figure 5. Duration of complete response curves for cervical adenopathy in the randomized RTOG mixed beam study.

A National Cancer Institute research program will shortly bring into operation four new hospital-based neutron generators (three cyclotrons and a D-T generator) in the United States. All prior neutron studies have of necessity utilized physics laboratory-based equipment, a condition which severely limited the scope of application for this form of cancer treatment. Limitations of beam flexibility, beam accessibility, and depth dose practically limited treatment to mixtures of neutrons and photons ('mixed beam').

Table 3. Results from the RTOG randomized head and neck study for patients with neck node metastasis

Stage	Mixed beam	Photon
N1	86%	75%
N2	62%	48%
N3	63%	53%
All patients*	69%	55%

* $p = .025$.

Table 4. Results from the RTOG randomized head and neck study for patients with neck node metastasis

Stage	Mixed beam		Photon	
N1	78%		55%	
N2	39%		39%	
N2A		22%		44%
N2B		56%		23%
N3	24%		13%	
N3A		42%		15%
N3B		23%		0%
N3C		—		100%
All patients:	46%		33%	

* $p = .03$.

A new generation of Phase III studies is currently being designed to exploit the potential of these new machines. Hopefully, with these new tools the excellent tumor control rates obtained by Dr. Catterall and her associates can be duplicated without the morbidity associated with a poorly penetrating radiation beam. Until randomized controlled trials are completed using the new hospital-based isocentric neutron generators, the place of fast neutron beam radiation therapy in the armamentarium of head and neck oncologists is yet to be defined.

References

1. Gray LH, Conger AD, Ebert M, Hornsey S, Scott OCA: Concentration of oxygen dissolved in tissues at time of irradiation as factor in radiotherapy. Br J Radiol 26:638, 1953.
2. Howlett JF, Thomlinson RH, Alper T: A marked dependence of the conformative effective causes of neutrons on tumor line and its implications for clinical trials. Br J Radiol 48:40, 1975.
3. Gragg RL, Humphrey RM, Thomas HT, Meyn RE: The response of Chinese hamster ovary cells to fast neutron radiotherapy beams. I. Variations in RBE with position in the cell cycle. Radiat Res 76:283, 1978.
4. Gragg RL, Humphrey RM, Meyn RE: The response of Chinese hamster ovary cells to fast neutron radiotherapy beams. II. Sublethal and potentially lethal damage recovery capabilities. Radiat Res 71:461, 1977.
5. Hall EJ, Kraljevic J: Repair of potentially lethal radiation damage: comparison of neutron and X-ray RBE and implications for radiation therapy. Radiology 121:731, 1976.
6. Stone RS: Neutron therapy and specific ionization. Amer J Roentgenol 59:771, 1948.
7. Brennan JT, Phillips TL: Evaluation of past experience with fast neutron teletherapy and its implications for future applications. Europ J Cancer 7:219, 1971.
8. Catterall M: The treatment of advanced cancer by fast neutrons from the Medical Research Council's cyclotron at Hammersmith Hospital, London. Europ J Cancer 10:343, 1974.

9. Catterall M, Bewley DK, Sutherland J: Second report on a randomized clinical trial of fast neutrons compared with X- or gamma rays in treatment of advanced cancers of the head and neck. Br Med J 1:19, 1977.
10. Maor MH, Hussey DH, Fletcher GH, Jesse RH: Fast neutron therapy for locally advanced head and neck tumors. Int J Rad Onc Biol Phys 7:155, 1981.
11. Griffin TW, Blasko JC, Laramore GE: Results of fast neutron beam pilot studies at the University of Washington. Europ J Cancer Suppl: 23, 1979.
12. Battermann JJ, Breuer K: Results of fast neutron teletherapy for locally advanced head and neck tumors. Int J Rad Onc Biol Phys 7:1045, 1981.
13. Henry LW, Blasko JC, Griffin TW, Parker RG: Evaluation of fast neutron therapy for advanced carcinomas of the major salivary glands. Cancer 44:814, 1979.
14. Kaul R, Hendrickson F, Cohen L, Rosenberg I, Ten Haken R, Awschalom M, Mansell J: Fast neutrons in the treatment of salivary gland tumors. Int J Rad Onc Biol Phys 7:1667, 1981.
15. Griffin TW, Davis R, Laramore GE, Hussey D, Hendrickson F, Rodriguez-Antunez A: Fast neutron irradiation of metastatic cervical adenopathy: the results of a randomized RTOG study. Int J Rad Onc Biol Phys (in press).

7. Chemical modifiers of radiation and chemotherapy: tumor sensitization and normal tissue protection

C. NORMAN COLEMAN and TODD H. WASSERMAN

1. Introduction

1.1. Radiosensitizers and protectors – clinical rationale

The need for effective radiosensitizers and protectors is well illustrated by the problem of treating tumors of the head and neck region. Although local control of early stage (T_1, T_2) tumors is excellent for all sites, control of larger (T_3, T_4) tumors, with the exception of the nasopharynx, is extremely poor and never above 50–60% [1–4]. Local control can be improved by the combination of radiotherapy with radical surgery however such treatment is extremely morbid and far from 100% effective. The use of an effective radiosensitizer or protector would be expected to improve local control probability without an increase in treatment morbidity.

The ability of radiotherapy to produce local control is limited by the tolerance of normal tissues. Doses in excess of 6500 rad in $6\frac{1}{2}$ weeks produce a rapidly increasing risk of soft tissue and bone injury [5]. Since increasing radiation dose increases the probability of local control [6, 7] due to increased killing of malignant cells, any process that enhances tumor cell killing for a given radiation dose (sensitization) or that decreases the relative amount of normal tissue injury (protection) will have significant therapeutic benefit.

1.2. Radioresistance of tumors

There are several possible mechanisms of tumor radioresistance: (a) an excess number of clonogenic cells; (b) oxygenated cells that are resistant by virtue of having too shallow a slope of the cell survival curve; (c) the presence of hypoxic cells and (d) the ability of tumor cells to repair potentially

Gregory T. Wolf (ed), Head and Neck Oncology.
© *1984 Martinus Nijhoff Publishers, Boston. ISBN 0-89838-657-8. Printed in The Netherlands.*

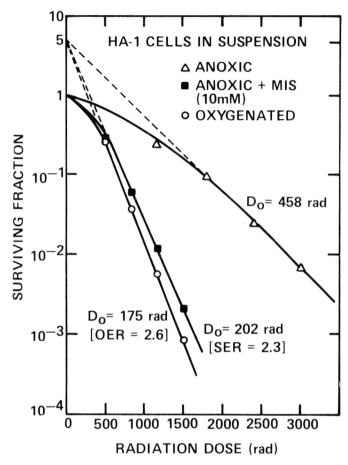

Figure 1. In vitro sensitization of hypoxic cells by oxygen and misonidazole (MIS). D_0 is the slope of the individual curve. The oxygen enhancement ratio is the ratio of the slope of the survival curve in hypoxic conditions ($D_0 = 458$) divided by the slope of the curve when the cells are oxygenated ($D_0 = 175$); OER = 2.6. The sensitizer enhancement ratio (SER) for MIS = 2.3. This SER is much higher than that possible with MIS clinically (SER approximately 1.2) due to the dose limiting toxicity of MIS (see text).

lethal damage. The latter is still uncertain and will not be discussed in this chapter [8].

The relationship between cell killing (or cell survival) and radiation dose is exponential. This means for a given dose of irradiation a certain fraction of cells is killed rather than a certain number [9, 10]. Figure 1 illustrates both the shape of the cell survival curve and the effect of hypoxia [9]. Note that the survival curve has an initial slope called the 'shoulder' that is less steep than the final slope. The dose per fraction used in therapeutic irradiation is 180–200 rad and cell killing is on the shoulder of the cell survival curve, therefore, if there are too many clonogenic cells or the slope is insufficiently steep the tumor will not be cured. In the presence of hypoxia the slope of the curve is even less steep. Consequently, for a given level of cell killing two to three times the dose of irradiation is needed when the cells are hypoxic compared to when the cells are well oxygenated.

1.3. Oxygen effect

The survival curves for oxygenated and hypoxic cells *in vitro* are shown in Fig. 1. The ratio of slopes, called the oxygen enhancement ratio (OER), for most tissues is 2.5 to 3.0. This means that to achieve a given level of cell killing, 2.5 to 3 times more dose is required when the cells are hypoxic. The level of hypoxia required for hypoxia induced radio resistance is quite low [9] and does not occur to any appreciable extent in normal tissues. The postulated mechanism of resistance of hypoxic cells is as follows. Therapeutic irradiation causes ionization in tissue. Free radicals are created primarily in water and to a lesser extent in biologically active molecules such as DNA. It is felt that DNA is the major target for cell killing, therefore DNA damage is important [9]. Free radicals are very unstable. In the presence of oxygen, peroxide radicals are formed, which are much more stable, and by persisting longer are able to do more permanent damage. This is particularly important if the free radicals are formed elsewhere than in the DNA such as in cellular water as they must be present for sufficient time to diffuse to the DNA. The current hypoxic cell radiosensitizers are drugs designed to act as oxygen mimics and take the place of oxygen in the hypoxic cells at the time of irradiation.

1.3.1. Reoxygenation

In general most tumors studied in the laboratory have a hypoxic fraction of approximately 10–30% [11]. If the cells that started out hypoxic remained so throughout treatment, after the first log of cells were killed the remaining 10% of the initial cell population would all be hypoxic and quite resistant to irradiation. Studies in animals have shown that within a few hours of a single dose of irradiation the percentage of hypoxic cells is similar to that prior to irradiation. For example if a tumor with 15% hypoxic cells is given a dose of 1000 rads essentially 100% of the remaining cells will be hypoxic immediately after the irradiation is given. However by six hours later the tumor will again have 15–20% hypoxic cells [9]. This phenomenon is called reoxygenation. Since reoxygenation occurs after each fraction of irradiation it would be best exploited using a treatment scheme with more, rather than fewer, fractions. As will be described below, many of the clinical trials using hyperbaric oxygen or radiosensitizers used few radiation fractions. Thus, the benefit of reoxygenation is decreased. It is, therefore, not possible to accurately compare the efficacy of the sensitized radiotherapy to standard frac-

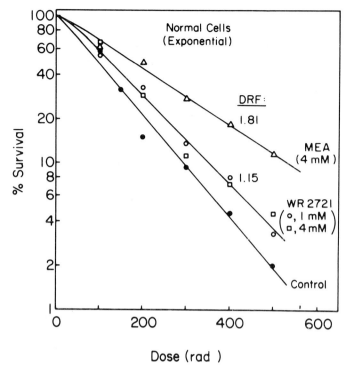

Figure 2. In vitro Protection by WR-2721 or MEA *in vitro* using CC105, a human fibroblast line. MEA (mercaptoethylamine) and WR-2721 are both a source of -SH (thiol) groups. The DRF, the dose reduction factor, is analogous to the enhancement ratio described in Fig. 1 (reprinted with permission from Ritter *et al.*, Int J Radiation Oncology Biol Phys 8:523 [12]).

tionated radiotherapy, when the treatment scheme used with the sensitizer employs different fractionation.

1.4. Radioprotectors

In a manner opposite to that of oxygen, thiols (SH groups) act as radioprotectors. Figure 2 illustrates that the addition of thiols will shift the radiation survival curve of oxygenated cells to the right, i.e. the cells become more resistant [12]. Protection of hypoxic cells does not occur [13] thus normal cells and oxygenated tumor cells will be protected. The current protector in clinical trials, WR-2721, is a phosphorothioate with the SH group being linked to a phosphate. The drug must be activated *in vivo* by phosphatases [14] and is felt to confer protection by chemically reducing free radicals.

1.5. Hyperbaric oxygen (HBO)

One of the earlier attempts to overcome tumor hypoxia was the use of high pressure oxygen. Patients were treated in special compression chambers with an oxygen pressure of three atmospheres. This required a lengthy compression and decompression phase. It was technically cumbersome to do these trials and in most trials only a few fractions of radiation were employed. As discussed in the reoxygenation section (1.3.1), these treatment schemae lessen the potential benefit of reoxygenation and tend to bias the results against the HBO when compared to standard treatment in air as the HBO treatment permitted only a few chances for tumor cells to reoxygenate.

Henk [15] recently summarized the difficulties with interpretation of the results of the HBO trials. Most of the trials contained small numbers of patients making it difficult to see small (20%) differences if they exist. The end point should be local control and not survival as the purpose was to augment radiotherapy, a local treatment. Technical logistics of the trials including radiotherapy technique were difficult. Finally, normal tissue injury appeared to be increased. Without better measures of normal tissue injury it was impossible to say precisely how much increase in normal tissue injury occurred in relation to increase in local tumor control.

Henk and his colleagues completed two head and neck HBO trials at Cardiff [16, 17]. In the first trial both HBO and control groups received 4500 rads in 10 fractions over three weeks. Local control was statistically superior in the HBO group in both primary site and nodes. A number of factors worked against there being a survival advantage: increase in complications in the HBO group, particularly of the laryngeal cartilage; the use of salvage surgery; and the occurrence of second primaries [16]. A second trial was done using HBO with a slightly lower total dose (4100 rads) than the first trial. This was compared to a standard fractionation regimen of 200 rads, five times a week for six weeks. There was a statistically improved survival in the HBO group vs the air group. For patients with larynx cancer there was an improvement in freedom from relapse [17]. Henk later pointed out that the major advantage was for the patients with T_3 (2 to 5 cm) tumors. Sause and Plenk [18] reported on a randomized trial using HBO with radiotherapy of 12 fractions of 400 rads (total 4800r) vs treatment in air using 250 rads in 25 fractions to a total dose of 6250. There were 46 patients in the study and the results were similar in both groups.

Therefore, with the limitations as outlined above, the results suggested that there may be some benefit using HBO for tumors of moderate size. The technical difficulties using HBO have made it less attractive than sensitizers. As will be discussed, some of these limitations of treatment regimens seen in the HBO trials have been a problem for the early sensitizer trials.

2. Radiosensitizers

For a good number of years various chemical compounds were studied to see whether they could sensitize cells to irradiation by acting as oxygen mimics. Since oxygen is the best sensitizer it is not expected that normal tissues will be sensitized. In 1974, the first of the nitroimidazoles entered clinical trials. The drug used was metronidazole, a compound that had been used as an antitrichomonad. Metronidazole is a 5-nitroimidazole which, in its Phase I trial, demonstrated nausea and vomiting as its dose limiting toxicity [19]. Later studies showed that neurologic toxicity, particularly a central neuropathy could occur [20].

This drug was used in a randomized trial for the treatment of malignant gliomas (grade III and IV) [21]. Due to the dose limiting neurotoxicity a reasonably high dose of drug could only be administered nine times. Additionally, at that time it was unknown whether or not normal tissue injury would be enhanced. Therefore, a radiotherapy schema was chosen using 330 rad, three times a week for three weeks. This is equivalent to a dose of 4000–4500 rad using standard fractionation of 200 rad, five times weekly [21]. The patients who received metronidazole had a statistically superior median survival compared to those not receiving drug. This demonstrated the biologic activity of the sensitizer. However, the sensitizer plus radiation group had survival equivalent to that of patients given standard fractionated high dose radiation, and there were no patients cured [21].

Thus, these results are similar to those seen with hyperbaric oxygen. There was benefit from using the sensitizer with the few-fraction radiation schema which was employed. As discussed above, to evaluate the therapeutic benefit of the sensitizer it must be tested with standard radiation fractionation so that it can be shown that hypoxia per se is a cause of tumor resistence during standard treatment.

2.1. Misonidazole (MISO)

It has been demonstrated in the laboratory that 2-nitroimidazoles are more efficient sensitizers compared to 5-nitroimidazoles [22]. The change in position of the nitro group increases the electron affinity of the compound, an important determinant in the ability of a compound to act as a hypoxic cell sensitizer [22]. The structure of MISO and some of its analogs are shown in Table 1. The analogs and the rationale for their use are discussed below.

Misonidazole initially underwent Phase I trials in the United States and England. Phase I trials are designed to determine the drug's toxicity, maximum tolerated dose (MTD), and pharmacology. Efficacy is not a goal of these trials. Patients on these trials have an advanced stage of disease but are physiologically well compensated with adequate hematopoietic, hepatic and renal function. MISO was initially used as an oral preparation, given four hours prior to radiotherapy. The general findings of the MISO Phase I trials are as follows [23–25]:

(a) The single dose MTD was 4–5 gm/m^2 due to nausea and vomiting.

(b) The multiple dose MTD was approximately 10–12 gm/m^2 due to the development of neuropathy. A peripheral neuropathy occurred in approximately 40 to 50% of the patients at this dose which was characterized by sensory dysesthesia and paresthesis with very occasional motor weakness. This could be quite debilitating and long lasting, particularly with the higher grade of toxicity [25, 26]. A central neuropathy characterized by confusion occurred in approximately 10% of patients as did mild hearing loss. Of interest it was noted that the MTD was not dependent on dose schedule, with various dose sizes being given over schedules ranging from three to seven weeks [23].

(c) The drug was well absorbed orally. The estimated bioavailability was 80–100% [27].

(d) The drug penetrated well into tumors. It was important to discern the morphology of the biopsy specimen as it would be expected that drug would not penetrate well into the necrotic centers. The tumor concentration near the necrotic center was approximately 70–80% that of the plasma level [28, 29].

(e) The drug had a prolonged terminal halflife of 13 hours after oral administration and 8–9 hours after intravenous (i.v.) administration. A

Table 1. Structure of 2-nitroimidazoles used in clinical trials MIS: Misonidazole, DMM: Desmethylmisonidazole. Partition coefficient is a measure of the relative drug solubility in octanol vs water. MIS is the most lipophilic and SR-2508 is the most hydrophilic of the group.

Compound	R	Mol Wt	Partition Coeff (P)
MIS	$CH_2CH(OH)CH_2OMe$	201	0.43
DMM	$CH_2CH(OH)CH_2OH$	187	0.13
SR-2508	$CH_2CONHCH_2CH_2OH$	214	0.046

patient's drug exposure per dose of drug could be defined by calculating the area under the curve (AUC) of plasma concentration versus time. The patients with neurotoxicity generally had a higher AUC than patients who did not have neurotoxicity [24, 26].

(f) Approximately 10% of the parent compound was excreted unchanged in the urine. An additional 20% of drug was excreted as the demethylated compound, desmethylmisonidazole (DMM). Using high performance liquid chromatography (HPLC) this metabolite was found in the plasma [23]. Being more water soluble than MISO, DMM was more rapidly cleared, producing a lower drug exposure for a given dose of drug. This factor led to the use of DMM in subsequent clinical trials.

(g) Dilantin and dexamethasone decrease the incidence of neuropathy [30, 31]. The dilantin effect is felt to be due to induction of hepatic enzymes that facilitated MISO metabolism. The mechanism of action of corticosteroids is not known. It appears that higher doses of MISO can be given if concomitant dexamethasone is used (Urtasun, personal communication).

2.1.1. MISO – Clinical trials in head and neck cancer

A number of phase II and phase III trials in patients with advanced head and neck cancers have been done or are ongoing using MISO with varying fractionation schemae of radiation (Table 2).

The RTOG conducted a phase I/II trial [32] to determine the toxicity and the potential value of MISO as an adjuvant to definitive radiation therapy in stage T3 and T4 cancers of the oral cavity, oropharynx or hypopharynx. The radiation was delivered in two separate treatments of 250 rad and 210 rad on each day of MISO while maintaining relatively standard fractionation of 5 total fractions and 1000 rad per week. Total radiation doses were in the range of 6500–7000 rad over $6\frac{1}{2}$ to 8 weeks. The MISO dose was initially 2.5 gm/m^2 once a week for 6 weeks, but because of toxicity after the first 30 patients, the dose was reduced to 2 gm/m^2 once a week for 6 weeks.

In the one year the study was ongoing, 50 patients were entered. Toxicity was confined to neurotoxicity, with one-third of the patients experiencing a mild or moderate peripheral neuropathy. Encephalopathy occurred in 10% of the 30 patients receiving the 2.5 gm/m^2 dose. Acute mucosal and skin reactions were not enhanced and unusual late normal tissue toxicities were not observed. Complete response of all tumor was noted in 67% of the 36 patients completing the prescribed radiation and at least three doses of MISO. Twenty-two percent of this group of 36 patients had a partial response of greater than 50% for an overall response of 89%. Complete response rate in all patients entered (n = 50) was 50% with partial response noted in an additional 28% of (n = 36) patients for a total response rate of

Table 2. Results of head and neck radiotherapy plus MISO trials

Head and neck trials using misonidazole

Type of trial	Population	XRT schedule	Miso schedule	Result
RTOG (78–02) Phase II, one arm [32]	T_3, T_4 tumors oral cavity oro-, hypo- pharynx	250+210r with MISO 180r 3/week = 1000r/wk – for total 6500–7000r	2.5 g/m² (re- duced to 2.0 g/m²) total 12–15 g/m²	CR = 67% at end of treatment; To phase III
RTOG (79–15) phase III, ran- domized	Inoperable	standard 180–200r/day to approx 7000 rads vs. same schedule as RTOG 78–02 (above)	No Miso vs. same schedule as RTOG 78–02 (above)	In analysis
RTOG (79–04) phase II ran- domized [33]	Stage III, IV or recurrent	400 rads daily × 11 to- tal 4400 rads	1.5 g/m² 3/wk total = 10.5 g/m	In analysis
Phase III, ran- domized (S. Africa) [34]	T_3, T_4, or N_3 all sites	600 twice weekly for 33 weeks total = 3600 rads	2 g/m² with XRT total = 12 g/m²	local control 1 yr = 22–23% no difference ±MISO
Phase II (Italy) [35]	Advanced	200+150+150r three fraction per day × 10 days	1.2 g/m² daily × 10 total = 12 g/m²	68% CR at end of treatment
EORTC phase II, randomized 1/3 had MISO [36, 37]	Advanced all sites	160r 3 times daily 4800r/2wks-split Boost to total about 7000r	1.5 g/m²/day total = 13– 14 g/m²	Local control MISO – 57% non-MISO – 48% $p = 0.38$; to phase III
MCR, England phase III, ran- domized, [38]	T_3, T_4 N_2, N_3 multiple sites	4000–4500r in 10 fractions 5000–5700r in 20 fractions	1.2 g/m² total = 12 g/m² or placebo 0.6 g/m² total = 12 g/m² or placebo	1yr. local control 10fxs+MISO – 37% 10fx+placebo – 42% 20fx+MISO – 50% 20fx+placebo – 53%
Danish, phase III random- ized [40]	Advanced	4000r in 20 fractions or 413r/2fxs/wk × 4 weeks	0.55 g/m² total = 11 g/m² or placebo 1.4 g/m² × 8 to- tal = 11.2 g/m² or placebo	2 yr local control MISO – 48% pla- cebo – 32% MISO – 56% pla- cebo – 45%

78% for all patients entered. The complete response rate was statistically better among the 30 patients receiving the higher dose of MISO, than 20 patients receiving a lower dose (55% vs 18%). The reduced dose of MISO would seem to lead to reduced tumor control with the fractionation scheme tested. It also, however, led to a reduction in the incidence and severity of neurotoxicity, particularly by the elimination of severe peripheral neuropathy (beyond grade 1) and central neurotoxicity (encephalopathy).

The overall good complete response rate observed coupled with the fact that the median survival was 18 months with several long term tumor free survivors (17/36 47% alive NED at 9–24+ months) was deemed sufficiently encouraging to warrant a phase III study described below. These data would support the notion that if an effective non-toxic sensitizer could be developed it would improve the therapeutic efficacy of radiation in advanced head and neck cancers.

The randomized, phase III, RTOG trial of advanced head and neck cancers, treated with irradiation with and without weekly MISO of 2 gm/m^2 orally [33], began in August 1979 and was closed in February 1983. The endpoints of this randomized trial were the evaluation of local control of primary tumor and regional nodes, and the assessment of tumor free interval and of normal tissue tolerance. The radiotherapy plus MISO schedule was modified to include two fractions once a week on the day of the MISO as used in the Phase II trial described above. The radiation therapy alone schedule was conventional fractionation. Both schedules used the same weekly total dose, and the final dose for the entire course of treatment was in the range of 6600–7380 rad. The study accrued a total of 360 patients in the $3\frac{1}{2}$ years and is undergoing continuing analysis. Preliminary data indicate that between 49 and 55% of the patients obtained a complete remission of their tumor. The MISO related toxicity has been quite minimal and acceptable.

The RTOG has concluded a limited institution randomized pilot study of high dose per fraction radiation with or without MISO [33]. The radiation dose used is 4800 rad in 12 fractions over 2.5 weeks plus a 400 rad boost. The MISO dose is 1.5 gm/m^2, 3 times per week, for 7 doses, for a total dose 10.5 gm/m^2. This study was completed in February, 1983 and is currently being analyzed.

Sealey *et al.* [34] of South Africa have studied MISO in a randomized study of advanced head and neck cancer in 97 patients. Radiation was given in large fractions of 600 rad, 2 fractions per week for 3 weeks (total dose 3600 rad) either alone or in conjunction with MISO 2 gm/m^2 (total dose 12 gm/m^2). The incidence of acute mucosal and other reactions were similar between the two groups. There was a 26% incidence of MISO induced peripheral neuropathy. Local tumor control was similar between the two groups with a one year local control rate of 22% in both groups. The authors concluded that this study showed no advantage to treatment with MISO, probably due to the inadequate frequency of drug administration due to dose-limiting neurotoxicity.

Arcangeli *et al.* [35] have piloted the use of MISO in association with multiple daily fractionated radiotherapy in patients with advanced head and neck cancers. These investigators have added MISO at a dose of $1.2 \, gm/m^2$ daily for ten doses (total dose $12 \, gm/m^2$) in conjunction with three daily fractions of radiation either alone or with the addition of hyperthermia. This pilot study included 22 patients with multiple daily fraction radiotherapy plus MISO and 20 patients with multiple daily fraction radiotherapy plus MISO plus hyperthermia. The complete response rate at the end of treatment was 68% for the former group and 80% for the latter group. This complete response rate was higher than that for conventional radiation or multiple daily fractionated radiation alone in a non-randomized comparative group. The complete response rate, was improved over that of the more conventional treatment at the time intervals of 6 months and 12 months post treatment. The toxicity of the MISO plus multiple daily fraction radiation was acceptable except for some increased mucositis necessitating a break in treatment in some patients. This group is currently doing a pilot randomized study of multiple daily fraction radiation with or without MISO.

The European Organization for Research on Treatment of Cancer (EORTC) Cooperative Group is conducting a randomized trial of conventional radiation vs three daily fractions of radiation vs three daily fractions of radiation plus MISO for patients with advanced head and neck cancers [36, 37]. This study accrued 300 patients during its first year (1981), and is still in analysis. Preliminary data indicate that the tolerance and toxicity of multiple daily fraction radiotherapy combined with MISO is acceptable.

The Medical Research Council (MRC) of England conducted a randomized, double blind trial of MISO or placebo with radiation [38]. This trial which included patients with T3, T4, N2, N3 cancers of mixed sites studied two schedules of radiation, the first was 4000–4500 rad, 10 fractions, 22 days, which was a schedule similar to the previous MRC experience with hyperbaric oxygen. The second radiation schedule was 5000–5700 rad in 20 fractions, 28 days. The radiation schedule employed was an institutional choice. MISO, given before each fraction of radiation, was given at a dose of $1.2 \, gm/m^2$ with the 10 fraction schedule or at $0.6 \, gm/m^2$ with the 20 fraction schedule, for a total dose of $12 \, gm/m^2$ for either schedule. The study, which is now closed and in analysis, accrued 168 patients in the 10 fraction schedule and 99 patients in the 20 fraction schedule. There was a high incidence of neurotoxicity: 50% in the 20 fraction dose schedule, and 65% in the 10 fraction dose schedule. This high incidence of toxicity was attributed to a lack of age exclusion, a lack of routine hydration of patients, and the fact that there was no monitoring of blood MISO levels. The study was closed because of the toxicity and the apparent lack of substantial efficacy. Local tumor control at 1 year was 37% with 10 fractions of radiation and MISO, 50% with the 20 fractions of radiation and placebo. Thus, there was apparently no difference in tumor control.

A randomized study using MISO with radiation in advanced head and neck cancer was conducted at the Institute Curie in Paris, from February, 1979 thru May, 1982 [39]. The radiation was given in one of two schedules: two fractions per day (similar to that of the RTOG study above) in conjunction with 2.5 gm/m^2 of MISO once weekly; or in a schedule of daily radiation with MISO at 0.7 gm/m^2 daily during the first and last two weeks of treatment for a total dose of 14 gm/m^2. Approximately 150 patients have been entered in the radiation alone or radiation plus MISO arms. Peripheral neuropathy has occurred in only 17% of the patients. No difference has yet been observed in the local control or survival in the patients receiving the MISO.

The Danish Head and Neck Study Group has an ongoing double blind, randomized, multicentered trial of radiotherapy plus MISO or placebo [40]. The study, which opened October, 1979 has accrued 296 patients as of June, 1982. A total dose of radiation of 4000 rad is given in 20 fractions over 4 weeks either with MISO (at 0.55 gm/m^2 with every fraction, total dose 11 gm/m^2) or with placebo. A second schedule of radiation employed is 413 rad, 2 fractions per week, for 4 weeks, with either MISO (1.4 gm/m^2 for 8 doses, total dose of 11.2 gm/m^2) or placebo. After a three week rest all patients received a boost radiation dose of 2400 rad in 12 fractions. The overall incidence of MISO induced neurotoxicity is 30%, with the females having a statistically higher incidence than males. The higher toxicity incidence in the females is attributed to a larger drug exposure as measured by the plasma pharmacokinetic profile. The local control rate at 2 years is as follows: two fractions per week with MISO (n = 85), 56%; two fractions per week with placebo (n = 68) 45%; five fractions per week MISO (n = 77) 48%; five fractions per week with placebo (n = 66) 32%; total MISO patients (N = 162) 52% (+/−5%); total placebo patients (n = 134) 40% (+/−6%).

The results of the studies described above provide no definitive proof as to the ability of MISO to alter the local control rate of tumors by radiation. In interpreting the radiosensitizer trials it should be remembered that the proper endpoints to measure would be the complete response rate at the end of treatment, and the actuarial freedom from local recurrence. It would not be anticipated that improved local treatment would necessarily influence survival rate as many of these patients succumb to distant metastases.

It may be that the results with large fraction intermittent radiation with

MISO will not be superior to, but only equivalent to that of conventional fractionated radiation. The logistical and economical advantages of fewer fractions particularly with patients with far advanced cancers would seem to favor the large fraction radiation. However, there may well be significantly more long term morbidity from the large fractions of radiation employed. As will be discussed below, the lack of positive clinical results with MISO does not mean that hypoxic cells are not important in the local control of advanced head and neck cancers treated with radiation or that a therapeutic gain could not be expected with an improved radiosensitizer.

2.1.2. Therapeutic efficacy of MISO

In general the use of MISO has not produced any major therapeutic advantage. The problem with the necessity of using unusual fractionation schemae has been discussed above. A second major consideration is the enhancement obtainable for a given tissue level of MISO. The previously defined term oxygen enhancement ratio (OER) is the ratio of the dose of radiation necessary to produce a given level of cell killing without oxygen compared to the dose of radiation needed to produce the same level of cell killing with oxygen (Fig. 1). A similar term using a sensitizer rather than oxygen can be calculated and is called the sensitizer enhancement ratio (SER). The OER is 2.5–3.0 for most animal tumors. It was initially felt that at a MISO dose of $2 \, g/m^2$ an SER of up to 1.6 could be obtained [41]. That is probably an optimistic number. The SER for this drug dose is more likely in the range of 1.1–1.2 [42, 43]. Thus, even if MISO had been effective it would be very unlikely to yield a statistically significant improvement in a limited sized clinical trial due to the small benefit that could have been provided by the dose employed.

2.2. Pharmacologic considerations in drug development

Since neuropathy was the dose limiting toxicity, it became desirable to produce a drug that would not cross the blood brain barrier. Additionally, a higher total drug exposure as measured by AUC correlated with toxicity. Brown, Lee, Workman and colleagues [44, 45] developed a series of 2-nitroimidazoles that had the same electron affinity but which differed in their pharmacologic properties. The rationale for drug development is illustrated in Fig. 3 which shows theoretical data for two drugs that are equal radiosensitizers. Drug A is more lipid soluble (lipophilic) than drug B. As illustrated, both achieve equal plasma and tumor levels however by being less lipophilic drug B does not penetrate the blood brain barrier and achieves a lower concentration in the neutral tissues. Figure 3 illustrates that drug B, being less lipophilic, requires less metabolism and is excreted more

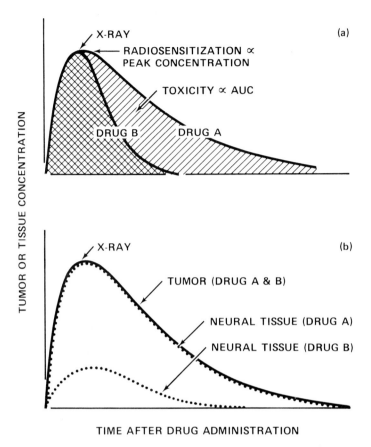

Figure 3. Theoretical pharmacokinetic considerations for sensitizer development. Drug A and B, when given orally produce an equal peak plasma and tumor concentration. The latter is the important factor for radiosensitization. Drug A is more lipophilic therefore it achieves a higher level in neural tissue than Drug B and it requires more hepatic metabolism than Drug B which is excreted predominantly by the kidney. Drug A has a larger area under the curve (AUC) which for many drugs correlates with toxicity. Drug B would theoretically be the superior drug (reprinted with permission by Brown in Cancer Treat Rep 65:95 [44]).

rapidly than drug A. This produces a lower AUC for drug B. Therefore, a less lipophilic drug is advantageous [44].

Figure 4 shows data from *in vivo* trials in mice using ten 2-nitroimidazoles that differ in lipophilicity. Lipophilicity is measured by octanol: water partition coefficient (*P*). The higher the *P* the more lipophilic the drug. For all but the most hydrophilic drug (SR-2530) the tumor: plasma ratio is one. As drugs become very hydrophilic they do not readily cross the cell membrane. As *P* decreases the brain: plasma ratio declines. The structures and *P* of the drugs used in clinical trials are in Table 1. In Fig. 4 it is seen the MISO has brain: plasma ratio of 1. DMM has a lower brain: plasma ratio however after a few hours this ratio will reach 1. SR2508 has a brain: plasma ratio of

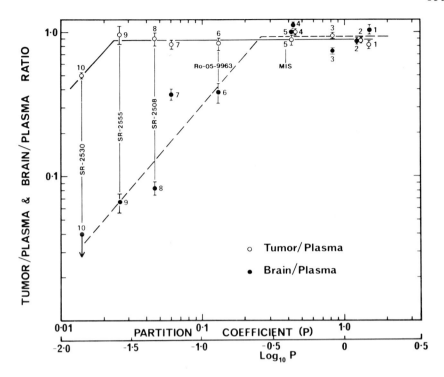

Figure 4. Tumor/Plasma (T/P) and Brain/Plasma (B/P) ratio of ten 2-nitroimidazole compounds in mice. The three drugs of interest Mis, RO-05-9963 (DMM) and SR-2508 all achieve a T/P ratio of one. The B/P ratio is 1.0 for MIS and 0.3 to DMM, However, within 2 hours it is 1.0 for DMM. The B/P ratio for SR-2508 is <0.1 and this is maintained for days, during a constant drug infusion. SR-2555, although having a T/P ratio of 1.0 is too hydrophilic to readily penetrate the cell membrane (reprinted with permission by Brown, in Int J Radiation Oncology Biol Phys 8:1491 [47]).

less than 0.1 and this remains at this ratio despite prolonged infusion (Eifel, personal communication). Thus, it is predicted that SR-2508 will be the optimal drugs of this group.

2.3. Desmethylmisonidazole (DMM)

Approximately three years ago SR-2508 was selected to proceed through the National Cancer Institute pre-clinical testing. Since DMM was an endogenously formed analog of MISO it was able to enter human trials more rapidly than a newly synthesized drug. A phase I trial of intravenous DMM was started by the Radiation Therapy Oncology Group (RTOG) [47], while oral DMM was tested by Dische and colleagues in England [48]. The data predicted that the total dose tolerable in humans would be approxiately 1.5 times that of MISO.

The RTOG trial has recently been closed. The results of the RTOG and English trials were as follows [47-50]:

(a) Neurotoxicity was the dose limiting toxicity. Unlike MISO there were no documented cases of central neuropathy. The peripheral neuropathy was qualitatively similar to that of MISO.
(b) The total dose of drug which produced a 30 to 50% incidence of neuropathy was between 13.5-15.0 g/m^2. Assuming a bioavailability of 80-90% for oral MISO [27] vs. 100% for IV DMM the total dose of DMM delivered to produce an incidence of neuropathy similar to that of MISO was about 1.5 times that of MISO, close to the prediction in animals.
(c) The pharmacokinetic parameters were as predicted [47]. Table 3 compares the pharmacokinetic parameters of MISO, given orally and IV, and IV DMM. Being more hydrophilic DMM is excreted more rapidly, and more of the parent compound is excreted unchanged in the urine47-49. Due to the toxicity of DMM, data on drug levels in tumors were not vigorously pursued as it was clear that it would not be a very useful drug clinically. What little data there were suggested that DMM did achieve a reasonable tumor:plasma ratio of a approximately 85% [51].
(d) The drug was not sufficiently better than MISO, so further trials of DMM were not planned.

2.4. Attemps to prevent or ameliorate neuropathy

It is known that the 2-nitro (NO_2) group can be reduced to an amine (NH_2). This can be seen to a small extent in various tissues but the predominant site would be in the gastrointestinal tract [52]. It had been shown previously that amino-MISO, the reduction product, is much more toxic than MISO [53]. Furthermore, other drugs containing amines, such as isoniazide, produce a neuropathy that is preventable by simultaneously administering pyridoxine (Vitamin B_6) [54]. Studies in mice by Eifel et al. supported the

Table 3. Pharmacokinetic compression. t 1/2 Beta = terminal half life of drug elimination

Pharmacokinetic comparison of MISO and DMM (normalized for a dose of 1.0 gm/m^2)

	DMM	IV MISO	Oral MISO
1 hr blood level (µg/ml)	41 (±9)	48 (±10)	30±9 (at 4–6 hrs)
t 1/2 Beta (hrs)	6 (±2)	9.3 (±1.0)	13.8±5.1)
% urine recovery in 24 hrs	62 (±12)	23 (±5)	30 (±13)
		(2/3 as DMM)	

Mean values ±1 standard deviation.

hypothesis that amino-MISO is neurotoxic and that the simultaneous administration of pyridoxine could lessen the neurotoxicity of MISO [55].

This laboratory observation was tested in the clinic. In the DMM trial it was shown that a dose of 1.5 g/m², three times a week for three weeks, (total 13.5 g/m²) produced an incidence of peripheral neuropathy of about 50%. As an amendment to the DMM trial nine patients were treated with oral pyridoxine in addition to DMM. Five patients developed neuropathy. However, while the plasma pharmacokinatic profile of DMM was unchanged by the addition of pyridoxine, the percentage of drug recovered was markedly reduced. This, although not preventing neuropathy, pyridoxine did have some impact on the excretion pattern of DMM. This is being studied further in the laboratory for potential clinical use (Coleman, in progress).

As mentioned above the use of corticosteroids in the prevention of the neuropathy of MISO is also being explored however the utility of this approach is as yet unknown (Urtasun, in progress).

2.5. Newer sensitizers in clinical trial

2.5.1. 2-nitroimidazoles
SR-2508, the structure of which is in Table 1, has now entered Phase I clinical trials. The rationale for its design has been described above (in Section 2.2).

A second compound in clinical trials, Ro-03-8799, is a 2-nitroimidazole that has a basic side chain [56, 57] and *in vitro* has electron affinity superior to that of MISO. No results are yet available from the early clinical trials being done in England [58].

2.5.2. Non-nitro compounds
A number of laboratories are investigating hypoxic cell radiosensitizers that are quire dissimilar in structure from MISO. At present no clinical trials are planned with these agents.

3. Radioprotectors

The basic rationale for development of these compounds, discussed in Section 1.4, is that thiol (SH) groups can chemically restore radiation induced free radicals. Therefore, no permanent radiation damage would be done to the critical targets in the cell. This would be important in oxygenated cells where oxygen and thiols 'compete' for the radicals. Much of the work in development of protectors has been accomplished by Yuhas and his colleagues [14]. Free thiols such as cysteamine are too toxic to administer in clin-

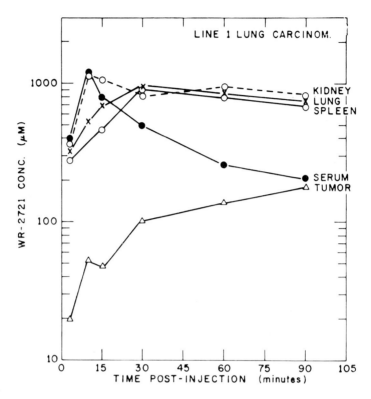

Figure 5. Tissue distribution of WR-2721 after intraperitoneal injection. The drug level in tumor slowly increases, therefore the timing of WR-2721 and radiation or chemotherapy may be critical in the effective use of this protector (reprinted with permission by Yuhas in Cancer Clin Trials 3:211 [62]).

ically useful doses. However a series of drugs were developed at the Walter Reed Institute in which the thiol group is covered by a phosphate thereby reducing toxicity. The drug must then be activated *in vivo* by phosphatases to become a protector. WR-2721 was the best protector *in vivo* and is now in clinical trials [59, 60].

Knowledge of the pharmacologic disposition of WR-2721 is crucial to its optimal use. The drug must be first desphosphorylated and can then be present in two forms, the thiol and the disulfide. An assay for this drug is being developed by Fahey *et al.* [61]. Yuhas *et al.* have performed distribution studies using WR-2721 labeled with radioactive sulfur. These studies showed that location of the drug but not the specific from in which it exists [62]. Figure 5 illustrates data from rat experiments. It can be seen that the drug rapidly reaches normal tissues but equilibrates more slowly with tumors. Thus, timing of the drug with irradiation can theoretically influence the relative amount of protection achieved in normal tissues and tumors.

Not all normal tissues are protected. The drug does not enter the nervous system. Since spinal cord tolerance to radiotherapy is relatively low, this is a drawback to the clinical use of WR-2721. The specific protection factor or dose modification factor (DMF) differs slightly in various experiments. This DMF is analogous to the enhancement ratio described above. A reduction factor of two means that twice the dose is needed to produce a given effect with protector than without it. In general good protection (DMF > 2) is seen for bone marrow, skin, salivary gland, and liver; moderate protection (DMF = 1.4–2.0) is seen for intestine and kidney; minimal (DMF = 1.2–1.4) for lung; and the brain and spinal cord are not protected (DMF = 1.0) [14, 63]. Protection of salivary gland function appears to be highly effective due to accumulation of WR-2721 in that organ and may therefore be of significant benefit to patients with head and neck cancer.

3.1. WR-2721

From the series of drugs studied by Yuhas, WR-2721 appeared to be the most promising. It is currently undergoing Phase I testing with radiotherapy and chemotherapy [59, 60]. The trials are designed to define the maximum tolerated single dose and to establish the tolerance of a multiple dose schedule. For radiotherapy the same problems exist as seen with sensitizers – the drug must be given in a sufficient individual dose to produce protection yet must be given with multiple daily treatments.

Administration of WR-2721 produces a variable incidence of hypotension, somnolence, nausea and vomiting [60]. It is as yet unknown what role this drug will have in clinical radiotherapy.

3.2. Other radioprotectors

There is no other new radioprotector that is scheduled for clinical trials. Other drugs are being investigated experimentally including diethydithiocarbomate (DDC) [64] which in preliminary data unfortunately protected not only all normal tissues but tumors as well (Evans, personal communication).

4. Nitroimidazoles as chemosensitizers

In 1979, Rose and colleagues first demonstrated that MISO could enhance cell killing of chemotherapy *in vivo*, particularly by alkylating agents [65]. His experiments utilized a large single dose of MISO with melphalan or cyclophosphamide. He demonstrated that (a) an enhancement ratio of approximately 2.0 was seen for tumors, (b) a smaller enhancement (approximately 1.3) was observed for normal tissue injury, and (c) when using a large single dose of MISO the timing of drug administration was important with the best enhancement seen when the drugs were given simultaneously.

Following those results a number of other groups began investigating the interaction between hypoxic sensitizers and chemotherapeutic drugs. Some of these findings will be summarized below, however two more comprehensive reviews are available [66, 67].

4.1. Possible mechanisms of action of chemosensitization by nitromidazoles

By attempting to understand the basic mechanism of interaction some of the empiric observations have been explained. The potential mechanisms of chemosensitization initially considered were [66, 67]:

(a) pharmacologic interaction of drugs,
(b) repair of chemotherapy induced potentially lethal damage (PLD),
(c) manifestation of the *in vivo* pre-incubation effect.

4.1.1. Pharmacologic interaction of drugs
Initial studies suggested that the sensitizer may be prolonging the half-life of the alkylating agent. It is known in mice that the administration of large single doses of MISO can reduce body temperature by 5 °C. Brown, Hirst and colleagues [68] gave multiple small doses of MISO to mice which duplicated the longer half life in humans and which, unlike a large single dose of MISO, had little effect on body temperature of the mice (Horsman, personal communication). In these multiple dose MISO experiments, which may be more predictive of what will be seen clinically, a tumor enhancement of 2.0 was obtained without any enhancement of alkylating agent damage to several normal tissues [68]. More recent work has shown that the plasma half life of melphalan is altered when a large single dose of MISO is used but is minimally changed when a multiple MISO dose schedule is employed (Horsman *et al.*, Coleman *et al.* in preparation). Therefore, pharmacologic interaction is at most a minor part of the enhancement.

4.1.2. Repair of chemotherapy induced potentially lethal damage
There is a phenomenon seen after cells are treated with radiotherapy or chemotherapy called potentially lethal damage repair [69, 70]. To demonstrate this effect, the cells must be kept in depleted medium or in crowded conditions. A certain level of cell survival is seen if cells are plated imme-

diately after treatment. However, if the cells are left alone for a number of hours and then plated a larger fraction of cells survive. This survival increase is operationally called repair of potentially lethal damage (PLDR). Some of the initial laboratory observations suggested that MISO inhibited the PLDR [67]. However, MISO enhancement of tumor killing was seen in cell lines that do not exhibit the phenomenon of PLDR. Therefore, this phenomenon is not the mechanism of chemosensitization.

4.1.3. Manifestation of the in vitro pre-incubation effect

It had been demonstrated *in vitro* that MISO itself can be cytotoxic. This requires incubation of cells for a number of hours with MISO under hypoxic conditions, during which time reduction of the nitro group of MISO occurs. Under these conditions no MISO cell killing is seen for the first few hours. After a certain amount of time has elapsed, cell killing is observed. However, changes in the cells are occurring during the early part of the MISO incubation as those cells are rendered more sensitive to treatment with radiation, drugs, or heat [71]. This effect has been called the preincubation effect. The magnitude of the effect *in vivo* is unknown. During this pre-incubation period thiols, particularly glutathione are being depleted by the nitro reduction process.

Taylor *et al.* investigated the possible mechanisms of chemosensitization to melphalan *in vitro* [72]. A drug diethylmaleate, that depletes glutathione, was used to study the role of thiol depletion by MISO when used for its chemosensitization. These results suggest:

(a) gluthathione depletion accounts for only a small part of the sensitization;
(b) alteration by MISO of the amount of melphalan that binds to cellular macromolecules is minimal;
(c) the amount of DNA cross-linking formed is greatly enhanced. The mechanism of enhancement of cross-link formed by MISO remains to be established, but this appears to be an important mechanism of chemo-enhancement.

Therefore, the 'pre-incubation effect' which requires some tumor hypoxia appears to best explain the chemosensitization.

4.2. Clinical trials

At present a number of groups are conducting phase I clinical trials of sensitizer with chemotherapy. The animal data suggested that the alkylating agents and nitrosoureas, particularly BCNU and CCNU would be enhanced [67]. There is little data as yet available from these trials.

Coleman *et al.* recently completed a trial using MISO plus melphalan (LPAM) as a Northern California Oncology Group Phase I study. Analysis suggests that melphalan bone marrow toxicity is not enhanced by MISO [73]. Pharmacologic analysis of LPAM was studied and the calculated pharmacokinetic parameters appear to be similar to that previously published when LPAM was administered alone. However the comparative pharmacokinetics of melphalan, with and without MISO, will be studied in a randomized trial soon to be done.

No therapeutic results are yet available. It is expected that a good deal of data using chemosensitizers in the clinic will appear in the next few years.

5. Thiol protectors with chemotherapy

In addition to its role as a radioprotector, WR-2721 can protect against cytotoxicity of cisplatin and alkylating agents [74–78]. Yuhas demonstrated that mouse lethality for nitrogen mustard can be lessened with WR-2721 [74]. Both acute lethality and renal damage of cisplatin can be reduced [75]. Wasserman *et al.* demonstrated bone marrow protection as measured by the CFUs assay [77]. The nitrogen mustard protection appears to be due to direct interaction of the thiol with the mustard. The mechanism of protection of cisplatin is less clear. Harris *et al.* demonstrated *in vitro* that giving WR-2721 before or after cisplatin can decrease cisplatin cytotoxicity. There did not appear to be direct interaction of drugs [76].

Phillips *et al.* in their recent summary of the chemoprotection data noted that either no or minimal tumor protection has been observed therefore, the use of WR-2721 plus chemotherapy would result in a therapeutic gain [78].

5.1. Clinical trials with WR-2721 as a chemoprotector

As was the case with sensitizers, clinical trials with WR-2721 as a chemoprotector were based on data derived from animal experiments. The current trials are Phase I/II trials. They are designed (a) to determine an optimal dose and schedule of WR-2721 and (b) to see if chemoprotection is observed. Glick *et al.* [60] are doing studies in which the single dose of WR-2721 has been escalated seeking a maximum tolerated dose (MTD). Having achieved a WR-2721 dose in the range of 1000 mg/m^2 chemotherapeutic agents have been given in escalating doses. Chemotherapy trials started included those with cisplatin, cyclophosphamide and nitrogen mustard.

Before deciding on the efficacy of WR-2721 as a protector a sufficiently high dose of protector must be delivered. Furthermore, the state of the drug at any given time, i.e. the phosphate, thiol, or disulfide must be known to maximize the chemoprotection to normal tissues and minimize the protection of tumors. The MTD of WR-2721 has not yet been achieved. As of now, the assay for WR-2721 in its three forms, is not yet available for use in the clinic.

At the present doses and schedules of WR-2721 being used, the preliminary clinical results do not yet suggest that chemoprotection occurs. It is expected that the role of WR-2721 as a chemoprotector will be clarified within the next one to two years.

5.2. Other chemoprotectors

Since cisplatin is a very useful drug in head and neck cancer it is worth mentioning other work being done with drugs that may lessen cisplatin nephrotoxicity. Howell *et al.* [79, 80] have reported that thiosulfate given systematically can reduce the nephrotoxicity of cisplatin, administered by the intraperitoneal route in patients with ovarian cancer. The interperitoneal concentration of drug is 21 times higher than the plasma concentration and dose of cisplatin up to 270 mg/kg have been given intraperitonealy without producing nephrotoxicity. Further work is being done by this group.

6. Summary and conclusions

At this point in time, there have been no major clinical improvements using the nitroimidazole sensitizers and thiol protectors for radiotherapy and chemotherapy. The toxicity of the previously used sensitizers, misonidazole and desmethylmisonidazole, have limited their use. SR-2508 which from animal data is predicted to be much less toxic is now undergoing a Phase I clinical trial. Since local failure is a problem with head and neck cancer, and since both external and interstitial radiotherapy are extremely important in treating head and neck tumors, the development of a good sensitizer would be very beneficial to these patients. It is expected that physicians involved with the treatment of these patients will be important participants in the clinical trials of the new sensitizers.

Clinical trials using WR-2721 as a radioprotector and chemoprotector, and employing MISO as a chemosensitizer are still early in development. Since radiotherapy can produce substantial morbidity in the head and neck area – dry mouth, ulceration, necrosis – a protector of normal tissues would improve the patients' long term functional results.

The current best chemotherapeutic agents for head and neck cancer are cisplatin, methotrexate and bleomycin. In animals, the nitroimidazoles sensitize only alkylating agents and nitrosoureas so the role of chemosensitizers in head and neck cancer chemotherapy may be limited. However, a great emphasis in chemoprotector research is on drugs that lessen cisplatin nephrotoxicity. Thus, head and neck patients will likely be involved in these clinical trials.

Although still early, the trials with these sensitizers and protectors are quite exciting. These new compounds, unlike other chemotherapeutic agents, are not active agents *per se* but rather modify the effect of active agents on both tumors and normal tissues. The study of these modifying drugs will not only potentially improve results of treatment but will add substantially to our knowledge of basic cancer biology. The ability to sensitize tumors while protecting normal tissues could greatly enhance the therapeutic ratio. This could be extremely useful particularly for patients with advanced head and neck cancers for whom current therapy can be quite morbid while providing only a modest rate of long term success.

Acknowledgements

The authors wish to thank Dr. Tony Howes for editorial assitance and Ms. Marge Keskin for secretarial assistance.

References

1. Fletcher GH, Lindberg RD, Caderao JB, Wharton JT: Hyperbaric oxygen as a radiotherapeutic adjuvant in advanced cancer of the uterine cervix. Preliminary results of a randomized trial. Cancer 39:617–623, 1977.
2. Fazekas JT, Sommer C, Kramer S: Adjuvant intravenous methotrexate or definitive radiotherapy alone for advanced squamous cancers of the oral cavity, oropharynx, supraglottic larynx or hypopharynx. Concluding report of an RTOG randomized trial on 638 patient. Int J Radiation Oncology Biol Phys 6:533–541, 1980.
3. Fletcher GH: Place of irradiation in the management of head and neck cancers. Semin Oncol 4:375–385, 1977.
4. Hoppe RT, Goffinet DR, Bagshaw MA: Carcinoma of the nasopharynx. Eighteen years experience with megavoltage radiation therapy. Cancer 37:2605–2612, 1976.
5. Rubin P, Cooper RA Jr (eds): Radiation Biology and Radiation Pathology Syllabus. Chicago, American College of Radiology, 1975, pp 207–216.
6. Fletcher GH: The third annual lectureship of the Juan A. Del Regato Foundation. Squamous cell carcinomas of the oropharynx. Int J Radiation Oncology Biol Phys 5:2075–2090, 1979.

7. Perez CA, Lee FA, Ackerman LV, Korba A, Purdy J, Powers WE: Carcinoma of the tonsillar fossa. significance of dose of irradiation and volume treated in the control of the primary tumor and matastatic neck nodes. Int J Radiation Oncology Biol Phys 1:817–827, 1976.
8. Weichselbaum RR, Schmit A, Little JB: Cellular repair factors influencing radiocurability of human malignant tumours. Br J Cancer 45:10–16, 1982.
9. Hall EJ: Radiobiology for the radiologist. 2nd edn. New York: Harper & Row, 1978, pp 3–12, 79–92.
10. Whithers HR, Peters LJ: In: Fletcher GH (ed) Textbook of Radiotherapy. Philadelphia: Lea & Febiger 1980, pp 103–148.
11. Denekamp J, Hirst DG, Stewart FA, Terry NHA: Is tumour radiosensitization by misonidazole a general phenomenon? Br J Cancer 41:1–9, 1980.
12. Ritter MA, Brown DQ, Glover DJ, Yuhas JM: In vitro studies on the absorption of WR-2721 by tumors and normal tissues. Int J Radiation Oncology Biol Phys 8:523–526, 1982.
13. Yuhas JM: On the potential application of radioprotective drugs in solid tumor radiotherapy. In: Sokol GH, Maickel RP (ed) Radiation-Drug Interactions in the Treatment of Cancer. New York: John Wiley & Sons, 1980, pp 113–135.
14. Yuhas JM, Spellman JM, Culo F: The role of WR-2721 in radiotherapy and/or chemotherapy. Cancer Clin Trials 3:211–216, 1980.
15. Henk JM: Does hyperbaric oxygen have a future in radiation therapy? Int J Radiation Oncology Biol Phys 7:1125–1128, 1981.
16. Henk JM, Kunkler PB, Smith CW: Radiotherapy and hyperbaric oxygen in head and neck cancer. Final report of first controlled clinical trial. Lancet 16:101–103, 1977.
17. Henk JM, Smith CW: Radiotherapy and hyperbaric oxygen in head and neck cancer. Interim report of second clinical trial. Lancet 16:104–105, 1977.
18. Sause WT, Plenk HP: Radiation therapy of head and neck tumors: A randomized study of treatment in air vs. treatment in hyperbaric oxygen. Int J Radiation Oncology Biol Phys 5:1833–1836, 1979.
19. Urtasun RC, Chapman JD, Band P, Rabin HR, Fryer CG, Sturmwind J: Phase I study of high-dose metronidazole: A specific in vivo and in vitro radiosensitizer of hypoxic cells. Radiology 117:129–133, 1975.
20. Frytak S, Moertel CG, Childs DS, Albers JW: Neurologic toxicity associated with high-dose metronidazole therapy. Ann Int Med 88:361–362, 1978.
21. Urtasun R, Band P, Chapman JD, Feldstein ML, Mielke B, Fryer C: Radiation and high-dose metronidazole in supratentorial glioblastomas. N Engl J Med 294:1364–1367, 1976.
22. Adams GE, Clarke ED, Flockhart IR, Jacobs RS, Sehmi DS, Stratford IJ, Wardman P, Watts ME: Structure-activity relationships in the development of hypoxic cell radiosensitizers. I. Sensitization efficiency. Int J Radiation Oncology Biol Phys 35:133–150, 1979.
23. Wasserman TH, Phillips TL, Johnson RJ, Gover CJ, Lawrence GA, Sadee W, Marques RA, Levin V, VanRaalte G: Initial clinical and pharmacologic evaluation of Misonidazole (ro-07-0582) an hypoxic cell radiosensitizer. Int J Radiation Oncology Biol Phys 5:775–786, 1979.
24. Dische S, Saunders MI, Flockhert IR, et al.: Misonidazole — A drug for trial in radiotherapy and oncology. Int J Radiation Oncology Biol Phys 5:851–860,. 1979.
25. Phillips TL, Wasserman TH, Johnson RJ, Levin VA, VanRaalte G: Final report on the United States phase I clinical trial of the hypoxic cell radiosensitizer, Misonidazole (Ro-07-0582; NSC #261037). Cancer 48:1697–1704, 1981.
26. Thomas GM, Rauth AM, Black RE, Cummings BJ, Norenti VL, Bush RS: A phase I study of misonidazole and pelvic irradiation in patients with carcinoma of cervix. Br J Cancer 45:860–868, 1982.
27. Schwade JG, Strong JM, Gangji D: I.V. Misonidazole (NSC 261037). Report of initial clin-

ical experience. In: Brady LW (ed) Radiation Sensitizers: Their use in the Clinical Management of Cancer. New York: Masson Publishing, 1980, pp 414–420.

28. Dische S: Hypoxic cell sensitisers in radiotherapy. Int J Radiation Oncology Biol Phys 4:157–160, 1978.

29. Ash DV, Smith MR, Bugden RD: Distribution of misonidazole in human tumours and normal tissues. Br J Cancer 39:503–509, 1979.

30. Gangji D, Schwade JG, Strong JM: Phenytoin-Misonidazole: Possible metabolic interaction. Cancer Treat Rep 64:155–156, 1980.

31. Walker MD, Strike TA: Misonidazole peripheral neuropathy. Its relationship to plasma concentration and other drugs. Cancer Clin Trials 3:105–109, 1980.

32. Fazekas JT, Goodman RL, McLean CJ: The value of adjuvant misonidazole in the definitive irradiation of advanced and neck squamous cancer: an RTOG pilot study (#78–02). Int J Radiation Oncology Biol Phys 7:1703–1708, 1981.

33. Wasserman TH, Stetz J, Phillips TL: Radiation Therapy Oncology Group clinical trials with misonidazole. Cancer 47:2382–2390, 1981.

34. Sealy R, Williams A, Cridland S, Stratford M, Minchinton A, Hallet C: A report on misonidazole in a randomized trial in locally advanced head and neck cancer. Int J Radiation Oncology Biol Phys 8:339–342, 1982.

35. Arcangeli G, Mauro F, Nervi C: Multiple daily fractionation (MDF) in association with misonidazole (MIS): A two-year experience with head and neck cancer. In: Breccia A, Kimondi C, Adams GE (eds) Advanced topics on radiosensitizers of hypoxic cells. Plenum Press, New York, 1982, pp 249–260.

36. Horiot JC, VanDenBogaert W, Ang KK, Chaplain G, VanDerSchueren E, Nabid A, Vessiere M: EORTC experience with misonidazole combined with multiple daily fractionated (MDF) radiotherapy. Proc of the European Society for Therapeutic Radiology and Oncology, June 1982.

37. VanDenBogaert W, VanDerSchueren E, Horiot JC, Chaplain G, Arcangeli G, Gonzalez D, Svoboda V: The feasibility of high-dose multiple daily fractionation and its combination with anoxic cell sensitizers in the treatment of head and neck cancer. Int J Radiation Oncology Biol Phys 8:1649–1655, 1982.

38. Henk Jm: Misonidazole: MRC trials – head and neck. Proc of the European Society for Therapeutic Radiology and Oncology, June 1982.

39. Bataini JP, Brunin F, AsselainB, Jaulerry C, Brugere J: Experience of using misonidazole in advanced head and neck cancer at the Institut Curie. Proc of the European Society for Therapeutic Radiology and Oncology, June 1982.

40. Overgaard J, Andersen AP, Jensen RH, Hjelm-Hansen M, Jorgensen K, Petersen M, Sandberg E, Sand-Hansen H: Misonidazole as an adjuvant to radiotherapy of carcinoma of the larynx and the pharynx – A preliminary report of the Danish head and neck cancer study. Proc of the European Society for Therapeutic Radiology and Oncology, June 1982.

41. Adams GE: Hypoxia-Mediated drugs for radiation and chemotherapy. Cancer 48:696–709, 1981.

42. Moulder JE: Dependence of misonidazole radiosensitization on drug and radiation schedules. Int J Radiation Oncology Biol Phys 8:75, 1982.

43. Brown JM: Clinical trials of radiosensitizers: What should we expect? Int J Radiation Oncology Biol Phys 10:475–479, 1984.

44. Brown JM, Lee WW: Pharmacokinetic considerations in radiosensitizer development. In: Bredy LW (ed) Radiation Sensitizers: Their Use in the Clinical Management of Cancer. New York: Masson Publishing, 1980, pp 2–13.

45. Brown JM, Workman P: Partition coefficient as a guide to the development of radiosensitizers which are less toxic than misonidazole. Radiat Res 82:171–190, 1980.

46. Brown JM: Clinical perspectives for the use of new hypoxic cell sensitizers. Int J Radiation Oncology Biol Phys 8:1491–1497, 1982.

47. Coleman CN, Wasserman TH, Phillips TL, *et al.*: Initial pharmacology and toxicology of intravenous desmethylmisonidazole. Int J Radiation Oncology Biol Phys 8:371-375, 1982.
48. Dische S, Saunders MI, Stratford MRL: Neurotoxicity with desmethylmisonidazole. Br J Radiol 1 54:156-157, 1981.
49. Wasserman TH, Coleman CN, Urtasun R, Phillips TL, Strong J: Final Report: Phase I trial of desmethylmisonidazole (DMM) – an hypoxic cell sensitizer. Int J Radiation Oncology Biol Phys 8:76, 1982.
50. Wasserman TH, Coleman Cn, Urtasun R, Phillips Tl, Nelson J, Von Gerichten D: Neuropathy of desmethylmisonidazole (DMM): Clinical and pathological description. Int J Radiation Oncology Biol Phys 8:77, 1982.
51. Dische S, Saunders MI, Riley PJ, Hauck J, Bennett MH, Stratford MRL, Minchinton AI: The concentration of desmethylmisonidazole in human tumours and in cerebrospinal fluid. Br J Cancer 43:344-349, 1981.
52. Chin JB, Rauth AM: The metabolism and pharmacokinetics of the hypoxic cell radiosensitizer and cytotoxic agent, misonidazole, in C3H mice. Radiation Res 86:341-357, 1981.
53. Born JL, Hadley WM, Anderson SL, Yuhas JM: Host and hypoxic cell toxicity studies with the terminal reduction product of misonidazole. In: Brady LW (ed) Radiation Sensitizers: Their Use in the Clinical Management of Cancer, New York: Masson Publishing, 1980, pp 79-82.
54. Stanulovic M: Metabolic and Drug-induced inactivation of vitamin B_6. In: Tryfiates GP (ed) Vitamin B_6 Metabolism and Role in Growth , Westport, Conn: Foods & Nutrition Press, Inc. 1980, pp 113-136.
55. Eifel PJ, Brown DM, Lee WW, Brown JM: Misonidazole neurotoxicity in mice decreased by administration with pyridoxine. Int J Radiation Oncology Biol Phys 9:1513-1519, 1983.
56. Williams MV, Chir B, Denekamp J, Minchinton AI, Stratford MRL: *In vivo* testing of a 2-nitroimidazole radiosensitizer (Ro 03-8799) using repeated administration. In: Sutherland RM (ed) Chemical Modification: Radiation and Cytotoxic Drugs. New York: Pergamon Press, 1982, p 593.
57. Stratford, Minchinton AI, Hill SA, McNally NJ, Williams MV, Chir B: Pharmacokinetic studies using multiple administration of RO 03-8799, A 2-nitroimidazole radiosensitizer. In: Sutherland RM (ed) Chemical Modification: Radiation and Cytotoxic Drugs. New York: Pergamon Press, 1982, p 469.
58. Saunders MI, Dische S, Fermont D, Bischop A, Lenox-Smith I, Allen JG, Malcolm SL: The radiosensitizer Ro-03-8799 and the concentrations which may be achieved in human tumours: A preliminary study. Br J Cancer 46:706-710, 1982.
59. Blumberg AL, Nelson DF, Gramkowski M, *et al.*: Clinical trials of WR2721 with radiation therapy. Int J Radiation Oncology Biol Phys 8:561-564, 1982.
60. Glick JH, Glover DJ, Weiler C, *et al.*: Phase I clinical trials of WR-2721 with alkylating agent chemotherapy. Int J Radiation Oncology Biol Phys 8:575-580, 1982.
61. Fahey RC, Dorian R, Utley JF: New Methods for analysis of WR-24721, WR-1065, and WR-33278. In: Conference on Chemical Modification: Radiation and Cytotoxic Drugs. Key Biscayne, FL, 107:81, 1981.
62. Yuhas JM, Spellman JM, Culo F: The role of WR-2721 in radiotherapy and/or chemotherapy. In: Brady LW (ed) Radiation Sensitizers: Their Use in the Clinical Management of Cancer. New York: Manor Publishing, 1980, pp 303-308.
63. Phillips TL: Rationale for initial clinical trials and future development of radioprotectors. Cancer Clin Trials 3:165-173, 1980.
64. Evans RG, Engel C, Wheatley C, Nielsen J: Modification of the sensitivity and repair of potentially lethal damage by diethyldithiocarbamate during and following exposure of plateau-Phase cultures of mammalian cells to radiation and cis-diamminedichloroplatinum (II). Cancer Res 42:3074-3078, 1982.

168

65. Rose CM, Millar JL, Peacock JH, Phelps TA, Stephens T: Differential enhancement of melphalan cytotoxicity in tumpour and normal tissue by misonidazole. In: Brady LW (ed) Radiation Sensitizers: Their Use in the Clinical Management of Cancer. New York: Manor Publishing, 1980, p 405.
66. McNally NJ: Enhancement of chemotherapy agents. In: Sutherland RM (ed) Chemical Modification: Radiation and Cytotoxic Drugs. New York: Pergamon Press, 1982, p 593.
67. Siemann DW: Potentiation of chemotherapy by hypoxic cell radiation sensitizers a review. Int J Radiation Oncology Biol Phys 8:1029–1034, 1982.
68. Brown JM, Hirst DG: The effect of clinically achievable exposure levels of misonidazole on the response of tumour and normal tissues in mouse to alkylating agents. Br J Cancer 45:700–708, 1982.
69. Nakatsugawa S, Sugahara T: Effects of inhibitors of radiation-induced potentially lethal damage repair on chemotherapy in murine tumors. Int J Radiation Oncology Biol Phys 8:1555–1559, 1982.
70. Weichselbaum RR, Little JB: Repair of potentially lethal × ray damage and possible applications to clinical radiotherapy. Int J Radiation Oncology Biol Phys 9:91–96, 1982.
71. Stratford IJ, Adams GE, Horsman MR, Kandaiya S, Rajaratnam S, Smith E, Williamson C: The interaction of misonidazole with radiation, chemotherapeutic agents or heat. A preliminary report. Cancer Clin Trials 3:231–236, 1980.
72. Taylor YC, Evans JW, Brown JM: Mechanism of sensitization of cells to melphalan by hypoxic treatment with misonidazole. Cancer Res 43:3175–3181, 1983.
73. Coleman CN, Friedman MK, Jacobs C, Halsey J, Ignoffo R, Leibel S, Hirst K, Gribble M, Carter SK, Phillips TL: Phase I trial of intravenous melphalan plus the sensitizer misonidazole. Cancer Res 1983 (in press).
74. Yuhas JM: Differential protection of normal and malignant tissues against the cytotoxic effects of mechlorethamine. Cancer Treat Rep 63:971–976, 1979.
75. Yuhas JM, Culo F: Selective inhibition of the nephrotoxicity of cis-dichlorodiammineplatinum (II) by WR-2721 without altering its antitumor properties. Cancer Treat Rep 64:57–64, 1980.
76. Shrieve DC, Harris JW: Protection against cis-dichlorodiammine pt (II) cytotoxicity in vitro by cysteamine. Int J Radiation Oncology Biol Phys 8:585–588, 1982.
77. Wasserman TH, Phillips sTL, Roxx G, Kane LJ: Differential protection against cytotoxic chemotherapeutic effects on bone marrow CFU's by WR-2721. Cancer Clin Trials 4:3–6, 1981.
78. Phillips TL, Yuhas JM, Wasserman TH: Differential protection against alkylating agent injury in tumors and normal tissues. In: Proc Natl Conference on Radioprotectors. Academic Press, 1983.
79. Howell SB, Pfeifle CL, Wung WE, Olshen RA, Lucas WE, Yon JL, Green M: Intraperitoneal cisplatin with systemic thiosulfate protection. Ann Int Med 97:845–851, 1982.
80. Howell SB, Pfeifle CE, Wung WE, Olshen RA: Intraperitoneal cis-diamminedichloroplatinum with systemic thiosulfate protection. Cancer Res 43:1426–1431, 1983.

8. The role of radiotherapy in the treatment of neck metastases from head and neck cancer

NEMETALLAH A. GHOSSEIN and PIERRE BATAINI

1. Introduction

Anyone who attempts to familiarize himself with the voluminous literature on head and neck cancer will soon realize that there is a lack of uniformity in the treatment policies for patients with metastatic neck nodes secondary to squamous cell carcinoma. This is due mainly to the fact that the treatment methods are based on the philosophy and experience of the team leader involved in the management of these patients. Evidently, the management of neck nodes should depend primarily on the location and stage of the primary lesion, the extent of the neck disease, and the age and medical condition of the patient. In many centers, neck dissection for either clinically obvious or occult metastasis remains the accepted policy; reserving ratiation therapy for the surgical failures.

Conventional radiotherapy that was used in the pre-megavoltage era, until the mid-fifties, has already proven its value in the control of neck metastasis. In a series of 534 carcinomas of the tonisllar region, treated from 1920 to 1948 at the Institut Curie in Paris, failure in the neck occurred in only 30 patients [1]. Also, tissue doses of the order of 4000–4500 rad given in 5–6 weeks proved their values in the 30's and 40's [2] in preventing nodal metastasis in clinically negative necks, setting the stage for the routine elective neck irradiation of patients who are at high risk of having subclinical or occult disease. It was not until the introduction of megavoltage irradiation (Cobalt 60, linear accelerator) and the convincing and excellent work of Dr. Gilbert Fletcher and his team at the M.D. Hospital and Tumor Institute in Houston, that the notion of elective irradiation for subclinical disease became well established [3–6]. In fact, recurrence in the neck from squamous cell carcinoma of the nasopharynx, tonsil and faucial arch, supraglottic larynx, and base of tongue, dropped to less than 2% from an expected incidence of 25–30% following elective treatment to the whole neck with doses of the order of 5000–5500 rad in 5–5½ weeks.

Gregory T. Wolf (ed), Head and Neck Oncology.
© *1984 Martinus Nijhoff Publishers, Boston. ISBN 0-89838-657-8. Printed in The Netherlands.*

The association of pre- or post-operative irradiation with radical neck dissection, for either occult or obvious neck disease, became necessary following the publication of surgical series showing the high incidence of homolateral or contralateral neck recurrences when nodal metastases were present in the pathological specimen [7]. As an example, in the Memorial Hospital series [8], a moderate dose of 2000 rad given in 5 fractions preoperatively to the neck, lowered the incidence of neck disease from 28.7% for patients who had surgery only, to 17.6% for those who had irradiation preoperatively and who had their primary lesion controlled. A more dramatic decrease in neck recurrences was obtained at the M.D. Anderson Hospital with doses of at least 5000 rad delivered either pre- or post-operatively. The recurrence rate dropped from 25.6% with surgery only, to 7.6% with the combined treatment [9]. Interestingly, pathologically negative nodes in patients who were treated with surgery only did not mean that these patients were not at risk of developing neck recurrences. In our own series of patients with cancer of the oral tongue [10], as well as that of the Memorial Hospital [8], 7% of those with pathologically negative nodes developed neck recurrences when surgery only was performed, whereas no patient who received preoperative irradiation and had histologically negative nodes developed neck disease. However, the incidence of recurrence following surgery alone is low enough to advise against routine post-operative irradiation in patients with negative specimens. Post-operative irradiation, becomes mandatory when major nodal involvement (>3 nodes positive, or invasion of the nodal capsule (R+), or the presence of nodal involvement at multiple levels) is present. These patients not only have a high incidence of failure (up to 70%) in the neck, but also their survival rate is lower [10, 11].

In order to define prognostic parameters for patients with metastatic neck disease, Cachin and his team at Gustave Roussy, have done extensive histological studies on a large number of radical neck specimens [12-15]. They found that capsular invasion (R+) was an indication of great tumor virulence and a most ominous finding in determining both local recurrence and long-term prognosis. Capsular invasion, that was associated with lowered survival by a factor of 2, was noted in half of those patients who had histologically positive nodes and in almost all N_3 cases. It was directly proportional to nodal size. At least 75% of nodes measuring 4–5 cm had invasion of the capsule. However, capsular invasion may also be present with nodes less than 1 cm.

In patients found to have capsular invasion, the classical post-operative dose of 5000 rad in 5 weeks will not prove sufficient to prevent neck recurrences. An additional dose of 1500–2000 rad should be delivered to the area of the neck where the capsule has been broken. It must be kept in mind that these high doses may cause important sequalae in an already dissected neck.

One of the controversial issues in head and neck oncology is the ability of radical radiotherapy to control clinically positive nodes. At the Institut Curie, in Paris, it has been the practice since 1958, to treat cancer of the oropharynx, nasopharynx, hypopharynx and supraglottic larynx, including nodal metastasis, by radical radiotherapy [16]. It is apparent that failures in the neck following irradiation of palpable nodes depend mainly on the location or origin of the primary tumor, the presence or absence of recurrence at the primary site, the possibility of delivering high radiation doses to the neck disease with an acceptable rate of complication, and the presence or absence of persistent adenopathy 6–12 weeks following radical irradiation [17, 18]. It is important to take into strong consideration the willingness of the surgeon to perform salvage neck surgery on radically irradiated nodes if the need arises. Although radical neck surgery following moderate preoperative radiation doses, may be performed with relative ease, salvage surgery following radical nodal irradiation, with doses of up to 7500–8500 rad, may be difficult and should only be performed by an experienced surgical team; otherwise the complication rate may be prohibitive [18].

2. Staging of neck disease

In the present study we have followed the UICC classification of 1973 [19] which is similar to the updated classification of the UICC, 1982 [20].

N_0 – Regional lymph nodes not palpable.
N_1 – Movable homolateral nodes.
   N_1a: Nodes not considered to contain growth.
   N_1b: Nodes considered to contain growth.
N_2 – Movable contralateral or bilateral nodes.
   N_2a: Nodes not considered to contain growth.
   N_2b: Nodes considered to contain growth.
N_3 – Fixed nodes unilateral or bilateral.

3. Management of patients with clinically negative nodes (N_0 stage)

The incidence of neck metastasis from squamous cell carcinoma of the head and neck has been recently reviewed at the Institut Curie [21, 22]. Patients with cancer of the lip, paranasal sinuses, or intrinsic larynx were not included, since nodal metastases are infrequently present at the time of initial presentation, (Table 1). Forty-five percent of patients had no palpable neck disease. The highest incidence of clinically negative necks was observed in patients with cancer of the oral tongue (64%). The lowest, as expected, in patients with nasopharyngeal (25%) and pyriform sinus carcinoma (28%).

It is now well established that 30–40% of patients with clinically negative necks do have occult metastasis on pathological examination of the radical neck specimen if surgery is performed without preoperative irradiation [7, 10, 23, 24]. Likewise, a similar number of patients with N_0 stage will present with neck metastasis at a later date if no treatment is applied to the neck [17, 25]. Because of this relatively high incidence of occult metastasis in the nodes the concept of elective neck irradiation is becoming widely accepted.

Occult metastasis essentially means that there is a relatively small number of clonogenic cancer cells in aggregates not exceeding 10^6 cells deposited in the lymph nodes. These cells are usually well oxygenated if no previous radical neck surgery was done and will require only a moderate radiation dose – of the order of 5000–5500 rad in $5-5\frac{1}{2}$ weeks – to be sterilized. These doses are well within the tolerance of the normal tissues of the neck if judicious techniques using megavoltage radiation (Cobalt 60, or 4–6 MEV accelerator) are employed. Obviously, a much larger number of viable cancer cells exists when palpable neck masses are present and in these cases definitely higher doses, of 7500 rad or more are needed to obtain sterilization [26–28].

There is evidence that the incidence of distant metastasis is increased if the cancer is not controlled in the neck [5, 24, 29] and that the 5 year survival is definitely better if there is no nodal recurrence [30, 31]. Thus the

Table 1. Squamous cell carcinoma of the head and neck; frequency of clinical neck disease at time of presentation according to primary site

Sites	Number of patients	Neck clinically	
		Negative	Positive
Oral tongue	602	383 (64%)	219 (36%)
Floor of mouth	490	253 (52%)	237 (48%)
Tonsil and faucial arch	661	274 (41%)	387 (59%)
Base of tongue (glosso-epiglottic)	359	117 (33%)	242 (67%)
Supraglottic larynx	218	115 (53%)	103 (47%)
Pyriform sinus (hypopharynx)	434	123 (28%)	311 (72%)
Marginal or lateral epilarynx	157	69 (44%)	88 (56%)
Nasopharynx	104	26 (25%)	78 (75%)
Totals	3025	1360 (45%)	1665 (55%)

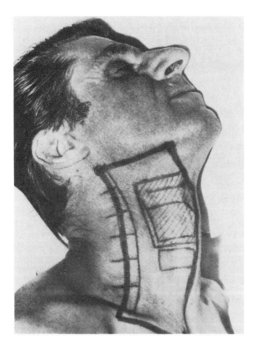

Figure 1. Treatment fields used for irradiation of N_0 stage supraglottic cancer. The thick line demonstrates the initial field used to deliver 5000 rads. The hatched area outlines the coned down portal to which an additional 1500–3000 rads is given to the primary lesion.
Reproduced by permission of Cancer, 1974 [36].

rationale for elective irradiation is to prevent neck recurrence and to diminish the occurrence of distant disease.

3.1. Treatment of N_0 neck for primaries other than oral cavity cancers

The incidence of nodal recurrence in patients with N_0 stage who received primarily, as a definitive form of treatment, routine elective whole neck irradiation to a dose of 5000 rad with high risk areas boosted to 5500 rad was examined (Fig. 1). Patients with oral cancer were excluded since surgery to the neck was often combined with radiotherapy in these instances. The result is shown in Table 2. Of the 724 patients studied, only 13 (1.8%) recurred in the neck when the primary lesion was controlled. When one considers neck recurrence in patients with uncontrolled cancer at the primary site, this incidence is double.

Our results, as well as those of others [5, 6] have demonstrated that elective neck irradiation for N_0 stage patients with cancer of the nasopharynx, base of tongue, tonsil and faucial arch, supraglottic larynx, and hypopharynx is extremely effective and resulted in less than 2% neck failure. Certainly,

174

prophylactic neck dissection for cancers originating at these sites is unjustified unless there are technical reasons preventing proper neck irradiation.

3.2. Treatment of N_0 stage in patients with oral cancer (mobile tongue and floor of mouth)

There is no general agreement regarding the use of prophylactic irradiation as the only treatment to the neck in patients with N_0 stage in cancers of the mobile tongue and floor of mouth. We consider the combination of radical neck dissection with pre- or post-operative irradiation, still to be the treatment of choice since the failure rate in the neck with radiotherapy only is significantly higher than the 2% reported above. Oral carcinomas are usually well differentiated and believed to be difficult to sterilize with the moderate radiation doses delivered in elective neck irradiation. Our policy has been, if the primary lesion is relatively small (T_1, T_2), to perform radical neck dissection following treatment of the primary lesion which is usually done using interstitial implantation. Patients who have >3 positive nodes or capsular involvement (R+) receive 5000 rad to the entire neck post-operatively and a boost of 1000–1500 rad to the area of the neck where the capsule has been broken. If the nodes are negative or minimally involved (≤ 3) and the capsule is intact (R−), no post-operative irradiation is given. Patients with large primary lesions receive either whole neck irradiation only, or preoperative neck irradiation followed by radical neck dissection, depending on the condition of the patient and response of the primary lesion.

Table 2. Site of failure for patients who received neck irradiation as primary treatment for N_0 stage* (minimum follow-up two years)

Sites	Number of patients	Failure in node only	Failure in primary and nodes
Tonsil and faucial arch	274	3 (1%)	9 (3%)
Base of tongue (glosso-epiglottic)	117	3 (2%)	9 (7.6%)
Pyriform sinus	123	3 (2.4%)	6 (5%)
Marginal or lateral epilarynx	69	3 (4%)	0 (−)
Supraglottic larynx	115	1 (1%)	7 (6%)
Nasopharynx	26	0 (−)	0 (−)
Total	724	13 (1.8%)	31 (4%)

* Excluding oral cavity.
Modified from Bataini JP et al. [21].

Recently the records of 315 patients with cancer of the oral tongue who had N_0 stage tumors were examined [10]. Two hundred and forty-four had neck dissection without preoperative irradiation. The findings are shown in Table 3. Sixty-six percent (160/244) had pathologically negative nodes and did not receive post-operative irradiation. Seven percent (11/160) developed neck recurrence; an incidence identical to that reported by Strong [8]. Thirty-four percent (84/244) had metastatic deposit in the nodes. Interestingly about 40% of those (33/84) with pathologically involved nodes had major nodal involvement (>3 N+ or R+). Although this group of patients was given post-operative irradiation the recurrence in the homolateral neck was relatively high (21%). This incidence, however, is definitely better than the 70% incidence of neck recurrences reported for patients who had surgery only and who were found to have positive nodes at multiple levels [8].

Sixty percent (51/84) of those patients with positive specimens had minimal nodal involvement (≤ 3 n+ and R−). These patients did not receive post-operative irradiation and 14% (7/51) experienced recurrences. Post-operative radiotherapy was not given to this group of patients since it was found that the incidence of local recurrence and survival was similar to those patients who had pathologically negative nodes [10]. Radiotherapy, therefore, was reserved for the not uncommon event that another primary cancer developed, that would require a radical radiotherapy course.

Of the 315 patients analyzed with N_0 stage tumors, 50 received neck irradiation only and 21 received preoperative irradiation followed by neck dissection. The incidence of neck recurrence in these patients is shown in

Table 3. Cancer of the oral tongue. Recurrence in neck alone in patients who initially had radical neck dissection with or without post-operative radiotherapy for a clinically negative neck (N_0) (minimum follow-up 2 years)

		Recurrence in neck only	
No. of patients	244		
Specimen negative	160/244 (66%)	11/160 (7%)	
Specimen positive	84/244 (34%)		25/244 (10%)
≤3N+ or R-ve[1] (No post-op RT)	51/84 (61%)	P* 7/51 (14%)	
>3N+ or R+ve[2] (post-op RT given)	33/84 (39%)	P* 7/33 (21%)	

* P = Not significant.
[1] R-ve = No capsular invasion.
[2] R+ve = Capsule is invaded.
Modified from Decroix Y and Ghossein NA [10].

Table 4. Fourteen percent (7/50) of those who had irradiation only developed neck recurrences. This incidence is definitely higher than the 2% observed for patients with head and neck cancer at sites other than the oral cavity and who received radiotherapy alone for an N_0 neck. The best group appears to be those patients who had preoperative neck irradiation followed by neck dissection. Only 5% (1/21) failed in the neck.

It has been shown, in a very small group of patients [32], that prophylactic neck irradiation alone is highly effective in controlling subclinical disease from oral tongue and floor of mouth primary tumors. This has not been our experience. Also, in a recent analysis of the results of elective neck irradiation for N_0 stage in 146 patients with squamous cell carcinoma of the oral tongue treated at the M.D. Anderson Hospital, Meor et al. [33] noted a neck recurrence rate of 33% for patients who had 2000 rad in 5 fractions. The recurrence rate was 16.6% for those patients who had the conventional 5000 rad to the upper neck by bilateral portals. This latter incidence is identical to that observed in our patients.

The reason for the discrepancy between the very low incidence of neck recurrences, following prophylactic irradiation of patients with primaries at sites other than the oral cavity and the relatively high incidence of neck disease for those treated for an oral cancer, is not apparent. As stated previously, one explanation may be that nodal deposits from well differentiated squamous cell carcinomas are usually more radio resistant and require higher doses than the 5000 rad conventionally given to the neck electively.

The policy for patients with small primary tumors (≤ 3 cm), and who therefore have a high chance of being controlled at the primary site, is to perform a conservative elective radical neck dissection with preservation of the sternocleidomastoid muscle and the jugular vein. Post-operative irradiation is only given in the presence of major nodal involvement. Those with a large primary tumor and who, therefore, have a high incidence of failure at the primary site receive electively 5500 rad in $5-5\frac{1}{2}$ weeks to the upper neck and 5000 rad to the lower neck without elective neck dissection. The reason

Table 4. Cancer of oral tongue. Recurrence in neck only in patients who had elective neck irradiation with or without neck dissection for N_0 stage (minimum follow-up two years)

	No. of patients	Number of recurrences in neck
Neck irradiation only	50	7 (14%)
Pre-op irradiation and neck dissection	21	1 (5%)

Modified from Decroix Y and Ghossein NA [10].

for not performing elective surgery is that salvage surgery, in the form of a composite resection, is often required at a later date.

In summary, patients with clinically negative neck (N_0 stage) who have a primary tumor located at a site other than the oral cavity should be treated primarily by elective neck irradiation, since moderate doses control the sub-clinical nodal disease in over 95% of these patients. Radical neck dissection is reserved for the unlikely event that there is tumor recurrence in the neck. Patients with cancer of the oral cavity have a definitely higher incidence of neck failure if treated by radiotherapy only. Therefore, the combination of radical neck surgery and radiotherapy is required and should be performed whenever possible.

4. Management of patients with clinically involved nodes (stage $N_1 b$, $N_2 b$, N_3)

In our present material of over 3000 cases, 55% of all patients with squamous cell carcinoma of the head and neck presented initially with cervical adenopathy. The frequency of neck metastasis is closely related to the site of the primary tumor (Table 1). For example, it is 36% in oral tongue cancer, but 75% in nasopharyngeal carcinoma. The frequency and location of neck disease according to the site of the primary has been extensively studied by other authors [34, 35] and need not be reviewed here.

Fine needle aspiration for cytological confirmation of nodal involvement was performed on those patients with $N_1 b$ and $N_2 b$ disease. Pathological involvement of the node was proven in about 75% of patients with carcinoma of the supraglottic larynx [36] and in almost 90% of those with hypopharyngeal cancer [28]. These findings are indicative of the high incidence of malignant involvement when a node is clinically palpable.

In the early 30's Regaud, at the Institute Curie [37] and later Baclesse, attempted to treat neck nodes with orthovoltage irradiation. Later on, radium needles and radon seeds were used either alone [38], or in combination with external irradiation [39, 40] to increase the local doses and to achieve better local control. It was not until the introduction of megavoltage in the mid 50's, that systematic attempts were made to control obvious neck disease with radical radiotherapy. The doses that are required are much higher than those used to control subclinical disease. Cobalt 60 gamma rays, and 4–6 MEV x-rays have the optimal energy to deliver a high radiation dose to the cervical nodes and at the same time have sufficient skin sparing effects. Also, electron beam therapy was found to be very useful in treating nodes and sparing the deeper structures such as the spinal cord.

At the Institut Curie, the treatment of cervical adenopathy has traditionally been with radical radiotherapy; the exception being metastases secondary to oral cancer where neck disease has been managed by either surgery alone or a combination of surgery and radiotherapy.

For the purpose of the present study we have reviewed the results obtained in over 1000 patients with clinically positive neck nodes treated primarily by radiotherapy.

4.1. Cervical adenopathies secondary to nasopharyngeal cancer

These adenopathies are radiosensitive and a high degree of control can be achieved by irradiation. In a series of 104 patients [41], 78 (75%) presented with cervical nodal metastasis. All were treated by radical irradiation. The results are shown in Table 5. Three patients (4%) required salvage surgery at 3, 8, and 12 months, respectively following radiotherapy. The pathological specimens were positive in only one instance. Uncontrolled neck disease was encountered in only 1 patient who also had uncontrolled disease at the primary site and distant metastasis. It is apparent that carcinomas of the nasopharynx, which are often poorly differentiated, are radiocurable and that the result of nodal irradiation is sufficiently satisfactory that neck surgery need be performed in only the rare instances where palpable neck nodes persist for at least 6 months after radiotherapy. It is common policy to treat the entire neck bilaterally to a dose of 5000 rad in 5 weeks, taking care to shield the spinal cord after a dose of 4000–4500 rad has been delivered. An additional dose of 1500–2500 rad is usually given to the nodal volume using shrinking tangential portals or electron beam (Fig. 2).

4.2. Cervical adenopathies secondary to cancer of the oropharynx (tonsils, faucial arch, and base of tongue)

Three hundred and eighty-seven of the 671 (59%) patients with cancer of the tonsil and faucial arch had clinically positive neck nodes at the time of presentation. Of the 359 patients with base of tongue carcinoma, 242 (67%) had neck involvement. In the majority of patients, their adenopathy was located in the upper neck at the same level as the primary disease. Of necessity, these adenopathies were included within the treatment portals covering the primary cancer and thus received a dose of at least 6500 rad. A booster dose of 1000–2500 rad was usually delivered to the nodal remnant; examples are shown in Figs. 3 and 4.

With radical radiotherapy, isolated neck failure was rare and was less than 10%, even when there were fixed nodes (N_3) (Table 6). There was a much higher incidence of neck failure (approximately 20%) when the primary disease was not controlled.

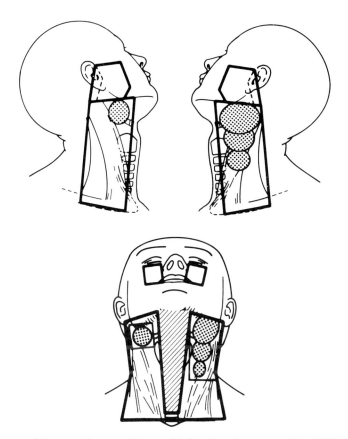

Figure 2. Cancer of the nasopharynx. 64-year-old female, who presented in 1959 with T_4N_3 stage. Received 2500 rad TD to the entire neck by lateral, and 2000 rad by anterior portals with midline shielding. The nodes were boosted by reduced tangential fields to bring the total dose to 7200 rad in 7½ weeks. Patient was NED in 1977 with no radiation sequalae.

Table 5. Nasopharyngeal carcinoma. Results of radiotherapy in controlling cervical adenopathy (stage N_1b, N_2b, N_3) (minimum follow up two years)

Total number of patients with cervical adenopathy	78/104 (75%)
Complete regression of nodes at end of radiotherapy	67/78 (86%)
Delayed clinical disappearance [1]	7/78 (9%)
Secondary nodal surgery [2]	3/78 (4%)
Specimen pathologically negative	2/3
Specimen pathologically positive	1/3
Nodal failure (with active primary and distant metastasis)	1/78 (1%)

[1] Between 3 and 15 months – average 6 months.
[2] At 3, 8, and 12 months following radiotherapy.
Modified from Brugére J *et al.* [41].

180

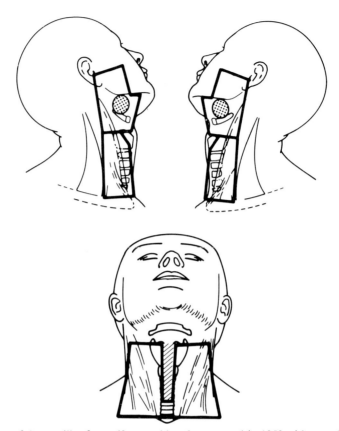

Figure 3. Cancer of the tonsillar fossa. 62-year-old male presented in 1958 with stage T_3N_2b of the right tonsil. The cervical adenopathies were included in the same portal as the primary lesion and received an estimated dose of 7000 rad in 5 weeks with reduced portals. The lower neck received a dose of 1500 rad by lateral portals and 4000 rad by anterior portals for a total given dose of 5500 rad. Patient was NED in 1975 with no radiation sequalae.

Table 6. Results of radical radiotherapy of cervical adenopathy secondary to squamous cell carcinoma of the oropharynx. Nodal failure in relation to initial stage (minimum follow-up two years)

Sites	Stage	No. of patients	Failure in node only	Failure in primary and nodes
Tonsil and faucial arch	N_1b, N_2b	172	12 (7%)	15 (9%)
	N_3	215	20 (9%)	50 (23%)
Total		387	32 (8%)	65 (17%)c
Base of tongue	N_1b, N_2b	128	4 (3%)	25 (19.5%)
(glosso-epiglottic)	N_3	114	7 (7%)	24 (21%)
Total		242	11 (5%)	49 (20%)

Modified from Bataini JP *et al.* [21].

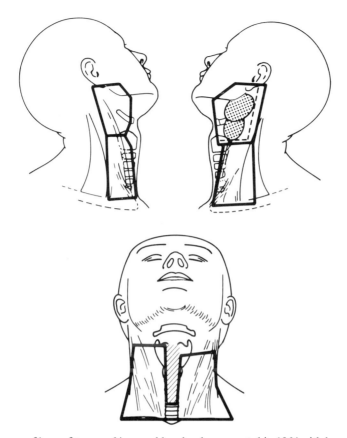

Figure 4. Cancer of base of tongue. 64-year-old male who presented in 1964 with large fixed neck nodes (N$_3$) from a T$_2$ lesion of base of tongue. The treatment portals to the primary lesion included the neck nodes and delivered 7500 rad in 7$\frac{1}{2}$ weeks. The portal was reduced (dotted lines) after a dose of 6700 rad had been delivered and a total dose of 8000 rad was given to the nodes. The left lower neck received 6400 rad (3000 bilateral and 3400 by anterior portals). The right lower neck received 5000 rad. The patient was NED in 1975. He had a moderate degree of subcutaneous fibrosis in the left upper neck.

4.3. Cervical adenopathies secondary to carcinoma of the supraglottic larynx, pyriform sinus, and marginal or lateral epilarynx

The incidence of palpable nodes from these cancers varied from 47% for primary tumors of the supraglottic larynx to 72% for the pyriform sinus. The entire neck was routinely irradiated to a dose of 4600–5000 rad with an additional booster dose of 2000–3000 rad delivered to palpable nodes (Figs. 5 and 6).

The rate of neck failure following radical radiotherapy in relation to the initial stage and site of the primary lesion is shown in Table 7. Again, it is noted that isolated neck failure occurred rarely, and in only about 10% of patients.

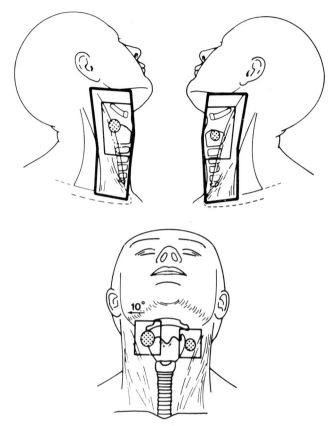

Figure 5. Supraglottic larynx. 30-year-old female with T_2N_2b stage, treated in 1965. The entire neck received 4000 rad by lateral portals. The fields were then reduced and an additional dose of 3000 rad was given. The nodes received further treatment by anterior reduced portals angled 10° laterally to avoid the midline structures. The left node received a total of 8000 rad and the right node a dose of 8500 rad. The patient was NED in 1982 with slight subcutaneous fibrosis in the right upper neck.

4.4. Overall results of radical neck irradiation for cervical adenopathies excluding metastasis from oral cancers

It has been our experience, as well as that of others, that recurrences in the neck following radiotherapy for cervical adenopathies secondary to squamous cell carcinoma of the oropharynx, nasopharynx, hypopharynx, and supraglottic larynx, are rare if the nodes are mobile and if an adequate radiation dose is given [5, 17, 42, 43]. The widely held belief in most centers, that nodal metastasis are neither radiosensitive nor radiocurable, as compared to the primary lesion, is not justified. This belief is certainly the cause for relying almost entirely on surgery (except for adenopathies secondary to nasopharyngeal cancer), for the treatment of cervical metastases. Of 584 patients who received radical neck irradiation for stage N_1b, N_2b, and

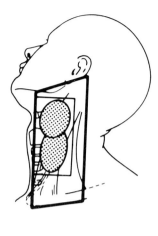
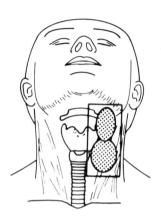

Figure 6. Cancer of epilarynx. 66-year-old male presented in 1961 with stage T_1N_3. Received by lateral opposing portals, to the entire neck, 4400 rad. The fields were then reduced and an additional 2000 rad was given. Treatment to the node was continued by an anterior portal until a total dose of 8000 rad was administered in 7 weeks. He died in 1967, following cholecystectomy and was free of cancer. He had slight fibrosis in the left upper neck.

Table 7. Results of radical radiotherapy of cervical adenopathy secondary to squamous cell carcinoma of supraglottic larynx, pyriform sinus, and marginal or lateral epilarynx. Nodal failure in relation to initial stage (minimum follow-up two years)

Site	Stage	No. of patients	Failure in node only	Failure in primary and nodes
Supraglottix larynx (36)	N_1b, N_2b	84	4 (5%)	10 (12%)
	N_3	19	4 (21%)	6 (31%)
Total		103	8 (8%)	16 (16%)
Pyriform sinus (28)	N_1b, N_2b	135	13 (10%)	17 (12%)
	N_3	176	24 (14%)	47 (27%)
Total		311	37 (12%)	64 (21%)
Marginal or lateral epilarynx [21]	N_1b, N_2b	37	2 (5%)	3 (8%)
	N_3	51	7 (14%)	13 (25%)
Total		88	9 (10%)	16 (18%)

who had a minimum follow up of two years, only 35 (6%) failed in the neck alone. In 625 patients with fixed nodes (N_3), the local control was 90% (Tables 8 and 9). The failure rate was at least double when the primary disease was not controlled. We considered two years as an adequate period of follow up, since very few recurrences are seen in a previously irradiated area more than two years after radiotherapy.

4.5. Cervical adenopathies secondary to cancer of the oral cavity

It is commonly accepted that adenopathies secondary to squamous cell carcinoma of the oral cavity are difficult to sterilize by radiotherapy alone and

Table 8. Overall results of radical radiotherapy for mobile unilateral or bilateral neck nodes (N_1b and N_2b), excluding oral cancers (minimum follow-up two years)

Sites	Number of patients	Failure in node only	Failure in primary + nodes
Tonsil and faucial arch	172	12 (7%)	15 (8%)
Base of tongue (glosso-epiglottic)	128	4 (3%)	25 (19.5%)
Pyriform sinus	135	13 (10%)	17 (12.5%)
Marginal or lateral epilarynx	37	2 (5%)	3 (8%)
Supraglottic larynx	84	4 (5%	10 (12%)
Nasopharynx	28	0 (−)	0 (−)
Total	584	35 (6%)	70 (12%)

Modified from Bataini JP et al. [21].

Table 9. Overall results of radical radiotherapy for fixed neck nodes (N_3) excluding oral cancers (minimum follow-up two years)

Sites	Number of patients	Failure in node only	Failure in primary and nodes
Tonsil and faucial arch	215	20 (9%)	50 (23%)
Base of tongue (glosso-epiglottic)	114	7 (7%)	24 (21%)
Pyriform Sinus	176	24 (13.6%)	47 (27%)
Marginal or Lateral epilarynx	51	7 (13.7%)	13 (25%)
Supraglottic larynx	19	4 (21%)	6 (31.5%)
Nasopharynx	50	0 (−)	1 (2%)
Total	625	62 (10%)	143 (23%)

Modified from Bataini JP et al. [21].

require neck surgery, either alone, or in combination with radiotherapy to obtain maximum local control.

Of the 602 patients with cancer of the oral tongue, treated at the Institut Curie between 1959 and 1972, 219 (36%) presented with clinically positive neck nodes [22]. Seventy-five percent of these patients had tumors staged as N_1b. Two hundred and sixty-seven of 490 patients (48%) with floor of mouth carcinoma likewise had positive neck nodes; 55% being classified N_1b [44]. As outlined previously in this chapter, it has been our policy to combine surgery and radiotherapy in the treatment of neck disease from oral cancers.

In our recent review of cancer of the oral tongue [10], 101 patients initially had a radical neck dissection followed by post-operative radiotherapy if there was major nodal involvement (>3 N+ or R+). Thirty-seven patients had negative specimens, and 8% of these patients developed neck recurrences. Of the 64 patients with positive specimens, 27 (41%) had major

Table 10. Cancer of oral tongue. Recurrence in neck alone in patients who had radical neck dissection initially for clinically positive nodes (minimum follow-up two years)

		Recurrence in neck only	
No. of patients	101		
Specimen negative	37/101 (37%)	3/37 (8%)	
Specimen positive	64/101 (63%)		11/101 (11%)
≤3N+ or R-ve [1] (No post-op RT)	37/64 (58%)	2/37 (5%)	
>3N+ or R+ve [2] (Post-op RT given)	27/64 (42%)	6/27 (22%)	

[1] R-ve = No capsular invasion.
[2] R+ve = Capsule is invaded.
Modified from Decroix Y and Ghossein NA [10].

Table 11. Cancer of oral tongue. Recurrence in neck alone in patients who had preoperative whole neck irradiation and radical neck dissection for clinically positive nodes (minimum follow up two years)

		Recurrence in neck only	
No. of patients	9		
Specimen negative	4/19 (21%)	0/4 (−)	
Specimen positive	15/19 (79%)		3/19 (16%)
≤3N+ or R-ve [1]	9/19 (47%)	1/9 (−)	
>3N+ or R+ve [2]	6/19 (32%)	2/6 (−)	

[1] R-ve = No capsular invasion.
[2] R+ve = Capsule is invaded.
Modified from Decroix Y and Ghossein NA [10].

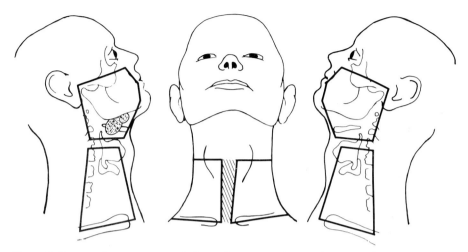

Figure 7. Preoperative treatment techniques for cancer of the oral tongue with cervical adenopathies. The primary lesion, including the upper neck (to the upper level of thyroid cartilage) receive, by lateral portals, a tumor dose of 5000–5500 rad in 5 to 5½ weeks. The lower neck is given a dose of 5000 rad (1500 by lateral portals and 3500 by anterior portals with midline shielding). A complete ipsilateral block dissection and a contralateral suprahyoid, which is completed to whole neck dissection if the subdigastric nodes are positive on frozen section, are usually performed 5–6 weeks after radiotherapy.

nodal involvement. Approximately 25% of these patients subsequently recurred in the neck. The recurrence rate in the neck for those patients with minimal nodal involvement was similar to those with a histologically negative specimen (5% vs. 8%) (Table 10).

Patients with locally advanced neck disease received 5000–5500 rad preoperatively to the neck. Results in this group are shown in Table 11. Despite the fact that these patients initially had more advanced neck disease, the incidence of recurrence was similar to the overall recurrence rate in the

Table 12. Overall results of treatment of cervical adenopathy secondary to squamous cell carcinoma of oral cavity (minimum follow-up two years)

Site	Stage	No. of patients	Failure in node only	Failure in primary and nodes
Oral tongue (22)	N_1b	164	18 (11%)	25 (15%)
	N_2b, N_3	55	5 (9%)	3 (6%)
Total		219	23 (11%)	28 (13%)
Floor of mouth (44)	N_1b	148	14 (10%)	22 (15%)
	N_2b, N_3	89	17 (19%)	13 (15%)
Total		237	31 (13%)	35 (15%)

group with lesser neck disease and who had surgery initially (16% vs. 11%).

Because of these results, and because a significant number of patients with clinically obvious neck diseases will ultimately be found to have major nodal involvement on historical examination, we have adopted a treatment policy of giving routine preoperative irradiation to the entire neck followed by radical neck dissection 5–6 weeks later (Fig. 7). The same policy is applied for cancers of the floor of mouth and other squamous cell carcinomas of the oral cavity. The overall results of our treatment of neck adenopathies in 456 patients with oral cancer, using mostly the combined modality demonstrates a failure rate in the neck alone of about 12% (Table 12).

5. Factors influencing the control of nodal metastases by radiation

In order to treat nodal disease with radiotherapy, a sufficiently high dose must be delivered to avoid unacceptably high recurrence rates.

Several factors influence the control of neck metastases by irradiation:

(1) The site of the primary tumor that may determine the inherent radiosensitivity of the metastasis.
(2) The nodal volume.
(3) The number of nodes and whether bilateral or unilateral.
(4) The rate of regression of the node during irradiation.
(5) The location of the node in relation to vital structures in the neck.
(6) The availability of sophisticated equipment and techniques (MegaVoltage, Electron beam, interstitial implant, etc.).

Table 13. Supraglottic carcinoma. Control of nodes according to size and given dose in patients with controlled primary site*

Dose in rad	Nodal size		
	2.5 cm	2.5–5.0 cm	5.0 cm
≤7000	7/7	1/1	—
7000–8700	18/18	—	—
8800–10,600	12/12	6/9	1/1
>10,600	1/1	1/2	1/3
Total	38/38 (100%)	8/12 (66.6%)	2/4

* Reproduced with slight modification by permission of Radiology [27].

Table 14. Pyriform sinus carcinoma. Nodal control according to size and radiation dose at two years in patients with controlled primary (determinate group)*

Dose in rad	≤3 cm		>3 cm	
	Number of patients	Control	Number of patients	Control
≤5500	2	0/2 ⎤	3	0/3 ⎤
≤6000	8	3/8 ⎥ 6/15 (40%)	4	1/4 ⎥ 3/13 (23%)
≤6500	5	3/5 ⎦	2	0/2 ⎥
≤7000	7	6/7 ⎤	4	2/4 ⎦
≤7500	11	10/11 ⎥	4	3/4 ⎤
≤8000	9	8/9 ⎥ 50/54 (93%)	3	2/3 ⎥
≤8500	8	7/8 ⎥	2	2/2 ⎥ 11/14 (79%)
≤9000	9	9/9 ⎥	3	2/3 ⎥
>9000	10	10/10 ⎦	2	2/2 ⎦
Total	69	56/69 (81%)	27	14/27 (52%)

≤3 cm Control: $P < 0.001$
>3 cm Control: $P < 0.01$
Total: $P < 0.01$

* Reproduced by permission of the Int J Radiation Onc Biol Phys [28].

(7) The experience of the radiotherapist in giving radical high doses using shrinking field techniques.

(8) Last, but not least, the experience of the surgeon in operating on patients following radical irradiation of the neck.

5.1. Nodal control in relation to size of node and radiation doses

We have analyzed nodal control according to the size of the adenopathy and radiation dose for patients with squamous cell carcinoma of the supraglottic larynx, pyriform sinus, tonsil and faucial arch, who were controlled at the primary site for at least two years. All metastatic nodes from supraglottic cancer that were less than 2.5 cm in diameter were controlled when the given dose was at least 7000 rad in 7 weeks. The control rate was 62% when the node was larger than 2.5 cm [27] (Table 13).

Nodes ≤3 cm in size from pyriform sinus cancers were controlled in 93% of patients when at least 7000 rad were given. Larger nodes were controlled in 80% of patients if the dose was ≥7500 rad [28] (Table 14). Similarly, adenopathies ≤3 cm in size that were from tonsillar or faucial arch carcinoma were controlled in over 90% of patients if the dose exceeded 6000 rad. Adenopathies larger than this size required at least 7500 rad to obtain control in about 85% of patients.

The higher cure rates obtained for nodes following radiotherapy compared to those obtained at the primary sites does not necessarily mean that metastases are more radiosensitive than primary tumors. Doses exceeding 7000–7500 rad could not be delivered, to primary areas, such as supraglottic larynx, hypopharynx, or oropharynx, without significant complication, whereas these doses could be given with relative ease for nodal remnants if the radiation portals were gradually reduced. Using cancer of the pyriform sinus as an example, it may be assumed that a similar number of cancer cells is present in small primary tumors (T_1, T_2) and small metastatic nodes (≤3 cm). The local control achieved with doses up to 6500 rad was similar for cancer at the primary site and adenopathy (36% and 40% respectively). A higher control rate was obtained for the nodes beyond this dose level, since a greater number of adenopathies received larger doses compared to the primary tumors (Fig. 8).

The limiting factor in these instances, therefore is the tolerance of normal tissues (cartilage, mucosa) at the site of the original tumor. This situation is exactly the reverse in cancer of the breast, treated by radical irradiation, where the dose given to the axillary lymphatics is the limiting critical factor.

Subcutaneous and muscle fibrosis that resulted from irradiation was never severe enough to limit neck movement. Asymptomatic cranial nerve pal-

190

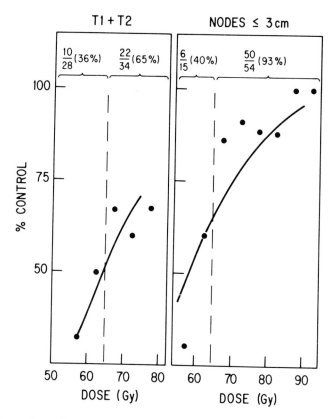

Figure 8. Comparison of local control for small tumors (T₁, T₂) and nodes ≤3 cm in squamous cell carcinoma of the pyriform sinus. Note that the control rate was similar for doses ≤6500 rads (36% vs. 40%), but higher for the nodes beyond this dose level (93% vs. 65%).
Reproduced with slight modification by permission of Int J Rad Onc Biol Phys, 1982 [28].

sy affecting mainly the 12th nerve in the submaxillary region was noted in 25 patients with advanced primary tumors who also had large adenopathies [45]. Other authors have also observed that severe complications from radical neck irradiation are rare [17]. However, it should be clearly understood that these large doses cannot be delivered to large volumes, and field shrinkage, as advocated by Baclesse many years ago, is indispensable for the prevention of undue fibrosis and complications. Bilateral nodes, or nodes at multiple levels, therefore are difficult to treat by this technique and neck surgery in these instances is often preferred.

6. Salvage surgery following neck irradiation

Except for oral cancer, salvage surgery is rarely needed for patients with initially N₀ stage, since the recurrence rate, after routine elective neck irradiation, does not exceed 2%. Surgery is usually performed because there is palpable nodal remnant persistent for at least 12 weeks following radiotherapy or because of neck recurrences that present several months to several years following complete disappearance of the initial neck disease. An extensive analysis was carried out recently by Brugére et al. [18] at the Institut Curie of over 1,100 patients treated primarily with irradiation for neck metastasis. Sixty-three percent had palpable nodal remnant at completion of treatment, however, two months later only 32% had palpable nodes.

Seven hundred and thirty-two patients treated between 1959 and 1974 were examined in order to determine the failure rate in the neck for those who had palpable nodes still remaining at the completion of irradiation. Despite the fact that very few of these patients were submitted to surgery following radiotherapy, the relapse rate in the neck was low and did not exceed 10%. Because several workers [17, 46, 47] have noted that there is a strong correlation between persistence of palpable nodes observed 6–12 weeks following irradiation and the incidence of recurrence in the neck, our present practice is to perform neck surgery routinely if palpable disease is present after an observation period of at least 12 weeks.

Since the establishment of this policy in 1974, 124 patients have been submitted to surgery. The histological findings are given in Table 15. Fifty-five percent had positive specimens and in 62% of those, the nodal capsule was involved (R+), indicating that these tumors are quite virulent. We do not yet know whether the policy of performing systematic neck surgery for nodal remnants will result in fewer neck recurrences or longer patient survival.

Neck disease may reappear several months or even, although very rarely, a few years following treatment. It is important in these instances, to be sure that there is no recurrence at the primary site or that a second primary has

Table 15. Histological results in 124 patients who had surgical resection for palpable nodes persistent 3 months after radical irradiation

Specimen	Number of patients	
Negative	56/124	(45%)
Positive	68/124	(55%)
N+ve and R−ve	14/68	⎤ (38%)
N+ve and R?	12/68	⎦
N+ve and R+ve	42/68	(62%)

R−ve − No capsular invasion.
R+ve = Capsular invasion present.
Modified from Brugére J et al. [18]

not developed – not an uncommon event. Eighty surgical resections were performed for recurrent disease. In two-thirds of these patients there was involvement of the node with rupture of the nodal capsule (R +). The survival of the whole group was poor; only 22% at 3 years. The prognosis was very grave for those who were found to have R +, since only 10% survived 3 years.

6.1. Type of surgery performed and complications

Complete neck dissection, either radical or conservative, remains the procedure of choice for patients with nodal recurrence or nodal remnant following radiation. This was done in two-thirds of such cases. Adenectomy, or resection of a limited group of nodes, was performed in about 30% of these patients (Table 16). Thirty-nine of the 204 (19%) patients operated upon experienced complication. In 5 (2.5%) these complications were fatal (Table 17). This incidence is not significantly higher than that reported for patients who had initial neck surgery without prior irradiation. These data indicate that neck surgery can be performed without excessive morbidity if the surgical team is experienced in operating on patients who have received radical neck irradiation, and if there is a close cooperation between the surgeon and the radiotherapist. Certainly this type of surgery should not be performed by physicians inexperienced in handling and avoiding the potential complications.

One approach to reducing potential risk of complication is to reduce the dose to the nodes when there is slow tumor regression during irradiation and to perform surgical resection after only 5500–6000 rad has been given. Often this is not possible because adenopathies are included within the treatment portal of the primary tumor.

Table 16. Type of neck surgery performed following radical neck irradiation

	Nodal remnant* (124 pts)	Nodal recurrence (80 pts)	Total (204 pts)
Adenectomy	7 (6%)	8 (10%)	15 (7%)
Limited neck dissection of one or more groups of lymph nodes	30 (24%)	15 (19%)	45 (22%)
Conservative neck dissection	12 (10%)	5 (6%)	17 (8%)
Radical neck dissection	75 (60%)	52 (65%)	127 (62%)

* Surgery performed 12 weeks following irradiation.
Modified from Brugére J et al. [18].

6. Survival of patients with nodal metastasis

It is generally accepted that long-term survival is influenced by the degree of nodal involvement. Since our patients, excluding those with oral cancers, were treated primarily by radiotherapy to the nodes, we have been able to determine their absolute survival at 3 years, according to the stage of the

Table 17. Post-operative complications of neck surgery following radical neck irradiation

Complication	Surgery for		
	Nodal Remnant* (124 patients)	Nodal recurrence (80 patients)	Total (204 patients)
Fatal			
Carotid rupture	1	2	3 (1.5%)
Post-operative intercurrent disease	—	2	2 (1%) ⎦ 5 (2.5%)
Non-fatal			
Skin necrosis (plastic repair)	4	0	4 (2%)
Wound dehiscence	19	5	24 (12%)
Lymphocyst	3	1	4 (2%)
Hematoma	5	4	9 (4%)
Total number of complications	32 (26%)	14 (17.5%)	46 (22.5%)
Total number of patients with complications	27 (22%)	12 (15%)	39 (19%)

* Surgery performed 12 weeks following irradiation.
Modified from Brugére J *et al.* [18].

Table 18. Absolute survival free of disease according to nodal stage for squamous cell cancer of the head and neck, excluding oral cancers (minimum follow-up 3 years)

Location	Number of patients	Survival according to stage (%)			
		N_0	N_1b	N_2b	N_3
Tonsil and faucial arch	661	50	40	29	25
Base of tongue	359	41	27	25	27
Supraglottic larynx	218	56	53	57	26
Pyriform sinus	434	36	34	(1/9)	15
Marginal or lateral epilarynx	157	59	36	(1/5)	23
Nasopharynx	104	38	44	50	34

Modified from Bataini JP *et al.* [21].

neck involvement. It should be noted that about 95% of the loco-regional failures occur within the first 3 years following treatment. The results are shown in Table 18.

Contrary to other types of head and neck cancer, the degree of nodal involvement in nasopharyngeal tumors does not significantly alter the long-term survival. For example, 10 of 26 patients with N_0 stage (38%) were free of disease at 3 years, while 30 of 78, or 38%, with clinical adenopathy, were alive [41]. It appears that the prognosis for patients with cancer of the supra-glottic larynx, hypopharynx, and oropharynx, who have mobile unilateral nodes (N_1b), was not significantly different from that of patients with no palpable disease in the neck. Radiation to the nodes has not only achieved control of the neck disease, but survival also appears to be similar to that of patients with initially N_0 stage. Large fixed lymph nodes (N_3), excluding those from nasopharyngeal primaries are associated with a grave prognosis and the survival rate in general does not exceed 25%.

Since neck disease in oral cancers is primarily treated by combined modality, we have examined the long-term survival in patients who had pathological staging of the neck for cancer of the oral tongue and floor of mouth. Those who had pathologically negative nodes had a five year survival of over 50%. The survival was somewhat worse for those who had minimal nodal disease ($\leq 3N+ R-$), and was quite poor when the disease extensively involved the neck ($>3N+ R+$) (Table 19).

7. Summary and conclusion

We have attempted in this chapter to present the experiences of the Institut Curie in the use of radiotherapy for the treatment of neck disease. It is clear that certain conclusions are warranted:

Table 19. Absolute survival free of disease of patients with oral cancers who had pathological staging of the neck (minimum follow up 5 years)

	Specimen		
		Positive	
	Negative	$\leq 3N+ R-$	$>3N+$ or $R+$
Oral Tongue (10)	115/214 (54%)	46/104 (44%)	16/67 (24%)
Floor of mouth (44)	100/190 (53%)	18/70 (26%)	1/11 (9%)
Total	215/404 (53%)	64/174 (37%)	17/78 (22%)

(1) Moderate radiation doses given electively for occult metastasis (N_0 stage), for patients with cancer of the nasopharynx, oropharynx, hypopharynx, and supraglottic larynx, will achieve about 98% local control when the primary lesion has been sterilized.

(2) Radical radiotherapy is very effective for controlling clinical adenopathies of relatively small volume ($\leq$3 cm). The failure rate in these instances is less than 10% and neck surgery may not be necessary. Larger adenopathies can be controlled by irradiation but require large doses that should be given only by an experienced team, if the sequalae are to be acceptable.

(3) Persistent nodes which remain palpable for at least 12 weeks after treatment should be treated surgically, since the majority of these patients will prove to have persistent viable tumor in the neck.

(4) There should be close cooperation between the radiotherapist and the surgeon, if radical nodal irradiation is to be successful. The surgeon should be experienced in operating on radically irradiated necks, if the complication rates from salvage surgery are to be acceptable.

(5) For oral cavity carcinoma, the treatment of neck disease, either occult or obvious, should be by a combined modality. Both surgery and radiotherapy are necessary in these instances.

We have not commented on the use of neutrons and other particle irradiation, (excluding electron beam), because this therapy is addressed in Chapter 6 and so far there is no evidence that these radiation modalities have achieved either higher local control rates, or improved survival as compared to conventional megavoltage radiotherapy. On the contrary, it appears that the complication rate from these modalities is higher [48]. Likewise it appears that neither radiosensitizers, nor the combination of chemotherapy with radiotherapy [49], for neck disease have improved the long-term local control or survival.

Acknowledgement

We are very grateful to the Attending and Technical staff of the Radiotherapy Department of the Institut Curie for their dedication in the treatment of these patients, and for their help in gathering the data used. We are also grateful to the Surgical Staff, without whose cooperation and support these studies could not have been done.

Our thanks also to Ms. Patricia Stacey for her help in preparing this manuscript and Mrs. Louise Mussolini for her secretarial assistance.

References

1. Ennuyer A, Bataini JP: Les tumeurs de l'Amygdale et de la region Velopalatine. Masson (Edit) Paris, 1956.
2. Leroux-Robert J, Ennuyer A, Calle R: Traitement des Cancers Hypopharyngés et Laryngopharyngés par l'Association Chirurgie-Radiotherapie. Bull Cancer 37:232–254, 1950.

3. Fletcher GH: Elective irradiation of subclinical disease in cancers of the head and neck. Cancer 29:1450–1454, 1972.

4. Fletcher GH, Jesse RH: Interaction of surgery and irradiation in head and neck cancers. Curr Probl Radiol 1:2–27, 1971.

5. Million RR, Fletcher GM, Jesse RH: Evaluation of elective irradiation of the neck for squamous cell carcinoma of the nasopharynx, tonsillar fossa, and base of tongue. Radiology 80:973–988, 1963.

6. Berger DS, Fletcher GH, Lindberg RD, Jesse RH: Elective irradiation of the neck lymphatics for squamous cell carcinomas of the nasopharynx and oropharynx. Amer J Roentgenol 111:66–72, 1971.

7. Beahrs OH, Barber KW: The value of radical dissection of structures of the neck in the management of carcinomas of the lip, mouth, and larynx. Arch Surg 85:49–72, 1952.

8. Strong EW: Preoperative radiation and radical neck dissection. Surg Clin North Am 49:271–276, 1969.

9. Fletcher GH: Radiation therapy and surgery. In: Murphy GP (ed) International Advances in Surgical Oncology. Vol. 2. New York, Alan R, Liss Inc,1979, pp 55–58.

10. Decroix Y, Ghossein NA: Experiences of the Curie Institut in treatment of cancer of the mobile tongue. II. Management of the neck nodes. Cancer 47:503–508, 1981.

11. Moyse P, Durand JC, Sadoul G: Le 'Envahissement ganglionnaire dans les cancers de la partie mobile de la langue. Bull Cancer 59:161–167, 1972.

12. Cachin Y, Eschwege F: Combinations of radiotherapy and surgery in the treatment of head and neck cancers. Cancer Treat Rev 2:177–191, 1975.

13. Cachin Y: Les modalites et la Valeur pronostique de l'envahissement ganglionnaire cervical dans les carcinomes des voies aerodigestives superieurs. Vie Med Can Fr 1:48–00, 1972.

14. Richard J: Orientation recentes de la Chiriugie ganglionnaire du cou. In: Pinel J, Leroux-Robert J (eds) Adenopathies Cervicales Malignes. Masson, Paris, 1982, pp 94–105.

15. Cachin Y, Guerrier Y, Pinel J: Les adenopathies cervicales metastatique. Nuovo Arch Italiano di ORL 5:207–220, 1977.

16. Ennuyer A, Bataini JP, Daudel R, Daudel P: A Propos de la Radiotherapie des Adenopathies Cervicales Secondaires aux Epitheliomas du Pharynx: Dose Ganglionnaire et Etalement. Bull Cancer 60:1–14, 1973.

17. Bartelink H, Breur K, Hart G: Radiotherapy of lymph node metastases in patients with squamous cell carcinoma of the head and neck region. Int J Rad Onc Biol Phys 8:983–989, 1982.

18. Brugére J, Point D, Laurent M, Bataini P: Chirurgie Ganglionnaire cervicale post-radiotherapique – Indications et resultats. In: Pinel J, Leroux-Robert J (eds) Adenopathies Cervicales Malignes. Masson, Paris, 1982, pp 151–156.

19. International Union Against Cancer: TNM Classification of malignant tumors, Geneva, International Union Against Cancer, 1973.

20. International Union Against Cancer. TMN Atlas. Spiessel B, Scheibe O, Wagner G (eds) Springer-Verlag, New York, 1982.

21. Bataini JP, Bernier J, Brugére J, Jaulerry Ch, Brunin F, Picco CH: Approche Radiotherapique des Adenopathies Cervicales secondaires aux Cancers Epidermiques du Larynx et du Pharynx. In: Pinel J, Leroux-Robert J (eds) Adenopathies Cervicales Maignes. Masson, Paris, 1982, pp 129–135.

22. Decroix Y, Ghossein NA: Experience of the Curie Institut in treatment of cancer of the mobile tongue. I. Treatment Policies and Results. Cancer 47:496–502, 1981.

23. Lee JG, Krause CJ: Radical neck dissection: Elective, therapeutic, and secondary. Arch Otolaryngol 101:656–659, 1975.

24. Nahum AM, Bone RC, Davidson TM: The case for elective prophylactive neck dissection. J Amer Acad Ophth and Otol 82:603–612, 1976.

25. Spiro RH, Strong EW: Epidermoid carcinoma of the mobile tongue. Treatment by partial

glossectomy alone. Am J Surg 122:707–710, 1971.

26. Fletcher GH: Textbook of Radiotherapy. Lea and Febiger, Philadelphia, 1980, pp 180–219.

27. Ghossein NA, Bataini JP, Ennuyer A, Stacey P, Krishnawamy V: Local control and site of failure in radically irradiated supraglottic laryngeal cancer. Radiology 112(1):187–192, 1974.

28. Bataini P, Brugere J, Bernier J, Jaulerry CH, Picot C, Ghossein NA: Results of radical radiotherapeutic treatment of carcinoma of the pyriform sinus: Experience of the Institut Curie. Int J Radiation Onc Biol Phys 8:1277–1286, 1982.

29. Jesse RM, Barkley MT Jr., Lindberg RD, Fletcher GH: Cancer of the oral cavity – is elective neck dissection beneficial? Am J Surg 120:505–508, 1970.

30. Fitspatrick PJ, Tepperman BS: Cervical Lymph node metastases: The place of radiotherapy. In: Kagan AR, Miles J (eds) Head and Neck Oncology – Controversies in Cancer Treatment. G.K. Hall, Publishers pp 233–245, 1981.

31. Fayos JV, Lampe I: The therapeutic problem of metastatic neck adenopathy. Am J Radiol 114:65–75, 1972.

32. Million RR: Elective neck irradiation for treatment of squamous carcinoma of the oral tongue and floor of mouth. Cancer 34:149–155, 1974.

33. Meor RT, Flatcher GH, Lindberg RD: Anatomical coverage in elective irradiation of the neck for squamous cell carcinoma of the oral tongue. Int J Rad Onc Biol Phys 8:1881–1885, 1982.

34. Lindberg RD: Distribution of cervical lymph node metastasis from squamous cell carcinoma of the upper respiratory and digestive tract. Cancer 29:1446–1449, 1972.

35. Fletcher GH: Textbook of Radiotherapy. Lea and Febiger, Philadelphia, 1980, pp 249–271.

36. Bataini JP, Ennuyer A, Poncet P, Ghossein NA: Treatment of supreglottic cancer by radical high dose radiotherapy. Cancer 33:1253–1262, 1974.

37. Regoud CEA: Les adenopathies consecutives aux cancers des levres, de la bouche; leurs indications therapeutique; leur traitement. Radiophysiologie et Radiotherapie 1, 1928.

38. Quick D: Radium in the treatment of metastatic epidermoid carcinoma of the cervical lymph nodes. Amer J Radiol 33:677–681, 1935.

39. Duffy SS: Treatment of cervical nodes in intra oral cancer. Surg Gynec Obst 664–671, 1940.

40. Martin HE, Sugarbaker E: Cancer of the tonsil. Am J Surg 52:158–196, 1941.

41. Brugére J, Bataini P, Point D, Jaulerry C: L'envalissment ganglionnaire cervical des epitheliomas du Naso-pharynx. Compte Rendue 74th Congres francais d'Orl, Paris, 1977, Arnette Ed. (Paris) pp 269–275.

42. Wizenberg MJ, Bloedorn FG, Weiner S, Garcia JR: Radiation therapy in the management of lymph node metastasis from head and neck cancers. Am J Radiol 114:76–82, 1972.

43. Schneider JJ, Fletcher GH, Barkley MT: Control by irradiation alone of non fixed clinically positive lymph nodes from squamous cell carcinoma of the oral cavity, oropharynx, supraglottic larynx, and hypopharynx. Am J Radiol 123:42–48, 1975.

44. Decroix Y: Personal communication.

45. Berger PS, Bataini JP: Radiation-induced cranial nerve palsy. Cancer 40:152–155, 1977.

46. Bataini JP: Meeting Groupe European Radiotherapie, Helsinki, 1979: Results of Radiotherapy of 1000 patients with pharynx tumors.

47. Sobel S, Rubin P, Keller B, Poulter C: Tumor persistence as a predictor of outcome after radiation therapy of head and neck cancers. Int J Rad Onc Biol Phys 1:873–880, 1976.

48. Laramore GE, Griffin TW, Tesh DW, Wong HH, Parker RG: Phase 1 pilot study of fast neutron teletherapy for advanced carcinomas of the head and neck. Cancer 25:192–199, 1983.

49. Hong WK, Bromer R: Current concepts: chemotherapy in head and neck cancer. New Engl J Med 308:75–79, 1983.

9. Immunopharmacologic effects of radiation therapy in head and neck cancers

J.B. DUBOIS

Introduction

Accompanying the therapeutic benefits of radiotherapy, neighboring healthy tissue is subjected to adverse effects. Moreover, ionizing radiation is a known immunosuppressor and thus can lead to dissemination of residual malignant cells after treatment. Do the benefits of radiotherapy on tumor evolution outweigh the suppressive action on host immune defense? Although the interaction between ionizing radiation and the immune system appears to be complex, the outcome is not always counterproductive and the mechanisms involved therefore merit thorough investigation. Numerous studies have shown that the changes in tumor immunity in the cancer patient are non specific whether they occur before (spontaneous), during or after treatment (more or less removed from the time of chemo- or radiotherapy). A more specifically oriented (and therefore more promising) approach would be to study cell mediated immunity based not only on T-lymphocytes but also macrophages and killer cell populations (natural and antibody dependent killer lymphocytes). Since the radiosensitivities of these populations differ, it would logically follow that their respective roles in post radiotherapeutic immunosuppression would depend on several variables. For many years, the only identified lymphocyte event following certain local irradiation was lymphopenia. Present day studies are much more refined and investigate various lymphocyte subpopulations thereby more realistically evaluating the repercussions of radiotherapy on immune response. The present study attempts to answer several questions dealing with radiotherapy of head and neck cancers. Does local radiotherapy of these cancers influence immune response? If so, what effect does it have on tumor evolution? Would a better understanding of the immunological mechanism of post-radiotherapeutic perturbations lead to a better control of these effects thereby providing a more efficacious therapy for head and neck can-

Gregory T. Wolf (ed), Head and Neck Oncology.
© *1984 Martinus Nijhoff Publishers, Boston. ISBN 0-89838-657-8. Printed in The Netherlands.*

cers, or at least offer a prognostic tool for this type of cancer based on immune response during and/or after irradiation?

The immune response

In order to understand the choice of criteria employed to judge the immune status of the cancer patient before or after treatment, it is first necessary to establish the mechanisms involved in the immune response and the methods available for the exploration of each of them.

The stem cells from which all immunocompetent cells arise are found in the liver during embryonic development and in bone marrow in the adult.

All such cells pass through the thymus where some undergo changes under the influence of thymic hormone leading to their maturity or differentiation and during which they acquire specific membrane antigens.

Cells that mature in this fashion are designated thymodependent and are referred to as T lymphocytes or thymocytes. These cells migrate into peripheral lymphoid tissue in the paracortical regions of lymph nodes, the white pulp of the spleen and Peyer's patches in the digestive tract. Other T lymphocytes pass into the peripheral blood to eventually be trapped by the thymus to become part of the corps of memory T cell. Non T lymphocytes probably mature at a site analogous to the bursus of Fabricius in birds designated bursa-dependent area of peripheral lymphoid organs: lymph nodes, spleen and digestive tract. The macrophage is also an immunocompetent cell that plays an important role in the immune response and is present in all lymphoid tissues. The immune response can be divided into three steps:

– an initiation phase which includes antigen recognition;
– a regulatory phase based on the various phenomena of cell cooperation;
– an effector stage involving different sensitized effector lymphocytes, immunoglobulin or antibody secretion.

In the initiation and antigen recognition step the macrophage, falsely labelled a 'helper cell' plays a major role. This cell represents the first basic cellular component of the immune response. The macrophage favors antigen capture by endocytosis and various transformations referred to as macrophage manipulation. The macrophage presents the antigen to the T memory lymphocyte which will either recognize or not recognize the antigen as either self or non-self.

The second step of the immune response (regulation) revolves around the interrelationships between the two major types of lymphocytes, the T and B lymphocytes. This step is based on cell cooperation which can be either positive (helper activity) or negative (suppressive activity). Helper activity is exercised by certain lymphocytes which 'help' B lymphocytes to secrete antibody. These cells are called helper T lymphocytes and carry Fc receptor for IgM (T_μ).

The T lymphocytes can function through direct contact with antigen transporter proteins when T lymphocytes react with hapten of the same antigen molecule thereby facilitating the transformation of B cells toward antibody synthesizing cells.

The cooperation between B and T lymphocytes can also occur indirectly when antigen stimulated T lymphocytes secrete specific and nonspecific soluble factors that in turn support the proliferation and differentiation of B lymphocytes into antibody producing cells – the plasmocytes.

Cell cooperation can also be negative in which case the process would include the participation of suppressor T lymphocytes bearing Fc receptor for IgG (T_γ). The result would effectively induce a suppression of immune response by means of several mechanisms: by actively permitting host tolerance to its own antigens; by permanently limiting antibody production; by limiting cell mediated immune response: graft versus host (G.V.H.) reaction or delayed hypersensitivity.

The final step in the immune response is the effector phase where the immune response is either carried out directly (cell mediated immunity) or indirectly through the intermediary of humoral mediators – the immunoglobulins or antibody (humoral immunity).

In humoral immunity, antibody secretion (IgG) is the end product of an effective and active immune defence.

In cell mediated immunity, a distinction must be made between:

(a) that part due to immunocompetent cells involved in cooperative cell suppression prior to activation or T cell inhibition which may or may not lend itself under certain circumstances and to certain degrees to a transformation into antibody secreting plasmocytes; and

(b) direct cell intervention by certain lymphocytes engaged in active immune response. Antigen-specific sensitized lymphocytes, in addition to participating in the previously described events, can also act through a direct cytotoxic property referred to as natural cytotoxicity. The cells responsible for this function are called natural killer cells. These cells have had no previous exposure to antigen and occupy a pivotal role in host immune surveillance vis a vis tumor antigen. Natural killer (NK) cells are morphologically indistinguishable from other lymphocytes but differ from T and B lymphocytes and macrophages in that they possess no specific membrane marker such as those associated with the function of these latter cell types.

Natural killer lymphocytes are involved in most antitumor immune mechanisms and exert a direct cytotoxic action against tumor cells. These same lymphocytes also play a role in delayed hypersensitivity leading to graft rejection and G.V.H. activity.

Other antigen-stimulated activated lymphocytes intervene in response to tumor aggression and secrete lymphokines that can facilitate NK activity or even T cell helper function.

The non-specific changes induced by cancer on humoral immunity and reflected by measurements of complement, complement fractions and immunoglobulin fractions are no longer indicated since they do not specifically truly reflect the immune status of the cancer patient either before or after treatment.

On the other hand, methods in oncology that explore cellular immunity have benefited from a growing interest in the intimate relationship between lymphocyte status and cancer evolution before and/or after treatment. Exploration aimed at each level of the immune response has been developed to more precisely pinpoint the respective responsibility attributed to each lymphocyte population or subpopulation and to investigate immune response as it relates to lymphocyte function. Numerous authors have already quantified the radiosensitivity of lymphocyte subpopulations using different methods of exploration of the immune response as it is shown in Table 1.

Our studies have employed the principle methods that offer a global indication of immune status: *in vivo* skin tests to assess delayed hypersensitivity that call into play several mechanisms of immune response and numerous *in vitro* tests offering a more analytical approach to the study of different lymphocyte populations and their sub-populations.

Table 1. Radiosensitivity of lymphocyte subpopulations as assessed in various systems[a]

System	D37 (r)	Reference
T dependent humoral response	70	Makinodan *et al.*, 1962
T dependent humoral response	80	Kennedy *et al.*, 1965
T dependent humoral response	214	Haskill *et al.*, 1970
T dependent humoral response	188	Petrov and Cheredeev, 1972
B cell responses (antibody production)	96	Addison, 1974
B cell responses (Ig production)	70–145	Anderson and Warner, 1975
B cell responses (cell-viability)	40	Anderson *et al.*, 1975
T cell responses (GVH)	100	Sprent *et al.*, 1974
T cell responses (proliferation)	64	Anderson *et al.*, 1972
T cell responses (cell viability)	100	Anderson *et al.*, 1974
T cell responses (allograft)	75	Celada and Carter, 1962
T cell responses (helper)	230	Janeway, 1975

[a] From Ref. [1].

Materials and methods

Immunological evaluation

Cell mediated immunity was evaluated by *in vivo* skin tests to explore delayed hypersensitivity and *in vitro* testing consisting of a total lymphocyte count, a study of spontaneous lymphocytotoxicity (NK activity), a study of lymphocyte markers in which we evaluated specific markers for T and B lymphocytes, a study of synthesis and selected protein transformation (lymphoblastic transformation) for both the total lymphocyte population as well as sub-populations. The latter was carried out using techniques developed in our laboratory and included a study with specific mitogens having different lymphocyte targets. The immune status of the head and neck cancer patients included in our study was evaluated before, during and at two month intervals after radiotherapy.

In vivo skin tests

This evaluation mostly focused on the *in vivo* response to 2, 4 dinitrochlorobenzene (DNCB) and involves a 2 step procedure. In the first step DNCB (20 mg/10 ml acetone) is applied to the skin (0.1 ml or 2,000 μg DNCB) to sensitize the patient. This application is evaluated two weeks later, after which a second sensitization (0.1 ml in 1.9 ml acetone) is performed. This second challenge is scored at the 48th hour and repeated in 5 days if the 48-hour result is negative. Each test is scored visually with no mechanical aids whatsoever. Results are reported as: no reaction ($-$) or anergy, erythematous reaction ($++$), phlyctenular reaction ($+++$), necrotic reaction ($++++$). DNCB was applied to the external surface of the upper arm and could be repeated with the second solution every month or 2 months during and after treatment.

Natural killer (NK) cell activity

A study of spontaneous cytotoxicity reflects natural killer cell activity and consists of placing tumor cells in contact with the patients lymphocytes. The tumor test cells were obtained from the K-562 non antigenic tumor cell line originating from blast cells extracted from pleural effusions of a patient with chronic myelogenous leukemia.

Patient blood was drawn into a heparinized syringe and diluted with an equal volume of MEM (Minimal Essential Medium). The mixture was then placed on a cushion of Ficoll-Metrizoate and centrifuged at room temperature for 30 min at 400 g. Lymphocytes were harvested from the sample

-Hypaque interface, washed twice in MEM and cultured in RPMI 1640 supplemented with 10% fetal calf serum (FCS) at the following lymphocyte concentrations: 10, 5, 2.5, and 1.25×10^6 lymphocytes per ml.

The K-562 cell preparation consisted of centrifugation (5 min at 200 g) in 0.2 ml TD buffer containing 200 μCi 51Cr. The cells were then placed in a shaker waterbath (37 °C) for one hour with slow but constant rocking. Labelling occurs over a period of 3 hours after which the cells were washed three times and centrifuged for 5 min at 200 g at room temperature in RPMI 1640. The cell concentration was adjusted to 10^5 cells per ml and 100 μl of this suspension was delivered to each test well.

To this, an equal volume of lymphocyte suspension was added. Wells were also included for control reactions as well as for maximum radio-activity release following the addition of 0.1 NHCl. The supernatants from all wells were counted in a gamma counter after a 4-h incubation in a 5% CO_2 atmosphere. The results are expressed as a percent based on the following formula:

$$\frac{\begin{array}{l}{}^{51}\text{Cr released in} \\ \text{the presence of} \quad - \quad \begin{array}{l}\text{Spontaneous} \\ {}^{51}\text{Cr} \\ \text{release}\end{array} \\ \text{lymphocytes}\end{array}}{\begin{array}{l}\text{Maximum } {}^{51}\text{Cr} \\ \text{release} \quad\quad - \quad \begin{array}{l}\text{Spontaneous} \\ {}^{51}\text{Cr} \\ \text{release}\end{array}\end{array}} \times 100$$

Normal cytotoxicity ranges from 80 to 90% of labeled marker activity when spontaneous release falls between 3 to 10% of maximum release (0.1 NHCl).

Lymphoblastic transformation tests

The lymphoblastic transformation test was carried out with the total lymphocyte population for all patients and with some lymphocyte subpopulations for certain patients. Three mitogens were used: phytohemagglutinin (PHA), pokeweed mitogen (PWM) and Concanavalin A (Con-A).

Blood was drawn under aseptic conditions on the same day in control subjects and in patients (disposable syringe previously heparinized with 0.2 ml of calcium heparinate or Calciparine). Total leukocytes and the differential leukocyte count were determined by the usual methods. Monocytes are eliminated by treatment with carbonyl iron. Fifty mg of carbonyl iron are added per 20 ml of whole blood and are incubated for 30 min at +37 °C, undergoing continuous agitation. The blood is then diluted in 5 ml

Hank's liquid (Pasteur Institute) for 15 ml of blood. The lymphocytes are separated on a Ficoll-metrizoate gradient at a density of 1.077. The monocytes having phagocytized the iron particles, cross the gradient. After centrifugation at 400 g for 30 min at the laboratory temperature, the lymphocyte ring is taken, washed 2 times in Hank's liquid completed by a molar solution of 4% Hepes, by a 5% decomplemented fetal calf serum (FCS) and by 5 units/ml of calcium heparinate, counted and adjusted to 2×10^7 cells/ml in RPMI 1640 containing 1% Hepes, 2% EDTA at 0.02% and 15% FCS.

The lymphocyte cultures were carried out with microtest 3040 plates. For each analysis, we placed, in 4 control wells and in 4 wells for each concentration of mitogen, 100 μl of lymphocyte suspension from the total lymphocyte population or from separated lymphocyte subpopulations at 1.000 lymphocytes/mm^3 (i.e. 1×10^5 lymphocytes/ml) and 50 μl of mitogen substance solution.

Three types of mitogens were used: phytohemagglutinin P (PHA-P) pokeweed mitogen (PWM) and Concanavalin A (Con-A). After determination of the concentration giving optimal stimulation we used the following concentrations of mitogen: for PHA-P, 3.75, 7.5, and 15 μg/well of pure PHA; for the PWM, 1 ml, 0.6 ml, and 0.3 ml of pure PWM; for the Con-A, 50 μg and 100 μg/ml.

Following addition of mitogen to the appropriate wells, the plates were placed in culture for 72 h in a CO2 incubator (5% CO2) at +37°C in a humid atmosphere. Sixteen hours prior to cell harvest, lymphocytes were tagged by addition of 50 μl of tritiated methyl thymidine (CEA, Saclay; specific activity 15 Ci/mM; 0.2 μCi/well). Cells were harvested with a MASH I (multiple apparatus sample harvester; O. Hiller, Madison, Wisconsin). Using the MASH I, thymidine-labeled, mitogen-stimulated lymphocytes were separated from the culture medium. Lymphocytes were then centrifuged, washed twice in 3% cold acetic acid, decolorized with hydrogen peroxide, and digested in one normal KOH. Radioactivity was measured in a beta liquid scintillation counter (Inter-technique) employing a 4-min count per sample. Results are expressed in desintegrations per minute (dpm) or as the stimulation index (dpm of stimulated lymphocytes/dpm of control lymphocytes). Each test run was accompanied by its own controls.

Separation of lymphocyte subpopulations

Glass wool column separation of lymphocytes
Following lymphocyte separation by Ficoll-Metrizoate, cells were passed through 250 mg of glass wool (1×10^8 lymphocytes/2.5 ml medium). Nonadherent cells were eluted with 30 ml of medium 199.

Preparative Separation of B and T lymphocytes

The technique was a modified version of that described by Schlossman and Hudson [2]. Rabbit anti-human (Fab')2 was prepared by successive injections of 5 mg of human (Fab')2 and complete Freund's adjuvant on Days 0, 7, 11 and 35. Blood samples were taken on Days 28, 42, and 44; rabbits were sacrificed on Day 46. Serums were pooled, purified by saturated ammonium sulfate precipitation, and passed over a column of Sepharose 4B coupled to Cohn Fraction II human gammaglobulin. Activation and conjugation of Sephadex G-200 was carried out over a 3 day period after allowing the G-200 to stand in distilled water adjusted to pH 10.2 by addition of 0.2N sodium hydroxide.

The Sephadex is then activated by adding 2 mg of cyanogen bromide per ml Sephadex, maintaining the pH between 10.2 and 10.5 for 10 min by addition of 0.2N NaOH. The activated Sephadex is washed with borate buffer at pH 8.4 until the Sephadex remains at pH 8.4. Conjugation takes place over 4 h at ambient temperature in the presence of human (anti-Fab')2 (1 mg of protein/ml Sephadex). The activated, conjugated Sephadex is then washed in PBS and kept at 4 °C following addition of sodium azide (1 %).

The column should be freshly prepared and consists of a 10-ml syringe containing a porous filter (Canson, 12-129) and a 3-way valve. The syringe is filled with the solution of activated conjugated Sephadex followed by 20 ml of complete separation medium and allowed to stand at +37 °C until use. At the same time, 300 mg Cohn fraction II gammaglobulins are slowly dissolved in 30 ml of complete separation medium, filtered through a millipore 0.45 μ filter, and kept at +37 °C until use.

After removing any bubbles from the colum, lymphocytes (cleared of monocytes by an iron carbonyl procedure) are introduced at 2×10^8 lymphocytes per 10-ml column. The flow rate of the cell solution is adjusted to 1 ml/min for the first 15 ml, after which the rate is increased.

Complete elution of T lymphocytes is carried out by passing 50 ml of complete separation medium over the column. B lymphocytes are eluted following a stabilization period of 10 min at ambient temperature by addition of 30 ml of gammaglobulins plus 10 ml of complete separation medium. The yield obtained for separation of normal, healthy donors is $71.87 \pm 5.03 \%$ for T lymphocytes and $13.17 \pm 4.22 \%$ for B lymphocytes.

Separation of lymphocyte subpopulations on a discontinuous bovine serum albumin gradient

A 20% fraction V bovine serum albumin (BSA) solution is dialyzed for 3 hr against distilled water at 4 °C, filtered through a 0.45 μ millipore filter, then lyophilized. A 30% solution is prepared from the lyophilisate and dilutions are adjusted to densities of 1.064, 1.072 and 1.096 at 4 °C. Densities were verified by refractometer at 25 °C using the following formula:

$$d_4^4 = 1.050 + 1.543 \, (n_{25}^D - 1.3670)$$

n_{25}^D	d_4^4
1.3735	1.064
1.3787	1.072
1.3936	1.095

(n = refractive index; d = density in g/cm^3)

All dilutions were made with Shortman's medium containing 121 volumes 0.147 M NaCl, 4 volumes 0.147 M KCl, 3 volumes 0.098 M CaCl2 and 1 volume 0.147 M MgSO4. These dilutions were all sterilized using 0.22 μ millipore filters and stored in 1-ml aliquots at 4 °C until use. The 4 fractions are gently introduced into 6 ml propylene tubes. Lymphocytes (10^8) in buffered medium 199 are layered onto the gradient. This is always carried out at 4 °C. The gradient is then centrifuged 30 min at 20,000 g at 4 °C in an MSE 25 equipped with a swinging bucket rotor. After centrifugation, each lymphocyte ring is removed, washed, and divided for use in different immunological tests. The repartition of different lymphocyte subpopulations in normal subjects in our laboratory is:

fraction 1.064: 13.45 ± 7.63 %
fraction 1.072: 61.83 ± 11.45 %
fraction 1.095: 15.75 ± 10.19 %.

Lymphocyte markers

E-rosettes
Thirty μl of lymphocyte suspension containing 5.10^5 cells is combined with 30 μl FCS (absorbed at +4 °C and +37 °C for 2 h at each temperature against sheep red blood cells (SRBC) which had been washed 3 times). Sixty μl of a suspension of SRBC (350.10^6/ml) were added to the lymphocytes in FCS. The ratio of SRBC/lymphocytes = 40.5.

The entire procedure is carried out in nonconical tubes. The final volume is 0.2 ml. The suspension is centrifuged for 5 min at 400 g after which the tubes are left at ambient temperature overnight. The following day, the cell pellets are very gently resuspended by a rotating wrist movement. After dilution, a drop of cell suspension is placed on a Thomas hemocytometer where the ruled surface facilitates counting. A rosette is defined as a lymphocyte associated with at least 3 SRBC. Two to three hundred cells are counted to establish a percentage of rosettes (where possible, results are given as absolute number of lymphocytes). In our laboratory the percent E-rosettes for normal healthy donors is: 66.61 ± 5.51 % (range: 52–75 %).

EAC-rosettes

This technique identifies cells bearing fraction 3 (C3) complement receptors. The technique involves purification of IgM from anti-sheep hemolytic serum. After titration to determine its agglutination titer, the serum is dialyzed for 24 h in 0.1 M Tris HCl at pH 8. The IgM fraction is recovered after separation on G200 Sephadex (Column: 93 cm high, 2.5 cm in diameter; flow rate 19 ml/h), then concentrated using an Amicon filter. Protein concentration and agglutination titer are noted for the final preparation. The first or second dilution under the agglutination titer was used for the EAC assay (determined after preliminary trials). The first step deals with the formation of EA complex. Fifty ml of 5% SRBC are mixed with 50 ml of IgM at the appropriate dilution. This solution is incubated for 30 min at 37 °C after which cells are washed 3 times. Control EA is prepared by adding SRBC (at 10×10^8 ml) and removing an aliquot. Complement is complexed in the following manner: 2 ml EA-IgM at 5×10^8 ml plus 2 ml of C57 B1/6 mouse complement diluted 1:5. This is followed by a 30-min incubation at $+37$ °C and 3 cell washes. Final cell concentration is adjusted to 10×10^8 SRBC/ml. Fifty μl of a 20×10^6 lymphocytes/ml suspension is added to 50 μl of EAC complex (10×10^8/ml) and incubated for 30 min at 37 °C. EAC-rosettes are counted after 500 μl of Hanks are added to the test suspension. EAC-rosettes are defined as a lymphocyte associated with a least 3 SRBC. A normal EAC value in our laboratory is: 16.44 ± 4.66% (range: 8 to 26.5%). Control tubes for E- and EA-rosettes are always negative).

Statistical analysis

All the results were interpreted with the X^2 distribution test and the Student-t test (significant level of 5%).

Patients

Our study included 54 oropharyngeal cancer patients: cancer of tonsillar tissue either contained or reaching to the anterior and posterior pillars of the faucial arch of the soft palate; cancer of tonsillar tissue and reaching to the amygdaloglossal sulcus and base of the tongue with or without vallecular involvement; isolated cancer of base of the tongue. We excluded from our study tumors that have reached structures beyond the oropharynx itself, e.g. those extending from the base of skull to the mouth of the esophagus.

All diagnoses for patients (treated between 1972 and 1979) were histologically confirmed spinocellular (differentiated), carcinomas (65% of patients);

slightly differentiated carcinomas (25% of patients) or undifferentiated carcinomas (10% of patients).

The age range of patients was between 24 and 75 years with a median age of 61. All tumors were staged according to the nomenclature adopted by the International Union Against Cancer (UICC), World Health Organization (WHO):

Primary tumor
T1 : Tumor less than or equal to 2 cm, measured across its greater diameter and limited anatomically.
T2 : Tumor diameter between 2 and 4 cm; may occupy two anatomically distinct sites; no infiltration of adjacent structures.
T3 : Tumor diameter greater than 4 cm.

Regional lymph nodes
N0 : Regional nodes not demonstratable.
N1 : Demonstratable, homolateral, cervical lymph nodes which are mobile; nodal metastases suspected.
N2 : Contralateral or bilateral, demonstratable, mobile, cervical lymph nodes; nodal metastases suspected.
N3 : Homolateral, contralateral or bilateral demonstratable, fixed cervical lymph nodes with a metastatic appearance.

All patients entered the study at the MO stage without distant metastatic evolution and were grouped as a function of primary tumor development and histological lymph node involvement (Table 2).

All patients were treated by external irradiation alone.

During the initial course of radiation therapy, the main target volume included the primary tumor and the first nodes draining this region (the posterior portion of the submaxillary group, the superior portion of the spinal and middle jugulocarotid groups to the subdigastric confluence). The entire volume was irradiated using two symmetric, transverse, lateral fields not exceeding 50 Gy/tumor.

Concurrently, a secondary target volume was irradiated which included the second nodal line of defense (the lower middle jugulo-carotid nodes and supraclavicular nodes). These nodes received between 55 and 60 Gy in the case of palpable nodes with the dose adjusted to the extent of node involve-

Table 2. Distribution of patients according to the TNM classification

	N0	N1	N2	N3	N
T1	—	—	—	—	0
T2	12	—	6	8	26
T3	—	4	5	19	28
T	12	4	11	27	54

ment. Patients with no palpable nodes received 45 to 50 Gy (5 × 2 Gy per week) delivered symmetrically and bilaterally to both upper and lower cervical nodes and to supraclavicular nodes.

During the second course of radiation therapy, a booster dose was delivered to the primary tumor as a function of tumor volume: 72 to 75 Gy for a large tumor mass which remained unchanged at the end of first course radiotherapy; 75 to 78 Gy for tumors which were initially small or reduced by the first 5 weeks of radiotherapy. The second course was administered by oblique anteroposterior fields with high energy X-photons delivered by a Sagittaire type linear accelerator.

Results

Skin tests

DNCB skin tests were performed before, during and after (every two months) radiotherapy. Of the 54 patients tested before radiotherapy 33% were DNCB positive (Table 3) compared with 92% of 29 normal control subjects.

Results of skin tests after 4 weeks of radiotherapy were statistically comparable to those before irradiation ($\chi^2 > 5\%$). This distribution of positive and negative reactions remained unchanged at the 2nd month post-radiotherapy ($\chi^2 > 5\%$). The results for all three periods (before, during and 2 months after radiotherapy) were statistically the same whether all 54 patients were taken as a whole (all stages together) or grouped according to tumor stage.

DNCB response correlated with both prognosis and tumor response to treatment.

There appears to be no prognostic significance for patients with negative DNCB tests after radiotherapy: 48.9% benefited from a favorable prognosis compared with 51.1% where prognosis was poor. For those patients whose DNCB remained positive or converted from a previously negative to a positive test, 80.2% demonstrated a favorable prognosis at 6 months versus

Table 3. DNCB skin test reactivity before, during and after radiation treatment

Before radiotherapy		During radiotherapy		2 months after radiotherapy	
+	−	+	−	+	−
18	36	12	42	15	39
33.3%	66.6%	22.2%	77.8%	27.7%	72.3%

only 19.8% with poor prognosis. Other patients with favorable prognosis were those with a positive DNCB at 2 months post-radiotherapy or those whose originally positive DNCB had become negative during therapy but then converted to positive during the first 2 months post-radiotherapy ($\chi^2 < 5\%$) (Table 4).

These same findings were not only true of the mixed patient population but were also true when analyzed by tumor stage.

NK activity

Spontaneous lymphocytotoxicity prior to irradiation was statistically lower for head and neck cancer patients compared to a group of 22 normal control subjects.

Moreover, NK activity at the completion of radiotherapy was very significantly ($p < 0.005$) lower than pretreatment levels (Table 5).

Lymphoblastic transformation

Total lymphocyte population
Tritiated thymidine uptake for the 54 head and neck cancer patients taken

Table 4. Post-radiotherapeutic DNCB skin test[a]

DNCB −

Good prognosis at 6 months:	48.9%	}N.S. $\chi^2 > 5\%$
Poor prognosis at 6 months:	51.1%	

DNCB +

Good prognosis at 6 months:	80.2%	}S.S. $\chi^2 < 5\%$
Poor prognosis at 6 months:	19.8%	

[a] The skin test was performed for each patient 2 months after completion of radiation treatment.

Table 5. Natural killer (NK) cell activity

Before irradiation	After completion of radiation treatment	Statistical analysis Student-t-test-X^2 test
A 87.2 ± 5.3		B/A : S.S. $p < 0.01$
B 55.2 ± 3.8	B1 28.1 ± 3.5	B1/B : S.S. $p < 0.005$

A: Percent of lymphocyte cytotoxicity in control subjects (22 cases).
B, B1: Percent of lymphocyte cytotoxicity in head and neck cancer patients (39 cases).

together is given in Table 6. Uptake was significantly lower immediately ($p<0.005$) following and at 2 months after radiotherapy ($p<0.01$). However, the proliferative ability of these lymphocytes seems to have been restored judging from thymidine uptake at 8 months postradiotherapy which was statistically the same as initial (pretreatment) levels. This held true for all three of the mitogens employed: PHA, PWM and Con A.

Thymidine uptake was also studied as a function of the extension of primary tumor and lymph node involvement.

The different stages of primary tumor evolution and lymph node participation did not significantly alter uptake patterns for any of the 3 mitogens employed ($p>0.2$).

We investigated a possible correlation between thymidine uptake at 2 months post-radiotherapy and prognosis. As seen in Table 7, prognosis was

Table 6. Total lymphocyte population response to the three mitogens

	A Before radiotherapy	B End of radiation treatment	C 2 months after completion of radiation treatment	D 8 months after completion of radiation treatment
PHA	$71,011\pm2,714$	$14,000\pm711$	$14,710\pm790$	$69,284\pm1,022$
PWM	$39,874\pm1,175$	$10,000\pm591$	$14,815\pm718$	$37,224\pm810$
Con A	$30,990\pm1,095$	$8,600\pm458$	$9,815\pm650$	$24,110\pm770$

A/B: $p<0.005$ (S.S.); A/C: $p<0.01$ (S.S.); A/D: $0.1<p<0.2$ (N.S.).
Mean values for 54 head and neck cancer patients (dpm$\pm$SE).

Table 7. Prognosis of patients according to lymphoblastic stimulation index (S.I.) 2 months after completion of radiation treatment*

	U.I.C.C. Stage	Evolutive disease	Deaths	NED
High S.I.	T2NO (11)	3	—	8
	T2N2 (5)	2	—	3
	T2N3 (6)	3	1	2
	T3N1 (2)	1	—	1
	T3N2 (2)	2	—	—
	T3N3 (5)	2	—	3
Low S.I.	T3N1 (2)	2	1	—
	T3N2 (3)	2	1	—
	T2N3 (2)	1	1	—
	T3N3 (14)	10	2	2
	T2N0 (1)	—	—	1
	T2N2 (1)	1	—	—

* 2 years data results.

inversely related to uptake where uptake was low at completion of radiotherapy and remained low for the 2 months which followed.

In contrast, a strong thymidine uptake was associated with non-evolving disease. Seventeen of thirty-one patients (51.6%) showed arrested tumor growth at 2 years post-therapy when uptake was high compared to only 3 of 23 patients (13%) with low thymidine uptake.

Moreover, patients whose low level of label incorporation returned to normal by the 8th month post-therapy carried a more favorable prognosis (77 NED out of 34 patients) than those whose values remained depressed (2 NED out of 20 patients) (Table 8).

Lymphocyte subpopulations

Lymphocyte subpopulations were separated on glass wool columns for 23 patients. These subpopulations underwent mitogen (PHA, PWM and Con A) stimulation immediately following and 3 weeks post-radiotherapy.

No difference in thymidine uptake was observed before radiotherapy for the lymphocyte population as a whole nor for the individual subpopulations including the glass wool non adherent lymphocytes (Table 9).

However, thymidine uptake was significantly ($p < 0.001$) impaired following radiotherapy for the combined lymphocyte population and to a lesser degree for the glass wool nonadherent subpopulation. The ratio of the thymidine uptakes for both these populations was approximately equal to 1 before radiotherapy. This strongly contrasts with elevated values of this ratio ($p < 0.01$) post-therapy, suggesting a selective radiosensitivity of the total lymphocyte population which the non-adherent cells do not possess. This sensitivity would therefore concern the cells retained on glass wool columns which are mostly monocytes. This finding was constant ($p < 0.01$, Table 9) for all three mitogens (PHA, PWM and Con A).

Lymphocyte subpopulations separated (after elimination of monocytes with iron carbonyl) on immuno-absorbant columns using conjugated anti-Fab human immunoglobulin were stimulated with all three mitogens: PHA,

Table 8. Lymphocyte response to mitogens 8 months after completion of radiation treatment

	A	B
PWA	38,115±1,001	78,770±709
PWM	25,014±711	40,110±1,245
Con A	20,010±1,127	27,811±1,800
NED	2/20	17/34

A: Low thymidine uptake 8 months after radiation treatment.
B: Normal thymidine uptake 8 months after radiation treatment.
Mean values (dpm±SE).

214

Table 9. Restoration of lymphocyte responses to mitogens in 23 head and neck cancer patients for non-adherent lymphocyte sub-populations after radiation treatment

	Before radiation treatment			After radiation treatment (21 days)		
	Total lymphocyte population	Non adherent lymphocytes	Ratio non adherent/total	Total lymphocyte population	Non adherent lymphocytes	Radio non adherent/total
PHA	82,824±1,800*	76,100±728	0.92	10,020±625	54,120±890	5.40
PWM	56,714±1,220	47,810±629	0.84	9,817±612	45,819±729	4.67
Con A	48,800±819	47,100±870	0.97	7,024±815	30,190±917	4.30

* Results expressed in dpm±SE.

Table 10. Lymphocyte subpopulations responses to the mitogens for the 3 BSA density fractions

	Before radiotherapy			1st post-radiotherapy week			3 months after radiotherapy		
	1.064	1.072	1.095	1.064	1.072	1.095	1.064	1.072	1.095
PHA	48,141±1015	80,815±1220	87,800±1710	7,800±415	8,922±491	10,815±701	9,815±620	30,800±794	40,800±710
PWM	28,170±1810	25,610±783	20,010±780	4,500±300	7,845±475	7,140±600	7,100±520	29,990±663	38,814±440
Con A	38,690±718	18,990±791	24,608±692	5,750±401	6,995±608	9,148±380	6,810±691	24,675±565	30,890±648

T 1.064, T 1.072, and T 1.095 (mean dpm±SE): mean values for 23 patients.

PWM, and Con A. Thymidine uptake for all three cell populations (1.064, 1.072 and 1.095) showed a significant ($p<0.01$, Table 10) and homogeneous decrease immediately after radiotherapy. Three months later, the mitogen response was dissociated. As shown in Table 10, thymidine uptake for the T 1.064 subpopulation remained low whereas the values for the 1.072 and 1.095 subpopulations returned to pretreatment levels for most patients. This latter event was strongly correlated with a favorable prognosis.

Lymphocyte markers (Rosette-forming cells, R.F.C.)
Table 11 shows non-significant changes in E.A.C.-rosette levels resulting from radiotherapy as opposed to the significant ($p<0.05$) reduction in E-Rosette values immediately after radiotherapy compared with control values. This decrease persisted for several weeks.

An analysis of rosette formation as a function of primary tumor stage or lymph node involvement led to the same conclusions. The different tumor stages of all 23 patients showed no change in EAC-rosette levels but a significant ($p<0.05$) fall in E-rosette values.

Discussion

In our study, as in numerous other studies [3] evaluation of immune response based on delayed hypersensitivity showed a weaker response in cancer patients following stimulation by various antigens, particularly

Table 11. Rosette-forming cells before, at the end, and 3 months after radiation treatment

	E-rosettes	EAC-rosettes
Beforeirradiation		
patients	60.5 ± 2.0 [a, c]	18.1 ± 5.8 [b]
controls	59.7 ± 3.6	19.8 ± 3.0
At completion of radiation treatment		
patients	50.1 ± 3.3 [c]	18.8 ± 2.0 [b]
controls	61.7 ± 3.8	20.5 ± 2.1
3 months after completion of radiation treatment		
patients	38.4 ± 4.9 [c]	19.9 ± 2.8 [b]
controls	60.4 ± 5.3	20.4 ± 3.2

[a] Mean values for 23 patients.
[b] No statistically significant difference ($p>0.1$).
[c] Statistically significant difference ($p<0.05$).

DNCB. The number of patients with a positive pretreatment DNCB was much less than the frequency encountered in a normal control population. As it was previously reported in literature [4-6], this finding was even more accentuated as tumor growth progressed. In contrast, other authors [7] do not find any correlation between a positive DNCB and tumor stage.

We found that positive response decreased during and following radiotherapy but these decreases were not found to be significant ($\chi^2 > 5\%$) when compared with pretreatment values. Certain authors such as Gross *et al.* [8] report that 85% of their patients convert to negative DNCB following radiotherapy [9]. However, other investigators [10] have found no impairment of cell mediated immunity after radiotherapy as determined by skin reactivity to established antigens or newly acquired antigens, such as DNCB.

Beyond a static evaluation of positive or negative DNCB tests, there appears to be a more interesting correlation between skin reactivity and prognosis. Our study clearly shows that, although a 6 month prognosis based on negative DNCB tests shows no correlation, there is a very significant correlation between positive DNCB results and a favorable prognosis at 6 months.

The results were the same whether taken for the patient population as a whole or based on tumor stage.

Numerous authors have confirmed these findings and have strongly promoted the use of this test as a pronostic indicator. Bosworth *et al.* [11] have shown that 96% of the patients responding favorably to radiotherapy demonstrated positive DNCB tests, 62% for patients with a moderate response to irradiation and 35% for patients with radioresistant tumors. A positive DNCB test appears to be an accepted endpoint of good short term prognosis for patients undergoing radiotherapy, surgery [12] or even chemotherapy [13].

The delayed hypersensitivity studies were intended to give a very broad appreciation of immune response [14]. Lymphocyte counts and functional exploration offered a more precise approach to a study of the different phases of the immune response and changes occuring as a result of radiotherapy.

Many authors [15-17] have shown that lymphocyte counts are valuable criteria for monitoring the immune status of patients undergoing radiation therapy. Lymphopenias, occasionally severe, have been reported during and after irradiation. Moreover, some authors have found a relationship between lymphopenia and prognosis whether the lymphopenia arises before [18-20] or after radiotherapy: the more marked the lymphopenia, the poorer the prognosis. However, it should be kept in mind that this simple numerical indicator says nothing about the functional state of the lymphocyte pool which may undergo extreme perturbations while displaying a normal lymphocyte count.

For this reason, additional information is needed and can be provided by a study of lymphocytotoxicity on cultured target cells, an appreciation of lymphocyte markers and by *in vitro* mitogen stimulation tests [21]. The results from these tests can provide a fuller understanding of cell mediated immunity. Our study of natural killer activity in head and neck cancers showed a statistically significant spontaneous fall in cytotoxicity and a decreased NK activity after radiotherapy for all head and neck cancers taken together.

The mechanism by which immunodepression appears following radiation treatment is still not completely elucidated. However, the modification of natural killer (NK) activity would imply an action on Fc receptor bearing cells involved in spontaneous lymphocytotoxicity. Some authors [22] believe that both T and T cells with IgG receptors mediate natural and antibody dependent lymphocyte cytotoxicity (ADCC). Wasserman *et al.* [23] noted that both cell types decrease following radiation treatment. TG cells (essentially radiosensitive suppressor cells) have been reported to mediate both NK and ADCC whereas TM cells (essentially helper cells shown to be less radiosensitive than TG cells) are considered to lack these activities. Opinion is divided on the nature of the effector cells in NK cell activity [24–27]. Several workers have characterized TG and TM cells using monoclonal antibodies specifically directed against helper (OKT4) and suppressor (OKT5) subsets. Reinherz *et al.* [28] have shown that there is no overlapping between OKT5 and TG cells. Gupta *et al.* [29] reported that 40 to 80% of TG cells react with monoclonal antibodies that identify cytotoxic-suppressor cells in man. Cordier *et al.* [30] reported that most of this type of reactivity resides in TG cells whereas Pilcher [31] found NK cell activity in both TG and TM fractions. Other authors [32] have shown that precursors of NK cells are more radiosensitive than the NK cells themselves but that this can be overcome by the introduction of interferon.

In the same way, lymphoblastic transformation with different antigens before, during and after radiotherapy of head and neck cancers shows a statistically significant immuno-deficiency (50–75% before treatment compared to normal controls). This effect would be added to the immunosuppressive effects already admitted for irradiation per se. This is a well established observation in the literature [33–46].

The decreasing variation noted for blastic stimulation following irradiation is due to the therapy itself and not spontaneous variation in thymidine uptake as suggested by some authors [47] for lymphocyte cultures of non irradiated normal subjects. In our study, tritiated thymidine uptake in response to the 3 mitogens after irradiation did not vary significantly between the different stages of tumor development. This is in direct contradiction with previously published findings [48] in which blastic stimulation after irradiation varied as a function of tumor evolution. Interpretation of the effects of ionizing radiation on tritiated thymidine uptake by lymphocytes stimulated with different antigens leads one to consider different possible mechanisms. To begin with, radiation may act by altering blastogenesis and lymphocyte differentiation. Different results such as those from Song *et al.* [49] indicate that the lymphocytes irradiated with doses of 10 Grays can transform to blast cells upon stimulation with PHA as do the control lymphocytes, but the blast cells transformed in this manner are unable to divide into small lymphocytes. If the response of T cells to antigens is similar to the response to PHA, we could conclude that irradiation of T cells would not prevent blastogenic transformation and DNA synthesis after antigen stimulation. Subsequent division of the antigen induced blast cells into small effector cells would be arrested by a minimal dose of 10 Gy.

The second possible mechanism deals with the effect of ionizing irradiation on lymphocyte cytotoxicity. This was evaluated by ^{51}Cr release using a cytotoxic assay with mouse (C57B1) splenocytes against P815 × 2 mastocytoma cells from DBA mice. The results show a very early (within a few hours) significant exponential decrease in lytic units as a function of irradiation dose. Numerous studies support the observation that not only do lethal cell changes occur which can cause humoral release of immunosuppressive cytotoxins, from irradiated tissues, but that marked lymphocyte metabolic perturbations also occur [50–54].

A third mechanism deals with potentially altered immunocompetency of irradiated lymphocytes which fail to stimulate allogenic lymphocytes in mixed lymphocyte cultures (MLC).

Radiotherapeutic immunosuppression during the treatment of head and neck cancers may arise from irradiation of different lymphoid organs (thymus, lymph nodes, bone marrow) [55]. However, radiosensitivity varies for each of these tissues. In this respect, bone marrow would be more affected than thymus [56]. Irradiation of circulating lymphocytes is probably a function of target volume. Most circulating lymphocytes are in Go phase. It is for this reason that the dose-response curve for irradiation versus tritiated thymidine uptake can be attributed to inhibition of induction of blast transformation. As other authors [57, 58] have pointed out, the role of certain serum factors should also be taken into account. Twomey *et al.* [59] found that serum from patients with head and neck cancers significantly suppressed lymphocyte response to PHA and Con A. Grant *et al.* [60] have demonstrated a circulating immunosuppressive factor found in higher concentrations in venous blood draining tumor tissue than in the systemic circulation. Currie *et al.* [61] have shown by lymphocytotoxic studies in cancer patients that serum factors act on lymphocytes and not on autologous tumor cells *in vitro*. Furthermore, if these same lymphocytes are washed prior to contact with target cells, the previously impaired cytotoxic function becomes quasi-normal. In contrast, Chee *et al.* [62] have shown that normal lymphocytes incubated with serum from irradiated patients demonstrate no change in cytotoxic function thereby suggesting that serum factors are not present. Other authors [63, 64] reported the presence of antibodies to herpes simplex virus-induced tumor-associated antigens in the serum of patients with head and neck cancer. In addition, there was a positive correlation between abnormal immune reactivity and the presence of these antibodies.

Recent data suggest that the capacity of either T lymphocyte subset depends on the nature of the target cell [65]. Other separation methods have been used for immunocompetent cells. Some authors [66–69] have shown that monocytes removed from the total lymphocyte population are very significantly immunosuppressive after radiotherapy. Prior to removal of monocytes by glass wool, tritiated thymidine uptake after irradiation was significantly lower ($p < 0.01$), whereas this same uptake reached preirradiation levels after monocyte elimination. It is as if irradiation stimulates an immunosuppressive cell population (monocytes which are retained on glass wool) thereby allowing monocyte-free lymphocytes to express normal tritiated thymidine uptake.

Blomgren et al. [70, 71] have shown in mixed lymphocyte cultures (MLC) that the response and stimulation capacities of cell preparation obtained at completion of radiation therapy were increased following depletion of phagocytic cells. This partially explains the immunosuppression observed shortly after radiation therapy which is associated with the appearance of nonspecific suppressor cells demonstrating monocyte characteristics. This selection of an immunosuppressive subpopulation by radiotherapy may be favored by cell repair and tumor cell growth [72]. However, one cannot neglect the possibility that radiotherapy may render tumor cells more vulnerable to the effects of immunocompetent cells. Moreover, it should be noted that the cell population thus separated and referred to as 'adherent' and 'nonadherent' are not homogenous populations and that the adherent fraction contains not only monocytes [73–78]. Before coming to a definite conclusion, other methods of separation should be considered. An alternative procedure consists of a Sephadex column technique where Sephadex is conjugated to human antiimmunoglobulin. The cells eluted from this column are essentially T cells which are then placed on a BSA gradient and separated on the basis of cell density. Stimulation of each subpopulation by the 3 mitogens immediately after radiotherapy, and 3 months after radiotherapy, demonstrated a change in cell response for the 23 patients investigated. Fractions 1.072 and 1.095 had significantly impaired tritiated thymidine uptake immediately after irradiation, whereas this value rose to almost normal when average uptake was reexamined at a much later time. For patients who reestablish normal uptake values, we noted a good prognosis whereas for the patients with persistent impaired immune response, the prognosis was poor with continued neoplastic evolution or relapse.

For patients in which the 1.064 fraction was decreased for several weeks after cessation of radiotherapy, no correlation was established between levels of this fraction and either evolution of the disease or prognosis.

The difference between the different cell fractions may be due to the fact that T 1.064 contains the youngest, most immature and undifferentiated cells, therefore the most radiosensitive. One can understand the profound effect of irradiation on highly undifferentiated marrow stem cells from which will ultimately evolve different myeloid and lymphoid lines. Their radiosensitivity involving almost irreversible radiolesions (long and difficult regeneration of stem cells) may be the origin of immunological consequences as a result of moderate and long term radiotherapy.

Our study of lymphocyte markers showed a significant drop in E-rosette forming cells (T cells) but no significant change for EAC-rosette (null or B cells), as others [79–85] have previously shown. T-cells appear to be considerably more radiosensitive than other lymphocyte subpopulations.

These results are in direct contradiction with those reported by Blomgren [86] who found a significantly lower EAC-rosette value and sightly increased E-rosettes for breast cancer patients treated by radiotherapy. Some in vitro studies [87], have also shown non-T cell radiosensitivity to be greater than that attributed to T cells.

These seemingly contradictory findings may be due to the fact that the non-T population is repopulated much faster than the T population which can remain at low levels for several months or even years. Some experimental results [88] suggest that this is due to a change in the chronology of the repair mechanism following radio-lesions in B and T splenocyte populations after whole body X irradiation. Since the non-T population recuperates more quickly, false radioresistance can be noted during testing which may have been performed too late to pick up the rapidly reversed modifications of the non-T population. The slight increase in T cells reported by Blomgren [71] which was not present in our results [89], was accompanied by a weaker PHA response.

The analysis of post-radiotherapeutic immunodeficiency should not only include studies of impaired lymphocyte function mechanism and of action involved, but also an appreciation of the time involved in repairing cellular damage observed under therapy as well as the duration of radiation effects. Many authors [90–92] have emphasized the prolonged weakening effect of radiation on the immune response. Thomas et al. [93] noted that decreased response lasts for about 1 year in patients with lung carcinoma. Similar observations have been reported by other authors [94] for patients with breast cancer treated by radiotherapy alone. Tarpley et al. [95] described the same phenomena in certain laryngeal cancers. Fuks et al. [96] using E-rosette and cytotoxicity assays, have shown that suppressed T lymphocyte function may last for over 2 years and that mixed lymphocyte cultures of cells from these patients in contact with allogenic lymphocytes reflect strongly impaired T cell function for at least 3 years. However, numerous authors [97–100] have stressed the opposite: repaired lymphocyte function with test values returning to normal.

Our correlative study of post-irradiation immunosuppression and prognosis is of definite interest since as in the literature [101] the return of normal function or the prolongation of post-radiotherapeutic immunosuppression can serve as a reliable indication of favorable or poor prognosis. A study at 8 months-post-irradiation showed a significant difference between patients where thymidine uptake had returned to normal in response to PHA, PWM and Con A and those where uptake remained impaired.

In the former group, the ratio of patients cured to total number of patients (17/34) was significantly higher than for the second group (2/20).

In recent years a correlation between prognosis and *in vitro* tests, as well as skin tests, has been demonstrated. Although there is no correlation between pretreatment levels and survival there is a significant correlation between elevated *in vitro* post-radiotherapeutic immune response and survival time.

Still other studies [9, 102] have demonstrated a prognostic indicator based on monitoring T lymphocyte changes, where a poor prognosis would correspond to prolonged T lymphocyte suppression following irradiation, with minimal prognostic potential attributed to B lymphocytes.

In conclusion, the essential points resulting from our study are:

(1) There is a clear immunosuppression in patients treated by radiotherapy.

(2) The different behavior of the various lymphocyte sub-populations (exaggerated post-irradiation monocyte suppressor function or predominance of T-lymphocyte suppression) demands that these different sub-populations be examined individually. This would therefore imply developing new, or perfecting existing techniques for quantitative and/or qualitative lymphocyte separation and testing of a given lymphocyte function.

(3) A prognostic parameter based on monitoring immune function during, and for a considerable time after radiotherapy by skin tests and *in vitro* tests with an emphasis on T lymphocytes.

(4) Additional studies will be necessary to further examine the correlation between functional laboratory test results and clinical evolution in order to better modulate immunological perturbation, either by reinforcing a beneficial disequilibrium or impeding negative radiotherapeutic immunological events that contribute to tumor evolution.

222

References

1. Anderson RE, Warner NL: Ionizing radiation and the immune response. Advances Immunol 24:215–335, 1976.
2. Schlossman SE, Hudson L: Specific purification of lymphocyte populations on a digestible immunoabsorbant. J Immunol 110:313, 1973.
3. Ghossein NA, Bosworth JL, Bases RE: The effect of radical radiotherapy on delayed hypersensitivity and the inflammatory response. Cancer 35:1616–1620, 1975.
4. Catalona WJ, Chretien PB: Abnormalities of quantitative dinitrochlorobenzene sensitization in cancer patients. Correlation with tumor stage and histology. Cancer 31:353–356, 1973.
5. Jenkins VK, Griffiths CM, Ray P, Perry RR, Olson MH: Radiotherapy and head and neck cancer. Role of lymphocyte response and clinical stage. Arch Otolaryngol 106:414, 1980.
6. Vetto RM, Burger DR, Vandenbark AA, Finke PE: Changes in tumor immunity during therapy, determined by leucocyte adherence inhibition and dermal testing. Cancer 41:1034–1039, 1973.
7. Eilber FR, Morton DL, Ketcham AS: Immunologic abnormalities in head and neck cancer. Amer J Surg 128:534, 1974.
8. Gross L, Manfredi OO, Protos A: Effect of Cobalt-60 irradiation upon cell-mediated immunity. Radiology 106:653–655, 1973.
9. Stefani S, Kerman R, Abbate J: Serial studies of immunocompetence in head and neck cancer patients undergoing radiation therapy. Amer J Roentgenol 126:880–886, 1976.
10. Clement JA, Kramer S: Immunocompetence in patients with solid tumors undergoing cobalt 60 irradiation. Cancer 34:193–196, 1974.
11. Bosworth JL, Ghossein NA, Brooks TL: Delayed hypersensitivity in patients treated by curative radiotherapy. Its relation to tumor response and short-term survival. Cancer 35:353–358, 1975.
12. Eilber FR, Morton DL: Impaired immunological reactivity and recurrence following cancer surgery. Cancer 25:362–367, 1970.
13. Hersh EM, Whitecar JP, Maccredie KB, Bodey GP, Freireich EJ: Chemotherapy, immunocompetence, immunosuppression and prognosis in acute leukemia. New Engl J Med 285:1211–1216, 1971.
14. Golub SH, O'Connell TX, Morton DL: Correlation of *in vivo* and *in vitro* assays of immunocompetence in cancer patients. Cancer Res 34:1833–1837, 1974.
15. Idestrom K, Petrini B, Blomgren H, Wasserman J, Wallgren A, Baral E: Changes of the peripheral lymphocyte population following radiation therapy to extended and limited fields. Int J Radiat Oncol Biol Phys 5:1761–1766, 1979.
16. Baral E, Blomgren H, Petrini B, Wasserman J: Blood lymphocytes in breast cancer patients following radiotherapy and surgery. Int J Radiat Oncol Biol Phys 2:289–295, 1977.
17. Stjernsward J, Jondal M, Vanky S, Wigzell H, Sealy R: Lymphopenia and change in distribution of human B and T lymphocytes in peripheral blood induced by irradiation for mammary carcinoma. Lancet 1:1352–1356, 1972.
18. Papatesta AE, Kark A: Peripheral lymphocyte counts in breast carcinoma. An index of immune competence. Cancer 34:2014–2017, 1974.
19. Reisco A: Five year cancer cure: Relation to total amount of peripheral lymphocytes and neutrophils. Cancer 25:135–140, 1970.
20. Hilal EY, Wanebo HJ, Pinsky CM, Oettgen HF: Immunologic evaluation and prognosis in patients with head and neck cancer. Am J Surg 134:469–473, 1977.
21. Doria G: Immunological effects of irradiation: Waiting for a model. Int J Radiat Oncol Biol Phys 5:1111–1116, 1979.
22. Herberman RB, Kjeu JY, Kay HD, Ortaldo JR, Riccardi C, Bonnard GD, Holden HT,

Fagnani R, Santoni A, Puccetti P: Natural Killer cells: Characteristics and regulation of activity. Immunol Rev 44:43, 1979.

23. Wasserman J, Baral E, Biberfeld G, Blomgren H, Petrini B, Von Stedingk LV, Strender LE: Effect of *in vitro* irradiation on lymphocyte subpopulations and cytotoxicity. In: Dubois JB *et al.* (eds) Immunopharmacologic Effects of Radiation Therapy. New York, Raven Press, 1981, pp 123–135.

24. Pross HF, Baines MG: Spontaneous Lymphocyte mediated cytotoxicity against tumor target cells. VI. A brief review. Cancer Immunol Immunother 3:75–85, 1977.

25. Dean DM, Pross HF, Kennedy JC: Spontaneous human lymphocyte-mediated cytotoxicity against tumor target cells. III. Stimulatory and inhibitory effects of ionizing radiation. Int J Radiat Oncol Biol Phys 4:633–641, 1978.

26. Moretta L, Webb SR, Grossi CE, Lydyard PM, Cooper MD: Functionnal analysis of two human T cell subpopulations: Help and suppression of B cell response by T cells bearing receptors for IgM (Tm) or IgG (Tg). J Exp Med 146:184–200, 1979.

27. Thorn RM, Henney CS: Studies on the mechanism of lymphocyte-mediated cytolysis. VI. A reappraisal of the requirement of protein synthesis during T cell-mediated lysis. J Immunol 116:146–155, 1976.

28. Reinherz EL, Moretta L, Roper M, Breard JM, Mingari MD, Cooper MD, Schlosman SF: Human T lymphocyte sub-populations defined by Fc receptors and monoclonal antibodies. J Exp Med 151:969–974, 1980.

29. Gupta S, Winchester RJ, Good RA: General orientation of human lymphocyte sub-populations. In: Bach F, Good R (eds) Clinical Immunology. New York, Academic Press, 1980, pp 2–31.

30. Cordier G, Samarut C, Revillard JP: Contribution of lymphocytes bearing Fcγ receptors to PHA induced cytotoxicity. Immunology 35:49–56, 1978.

31. Pichler WJ, Gendelman FW, Nelson DL: Fc receptors on human T lymphocytes. II. Cytotoxic capabilities of human Tγ, Tμ, B and L cells. Cell Immunol 42:410–417, 1979.

32. Ghossein NA, Kadish AS, Rubinstein A: Effects of radiotherapy on the immune system of patients with localized cancer. In: Dubois JB *et al.* (eds) Immuno Pharmacologic Effects of Radiation Therapy. New York, Raven Press, 1981, pp 207–217.

33. Wanebo HJ, Jun My, Strong EW, Oettgen H: T cell deficiency in patients with squamous cell cancer of the head and neck. Am J Surg 130:445–451, 1975.

34. Wanebo HJ: Observations on the effects of adjuvant Radiation on immune tests of patients with colorectal cancer and head and neck cancer. In: Dubois JB *et al.* (eds) Immunopharmacologic Effects of Radiation Therapy. New York, Raven Press, 1981, pp 241–252.

35. Rafla S, Yang SJ, Meleka F: Changes in cell-mediated immunity in patients undergoing radiotherapy. Cancer 41:1076–1086, 1978.

36. Nordman E, Toivanen A: Effects of irradiation on the immune function in patients with mammary, pulmonary or head and neck carcinoma. Acta Radiol Oncol Biol Phys 17:3–9, 1978.

37. Mason JM, Kitchens GG, Eastham RJ, Jennings BR: T lymphocytes and survival of head and neck squamous cell carcinomas. Arch Otolaryngol 103:223–227, 1977.

38. Dellon A, Potvin C, Chretien P: Thymus dependent lymphocyte levels during radiation therapy for bronchogenic and esophageal carcinoma. Am J Roentgenol 123:500–511, 1975.

39. Maclaren JR, Olkowski ZL, Skeen MJ, MacConnell FMS, Benigno B, Mansour K, Nixon DW, EElls R, Shah NK: Response of immune parameters to irradiation of patients with head and neck, bronchogenic, and uterine cervical cancers and to subsequent immunotherapy. In: Dubois JB *et al.* (eds) Immunopharmacologic Effects of Radiation Therapy. New York, Raven Press, 1981, pp 253–274.

40. Blomgren H, Baral E, Jarstrand C, Petrini B, Strender LE, Wallgren A, Wasserman J:

Effect of external radiation therapy on the peripheral lymphocyte population. In: Dubois JB *et al.* (eds) immunopharmacologic Effects of Radiation Therapy. New York, Raven Press, 1981, pp 299–319.

41. Wara WM, Phillips TL, Wara DW, Ammann AJ, Smith V: Immunosuppression after radiation therapy for carcinoma of the nasopharynx. Am J Roentgenol 123:482–485, 1975.

42. Deegan MJ, Coulthard SW, Qualman SJ, Schork MA: A correlative analysis of *in vitro* parameters of cellular immunity in patients with squamous cell carcinoma of the head and neck. Cancer Res 37:4475–4481, 1977.

43. Order SE: The effects of therapeutic irradiations on lymphocytes and immunity. Cancer 39:737–743, 1977.

44. Merz T, Hazra T, Ross M, Ciborowski L: Transformation delay of lymphocytes in patients undergoing radiation therapy. Amer J Roentgenol 127:337–339, 1976.

45. Slater JM, Ngo E, Lau BHS: Effects of therapeutic irradiation on the immune response. Amer J Roentgenol 126:313–320, 1976.

46. Davies AJS, Wallis VJ, Peckham MJ: Suppression of the immune response by ionizing radiation. In: Dubois JB *et al.* (eds) Immunopharmacologic Effects of Radiation Therapy. New York, Raven Press, 1981, pp 1–6.

47. Diomigi R, Zonta A, Albertario F, Galeazzi R, Bellinzona G: Cyclic variation in the response of lymphocytes to phytohemagglutinin in healthy individuals. Transplantation 16:500–559, 1973.

48. Han T, Takita H: Immunologic impairment in bronchogenic carcinoma: a study of lymphocyte response to phytohemagglutinin. Cancer 30:616–621, 1972.

49. Song CW, Rhee JG, Kim T, Kersey JH, Levitt SH: Effect of X-Irradiation on immunocompetency of T-lymphocytes. In: Dubois JB *et al.* (eds) Immunopharmacologic Effects of Radiation Therapy. New York, Raven Press, 1981, pp 75–91.

50. Cantor H, Boyse EA: Functional subclasses of T lymphocytes bearing different Ly antigens. I. The generation of functionally distinct T cell subclasses is a differentiative process independent of antigen. J Exp Med 141:1376–1389, 1975.

51. Cantor H, Boyse EA: Functional subclasses of T lymphocytes bearing different Ly antigens. II. Cooperation between subclasses of Ly^+ cells in the generation of Killer activity. J Exp Med 141:1390–1399, 1975.

52. Huber B, Cantor H, Shen FW, Boyse EA: Independent differentiative pathways of Ly 1 and Ly 23 subclasses of T cells experimental production of mice deprived of selected T cell subclasses. J Exp Med 144:1128–1133, 1976.

53. Baskies AM, Chretien PB, Weiss JF, Makuch RW, Kenady DE, Spiegel HE: Improvements in circulating levels of immune reactive proteins simultaneous with depression of thymus-dependent lymphocytes during radiation therapy for solid malignancies. In: Dubois JB *et al.* (eds) Immunopharmacologic Effects of Radiation Therapy. New York, Raven Press, 1981, pp 347–363.

54. Cerottini JC, Brunner KT: Cell-mediated cytotoxicity, allograft rejection and tumor immunity. Adv Immunol 18:67–132, 1974.

55. Sharp JG, Watkins EB: Cellular and Immunological consequences of thymic irradiation. In: Dubois JB *et al.* (eds) Immunopharmacologic Effects of Radiation Therapy. New York, Raven Press, 1981, pp 137–179.

56. Stratton JA, Byfield PE, Byfield JE, Small RC, Benfield J, Pilch Y: A comparison of the acute effects of radiation therapy including or excluding the thymus on the lymphocyte sub-populations of cancer patients. J Clin Invest 56:88–97, 1975.

57. Einhorn N: Effect of local radiotherapy on the level of EBV associated membrane – reactive antibodies in the sera of patients with certain malignant tumor. Cancer 29:714–723, 1972.

58. Moroson H, Abithol A, Madden R: Reversal by serum of the immunosuppressive effect of

total body irradiation in rats. In: Dubois JB *et al.* (eds) Immunopharmacologic effects of Radiation Therapy. New York, Raven Press, 1981, pp 181–193.

59. Twomey PL, Catalona WJ, Chretien PB: Cellular immunity in cured cancer patients. Cancer, 33:435–440, 1974.

60. Grant RM, Harris C, Mathieson W, Norman JN: The influence of serum and cellular factors in the depression of phytohemagglutinin (PHA) induced transformation of lymphocytes in gastro.intestinal carcinoma. Brit J Surg 60:322–327, 1973.

61. Currie GA, Basham C: Serum mediated inhibition of the immunological reactions of the patient to his own tumor: a possible role for circulating antigen. Brit J Cancer 26:427–431, 1972.

62. Chee CA, Illbery PLT, Rickenson AB: Depression of Lymphocyte replicating ability in radiotherapy patients. Brit J Radiol 47:37–43, 1974.

63. Silverman NA, Alexander JC, Hollinshead AC, Chretien PB: Correlation of tumor burden with *in vitro* lymphocyte reactivity and antibodies to Herpes virus tumor associated antigens in head and neck squamous carcinoma. Cancer 37:135–140, 1976.

64. Hollinshead AC, Chretien PB, Lee O, Tarpley JL, Kerney SE, Silverman NA, Alexander JC: *In vivo* and *in vitro* measurement of the relationship of human squamous carcinomas to Herpes Simplex virus tumor associated antigens. Cancer Res 36:3274–3278, 1976.

65. Lum LG, Muchmore AV, Decker JM, Blaese RM: MICC Cytotoxic effector function of human T. Lymphocyte sub-populations bearing Fc receptors for IgG and IgM. Clin Exp Immunol 37:558–561, 1979.

66. Pierce CW: Macrophages: modulators of immunity. Amer J Pathol 98:10–28, 1980.

67. Wasserman J, Blomgren H, Petrini B, Baral E, Strender LE, Jarstrand C, Von Stedingk LV: Effect of Radiation Therapy and *in vitro* X-Ray exposure on Lymphocyte sub-populations and their functions. Amer J Clin Oncol 5:195–208, 1982.

68. Moroson H, Nowakowski J, Schechter M: Enhanced lymphocyte-mediated Killing of tumor cells after tumor irradiation*in vivo*. Int J Radiat Oncol Biol Phys 33:473–482, 1978.

69. Jerrells TR, Dean JH, Richardson GL, Mac Coy JL, Herberman RB: Role of suppressor cells in depression of *in vitro* lymphoproliferative responses of lung cancer and breast cancer patients. J Natl Cancer Inst 61:1001–1009, 1978.

70. Blomgren H, Wasserman J, Baral E, Petrini B: Evidence for the appearance of non-specific suppressor cells in the blood after local radiation therapy. Int J Radiat Oncol Biol Phys 4:249–253, 1978.

71. Blomgren H, Wasserman J, Wallgren A, Idestrom K, Baral E, Petrini B: Changes in mixed lymphocyte culture (MLC) functions of peripheral lymphoid cells after radiation therapy for breast carcinoma. Int J Radiat Oncol Biol Phys 5:49–53, 1979.

72. Fujimoto S, Greene MI, Sehon AH: Regulation of the immune response to tumor antigens. I. Immunosuppressor cells in tumor bearing hosts. J Immunol 116:791–799, 1976.

73. Unanue ER: The regulation of lymphocyte functions by the macophage. Immunol Rev 40:227–255, 1978.

74. Jandinski T, Cantor H, Tadakuma T, Peavy DL, Pierce CW: Separation of helper T-cells from suppressor T-cell expressing different Ly component. I. Polyclonal activation: suppressor and helper activities are inherent properties of distinct T-cell subclasses. J Exp Med 143:1382–1390, 1976.

75. Ryoyama K, Ehrke MJ, Mihich E: Cell-cell interactions in the generation of 'non-specific' suppressor cells in culture and its modification by Adriamycin. In: Dubois JB *et al.* (eds) Immunopharmacologic Effects of Radiation Therapy. New York, Raven Press, 1981, pp 23–37.

76. Gershon RK: The importance of suppressor cells in immunoregulation. In: Singhal SK, Sinclair NR (eds) Suppressor Cells in Immunity. London , Ontario, University of Western Ontario Press, 1975, pp 1–11.

226

77. Waldmann TA, Broder S: Suppressor cells in the regulation of the immune response. Prog Clin Immunol 3:155–199, 1977.
78. Greene MI, Fujimoto S, Sehon AH: Regulation of the immune response of the tumor antigens. II. Characterization of thymic suppressor factors produced by tumor-bearing hosts. J Immunol 119:757–764, 1977.
79. Agarossi G, Pozzi L, Mancini C, Doria G: Radiosensitivity of the helper cell function. J Immunol 121:2118–2121, 1978.
80. Lajtha LG: Stem cell concepts. Differentiation 14:23–34, 1979.
81. Alexander P: The bogey of the immunosuppressive action of local radiotherapy. Int J Radiat Oncol Biol Phys 1:369–371, 1976.
82. Anderson RE, Olson GB, Autry JR, Howarth JL, Troup GM, Bartels PH: Radiosensitivity of T and B lymphocytes. IV. Effects of whole body irradiation upon various lympoid tissues and number of recirculating lymphocytes. J Immunol 118:1191–1200, 1977.
83. Birkeland SA: Influence of irradiation on the capacity of human T and B lymphocytes to form E and HEAC Rosettes. Transplantation 29:23–24, 1980.
84. Fudenberg HH, Wybran J, Robbins D: T-Rosette forming cells, cellular immunity and cancer. New Engl J Med 292:475, 1975.
85. Raben M, Heise er, Kucera LS, Hale A, Witcofski R, Plunkett S: Effects of irradiation on lymphocyte subpopulation. In: Dubois JB et al. (eds) Immunopharmacologic Effects of Radiation Therapy. New York, Raven Press, 1981, pp 321–328.
86. Blomgren H, Glas U, Melen B, Wasserman J: Blood lymphocytes after radiation therapy of mammary carcinoma. Acta Radiol Ther Biol Phys 13:185–200, 1974.
87. Wasserman J, Baral E, Blomgren H, Petrini B: The effect of in vitro irradiation on lymphocyte subpopulations and cytotoxicity. J Clin Lab Immunol 1:147–150, 1978.
88. Smith DM, Gross RL, Baron P, Thomas RG: The effect of low level, whole body X-irradiation on splenic immunologic function. Radiat Res 74:469–470, 1978.
89. Dubois JB, Serrou B: Effects of ionizing radiation on cell-mediated immunity in cancer patients. In Dubois JB et al. (eds) Immunopharmacologic Effects of Radiation Therapy. New York, Raven Press, 1981, pp 275–298.
90. Gerber M, Dubois JB, Pioch Y, Serrou B: Effects of localized radiotherapy upon the cellular immune response. Radiat Res 85:390–398, 1981.
91. Hoppe RT, Fuks ZY, Strober S, Kaplan HS: Immunosuppressive effects of ionizing radiation. In: Dubois JB et al. (eds) Immunopharmacologic Effects of Radiation Therapy. New York, Raven Press, 1981, pp 195–206.
92. Wara WM, Ammann AJ, Wara DW: Effects of thymosin and irradiation on immune modulation in head and neck and esophageal cancer patients. Cancer Treat Rep 62:1775–1778, 1978.
93. Thomas JE, Coy P, Lewis HS, Yven A: Effect of therapeutic irradiation on lymphocyte transformation in lung cancer. Cancer 27:1046–1050, 1971.
94. Stjernsward J: Radiotherapy, host immunity and cancer spread. In: Stoll BA (ed) Secondary Spread in Breast Cancer. Chicago Heinemann Medical and Year Book Medical, 1977, pp 139–167.
95. Tarpley JL, Potvin C, Chretien PB: Prolonged depression of cellular immunity in cured laryngopharyngeal cancer patients treated with radiation therapy. Cancer 35:638–644, 1975.
96. Fuks ZY, Strober S, Bobrove A, Sasazuki T, Mac Michael A, Kaplan HS: Long term effects of radiation on T and B lymphocytes in peripheral blood of patients with Hodgkin's disease. J Clin Invest 58:803–814, 1976.
97. Sharp JG, Thomas DB: Origins of the radioresistant precursor cells responsible for the initial phase of thymic regeneration after X-irradiation. J Reticuloendothel Soc 22:169–176, 1977.
98. Song CW, Guertin DP: Combined effect of X-irradiation and cell-mediated immune reac-

tion. Radiat Res 75:586–592, 1978.

99. Suit HD, Batten GW Jr: Theoretical considerations of the effect of an immunological rejection response on the growth of tumor. In: Chicago, Year Book Medical (eds) Neoplasia in Childhood. 1979, pp 51–59.

100. Wara WM, Wara DW, Ammann AJ: Immunosuppression and reconstitution after Radiation Therapy. In: Dubois JB *et al.* (eds) Immunopharmacologic Effects of Radiation Therapy. New York, Raven Press, 1981, pp 219–229.

101. Jenkins VK: Immunocompetence in head and neck cancer patients undergoing radiotherapy. In: Prasad N (ed) Radiotherapy and Cancer Immunology. Boca Raton, Florida, CRC Press Inc, 1981, pp 51–64.

102. Olkowski SL, Wilkins SA: T-lymphocyte levels in the peripheral blood of patients with cancer of the head and neck. Amer J Surg 130:440–444, 1975.

10. Cell kinetics in the study and treatment of head and neck cancer

ROBERTO MOLINARI, AURORA COSTA, ROSELLA
SILVESTRINI, FRANCO MATTAVELLI,
GIULIO CANTÙ, FAUSTO CHIESA and FABIO VOLTERRANI

1. Cell proliferation

Every cell able to reproduce itself passes through a cell cycle composed of
four successive phases (Fig. 1), and each one is characterized by a series of
biochemical events that prepare the following phase and that are governed
by specific enzymes. The first one is the mitotic phase (M), which has been
well known for a long time because it is morphologically identifiable under
light microscopy. Another characteristic phase is that in which the cell syn-
thesizes its DNA for replication (S). Between these phases two other time
intervals are intercalated: a postmitotic (G_1) and a premitotic (G_2) phase,
where G stands for gap. In fact, during these phases, RNA and proteins are
synthesized, but biochemical events have not yet been well defined. In every
tissue, either normal or neoplastic, the duration of the S phase, G_2 and M
are quite constant, accounting respectively for 8–30 h, 1–2 h, and 30–
90 min. The widest variation (from hours to months) occurs in the G_1
phase.

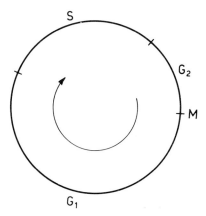

Figure 1. The cell cycle.

Gregory T. Wolf (ed), Head and Neck Oncology.
© *1984 Martinus Nijhoff Publishers, Boston. ISBN 0-89838-657-8. Printed in The Netherlands.*

230

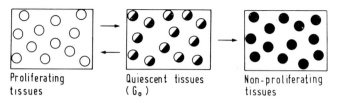

Proliferating
tissues

Quiescent tissues
(G₀)

Non-proliferating
tissues

Figure 2. Compartments of cell proliferation in normal tissues.

1.1. Normal tissues

From a kinetic standpoint, three main groups of normal tissues can be considered (Fig. 2). (1) Nonproliferating tissues, which have definitely lost the ability to proliferate, i.e., neuronic cells, striated muscle. (2) Normally non-proliferating tissues (G_0), which still conserve their potential capacity to proliferate as a response to physiological stimuli, i.e., periosteum and hepatic cells after partial hepatectomy. (3) Proliferating tissues, in which cell proliferation maintains the population constant. They can exhibit a very low basic proliferative rate (hepatic parenchyma, smooth muscle, connective tissue) or a moderate to high proliferative rate. The latter is the case for tissues whose cells have a very short life span, such as bone marrow, mucosal cells of the gastrointestinal system, oral cavity, bladder or vagina, and exocrine glands under particular stimuli.

In summary, apart from the first group, all normal tissues are thought to be constituted of potentially proliferating cells or resting cells that can be stimulated to proliferate as a consequence of a decreased cell pool. The condition of steady state is controlled by enzymes and chalones, which assure an exact balance between dead cells and newly produced cells. Normal tissues with high cell renewal rates constitute an important problem for the oncologist, both chemotherapists and radiotherapists, since their proliferative state is generally more susceptible to ionizing radiations and cytotoxic drug effects [1–4].

1.2. Neoplastic tissues

The essential difference between normal and neoplastic cells has been repeatedly shown to be a function of the perturbation of very subtle mechanisms of control of their main activities: proliferation and functional differentiation. These activities are strictly controlled in normal organs and tissues so that a correct cell function is the absolutely prevalent end point, whereas proliferation occurs only to reconstitute the amount of lost differentiated cells in a balanced way. From this point of view, tumor cells can be defined as cells in which these mechanisms are not necessarily completely lost, but certainly altered. Their perturbation involves both differentiation and proliferation to various degrees, and this can partially explain the behavioral differences that exist among different tumor types. However, whereas the loss of differentiation can also happen in several diseases other than cancer, uncontrolled proliferation is peculiar of malignancy and is the main mechanism that causes the host's death. Both normal and neoplastic tissues can be highly proliferative, but tumor cells do not necessarily proliferate faster than normal cells. In fact, the cell cycle duration is generally reported to be shorter in tumor cells than in the normal cells of the tissue of origin, but there are also normal tissues in which cell duplication time is shorter than the malignant counterpart [1].

In tumor cell lines or in animal ascitic tumors, all cells are continuously proliferating and their number increases exponentially. Conversely, in solid tumors of animals and humans, growth is thought to be exponential only in the preclinical phase of development, whereas during clinical life some factors cause a progressive decrease in tumor growth rate [4]. In this way, at any time only a fraction of cells is actually proliferating, whereas the other cells are not proliferating for a number of reasons. A certain amount of the new cells are inherently sterile or reach a certain degree of differentiation; moreover, a number of cells are simply resting or quiescent (G_0 cells), and their number can markedly expand the G_1 phase. These cells represent a sort of stem cell, which can be stimulated to enter the reproductive cycle by a reduction in the proliferating pool or by other still unknown stimuli (recruitment).

The negative contribution to growth by cell death and cell loss must also be considered. A large fraction of cells meet death by nutritional deficiency, DNA alteration, or immunological host reaction. Dead cells may autolyse and be resorbed or removed by phagocytosis. Moreover, cells can leave the tumor by exfoliation at a surface (and this is typical for mucosal cancers) or via the lymphatics or the bloodstream (metastases). A combination of all these events results in a tumor mass and can explain the various patterns of natural history of different tumor types and also of different tumors of the same type.

2. Methodologic approaches

Growth of a tumor mass can be determined by clinical or radiological evaluation [5, 6] of its size at various intervals, but this is possible only for lesions accessible for the different types of measurement. Tumor growth may also be estimated on the basis of the proliferative activity of the cell population, which can be evaluated by means of more or less sophisticated experimental approaches. One of these approaches is based on the fact that cells in the S phase specifically incorporate a metabolic precursor of DNA synthesis, [^{3}H]thymidine. The cells that become labeled can be detected by autoradiographic techniques [4], that give images composed of black grains visible under light microscopy.

Complete knowledge of kinetic status of a tumor would require the determination of the length of the cell cycle and of the four phases, together with an assessment of cell distribution in the various phases. This information can be obtained by use of a technique that evaluates the percentage of labeled mitoses (PLM) [7] at successive times after a single injection of labeled precursor in *in vivo* experiments or after a pulse labeling in *in vitro* experiments. However, this methodology, which is largely feasible in experimental systems, is often not applicable to human tumors for logistic and ethical limitations mainly related to the need for serial biopsies.

These constraints, which are responsible for the few studies performed in the past on human tumors, have been overcome by the introduction of very simplified methodology that requires a tumor sample at only one time. This approach evaluates the number of cells that are labeled as compared to the total population of cells 1 h after the injection of [^{3}H] thymidine in the patient or after 1 h of *in vitro* contact of the tumor biopsy with the ^{3}H labeled precursor. This kinetic parameter is called the labeling index (LI); it does not represent the total number of proliferating cells but the fraction that is in the S phase at a precise time. However, the LI is generally used as an indicator of potential proliferative rate.

Owing to the heterogeneity of the cell population within a tumor mass, an accurate evaluation needs to score many specimens sampled from different areas of each tumor. Moreover, the strict relation of *in vivo* to *in vitro* determinations of the LI [8] has resulted in a preference of the latter for ethical and economic reasons. This simplified methodology allows cell kinetic determination on a large series of tumors with results obtained in 3 to 10 days.

Another type of approach is represented by a more recent and sophisticated methodology, flow cytometry (FCM). This technique is based on the binding of fluorescent dyes to cell macromolecules (DNA, RNA, proteins) and on their activation by a laser beam [9–11]. In such a way, the distribution of cells in the different cycle phases can be analyzed and quantified by mathematical procedures [12–15]. The results are obtained very quickly, but this methodology, which requires cell suspensions, still has some intrinsic problems related to the possibility of a selection of cell subpopulations during disaggregation procedures of solid tumors.

Prospectives and limits of the different experimental approaches has led to the reservation of the application of FCM and PLM to a restricted number of cases, and to use the LI procedure for routine use. In the last few years, a renewed interest in the cell proliferative status of human tumors, promoted by this simplified technical procedure, has resulted in the collection of much information for several tumor types [16–19].

3. Kinetics of epidermoid carcinoma

Most cell kinetic investigations of human epidermoid carcinoma have been carried out on small series of patients [20–23], and relatively few data have been obtained by the estimation of LI [24–26]. A complete investigation with speculative and clinical purposes should include the analysis of the relationship between the proliferative activity of the primary tumor and different clinical (sex, age, anatomical site) and pathologic (stage, histological differentiation) features, the evaluation of the relationship between the proliferative activity of the primary tumor and that of lymph node metastases, the assessment of the relevance of proliferative activity to clinical outcome in patients homogeneously treated, and the definition of the predictive role of proliferative activity on response to chemo- or radiotherapy. The final aims should be to gain information for a better understanding of the biology of this neoplasm, and to identify new biological features or to define experimental approaches of potential prognostic or therapeutic use.

A systematic evaluation of cell kinetics of head and neck carcinomas was planned in 1978 at the Istituto Nazionale Tumori of Milan. Most data obtained from this study are already available for useful interpretation and can be used to draw some conclusions. Other findings are still insufficient and can only suggest some trends or new working hypotheses. We will make an effort to refer to the latter as a component of the emerging literature.

3.1. Relationship with different morphological, clinical and pathological features

Kinetic studies were performed on a series of untreated patients with epidermoid carcinoma located in various sites of the oral cavity, oropharynx and larynx. The LI was determined on samples of fresh tumor material incubated *in vitro* for 1 h with [^{3}H] thymidine. From a comparison with other human tumors examined, head and neck cancers showed a median proliferative activity (12.4%) similar to that observed for lung cancer, less than that for testicular tumors and markedly higher than that observed for non-Hodgkin lymphomas (NHL), melanoma and breast cancer (Table 1). Notwithstanding the gradient of median proliferative rates observed for the different tumor types, a wide range of proliferative rates were associated with head and neck cancers as well as with all tumor types. Nonetheless, epidermoid carcinoma can be defined as a highly proliferative tumor; this is

Table 1. Cell kinetics of human solid tumors

Tumor type	No. of cases	Labeling index (%)		Authors
		Median	Range	
Testis	78	27.0	0.1 –77.3	Silvestrini *et al.* 1981 [27]
Head & neck	21	13.0*	1.0 –30.0	Cinberg 1980 [23]
	90	12.4*	0.01–50.0	Costa *et al.* 1982 [28]
Lung	28	10.1†	0.9 –23.8	Muggia 1973 [29]
	10	11.5	3.0 –30.0	Livingston *et al.* 1974 [30]
Lymphoma	88	4.1	0.01–30.0	Costa *et al.* 1981 [18]
	69	2.0	0.1 –34.0	Scarffe *et al.* 1980 [17]
	28	3.0	0.4 –46.0	Cooper *et al.* 1968 [31]
Melanoma	25	3.3	0.5 –12.0	Livingston *et al.*1974 [30]
Breast	541	2.8	0.01–40.7	Gentili *et al.* 1981 [16]
	133	2.21	0.04–18.6	Meyer & Hixon 1979 [32]
	128	1.04*	0.06–16.84	Tubiana *et al.*1981 [33]
	67	4.7‡	0.5 –34.3	Schiffer *et al.*1979 [34]

* Geometric mean.
† *In vivo.*
‡ Cell suspension.

in agreement with concurrent studies on the clinical doubling time of these tumors [6], which showed median times to be as low as 7 to 8 days.

Proliferative activity was not *sex* related, whereas some differences emerged as far as *age* is concerned. An inverse type of relation was observed, with a significantly higher proliferative activity ($p<0.05$) in patients under 60 years of age than in older patients (Fig. 3). The lowest LI values (geometric mean, 8.4%) were observed in patients over 60 years. This finding corresponds to the clinical observation of a higher incidence of slow-growing cancers in the oldest patients. The highest LI values were observed for tumors from patients aged 50 to 60 years (geometric mean, 13.0%), in agreement with the high rate of clinical malignancy observed for this age subgroup, and may be related to a particular concentration of these cancers arising in alcoholics (hepatic failure of cirrhosis, dysmetabolism, immunological deficiency).

Proliferative activity does not appear to be related to *size* of the primary tumor. In fact, no relevant differences were observed among subgroups with T1, T2, T3 and T4 tumors. In contrast, a trend of higher proliferative activity was observed for tumors with neck node *metastases*. This finding was more evident when relatively smaller tumors were considered (Table 2). In a series of 55 cases, the analysis of the relationship between cell kinetics and histological grading showed only a trend of higher proliferative activity in poorly differentiated than in well-differentiated carcinomas, but without any

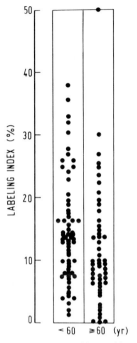

Figure 3. Proliferative activity of primary epidermoid carcinoma in relation to patient age.

Table 2. Proliferative activity of the primary tumor in relation to clinical stage

| | No. of cases | Labeling index (%) | |
		Mean*	Range
T2N0, 1a	29	9.9	0.8 –27.0
T2N1b, 2, 3	13	13.1	0.01–30.6
T3N0, 1a	27	10.6	1.2 –50.0
T3N1b, 2, 3	33	12.6	0.4 –35.8

* Geometric mean.

Table 3. Proliferative activity of the primary tumor in relation to histological differentiation

| Histology | No. of cases | Labeling index (%) | |
		Mean*	Range
Well differentiated	27	11.4	0.8–32.0
Moderately differentiated	20	12.9	1.2–35.8
Poorly differentiated	8	13.0	1.5–30.0

* Geometric mean.

Table 4. Proliferative activity of the primary cancer in relation to different sites of the head and neck

Anatomical sites	No. of cases	Labeling index (%)	
		Mean*	Range
Tongue	33	8.4	0.01–23.8
Alveolus & gingiva	9	9.0	1.1 –30.0
Retromolar area	19	9.3	0.01–38.0
Tonsil	9	11.0	0.01–50.0
Larynx	12	11.2	3.2 –16.4
Palate, hard	5	12.0	1.2 –35.8
Palate, soft	3		1.5, 8.7, 13.9
Cheek	7	12.4	4.7 –24.9
Oropharynx	10	14.4	2.9 –33.0
Floor of mouth	24	15.3	4.7 –26.0

* Geometric mean.

statistical difference among the three histopathological subgroups considered (poorly, moderately, well-differentiated). Moreover, similar ranges were observed for different morphological patterns (Table 3).

Different *locations* of epidermoid carcinoma showed different degrees of proliferative activity (Table 4). The lowest rate was observed in the mobile tongue, gingiva and retromolar area (8.4 and 9.3), and the highest one in the oropharynx and floor of the mouth (14.4 to 15.3); tonsil, larynx, palate and cheek mucosa showed intermediate proliferative rates. However, in all of the sites a wide range of LI values was consistently observed.

In 24 cases operated on with composite resection, the proliferative activity was determined on both primary tumor and *lymph node metastases* (Fig. 4), and a slightly positive correlation coefficient ($r = 0.48$; $p = 0.10$) was

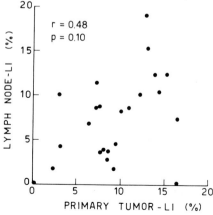

Figure 4. Relation between proliferative activity of the primary tumor and lymph node metastases.

observed. However, the LI in metastases tended to be lower than in the primary. In agreement with this finding, a lower doubling time of lung metastases than of the primary tumor has been observed for epidermoid carcinomas [6]. This appears to be in contrast with most observations in other tumor types [5, 35].

3.2. Predictive role of pretreatment proliferative activity

The relevance of potential malignancy markers of epidermoid carcinoma has been repeatedly analyzed in series of patients submitted to different clinical treatments. Most studies deal with the possible correlation between histopathological grading and response to radiotherapy, whereas such an analysis was seldom carried out in patients treated only with surgery. An up-to-date comprehensive conclusion is difficult, since patient selection and composition of the published series varies widely as far as the analysis of prognostic factors is concerned.

3.2.1. Prognostic relevance on clinical outcome after surgery

It is known that patients with histologically highly malignant tumors have a worse prognosis after surgical treatment, and this finding is still considered in planning therapy. However, precise markers of malignancy are still being sought. In fact, whatever the morphological variable considered, histological grading appears to be quite an important predictor of survival, but the difference is significant only between patients with well or poorly differentiated tumors, illustrating the lack of sensitivity of this variable.

The pretreatment LI has recently been related to prognosis in a series of 60 patients with cancer of the larynx and pharynx submitted to surgery or combined-modality therapies including surgery [24]. After a minimum 2-year follow-up, significant differences in disease-free or overall survival were found among three kinetic subgroups (i.e., slow, intermediate and high), with a pretreatment LI respectively lower than 6%, from 6 to 14%, and higher than 14%.

Similarly, we analyzed the relevance of pretreatment LI on disease-free survival in a group of 22 patients with locally advanced oral and pharyngeal carcinomas treated with surgery alone. The median LI value of 12.4% found for the total series was used as cutoff. Tumors had different locations, and the follow-up is still too short to allow any conclusion. However, preliminary results show a trend for patients with fast-proliferating tumors to relapse more frequently than patients with slow-proliferating tumors (Fig. 5).

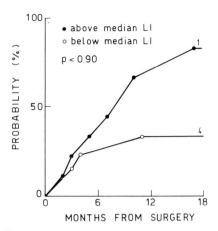

Figure 5. Probability of local recurrence of patients according to proliferative activity of primary epidermoid carcinoma.

3.2.2. Predictability of response to radiotherapy

The finding that less differentiated tumors are more likely to be radio-responsive was first reported by Bergonié and Tribondeau in 1906 [36]. Since that time, much effort has been made to identify some measurable markers of radiosensitivity. Pathologists have supplied clinicians with morphological classifications based on criteria of malignancy, but the actual relevance of morphological *grading* as a predictor of radiosensitivity can be confirmed only for very poorly differentiated carcinoma, and only for the immediate response. If long-term clinical results are considered, reliability of the histological grading is controversial and questionable, particularly when different series are compared. As a matter of fact, morphological grading is a subjective method, so that several authors deny its substantial value in practice. Subsequently, tumor growth was investigated. Doubling time was found to be related to the immediate radiation response [37], but its determination presents some practical problems in patients with squamous cell carcinoma, so that it has no practical use.

Mitotic index was the basis for histological malignancy grading. However, it does not allow a precise evaluation of the proliferative activity, because mitosis is a very brief event in the cell cycle and can seldom be determined at the moment of the examination. It is thus of little help for a correct measurement of tumor proliferation.

The pretreatment proliferative activity evaluated as LI has been consistently shown to be a predictor of early response to radiotherapy [38]. Patients with fast-proliferating tumors more frequently reach complete remission. However, when long-term response or overall survival is considered, the predictive accuracy of this kinetic marker decreases, so that most studies have concluded that there is no statistically significant correlation between pretreatment proliferative activity and clinical outcome [39–41].

Our experience fully confirms these findings for epidermoid carcinoma of the head and neck. In our study, the achievement of a complete tumor regression was analyzed for three kinetic subgroups in 28 patients with advanced cancer treated with external radiotherapy alone (Table 5). A complete remission was achieved in most of the cases, independent of the initial LI value (75%, 54%, and 82% complete remission rates respectively for low, intermediate, and high LI). Radioresponsiveness seems to depend mainly on tumor size or on certain characteristics of the lesion (infiltration, necrosis, bone involvement). Moreover, long-term clinical outcome is correlated with the pretreatment LI only in patients with slow-proliferating tumors, since disease-free survival was 0% when LI was ≤2% and nearly 50% in cases with a higher LI.

3.2.3. Predictability of response to chemotherapy

The correlation between proliferative activity and sensitivity to drugs has been consistently reported for different experimental tumors. A more frequent short-term response to chemotherapy of fast-proliferating tumors has also been reported for some human tumor types [42–46], but it has not been confirmed by others [18, 47, 48]. There is even stronger evidence that clinically similar tumors can respond differently to chemotherapy, and it is now generally believed that chemosensitivity is peculiar of the individual tumor and cannot be predicted on the basis of known biological, morphological or clinical variables.

An attempt was made to assess the ability of pretreatment LI, as well as the early variation of LI after partial chemotherapy, to predict short-term clinical outcome. Patients were submitted to presurgical intra-arterial regional administration of vincristine and bleomycin (VB), or of vincristine, bleomycin and methotrexate (VBM). The proliferative activity was determined before and after one-third of the full chemotherapy course. Pretreatment LI failed to correlate with clinical response. Moreover, although a decrease in LI was always observed, the degree in early inhibition was not related to pretreatment LI or to clinical response after the full course of chemotherapy. However, when the two treatment schedules (VB and VBM)

Table 5. Relationship between pretreatment proliferative activity and response to radiotherapy

Kinetic groups (LI range, %)	No. of patients	Complete remission (%)	Disease-free survival (%, actuarial at 36 mo)
0.01– 1.9	4	75	0
2.0 –13.9	13	54	47
14.0 –50.0	11	82	54

were compared (Table 6), a higher median LI inhibition was found for the VBM than for the VB regimen (81% and 49%, respectively), in spite of the very similar pretreatment LI values.

3.3. Predictive role of variations in proliferative activity

3.3.1. Predictability of response to radiotherapy
Several parameters have been considered in this regard. Objective reduction in tumor size during radiotherapy of epidermoid carcinoma was found to represent a useful predictor of radioresponsiveness, and this criterion is still widely used. As a rule, the response achieved after 40–45 Gy is assumed by several authors as a decisional point for going on with radiotherapy or changing the treatment. More recently, it has been proposed to anticipate this decision at 10 Gy and to consider a clinical regression greater than 10% as an indication of radioresponsiveness [49]. However, by using these different criteria, initial tumor regression has also been found to be correlated with short-term complete remission but not with long-term survival. Nevertheless, the habit of referring to the immediate response for judgment of radiosensitivity is quite widespread; in spite of that, radioresponsiveness and radiocurability are different phenomena. In our experience, we noticed that many tumors recurred after a complete regression, whereas in several cases operated on for gross persistent disease, the specimens did not reveal viable tumor cells on histological examination.

More sophisticated approaches to predict radiosensitivity have recently been used. Some authors observed a good correlation between change in LI and clinical response [39, 50]. When the LI was reduced by more than two-thirds partial radiotherapy, a sharp reduction or disappearance of cancer

Table 6. Inhibiting effect on proliferative activity after one cycle of chemotherapy

	Chemotherapy schedule	
	VB* (11 cases)	VBM † (8 cases)
Pretreatment LI (%)		
Median	18.0	17.0
Range	5.8–32.0	5.8–35.8
LI Inhibition (%)		
Median	49	81
Range	0–100	18–99

* VB, vincristine and bleomycin.
† VBM, vincristine, bleomycin and methotrexate.

occurred with a higher frequency, and the larger the decrease in LI, the greater the decrease in tumor volume. Others have observed a progressive decrease in LI and cell density after one or several sessions of radiotherapy [40]. However, the fall in LI was significantly higher in patients who did not show important tumor regression and appeared to be inversely related to long-term survival. These controversial results could be explained by the diferent doses of radiotherapy, the different time that the LI determination was performed, and the use of other treatments in combination.

We analyzed the relevance of LI variations during radiotherapy on the immediate and long-term response to a full course of treatment in patients with locally advanced epidermoid carcinoma of the oral cavity and oropharynx. Preliminary determinations performed at successive times during radiotherapy indicated a 10 Gy course as the most suitable point to guarantee a correct biological determination; LI variations were thus routinely evaluated 48 h after the last session of radiotherapy that reached a cumulative dose of 10 Gy. A wide range of variations, not related to pretreatment LI, was observed, except for very low LI ($<2\%$), which always showed an increase in proliferative activity [41]. LI variations proved to be indicative of the immediate response, since a higher complete regression rate was observed in patients whose tumor proliferative activity was reduced by 70% or more than in those in which an LI reduction of less than 70% or an enhancement occurred [41]. However, the most striking finding was the correlation between LI variations and long-term response (Table 7). In fact, a fall in LI to more than two-thirds of the initial value corresponded to 82% 3-year disease-free survival, whereas when LI did not reach such an inhibition, or was enhanced, all patients relapsed within 19 months. Similarly, a significantly higher probability of 3-year survival (65%) was observed in those patients whose tumors have shown an LI reduction greater than 70% than in those with a lower LI reduction (20%).

In conclusion, the variation of LI after 10 Gy seems to represent an extremely sensitive test to predict intrinsic radioresistance, even for tumors that show a short-term complete clinical response. Accuracy in predicting radiosensitivity is slightly lower; in fact, 18% had recurrences, and in 15%

Table 7. Relevance of LI variations on long-term response to radiotherapy

LI variation	Long-term response (actuarial at 36 mo)	
	Disease-free survival (%)	Survival (%)
Reduction $<70\%$+enhancement	0 (8)	21 (15)
Reduction $\geq 70\%$	82 (11)	65 (13)

In parenthesis, number of patients at the beginning of treatment.

of the cases no complete regression occurred, in spite of a significant fall in LI. However, it must be stressed that all these patients had very extended lesions, so that the heterogeneity within the tumor could have played an important role in making the samples not adequately representative of the whole cell population.

4. Cell kinetics in cycle manipulation for scheduling combined treatments

Tumors are asynchronous cell populations with cells distributed in all phases of the cell cycle and in G_0. Radiation and most anticancer drugs are more active on proliferating than resting cells and show a phase- or cycle-specific mechanism of action. However, lack of specificity for tumor cells and toxic effects on normal tissues make it impossible to achieve in every case the eradication of the proliferating component. Moreover, resting cells (G_0) are practically unaffected by physical and chemical antitumor agents.

Combination of drugs with different mechanisms of action and different toxicities may increase their therapeutic efficiency. Unfortunately, the mechanisms of action of most drugs have been extensively investigated only in experimental *in vivo* and *in vitro* systems and seldomly in human tumors. Simultaneous administration of several drugs could also result in a mixture of actions that interfere with each other, and this could reduce instead of increase antitumor activity. The blocking mechanism of some drugs can be used to gain cohorts of cells in a particular phase and to increase cell killing by using a drug specifically active on the same phase. Although it has been assumed that reversibly arrested cells will proceed in a kind of synchronous wave into the next phase once the effect of the blocking agent has been removed and that suitable drugs administered at that moment could strike the cells in a particularly sensitive situation, the progression after block is not compulsory.

Agents more frequently used are vinca alkaloids, such as vincristine and vinblastine, to block cells in early M phase, or bleomycin in the S phase [51]. Cell killing in a successive time can be achieved by using S-phase-specific drugs, such as methotrexate, cytosine arabinoside, and hydroxyurea [52]. However, even though synchronization of cells has been possible in experimental systems with this approach, an attempt performed on squamous cell carcinoma showed only a poor degree of synchronization following intra-arterial administration of vincristine [53].

This negative result, which could be ascribed to different factors, such as heterogeneity of the cell population, could lead to the conclusion that a therapeutically useful level of synchronization cannot be achieved in epidermoid carcinomas of the head and neck. Nevertheless, improvement of clinical results by using combinations of vincristine, bleomycin and methotrexate in particular sequences according to a theoretical synchronization schedule has been consistently reported from clinical studies [54–56]. These results can probably be ascribed to a recruitment in the cell cycle of resting cells as a consequence of a progressive decrease in the cell proliferating pool.

A new approach in cell cycle manipulation [57] is aimed at synchronizing the normal proliferating cells (bone marrow, gastrointestinal mucosal cells, etc.), that are more sensitive than neoplastic cells to drugs, and administering the drugs at suitable intervals to cause the maximum damage to neoplastic cells while sparing normal ones. This goal could be reached by using substances, such as chalones, which may represent the ultimate regulators of cell passage from one phase to the next. The use of a G_1 chalone at high dose for a short time could induce the arrest of all susceptible cells, either normal or neoplastic, in phase G_1; but tumor cells should be less chalone-sensitive than the normal ones and escape the block earlier than the latter, and thus become a good target for S-phase-specific agents. However, this is still a tentative field and further work is needed.

A promising application of kinetic information is for defining optimum schedules for combinations of chemo- and radiotherapy. Both modalities can induce important variation in the composition of cell populations in epidermoid cancer, and this could be opportunely used to schedule simultaneous administration of drugs and external radiotherapy. Several studies have shown that the addition of single drugs (bleomycin, methotrexate) immediately before and/or during radiotherapy produces a very small change, if any, on immediate response rate and survival in comparison to radiotherapy alone. Intra-arterial single drug chemotherapy before radiotherapy led us to the same conclusion.

More recent clinical trials [54] including polychemotherapy (vincristine, bleomycin, methotrexate) before and at successive intervals during radiotherapy have shown an increased response rate in comparison to those obtained with radiotherapy alone. Intervals were defined suite empirically, and it is reasonable to believe that a more appropriate scheduling of chemotherapy through the monitoring of cell kinetics on individual patients could lead to an improvement in clinical results.

5. Present and future clinical use of cell kinetics

The impact of cell kinetics on prognosis and treatment becomes clear and, without becoming too enthusiastic, some conclusions can already be drawn. Epidermoid carcinoma of the head and neck is one of the fastest proliferating solid tumors, although its actual growth is constantly decreased by substantial cell death and cell loss. Not only is higher proliferative activity associated with hither lymphatic and hematogenous spread, but it can also markedly affect the outcome of local treatments. Kinetic patterns represent a more reliable biological variable than histopathological grading to measure the potential of malignancy.

High proliferative activity of a cell population correlates with higher probability of recurrence and lower survival rate in patients treated with surgery alone. Conversely, very low proliferative activity is associated with very poor long-term prognosis in patients who receive external radiotherapy as the only treatment, in spite of high immediate response rates. Both findings could be already assumed as discriminant factors for a better choice of the initial therapeutic approach in extreme situations. While there is no doubt that very slowly proliferating cancers are to be primarily treated with surgery when possible, it has not yet been clearly verified whether induction radiotherapy or chemotherapy will improve the outcome of combined modalities including surgery as the final procedure in fast-proliferating tumors. In contrast, the achievement of immediate complete regression after radiotherapy in 82%, with nearly 50% 3-year disease-free survival in patients with fast-proliferating tumors, strongly indicates that a large fraction of proliferating cells can actually be destroyed. Thus, a therapeutic approach that includes preoperative radiotherapy appears quite reasonable in these cases.

Chemotherapy can also induce a significant decrease in proliferative activity when given as first treatment, with the advantage of reduced postoperative complications. Although no definite conclusions have been reached on the impact of preoperative chemotherapy on survival in head and neck cancer, its application can be considered theoretically useful at least with regard to cell kinetic manipulation. Preoperative intra-arterial chemotherapy has been used extensively by us in advanced lesions, and long-term results are strongly suggestive of a marked improvement over those obtained with surgery alone.

Further indications can derive from the analysis of variations induced on the kinetic pattern by fractional doses (10 Gy) of radiotherapy. In fact, an inhibition in proliferative activity of less than 70% is highly indicative of failure of response to radiotherapy alone. Such monitoring could be used to decide whether to go on with radiotherapy up to full doses or to switch to an alternative type of treatment. This attitude is supported by sufficient clinical evidence and could already be applied in clinical practice. In fact, the only technical constraint, i.e., the time required by the autoradiographic procedure for LI determination (6–10 days), does not seem to be determinant on the full course of radiotherapy. If an inhibition of LI of more or less than 70% is assumed as discriminant of radioresponsiveness or radioresistance, lower doses of radiotherapy given with different fractions in a shorter time are likely to be equally predictive.

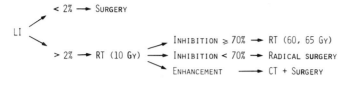

Figure 6. Treatment schedules of epidermoid carcinoma of the head and neck according to tumor cell kinetics. LI, labeling index; RT, radiotherapy; CT, chemotherapy.

Further studies could also lead to a better knowledge on cell kinetic modifications induced by different antiproliferative drugs or combined chemotherapy regimens, to identify the most active ones. Moreover, analysis of cell kinetics could be used to better combine chemotherapy and radiotherapy, in order to achieve the maximum LI inhibition from the beginning of the treatment.

However, more rapid laboratory procedures are needed for this purpose. New promising techniques, such as FCM, are less time-consuming and can give additional information about cell distribution in the different phases of the cell cycle. Due to these biological and technical advances, it is likely that in the near future cell kinetic determinations will be used not only as a prognostic factor but also as a powerful tool to plan treatment of epidermoid carcinoma of the head and neck. In this regard, it will probably supercede, if not completely replace, the usual clinical classifications of the primary tumor.

Consequent to these findings, a resonable approach to plan treatment of epidermoid carcinoma of the head and neck should always include pretreatment LI determination. Tumors with an original LI lower than 2% should be considered for primary surgical treatment, the others should receive 10 Gy of external radiotherapy. Patients with tumors that show an LI inhibition of at least 70% after 10 Gy should complete radiotherapy; for the others, the therapeutic strategy should be changed. A simple surgical treatment should be used for those tumors whose proliferative activity is not sufficiently inhibited by radiation, whereas chemotherapy should be planned in association with surgery when radiation has produced an increase in the LI (Fig. 6).

Acknowledgments

Supported in part by Progetto Finalizzato, Controllo della Crescita Neoplastica, grant no. 82.01335.96, from the Consiglio Nazionale delle Ricerche, Rome. The authors thank Lorena Ventura and Rosita Motta for technical assistance and Ms. B. Johnston for editing and preparing the manuscript.

246

References

1. Denekamp J: Cell kinetics and cancer therapy, Springfield, CC Thomas, 1982.
2. Lamerton LF, Steel GG: Cell population kinetics in normal and malignant tissue. Prog Biophys mol Biol 18:247–283, 1968.
3. Lamerton LF: Cell proliferation kinetics and the differential response of normal and malignant tissues. Br J Radiol 45:161–170, 1972.
4. Steel GC (1977): Growth kinetics of tumours. Cell population kinetics in relation to the growth and treatment of cancer, Oxford, Oxford University Press, 1977.
5. Malaise EP, Chavaudra N, Courdi A, Vazquez T: Tumor growth rate of pulmonary metastasis. In: Weiss L, Gilbert MA (eds) Pulmonary metastasis. Boston, GK Hall Medical Publications Division, 1978, pp 200–220.
6. Galante E, Gallus G, Chiesa F, Bono A, Bettoni I, Molinari R: Growth rate of head and neck tumors. Eur J Cancer Clin Oncol 18:707–712, 1982.
7. Quastler H, Sherman FG: Cell population kinetics in the intestinal epithelium of the mouse. Exp Cell Res 17:428–438, 1959.
8. Chavaudra N, Richard JM, Malaise EP: Labelling index of human squamous cell carcinomas. Comparison of in vivo and in vitro labelling methods. Cell Tissue Kinet 12:145–152, 1979.
9. Fried J, Perez AG, Clarkson BD: Flow cytofluorometric analysis of cell cycle distribution using propidium iodide. J Cell Biol 71:172–181, 1976.
10. Barlogie B, Göhde W, Johnston DA, Smallwood L, Schumann J, Drewinko B, Freireich EJ: Determination of ploidy and proliferative characteristics of human solid tumors by pulse cytophotometry. Cancer Res 38:3333–3339, 1978.
11. Crissman HA, Steinkamp JA: Rapid, one step staining procedures for analysis of cellular DNA and protein by single and dual laser flow cytometry. Cytometry 3:84–90, 1982.
12. Baisch H: Evaluation of pulse-cytophotometric data by mathematical analysis of DNA distribution. In: Valleron AJ (ed) Mathematical models in cell kinetics. Ghent, European Press Medikon, 1975, pp 65–67.
13. Fried J: Method for the quantitative evaluation of data from flow microfluorometry. Comput Biol Res 9:263–276, 1976.
14. Dean N: Quantitative analysis of flow system data. In: Lutz D (ed) Third international symposium on pulse cytophotometry. Ghent, European Press Medikon, 1978, pp 63–68.
15. Jett JH: Mathematical analysis of DNA histograms from asynchronous and synchronous cell populations. In: Luts D (ed) Third international symposium on pulse cytophotometry. Ghent, European Press Medikon, 1978, pp 93–102.
16. Gentili C, Sanfilippo O, Silvestrini R: Cell proliferation and its relationship to clinical features and relapse in breast cancers. Cancer 48:974–979, 1981.
17. Scarffe JH, Hann IM, Evans DIK, Morris Jones P, Palmer MK, Lelleyman JS, Crowther D: Relationship between the pretreatment proliferative activity of marrow blast cells and prognosis of acute lymphoblastic leukemia of childhood. Br J Cancer 41:764–771, 1980.
18. Costa A, Bonadonna G, Villa E, Valagussa P, Silvestrini R: Labeling index as a prognostic marker in non-Hodgkin's lymphomas. J Natl Cancer Inst 66:1–5, 1981.
19. Meyer JS, Friedman E, McCrate MM, Bauer WC: Prediction of early course of breast carcinoma by thymidine labeling. Cancer 51:1879–1886, 1983.
20. Bresciani F, Paoluzi R, Benassi M, Nervi C, Casale C, Ziparo E: Cell kinetics and growth of squamous cell carcinomas in man. Cancer Res 34:2405–2415, 1974.
21. Tejada F, McKenzie R, Leung I, Zubrod CG: Cell kinetics of primary head and neck cancer (abstract). Proc AACR ASCO 212, 1978.
22. Nervi C, Badaracco G, Morelli M, Starace G: Cytokinetic evaluation in human head and neck cancer by autoradiography and DNA cytofluorometry. Cancer 45:452–459, 1980.
23. Cinberg JZ: The percentage of cells in DNA synthesis in epidermoid carcinoma of the head

and neck: a preliminary report (abstract). International head and neck oncology research conference, Rosslyn, Virginia, September 8–10, 1980.

24. Chauvel P, Demard F, Gioanni S, Vallicioni S: Valeur pronostique de l'index de marquage dans les cancers des voies aéro-digestives supérieures (à propos de 60 observations). Forum de Cancérologie, Association Française pour l'Etude du Cancer, 1st Juin 1981.

25. Chauvel P, Demard F, Gioanni J, Vallicioni J, Schneider M, Lalanne CM: Comparison between the labelling index and other prognostic factors in head and neck cancers (abstract). UICC Conference on clinical oncology, 1981.

26. Cinberg JZ, Chang TH, Hebbard P, Bases R, Vogl SE: An application of immunocytology to the analysis of the cell kinetics of upper respiratory and digestive tract squamous carcinoma. Cancer 51:1843–1846, 1983.

27. Silvestrini R, Pilotti S, Costa A: Kinetic characterization of germ cell testicular tumors (abstract). UICC Conference on clinical oncology, Lausanne, October 28–31, 1981.

28. Costa A, Molinari R, Cantù G, Silvestrini R: The kinetic characteristic of the cell population in head and neck cancers and its clinical relevance (abstract). Proc 13th Int Cancer Congress, Seattle, September 8–15, 1982.

29. Muggia FM: Correlation of histologic types with cell kinetic studies in lung cancer. Cancer Chemother Rep 4:69–71, 1973.

30. Livingston RB, Ambrus U, George SL, Freireich EJ, Hart SS: In vitro determination of thymidine-^{3}H labeling index in human solid tumors. Cancer Res 34:1376–1380, 1974.

31. Cooper EH, Peckham MJ, Millard RE, Hamlin INE, Gérard-Marchant R: Cell proliferation in human malignant lymphomas. Eur J Cancer 4:287–296, 1968.

32. Meyer JS, Hixon B: Advanced stage and early relapse of breast carcinomas associated with high thymidine labeling indices. Cancer Res 39:4042–4047, 1979.

33. Tubiana M, Pejovic MJ, Renaud A, Contesso G, Chavaudra N, Gioanni J, Malaise EP: Kinetic parameters and the course of the disease in breast cancer. Cancer 47:937–943, 1981.

34. Schiffer LM, Braunschweiger PG, Stragand JJ, Poulakos L: The cell kinetics of human mammary cancers. Cancer 43:1707–1719, 1979.

35. Charbit A, Malaise E, Tubiana M: Relation between the pathological nature and the growth rate of human tumours. Eur J Cancer 7:307–315, 1971.

36. Fletcher G (translated by Bergonié J and Tribondeau L, 1906): Interpretation of some results of radiotherapy and an attempt at determining a logical technique of treatment. Radiat Res 11:587, 1959.

37. Breur K: Growth rate and radiosensitivity of human tumours. II. Radiosensitivity of human tumours. Eur J Cancer 2:173–188, 1966.

38. Dixon B, Ward AJ, Joslin CAF: Pretreatment ^{3}H-TdR labelling of cervical biopsies: histology, staging and tumour response to radiotherapy. Clin Radiol 28:491–497, 1977.

39. Elequin FT, Muggia FM, Ghossein NA, Ager PJ, Krishnaswamy V: Correlation between in vitro labeling indices (LIs) and tumor regression following radiotherapy. Int J Radiat Oncol Biol Phys 4:207–213, 1978.

40. Courdi A, Tubiana M, Chavaudra N, Malaise EP: Changes in labeling indices of human tumors after irradiation. Int J Radiat Oncol Biol Phys 6:1639–1644, 1980.

41. Costa A, Molinari R: The proliferative activity as a potential tool for monitoring kinetic characteristics of oral carcinoma and their potential use for monitoring radiosensitivity (abstract). Proc AACR 193, 1981.

42. Thirlwell MP, Livingston RB, Murphy WK, Hart JS: A rapid in vitro labeling index method for predicting response of human solid tumours to chemotherapy. Cancer Res 36:3279–3283.

43. Thirlwell MP, Mansell PWA: A correlation of clinical response with in vitro prechemotherapy labeling index percentage (PLI) in human solid tumors. Proc AACR, ASCO 17:307, 1976.

248

44. Livingston RB, Sulkes A, Thirlwell MP, Murphy WK, Hart JS: Cell kinetic parameters: correlations with clinical response. In: Drewinko B, Humphrey RM (eds) Growth kinetics and biochemical regulation of normal and malignant cells. Baltimore, Williams & Wilkins, 1977, pp 767–785.

45. Hayes FA, Green AA, Mauer AM: Correlation of cell kinetic and clinical response to chemotherapy in disseminated neuroblastoma. Cancer Res 37:3766–3770, 1977.

46. Livingston RB, Titus GA, Heilbrun LK: In vitro effects on DNA synthesis as a predictor of biological effect from chemotherapy. Cancer Res 40:2209–2212, 1980.

47. Silvestrini R: Experimental approaches to improve the clinical management of tumors. Chemioter Oncol 5:14–20, 1981.

48. Sanfilippo O, Daidone MG, Costa A, Canetta R, Silvestrini R: Estimation of differential in vitro sensitivity of non-Hodgkin lymphomas to anticancer drugs. Eur J Cancer 17:217–226, 1981.

49. Arcangeli G, Mauro F, Nervi C, Starace G: A critical appraisal of the usefulness of some biological parameters in predicting tumour radiation response of human head and neck cancer. Br J Cancer 41:39–44, 1980.

50. Helpap B, Herberhold C, Thelen M, Stiens R, Koch U: Cell-kinetical analyses of squamous cell carcinomas of the oral region and the effect of a combined therapy of 5-fluorouracil and irradiation. A contribution to the discussion about tumor cell synchronization. Strahlentherapie 153:774–780.

51. Klein HO: Cell kinetic alterations in normal and neoplastic cell populations in vitro and in vivo following vincristine. A reply to Dr. Camplejohn's review article. Cell Tissue Kinet 13:425–434, 1980.

52. Barranco SC: Drug effects on the cell cycle. In: Busch H (ed) Effects of drugs on the cell nucleus. New York, Academic Press, 1979, pp 455–473.

53. Badaracco G, Morelli M, Nervi C, Starace G: Cytokinetic effects of combined infusion of vincristine in head and neck carcinoma. Eur J Cancer 15:17–26, 1979.

54. Price LA, Hill Bt, Calvert AH, Shaw HJ, Hughes KB: Kinetically-based multiple drug treatment for advanced head and neck cancer. Br Med J 3:10–11, 1975.

55. Costanzi J: Bleomycin (Bleo) infusion as a potential synchronizing agent in carcinoma of the head and neck. Proc AACR, ASCO 17:10, 1976.

56. Molinari R, Mattavelli F, Cantù G, Chiesa F, Costa L, Tancini G: Results of a low-dose combination chemotherapy with vincristine, bleomycin and methotrexate (VBM) based on cell kinetics in the palliative treatment of head and neck squamous cell carcinoma. Eur J Cancer 16:469–472, 1980.

57. Tannock I: Cell kinetics and chemotherapy: a critical review. Cancer Treat Rep 62:1117–1133, 1978.

11. Local hyperthermia for advanced squamous carcinoma of the head and neck

PADMAKAR P. LELE

1. Introduction

A large number of patients with primary cancers arising in the head and neck region have residual or locally recurrent disease following intensive treatment with conventional modalities. Such tumors are often painful and are secondarily infected, and may erode into neurovascular bundles or compromise swallowing or airway functions. In many instances the combination of tumor location, extent, size, prior treatment and the general condition of the patient severely restrict the therapeutic avenues available, and result in a grim prognosis. In such patients, non-invasive cytoreduction should provide palliation by alleviating local tumor effects and may enhance local tumor control.

Hyperthermia, the elevation of tumor temperature to 42 °C or higher, is presently under intensive investigation in the management of patients who have failed all conventional anticancer therapy. Depending on the previous treatment, hyperthermia may be given in combination with radiation therapy or/and chemotherapy, or may be used alone. Mounting experimental and clinical evidence, indicates that hyperthermia will have a substantive role in cancer therapy. In this chapter, the biological basis for the tumoricidal action of hyperthermia is briefly summarized and clinical results are discussed from a preliminary study conducted collaboratively with Dr. T.J. Ervin, Division of Medicine, Sidney Farber Cancer Institute, Boston, MA; Dr. M.I. Feldman, Department of Radiotherapy, Boston University Medical Center, Boston, MA; Dr. C.W. Kaiser*, Department of Surgery, Pondville Hospital, Walpole, MA and Dr. C.D. Kowal**, Department of Internal Medicine, Section of Medical Oncology, Yale University School of Medicine, New Haven, CT.

The study was notable in the fact that significant antitumor effects were obtained in tumors that had failed conventional therapy without producing any significant toxicity. Further information on the biological basis and the

Gregory T. Wolf (ed), Head and Neck Oncology.
© *1984 Martinus Nijhoff Publishers, Boston. ISBN 0-89838-657-8. Printed in The Netherlands.*

rationale for the use of heat as an anticancer modality, studies and results on cell cultures *in vitro* and in experimental animals, various methods and instrumentation for delivery of hyperthermia and the clinical results can be found in the several publications now available [1–6].

2. Biologic rationale

Hyperthermia, in the range of 42.5° to 44 °C and sustained for 30 min or less, is demonstrably cytotoxic to cells in tumors and *in vitro*. The site of primary damage is not known with certainty but is believed to be either the cell membrane, cell nucleus or lysosomes. Hyperthermia has a greater effect on transformed and malignant cells than on normal cells, and thus is tumoricidal without significant or unacceptable toxicity to normal tissues. This is the basis for the use of whole body or regional hyperthermia. The relatively high sensitivity of the central nervous system, however mitigates against the use of whole body or regional hyperthermia for treatment of head and neck cancer because of the proximity of the tumors to the brain. For such tumors, hyperthermia localized to the tumor is to be preferred.

Cells in S phase, which are relatively radioresistant, are more sensitive to heat than cells in M or G phases of the cell cycle. This could have a selective effect on killing of radioresistant cells and cycling tumor cells. Furthermore, heat has greater effect on hypoxic cells, malnourished cells and those at low pH, which all tend to be radioresistant, than on normal cells. Thus the effects of heat and radiation are complementary to each other. Hyperthermia can also inhibit recovery from sub-lethal or potentially lethal radiation damage. Although this may not be selective for tumor in relation to normal tissue, the fact that with proper techniques heating can be localized to a preselected target volume enables localization of radiosensitization and substantial enhancement of the therapeutic ratio.

Experimental and clinical studies have demonstrated augmentation of cytotoxicities of certain chemotherapeutic agents at hyperthermia temperatures. Local hyperthermia can thus be used effectively to enhance the local cytotoxic effects of systemic chemotherapy on bulky tumor masses, without augmentation of bone marrow or other systemic toxicity.

3. Instrumentation

A variety of radiofrequency (RF), microwave (MW), and ultrasound (US) systems, are currently being tested as means of producing local/regional hyperthermia (LHT) in humans. Reports of these studies [7–16], have documented significant antitumor effects for recurrent squamous carcinoma of the head and neck, using a variety of treatment temperatures, fractionation schedules, and energy sources. From a summary of these reports and their findings, it is obvious that most of the investigators have used either RF or MW as their energy source (Table 1). Marmor *et al.* [10, 13] alone have reported on the use of US for LHT.

Ultrasound has several potential advantages for heating subcutaneous tumors when compared with RF or MW. Earlier laboratory and animal studies by Lele *et al.* [17–25] have demonstrated that US can be focused (FUS) at depth within tissues to maximize energy deposition and heating within the desired target volume without significant heating of intervening or adjacent normal tissues. This enables a more precise control of the depth and boundaries of the tissue volume heated and sparing of any surrounding critical normal tissues than is possible with RF or MW techniques. Tumor tissues also attenuate US to a greater extent than normal tissue, leading to their preferential heating. Accumulated data [24, 25] demonstrate that appropriate focusing and pattern of energy deposition permit the development of the desired temperature distribution within the treatment field. For example, the entire treatment volume can be held at a desired temperature without areas of excessively high or low temperatures. This ensures that *all* of the tumor is heated to a specified temperature and that valid and meaningful correlation can be made between the tumor heat dose and the bio-

Table 1. Clinical hyperthermia pilot studies head and neck cancer

Investigator	Energy source	Temp/Time	# Pts	Results
LeVeen [7]	RF/13.56 MHz	>46 °C × 30 min	7	Tumor regression
Arcangeli [8]	MW/500 MHz	42–43 °C × 45 min	20	Radiotherapy antitumor effect
Arcangeli [9]	MW/500 MHz	42–43 °C × 45 min	15	Adriamycin antitumor effect
				Bleomycin antitumor effect
Marmor [10]	US/2.05 MHz	43 °C	12	Radiation antitumor effect
Stehlin [11]	RF/13.56 MHz	? × 180 min	1	Tumor regression
Hornbach [12]	MW/433.92 MHz	? × 30 min	23	Radiation antitumor effect
Marmor [13]	US/1–3 MHz	43–45 °C × 30 min	12	1 CR, 7 PR
Caldwell [14]	MW/434 MHz	40 °C × 20 min	37	18/37 NED, 2 yrs
Perez [15]	MW/2450 or	42.5–43 °C × 90 min	2	2/2 CR
	915 MHz	42.5–43 °C + RT	6	4/6 CR
Fazekas [16]	MW/2450 MHz	42.5–43.5 °C × 40 min	1	No response
		42.5–43.5 °C + RT	2	1/2 PR

logical response. Of special importance is the fact that with FUS, it is possible to heat the well vascularized, growing edge of the tumor to the temperature necessary for therapeutic effect without placing adjacent or intervening tissues at risk. The inability to heat the periphery of the tumors to adequately high temperatures by RF, MW or unfocused US techniques, may account for recurrence of tumors at their periphery and the development of a necrotic crater in the center as reported by Marmor *et al.* [10, 13]. Additionally, US hyperthermia has a further advantage in that temperature measurement is easily accomplished by using commonly available, relatively inexpensive fine thermocouples. RF and MW require the use of specialized, expensive probes of significantly larger dimensions. Clearly FUS techniques seem to offer considerable and important advantages over RF and MW techniques for selective, controllable heating of tumors.

Although there have been several other LHT studies in head and neck cancer [7–16], the present study was undertaken since FUS had not previously been evaluated in the treatment of malignancies in this region. The characteristics of FUS should be expected to reduce normal tissue toxicity, permit uniform heating of the tumor target volume to a specified temperature and thus enable a definitive and clear evaluation of antitumor effects.

4. Focused ultrasound hyperthermia for head and neck cancers

4.1. Technique

From 10/79 to 4/80, 27 ambulatory patients with biopsy proven, advanced, recurrent or metastatic, previously treated squamous cell carcinoma of the head and neck were entered into a Phase I Hyperthermia Study.

Patients were initially evaluated at referring institutions and then were seen in the Hyperthermia Center at the Massachusetts Institute of Technology for LHT planning. All patients had histologically proven squamous cell carcinoma, ECOG performance status of <2 (>50% ambulatory), an estimated minimum survival of two months, and hematologic parameters of WBC >4000/mm^3, and platelet count >100,000/mm^3. Of the 27 patients interviewed and examined for entry into the study, 26 gave informed consent to the treatment. One patient refused treatment because of the need for thermocouple placement. The characteristics of the 26 patients entered into this study are shown in Table 2. Each of the patients had previously received intensive treatment by one or more of the conventional anticancer modalities: surgery 22/26 (85%); radiation 25/26 (96%) and chemotherapy 16/26 (62%).

During an initial treatment planning session, the ultrasonic frequency and

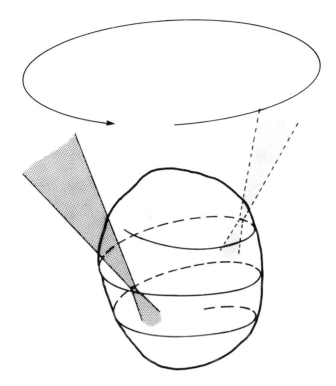

Figure 1. Mode of operation of Dynamically Scanned Focused Ultrasound with Intensity Modulation. Focusing ensures sparing of surrounding tissues. Dynamic scanning and Intensity Modulation enable precise 'tailoring' of heat-dose for the different parts of each tumor. Details are given in Ref. [24] and [25]. A Phased Array, capable of electronic focusing and steering is under evaluation.

the lens focal length were determined for the specific tumor. Coupling equipment was fabricated, if needed for the particular location and contours of the tumor. Temperature sensitivity of the skin overlying the tumor was determined since the disease or previous therapy (surgery or X-radiation)

Table 2. Patient characteristics

# Patients entered	27
# Patients treated	26
Sex: Male	21
Female	5
Age: 63 yr median (33–84 range)	
Previous treatment:	
Surgery	22
Radiotherapy	25
Chemotherapy	16

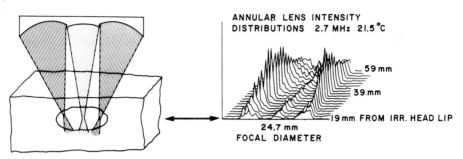

ANNULAR LENS INTENSITY
DISTRIBUTIONS 2.7 MHz 21.5 °C

59 mm

39 mm

19 mm FROM IRR. HEAD LIP

24.7 mm
FOCAL DIAMETER

Figure 2. Annular-focus Lens with a central 'leak': diagrammatic cross section and intensity distribution. Details are given in Ref. [22]. As shown in Fig. 4 (1), the system was mounted from a spring-loaded support which enabled it to follow respiratory or other movements.

could render it partially or wholly anesthetic. The thresholds of thermal sensibility were measured in terms of the minimum temperature differences from the resting skin temperature that could be perceived as cool, warm, hot or stinging, by using an electrothermal stimulator designed for such measurement [26], and were compared with those on contralateral side. As these thresholds are known to vary with the skin temperature [27, 28], they were measured after skin cooling, if this was necessary during hyperthermia treatment, as discussed below. Tumor dimensions were measured or estimated independently by two investigators and X-rays were reviewed for accurate treatment planning.

Hyperthermia for all treated lesions was achieved by use of FUS either in dynamically scanned mode [24, 25], or as a stationary annular focus system [22, 24] as shown in Figs. 1 and 2. Note that the coupling cone of the latter rested directly on the skin over the tumor. With the aid of a detachable pointer that indicated the location of the focal plane, the insonation head was positioned over the tumor and was coupled to the skin through degassed water and ultrasonic coupling gel to ensure unimpeded transmission of ultrasound into the tissues. The temperature of the degassed water in the coupling bag could be altered rapidly and maintained at any desired level between 10° and 45 °C and enabled precise control of the temperature of the skin in the portal. If the skin was infiltrated by the tumor it was kept at the therapeutic temperature. When the tumor was subcutaneous, or the skin was stretched thin and was likely to break down, the skin temperature could be held below 30 °C if necessary to obviate any heat pain or injury. Prior to treatment, a 22 gauge hypodermic needle – temperature probe was inserted into the tumor under local anesthesia. The site of insertion was placed well outside the portal of ultrasound to prevent any reduction in the heat sensibility of the skin within the portal and to preclude the modification of tumor response to hyperthermia by the local anesthetic, since Yatvin *et al.* [29] have demonstrated that local anesthetics potentiate the effects of

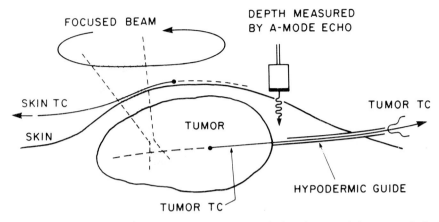

Figure 3. Diagram of the thermometry procedure. For clarity, the second thermocouple in the hypodermic needle, and the coupling water bag are not shown.

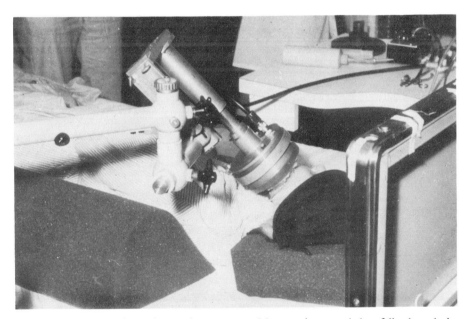

Figure 4. Photograph of a patient under treatment. Many patients tended to fall asleep during treatment and had to be kept awake to prevent unconscious movements.

heat on cell membranes. The probe contained two microthermocouples with their junctions spaced 10 to 20 mm apart. The needle was placed so that one thermocouple was centered well within the tumor and the second was located at the edge of the tumor. Additionally a third thermocouple was placed on the skin to record the skin temperature during treatment (Figs. 3 and 4). The depth of the temperature probe within the tumor was measured by A-mode ultrasound at a frequency of 15 MHz, yielding axial resolution of 0.2 mm. Temperatures at all three sites were recorded continuously on a strip-chart recorder.

To induce hyperthermia, a frequency of 2.7, 3.6 or 4.5 MHz was used depending on the thickness or subcutaneous extent of the tumor. During the induction of hyperthermia, the ultrasonic power level was controlled manually until the desired intratumoral temperature (as measured by the thermocouple placed at the edge) was achieved. This temperature was maintained either under manual or computer control. Intratumoral temperature distributions were determined in an initial group of patients by pulling out the thermocouple probe, in steps of 1 or 2 mm, prior to the end of the LHT. Such temperature distribution measurements were also made subsequently in tumors at different anatomical locations and also whenever any alterations were made in the hyperthermia delivery system.

Hyperthermia treatments, as outlined in Table 3, were administered at weekly intervals. Each patient received an initial trial of hyperthermia at 42 °C for 20 min. If no toxicity was seen, subsequent weekly treatments were at 42.5 °C. Toxicity as well as antitumor response were recorded before and after each treatment. Antitumor response criteria were defined as:

Complete response   — disappearance of all clinically detectable disease within the treatment field.

Partial response   — a >50% decrease in all measurable disease within the treatment field for >1 month.

Table 3. Treatment plan

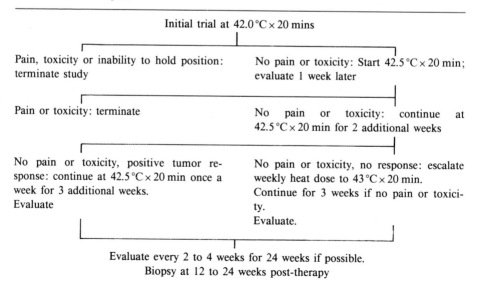

Initial trial at 42.0 °C × 20 mins

Pain, toxicity or inability to hold position: terminate study

No pain or toxicity: Start 42.5 °C × 20 min; evaluate 1 week later

Pain or toxicity: terminate

No pain or toxicity: continue at 42.5 °C × 20 min for 2 additional weeks

No pain or toxicity, positive tumor response: continue at 42.5 °C × 20 min once a week for 3 additional weeks. Evaluate

No pain or toxicity, no response: escalate weekly heat dose to 43 °C × 20 min. Continue for 3 weeks if no pain or toxicity. Evaluate.

Evaluate every 2 to 4 weeks for 24 weeks if possible.
Biopsy at 12 to 24 weeks post-therapy

Stable disease — a <25% change in tumor size stable over 1 month.

Disease progression — An objective increase of >25% of existing disease or the appearance of new tumor lesions within the treatment field.

4.2. Clinical results

Heat sensibility of skin over superficial tumors was found to be diminished to a variable extent in almost all cases. Some patients, with tumors infiltrating the skin, volunteered the statement to the effect that the skin felt 'both very sensitive and numb at the same time', which is indicative of partial cutaneous denervation.

Treatment data and specifics for the 26 patients who received hyperthermia treatment are tabulated in Table 4. Patients received six treatments on the average but with some variation. The tumor temperature during treatment as measured by the intratumoral thermocouple was 42–42.5 °C. In each case, the temperature was maintained at a constant level throughout the 20-min treatment sessions as shown in Fig. 5, which is typical of the data obtained in most patients except that the temperature in this instance was raised to 43.5 °C. The intratumoral temperature rose rapidly – within 4 min – from 33.5 °C to the desired therapeutic temperature of 43.5 °C and then leveled off. The rate of rise of temperature was dependent on the acoustic (ultrasonic) power level and thus could be controlled during the induction period. The temperature could be maintained to within ±0.25 °C of the preselected level of 42.0°, 42.5° or 43.0 °C automatically through the feed-back temperature control or manually with occasional adjustments to the ultrasonic power level. At temperatures of 43.0° or 43.5 °C for 3 to 5 min, in many tumors, there was sudden drop in temperature, requiring an increase in the ultrasonic power for its restitution. This is believed to be due to the cooling of the tumor by an increase in the local blood flow. The tumor temperature decayed rather slowly when the power was turned off.

Figure 6 shows a typical plot of the temperature across a treatment volume 15 min after induction of LHT. One can see a uniform temperature (±0.25 °C) within the tumor, but at the edge of tumor there is a sharp drop

Table 4. Treatment data

# Patients	26
# Treatment †/Patient	5.8 mean (3–10 range)
Treatment temperature	42–42.5 °C**
Maximum skin temperature*	26–39 °C

† Treatments given at weekly intervals.

* During treatment at maximum treatment temperature.

** In one patient treatment temperature was escalated to 45 °C at one session.

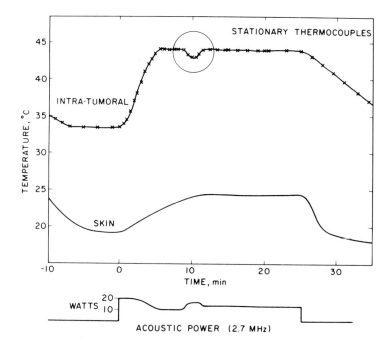

Figure 5. Temporal course of intratumoral and cutaneous temperatures and the ultrasonic (acoustic) power, during a session in a patient. The temperature was raised to 43.5 °C to elicit the thermovascular response which is encircled.

off to near normal temperatures in the tumor bed tissue. This uniformity of treatment to ± 0.25 °C was achieved for large tumors as well as small tumors measuring less than two cm.

Specific toxicity as related to the hyperthermia treatment is shown in Table 5. The 26 patients received 151 treatment sessions. The toxicity is tabulated per patient. No toxicity was seen in 20 of the 26 treated patients. Subjective symptoms of burning (1), stinging (1), and pressure (2) were seen in 4 of the 26 patients. The symptoms occurred early during their treatment, were transient, and were relieved by simple adjustments of power or position and in no case were dose-limiting. Burning and stinging were evoked at temperatures below 25 °C and were related to rate of rise of skin (and intratumoral) temperature and thus could be relieved immediately by reducing the ultrasonic power. The sensation of pressure was reported by two patients who were being treated using the stationary annular-focus system. In each, the sensation of pressure was traced to the pressure of the edge of the coupling cone on the hypodermic needle-temperature probe and was relieved by raising the cone one or two mm. Two objective toxicities were seen. One patient developed slight erythema of the skin overlying a large subcutaneous soft tissue sarcoma which had previously stretched the skin extensively. A second patient developed mild desquamation of the superficial epithelial

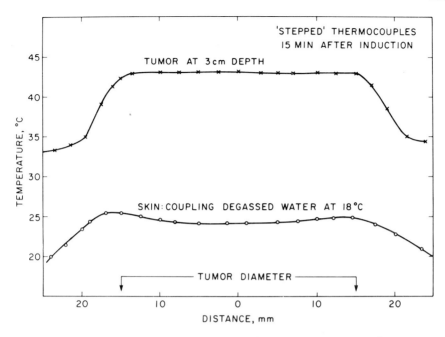

Figure 6. Intratumoral and cutaneous temperature distributions during a hyperthermia session in a patient. The thermocouple probes were pulled out in steps of approximately 2 mm 15 min after induction of LHT.

layers of the skin overlying a large soft tissue mass which was closely approximating the underlying dermis. Neither of the objective toxicities noted were dose-limiting and cleared without any intervention within 3 to 4 days. No objective toxicity was encountered when the skin in the treatment portal was normal.

Table 5. Incidence of toxicity

	Total	
	Patients (26)	Sessions (151)
*Toxicity**		
No toxicity	20	145
Subjective		
Burning	1	1
Stinging	1	1
Pressure	2	2
Objective		
Erythema	1	1
Desquamation	1	1

* Per patient.

The antitumor response to the hyperthermia treatment is noted in Table 6. Seven of the 26 patients were receiving concurrent chemotherapy and had multiple tumors, one of which was treated with LHT, the remaining ones being studied as controls. Two patients had lesions which were clinically inevaluable, the other twenty four patients were evaluable for response. Complete response was seen in three patients (13%), partial response in twelve patients (50%), and nine patients (37%) showed no response to hyperthermia treatments. Of the nine non-responding patients, seven showed a diminution in measurable disease in the treatment field but this was less than 50% and therefore could not be classified as Partial Response. Moreover, two of these seven patients and three of the twelve patients achieving partial tumor responses were subsequently biopsied and showed no evidence of tumor, but only fibrotic scar tissue or granulation tissue. One patient that did not achieve a partial response was biopsied and showed residual tumor. The exact duration of response beyond one month was not assessable since most of these patients had subsequent systemic treatment following the hyperthermia treatment course. The data on the seven patients with multiple tumors who were on chemotherapy are shown in Table 7. Note that addition of hyperthermia to chemotherapy improved the response in all the cases. Thus, if there was no response with chemotherapy alone in control tumors, the tumor receiving LHT in addition to chemotherapy

Table 6. Response to treatment

# Patients	26	
Evaluable lesions	24	
Response		
Complete response	3	13%
Partial response	12	50%
No response	9	37%

Table 7. Enhancement of local chemotherapeutic effects by LHT

Drug(s)	Control tumor	Tumor with LHT
Cyclophosphamide	NR	PR
Cis-Platinum-Bleomycin	NR	PR
Methotrexate	PR	CR
Cis-Platinum	NR	PR
Cis-Platinum-Bleomycin	NR	PR
Cyclophosphamide	NR	PR
Methotrexate	PR	CR

showed a Partial Response, and similarly LHT converted Partial Responses to Complete Responses.

5. Future prospects

The results presented above clearly demonstrate that FUS can heat a predetermined tissue volume in the head and neck region to a uniform temperature. This is rather remarkable in view of the fact that all of the tumors treated lay over either a bone or the air cavities of the aero-digestive tract and both of these reflect and/or scatter ultrasonic energy almost totally. The importance of careful selection of the ultrasonic frequency and optimization of the geometry of insonation for each individual tumor in order to produce uniform heating cannot be overemphasized. Such uniformity of dose distribution not only enables correlation of the 'heat-dose' (temperature × time) with the tumor response and toxicity, but apparently yields significant anti-tumor effects at a relatively modest heat dose level: 42.5 °C for 20 min weekly for 3 to 6 weeks which is a low heat-dose by current standards. The ability of FUS to heat the entire tumor, specially its proliferating, well vascularized margins, to a therapeutic temperature would seem to be responsible for the low heat-dose requirements for squamous cell carcinoma of the head and neck. Tissue response is obviously a function of both temperature and time [30], and further studies are clearly required to determine whether higher temperatures for shorter times or lower temperatures for longer times are optimal.

The results are also notable for lack of any significant toxicity to overlying soft tissues or skin. They thus contrast the results obtained by Marmor *et al.* [10, 13] using unfocused ultrasound in which up to 40% of the patients sustained pain, burns and central tumor necrosis and also contrast the results of other investigators using electromagnetic heating (MW and RF) techniques. The lack of toxicity with FUS cannot be attributed to any known differences in the patient population since 25/26 patients in this study had received prior radiation therapy and 16/26 had received prior chemotherapy. The lack of toxicity therefore must be related to the sparing of tissues outside the target volume by focusing of the ultrasonic energy into the tumor.

The objective response rate achieved with FUS compares favorably with those of other LHT studies in which significantly higher rates of toxicity and significantly higher heat-doses (temperatures and time) were reported. The numbers of complete and partial responses presented in Table 6 were determined in the conventional manner from changes in the dimensions of the tumor, and may be understated since tumor biopsies from some of the patients achieving a partial response failed to show any residual tumor.

Similar observations of residual masses, consisting of fibrous or granulation tissue, have been made with respect to deeper tumors and also have been noted by Parks and Smith [31], and Storm and Morton [32] following whole body hyperthermia. This suggests that 'histologically' complete responses might have been achieved in a larger proportion of patients than reported in Table 6. Further studies and biopsies to confirm these observations are essential to demonstrate the need for a re-definition of response criteria.

However, even the conventionally determined (and thus conservative) response rate to LHT compares favorably with response rates to combination chemotherapy in head and neck cancer. These results are remarkable since they were obtained in patients in whom prior chemotherapy and/or radiation therapy had failed. Importantly, local hyperthermia does not produce marrow toxicity, and with the use of a precise techniques, negligible local toxicity. Most reported data also indicate that LHT does not enhance or recall toxicities related to prior chemotherapy or radiation therapy. Results of Arcangeli et al. [9], Babayan et al. [32] and our own studies, clearly demonstrate that use of LHT can enhance the local tumoricidal effects of chemotherapy without increasing systemic toxicity. LHT potentiates the effects of radiation therapy and is an effective local radiosensitizer [1–6]. Local hyperthermia is thus an attractive candidate for combined modality studies in head and neck cancer.

Acknowledgements

Parts of this research were supported by USPHS Grants RR00088, CA30944 and CA31303. The author wishes to acknowledge the collaboration of Drs. Bertino, Ervin, Feldman, Frei, Kaiser* and Kowal** in the studies conducted and to thank Dr. Ervin and Dr. Kowal for their assistance in the preparation of this chapter.

* Dr. Kaiser is presently in Department of Surgery, VA Hospital, Manchester, N.H.
** Dr. Kowal is presently in Departments of Medicine and Pharmacology, University of Pittsburg, Pittsburg, PA.

References

1. Streffer C, van Beuningen D, Dietzel F, Rottinger E, Robinson JE, Scherer E, Seeber S, Trott K-R (eds): Cancer Therapy by Hyperthermia and Radiation (Proceedings of the 2nd International Symposium, Essen, June 2–4, 1977). Baltimore-Munich, Urban & Schwarzenberg, Inc., 1978.

2. Milder JW (ed): Conference on hyperthermia in cancer treatment. Cancer Research 39:6 (June, 1979).

3. Dethlefsen LA, Dewey WC (eds): Third International Symposium: Cancer Therapy by Hyperthermia, Drugs, and Radiation. (Symposium held at Colorado State University, June 22–26, 1980). National Cancer Institute Monograph 61, Bethesda (MD), US Dept of Health & Human Services, Public Health Service, National Institutes of Health, 1982.

4. Nussbaum GH (ed): Physical Aspects of Hyperthermia. American Association of Physicists in Medicine, Medical Physics, Monograph No. 8, New York, American Institute of Physics, Inc, 1982.

5. Hahn M: Hyperthermia and Cancer. New York, Plenum Publishing Corporation, 1982.

6. Storm FK (ed): Hyperthermia in Cancer Therapy. Boston, G.K. Hall Medical Publishers, 1983.

7. LeVeen HH, Wapnick S, Piccone V, et al.: Tumor eradication by radiofrequency therapy. JAMA 235:2198–2200, 1976.

8. Arcangeli G, Barocas A, Mauro F, et al.: Multiple daily fractionation (MDF) radiotherapy in association with hyperthermia and/or misonidazole: experimental and clinical results. Cancer 45:2707–2711, 1980.

9. Arcangeli G, Cividalli A, Mauro F, et al.: Enhanced effectiveness of adriamycin and bleomycin combined with local hyperthermia in neck node metastases from head and neck cancer. Tumori 65:481–486, 1979.

10. Marmor JB, Hahn GM: Radiation (XRT) with ultrasound-induced hyperthermia (ht) for superficial human neoplasms. ASCO Abstracts C404:389, 1979.

11. Stehlin JS, Freeff PJ, Giovanella BC, et al.: Dramatic response of cancer to localized hyperthermia. New York State Journal of Medicine January 1980, pp 70–72.

12. Hornback NB, Shupe R, Shidnia H, et al.: Radiation and microwave therapy in the treatment of advanced cancer. Radiology 130:459–464, 1979.

13. Marmor JB, Pounds D, Postic TB, et al.: Treatment of superficial human neoplasms by local hyperthermia induced by ultrasound. Cancer 43:188–197, 1979.

14. Caldwell WL: Evaluation of the Perth experience in treating with ionizing radiations and VHF 9434 megahertz radiations. Int J Radiat Oncol Biol Phys 5:1919–1921, 1979.

15. Perez CQ, Kopecky W, Baglan R, et al.: Local microwave hyperthermia in cancer therapy. Preliminary Report. (Proceedings of the Henry Ford Hospital Symposium 'Clinical Hyperthermia Today' Detroit, Michigan, June). 1980.

16. Fazekas J, Nerlinger T: Clinical hyperthermia pilot studies. Thomas Jefferson University Hospital (Proceedings of the Henry Ford Hospital Symposium. 'Clinical Hyperthermia Today', Detroit, Michigan, June). 1980.

17. Lele PP: Hyperthermia by ultrasound. (Proceedings of the International Symposium on Cancer Therapy by Hyperthermia and Radiation, Amer Coll of Radiology, Washington D.C., April 28–30, 1975). 1975, pp 168–178.

18. Lele PP, Parker KJ, Castro EP: Deep local hyperthermia by focused ultrasound. Int J Rad Oncol 4:118, 1978.

19. Lele PP, Frere RJ, Parker KJ, Greenwald RC, Shalev M, Greene KE: Local hyperthermia by focused ultrasound: technique and results in spontaneous tumors in dogs. (Third Int Symp: Cancer Therapy by Hyperthermia, Drugs and Radiation, June 22–26, 1980, Ft Collins, Colo), 1980.

20. Lele PP, Bertino JR, Ervin TJ, Feldman MI, Frei E, III, Kowal CD: Clinical evaluation of local hyperthermia by focused ultrasound. (Third Int Symp: Cancer Therapy by Hyperthermia, Drugs and Radiation, June 22–26, 1980, Ft Collins, Colo.) 1980.

21. Lele PP, Bertino JR, Ervin TJ, Feldman MI, Frei E, III, Kowal CD: Treatment of advanced squamous cell cancers of the head and neck, (Int Head and Neck Oncology Research Conference, National Cancer Institute, Sept 8–10, 1980, Rosslyn, Va.) 1980.

22. Lele PP: An annular-focus ultrasonic lens for production of uniform hyperthermia in cancer Therapy, Ultrasound in Med & Biol 7:191–193, 1981.

23. Lele PP: Local hyperthermia by ultrasound. physical aspects of hyperthermia. (American

264

Association of Physicists in Medicine, Summer School, Aug 3–7, 1981, Dartmouth College, Hanover, N.H.) 1981.

24. Lele PP: Physical aspects and clinical trials with localized ultrasonic hyperthermia. In: Storm FK (ed) Hyperthermia in Cancer Therapy. Boston, G.K. Hall Publishers, 1983.

25. Lele PP, Parker KJ: Temperature distributions in tissues during local hyperthermia by stationary or steered beams of unfocused or focused ultrasound. British Journal of Cancer 45:108–121, 1982.

26. Lele PP: An electrothermal stimulator for sensory tests. J Neurol, Neurosurg & Psychiat 25:329–331, 1962.

27. Lele PP: Relationship between cutaneous thermal thresholds, skin temperature and cross-sectional area of the stimulus. J Physiol 126:191–205, 1954.

28. Lele PP, Weddell G, Williams CM: The relationship between heat transfer, skin temperature and cutaneous sensibility. J Physiol 126:206–234, 1954.

29. Yatvin MB, Clifton KH, Dennis WH: Hyperthermia and local anesthetics: potentiation of survival of tumor-bearing mice. Science 205:195–196, 1979.

30. Lele PP: Temperature-duration thresholds for irreversible histologic and/or ultrastructural damage to normal mammalian tissues and tumors In Vivo. (Proc of the 7th Int Cong of Radiation Res, July 3–8, 1983, Amsterdam) 1983, pp D6–30.

31. Parks LC, Smith GV: Systemic hyperthermia by extracorporeal induction: techniques and results. In: Storm FK (ed) Hyperthermia In Cancer Therapy. Boston, G.K. Hall Publishers, 1983, Chapter 19.

32. Storm FK, Morton DL: Animal and clinical studies with microwave and radiowave hyperthermia. In: Storm FK (ed) Hyperthermia In Cancer Therapy. Boston, G.K. Hall Publishers, 1983, Chapter 15.

33. Babayan RK, Lele PP, Krane RJ: Thermochemotherapy of renal adenocarcinoma in Wistar-Lewis rats. (Presented at the American Urological Assoc, Inc, 77th Annual Meeting, May 16–20, 1982, Bartle Hall & Radisson-Muehlebach, Kansas City, Missouri.) 1982, p 142.

12. The use of chemotherapy in combination with radiotherapy in the treatment of head and neck squamous cancers

CHARLOTTE JACOBS

1. Introduction

Radiation therapy has excellent cure rates for patients with stage I and II, and some stage III squamous cell cancers of the head and neck. However, the results in patients with advanced inoperable cancers are often poor with radiotherapy alone [1]. In an attempt to improve these poor results, chemotherapy is currently being evaluated as part of a combined modality approach for these patients [2].

There are three theoretical ways in which chemotherapy and radiotherapy can be combined to improve cure rates:

1. Chemotherapy may be given prior to radiotherapy to decrease tumor bulk and therefore decrease the number of hypoxic cells.
2. Chemotherapy may be given simultaneously with radiotherapy to increase sensitization to irradiation.
3. Chemotherapy may be given following radiotherapy to irradicate residual microscopic disease either locally or distally.

The first two approaches might be expected to decrease local recurrence, while the third might have more impact on distant metastases. However, there are some potential disadvantages to the combined modality approach. When chemotherapy is used as the initial therapy, there is a delay in administering radiotherapy, and if patients do not respond to chemotherapy, tumor growth may occur prior to initiation of irradiation. Patients who have had a complete response to pretreatment chemotherapy may decline subsequent radiotherapy. From model systems, one would not expect chemotherapy alone to effectively eradicate malignant cells in these large solid tumors [3]. Chemotherapy used concurrently with radiotherapy may result in increased normal tissue destruction leading to less effective dose delivery. Finally, the acute and long term toxicities of chemotherapy need to be evaluated when used in conjunction with radiotherapy.

Gregory T. Wolf (ed), Head and Neck Oncology.
© *1984 Martinus Nijhoff Publishers, Boston. ISBN 0-89838-657-8. Printed in The Netherlands.*

This chapter will evaluate the current status of chemotherapy given prior to or concurrently with radiotherapy. Response rates, survival and toxicity data will be used to determine the therapeutic gain of the combined modality approach.

2. Chemotherapy prior to radiotherapy

2.1. Cisplatin + bleomycin

The combination of cisplatin followed by an infusion of bleomycin is one of the most commonly used pretreatment chemotherapy regimens (Table 1). Randolph et al. treated 21 patients with stage IV squamous carcinoma of multiple sites with cisplatin (3 mg/kg on day 1), followed by bleomycin (0.25 mg/kg days 3–10) [4]. On day 22 patients were evaluated for response.

Table 1. Chemotherapy prior to radiotherapy

| Author | # Patients | Chemotherapy | Response | | % Complete response following radiotherapy |
			% Complete	% Partial	
Randolph [4]	21	Cisplatin (CP) – 3 mg/kg Bleomycin (Bleo) – 0.25 mg/kg/d, 3–10	19%	52%	33%
Glick [5]	29	CP-80 – 100 mg/m^2 Bleo-15 u/m^2/d, 3–7	–	48%	48%
Brown [6]	23	Vinblastine – 4 mg/m^{2}dl Bleo – 15 mg/d, 1–7 CP – 50 mg/m^{2}d8	22%	52%	63%
Al-Sarraf [7]	77	Vincristine (VCR) – .5 mg/m^{2}dl, 4 Bleo – 30 u/d, 1–4 CP – 120 mg/m^{2}d6	29%	51%	–
Tannock [8]	33	Methotrexate (Mtx) – 100 mg/m^2 × 3, dl Leucovorin Bleo – 20 u/m^{2}dl-4 CP – 60 mg/m^{2}d5	9%	51%	36%
Marcial [9]	40	VCR – 1.5 mg/m^2 Bleo – 15 u/dX2 Mtx – 200 mg/m^2 Leucovorin	6%	54%	46%

They then received a second dose of cisplatin followed immediately by standard radiotherapy. On day 22, 19% had achieved a complete clinical response and 52% a partial response. At the end of radiation therapy 33% had achieved a complete response. Toxicity from chemotherapy was tolerable and included nausea and vomiting, alopecia, mucositis and renal dysfunction (creatinine greater than 2 mg % in 15% of patients). The authors felt that the 33% complete response rate at the end of radiotherapy was higher than previously observed with radiotherapy alone in this particular patient population. However, they concluded that the role of initial chemotherapy in producing improved survival was not yet evaluable.

Glick *et al.* treated a similar group of patients with cisplatin and bleomycin infusion followed by 6500–7500 rad of radiation therapy, over 7 weeks [5]. They reported no complete responses to initial chemotherapy and 48% partial responses. This is lower than the response rate reported by Randolph [4] and may be due to lower doses of cisplatin and bleomycin. Of interest is that following radiation therapy, 48% achieved a complete response. The authors noted that following chemotherapy, radiotherapy was completed on schedule without increased toxicity.

2.2. Cisplatin + bleomycin + other agents

Brown *et al.* treated 23 patients with advanced squamous cell cancers with a combination of vinblastine (4 mg/m² day 1), bleomycin (15 mg/day days 1–7), and cisplatin (60 mg/m² on day 8), repeated every 3 weeks for 3 cycles [6]. Twenty-two per cent of patients achieved a complete response and 52% a partial response. Nineteen patients received subsequent radiotherapy, and 63% were still free of disease at a followup of 10 months. Toxicity was acceptable. Despite the lower dose of cisplatin, a high complete response was reported. This may be due to the addition of a third drug, the delivery of 3 cycles of chemotherapy, or perhaps a patient population having better prognostic factors.

Al-Sarraf *et al.* treated 77 patients with advanced head and neck cancer with vincristine (0.5 mg/m² days 1, 4), bleomycin (30 units days 1–4), and cisplatin (120 mg/m² day 6) [7]. Twenty-nine per cent achieved a complete response and 51% a partial response. There was no influence of primary site or tumor differentiation on response rate. Following chemotherapy 32 patients underwent primary radiotherapy to 6600 rads. Chemotherapy was well tolerated and did not interfere with the planned radiotherapy. The authors evaluated the influence of several prognostic factors on survival. Stage IV tumors, grade III histology, and lack of response to chemotherapy were all associated with worse survival.

Tannock *et al.* treated 33 patients with a combination of cisplatin, bleomycin, and moderate-dose methotrexate for two cycles prior to definitive radiotherapy [8]. They achieved a complete response rate of 9% and a partial response rate of 51%. Following completion of radiation therapy 36% had a complete response. Toxicity was not excessive, and the loss of weight and mucosal reactions were similar to a comparison group receiving radiotherapy alone. However, at 16 months median followup only 24% were disease-free. These observations suggest that benefit from pretreatment chemotherapy may be related to the complete response rate, and a regimen that produces a low complete response rate will not ultimately affect survival.

2.3. Other agents

Marcial reported the Radiation Therapy Oncology Group (RTOG) experience with 40 patients treated with vincristine (1.5 mg/m^2), bleomycin (15 units/day $\times$ 2), and methotrexate (200 mg/m^2), repeated following a one week rest, followed by radiotherapy (6600 to 7000 rad in 6 to 7 weeks) [9]. Six per cent of patients achieved a complete response with chemotherapy which increased to 46% at completion of radiotherapy. Chemotherapy toxicity was acceptable, and 89% had no severe toxicity from radiotherapy.

2.4. Comparative studies of pretreatment chemotherapy + radiotherapy

There are few randomized studies of pretreatment chemotherapy followed by radiotherapy in head and neck cancer. Petrovich et al. randomized 23 patients with stage IV unresectable cancer to receive radiotherapy alone to 7000 rads in 7 weeks or methotrexate – 50–100 mg/kg over 6 h followed by leucovorin rescue repeated at 3 weeks [10]. Unfortunately, 34% of patients had protocol deviations, and most radiotherapy deviations were in the control arm. Thirty-three per cent of patients in the combination arm had a complete response as compared to 9% in the control arm. The median survival of the combination group was 12 months as compared to 5.6 months for the control group ($p = 0.13$). At followup of 30 months only 1 patient was alive in each arm. Thus, in this very small randomized study, pretreatment chemotherapy did improve overall response rate, however, it had no significant impact on survival. In addition, the authors noted that chemotherapy did not change the pattern of failure in these patients.

2.5. Conclusions

Pretreatment chemotherapy can achieve partial tumor responses in up to half of patients, with complete clinical responses in as many as 30%. Toxicity is tolerable, and pretreatment chemotherapy doesn't appear to enhance toxicity of subsequent irradiation. Several authors have identified subgroups who are more likely to benefit from pretreatment chemotherapy. However, even these pilot studies do not yet indicate a major improvement in eventual outcome. Regimens that are capable of achieving a higher complete response rate may prove to provide greater survival benefit.

3. Concurrent chemotherapy/radiotherapy

3.1. Methotrexate combined with radiation therapy

Methotexate (Mtx) blocks the generation of reduced folates by inhibition of dihydrofolate reductase. This interferes with the synthesis of thymidilic acid, and the resultant S-phase block of the cell cycle causes a high proportion of cells to accumulate in G-1 phase of the cell cycle. Cells in G-1 have increased sensitivity to irradiation [11]. In 1959 it was reported that mammary carcinomas in mice treated with combined irradiation and folic acid antagonists had a greater regression than those treated with irradiation alone [12]. *In vitro* studies have shown a therapeutic gain of anoxic tumor cells for the combination compared to irradiation alone [13]. The major toxicities of Mtx are myelosuppression and mucositis. Nausea, vomiting, diarrhea, and rash occur rarely.

3.1.1. Early trials
In 1960 Friedman treated his first patient with a combination of irradiation and Mtx [14]. This 84-year old female had a recurrence in a previously irradiated field. She received daily Mtx for one month followed by 3600 rad with complete resolution of tumor. Encouraged by this early result, he proceeded to treat 200 cases, 110 of which were primary tumors. The treatment involved sequential Mtx (7.5 mg daily × 7–14 days or 25 mg intravenous (IV) every 3 days × 5) followed by full-dose irradiation. Of 168 evaluable cases, the complete and partial response rate was 33% at the primary and 31% in nodes. Although the survival at two years was not improved, the local control rate was much improved for stage III (67%) and for stage IV (42%) cancers compared to previously observed local control rates.

The mucositis resulting from combined therapy was more intense and longer lasting than previously seen. Seventeen patients were treated with sublethal doses of irradiation following chemotherapy. There was a high failure rate, and the investigator abandoned this approach, concluding that following even an excellent chemotherapy response, full dose irradiation must be given. Finally, it was concluded that although Mtx induced a marked tumor shrinkage in many patients, an enhancement effect or an increased cure rate from this approach had not yet been proved.

Kramer began treating patients with Mtx prior to and then concurrent with irradiation [15]. His treatment plan was based on the following: it is well-known in head and neck cancer that there are differences in tumor regression based on tumor size. This could be a result of large numbers of hypoxic tumor cells or a decreased chance of cell kill based on cell number. Thus, if tumor cell volume could be decreased prior to irradiation, the cure rate might be increased. Patients were treated with Mtx (7.5 mg orally daily) with concurrent irradiation beginning on day 6. At toxicity, Mtx was discontinued and irradiation was continued to a total dose of 6500 rad.

Fifty-seven patients with stages III and IV cancers were treated with this regimen, and 61% obtained complete tumor clearance. At 3 years, 32% of patients were tumor free, and 44% of those who died had no evidence of local recurrence. However, this regimen was associated with a high incidence of severe mucositis (66%) and myelosuppression (50%). Different schedules of intermittent Mtx were utilized with a reduction of toxicity without change in tumor response. The author concluded that a randomized trial would be necessary to confirm the usefulness of combined therapy.

Others have noted that Mtx given prior to radiation therapy resulted in a high percentage of complete responders [16, 17]. Klimo and Danko [16] treated 48 patients with Mtx, either orally or IV prior to standard therapy. They noted significantly more toxicity with oral Mtx, even though the total dose was less, and therefore recommended the IV route of administration.

It should be noted that in most of the above studies, Mtx was given prior to irradiation. It may be that the optimal combination would involve Mtx used during irradiation. Pointon treated 34 patients with Mtx – 100 mg/m^2 IV 24 h prior to initiation of radiotherapy and at 14 days [18]. Radiation doses ranged from 4500 to 5500 rad. Eighty per cent of their patients had stage IV disease and 20% had stage III disease. At completion of therapy, 53% had a complete response, and the overall survival at 21 months was 63%. In 50% of the patients, the healing of mucosal reactions was delayed. Two patients had neutropenia, 1 resulting in death. The authors felt that if Mtx was to act as a sensitizer, it should be given concurrent with irradiation and that their regimen had acceptable toxicity.

3.1.2. Randomized trials

Randomized trials have failed to confirm these initially encouraging results (Table 2). Kligerman *et al.* randomized 22 patients to irradiation alone or Mtx prior to irradiation [19]. Although those who responded to Mtx appeared to have a better response to irradiation, the numbers were too small to draw conclusions. Von Essen *et al.*, as part of 4-arm study, randomized

Table 2. Randomized studies of methotrexate combined with radiotherapy

Author	Von Essen [20]	Knowlton [21]	Richard [22]	Lustig [23]	Fazekas [24]
# Patients:	42	96	39	75	712
Primary sites	Oral cavity oropharynx	All	Oral cavity	All*	All
Stages	III, IV	III, IV	IV	III, IV	III, IV
Radiation dose (rad)	6500	6000–6600	3000–6000	6400	5500–8000
Chemotherapy	7 mg/m²d × 5	.2 mg/kg/d × 4 240 mg/m² × 3	50 mg/d × 6–12	25 mgq3d × 5	25 mgq3d × 5
% complete response:					
Radiation Alone	53%	20–35%	–	–	–
Radiation+Chemotherapy	82%				
% Survival:					
Follow-up (months)	2–14	60	18	36	60
Radiation alone	23%	10%	17%	10%	5–21%
Radiation+Chemotherapy	15%	9%	20%	20%	12–27%

* Except sinuses, nasopharynx.

42 patients with cancers of the buccal mucosa and gingiva to irradiation alone or irradiation preceeded by Mtx [20]. Although the response rate for those completing therapy was 82% in the combination group compared to 53% for irradiation alone group, there was no difference in disease-free survival. At 2–14 months follow-up, 15% of patients with combined treatment were disease-free, compared to 23% for the control group. This study points out the problems associated with lack of stratification for important prognostic variables, since the combined therapy group had more T4 patients, more N3 patients, and more patients with bone involvement than the control group.

Knowlton et al. randomized 96 patients with stage III and IV cancer of the head and neck to irradiation alone or irradiation plus Mtx (0.2 mg/kg/day × 5 in the first 56 patients; 240 mg/m^2 on days 1, 5, and 9 in subsequent patients) [21]. At one month following completion of therapy, the complete response rate was 20–35%, and at 5 years the disease-free survival was approximately 10% in both groups. There was no difference between low and high-dose Mtx, except that the latter was more toxic.

Richards et al. randomized 39 patients with stage IV tumors of the oral cavity and oropharynx to radiation therapy or irradiation plus intra-arterial Mtx [22]. There was no significant difference in survival between the two groups (20% at 18 months). Only half of the patients received 6000 rad and half received 3000 rad, making subgroups too small for conclusions.

Following Kramer's original study [15], Lustig et al. randomized 75 patients with stage IV cancers to either radiation therapy alone or Mtx (25 mg IV q 3 days × 5) followed by irradiation [23]. The 3-year survival for the combined group was 20% and for the group receiving radiation therapy alone was 10%. From 1961 to 1965 the authors had previously treated a similar group of patients with oral Mtx (2.5 mg thrice daily × 5) prior to initiation of irradiation and continued concurrently until toxicity. Fifty per cent of these patients had a partial response from chemotherapy alone with oral Mtx as opposed to only 14% with IV Mtx. This non-randomized group of patients who received oral Mtx and irradiation had a 3-year survival of 33% which was significantly better than the radiation therapy alone group from the randomized trial. Patients with oral Mtx had significantly more mucositis and myelosuppression than those receiving IV Mtx. The improved survival in the group that received oral Mtx could not be attributed to differences in total Mtx dose or radiation dose. The development of distant metastases was lower in both chemotherapy groups, but this did not reach statistical significance.

A similar study of 712 randomized patients was reported by the Radiation Therapy Oncology Group [24]. In this study, 18% of patients had a delay of radiotherapy, and 9% of patients failed to complete the prescribed radiation treatment in the combined arm as opposed to 4% in the radiation alone group. There was no difference in the 5-year survival between the combined treatment and radiation alone groups for any tumor site. The overall 5-year survival was 18%. Patients in both groups had a similar failure rate at the primary site (32%).

Thus, despite early encouraging results with the combination of Mtx and irradiation, this approach has never proven to be superior to standard treatment in randomized trials. Most randomized trials utilized Mtx prior to irradiation, and the failure to detect benefit may be related to dose, scheduling, or drug activity.

3.2. Hydroxyurea combined with radiation therapy

Hydroxyurea inhibits ribonucleotide reductase, thus interfering with DNA synthesis. Following exposure to hydroxyurea, it has been demonstrated *in vitro* that cells in S-phase are killed and synchronized in the radiosensitive G-1 stage [25]. Phillips has shown *in vitro* that hydroxyurea enhances cell kill by inhibiting repair in cells that have received potentially lethal irradiation [26]. Toxicities of this drug include myelosuppression and nausea.

Lerner was one of the first to use hydroxyurea in combination with irradiation for head and neck cancer [27]. He treated 24 patients with advanced disease with hydroxyurea (80 mg/kg q 3 day) for 1 week prior to and then concurrent with irradiation. Some patients had subsequent surgery. Com-

Table 3. Randomized studies of hydroxyurea combined with radiotherapy

Author	Richards [28]	Hussey [32]	Stefani [33]
# Patients	40	42	126
Primary sites	All	All	All
Stages	All	IV	All
Radiation dose(rad)	5000–9000	4500–7500	6000
Chemotherapy	80 mg/kgq3d	16 mg/kg thrice weekly	80 mg/kg twice weekly
% Complete response:			
Radiation alone	17% *	56%	47%
Radiation + Chemotherapy	55%	67%	42%
% Survival:			
Follow-up (months)	–	24	6–33
Radiation alone	14%	27%	31%
Radiation + Chemotherapy	33%	30%	22%

* % Complete response in primary at surgery.

plete regression occurred in 79% of patients, and 63% were disease-free at 4–20 months. Toxicities of mucositis and leukopenia were acceptable.

Richards and Chambers (Table 3) randomized 20 patients with all stages of head and neck cancer to radiation therapy alone or irradiation plus hydroxyurea (80 mg/kg q 3 day during irradiation and up to 8 weeks following irradiation) [28]. They noted that following irradiation, many patients went on to surgical resection. In the radiation alone group, of 12 surgical cases, 2 were histologically negative for tumor at the primary site, and 5 were negative in the lymph nodes. Of the 11 patients treated with combined therapy prior to surgery, 6 were histologically negative at the primary and all were negative in the neck. Three of 7 patients in the radiation alone group developed distant metastases, whereas none in the group that received hydroxyurea developed distant metastases. At a later date, Richards and Chambers updated their initial study and found that survival was related to treatment: radiation therapy alone – 14%; irradiation plus hydroxyurea – 33%; irradiation plus surgery – 46%; irradiation plus surgery plus hydroxyurea – 67% [28]. Although these reports suggested an enhanced response to irradiation with the addition of hydroxyurea, the numbers were small, and there was variability in tumor site, stage, and treatment, so that definite conclusions could not be drawn. Of their next 610 patients, 69% were treated with concurrent irradiation and hydroxyurea (1500 mg daily) [29]. This was a nonrandomized study, and irradiation was given alone, prior to, or following surgery. All stages and sites of disease were included. When analyzed by site or treatment, the survival of the group treated with hydroxyurea was always superior to those groups not receiving hydroxyurea. However, because this was not a randomized study, it is unclear whether the different treatment groups are comparable with regard to tumor stage, site, irradiation, and surgical technique.

Several other reports of uncontrolled trials have noted an enhanced effect with irradiation and the use of concurrent hydroxyurea [30, 31]. Increased stomatitis, often causing delays in irradiation, was frequently noted.

Hussey and Abrams randomized 42 patients with stage IV disease to irradiation alone (4500–7500 rad) or irradiation plus concurrent hydroxyurea (16 mg/kg thrice weekly) [32]. The major toxicities were mucositis (41%) and neutropenia (43%). In the control group, 56% of patients had complete regression of tumor as compared to 67% in the combined therapy group. At 24 months, 27% of patients in the control group were free of disease as compared to 30% in the combined therapy group. Both groups had a local control rate of 38% at 6–24 months.

Stefani et al. performed a randomized trial with 126 patients with tumors of various sites and stages in which irradiation alone or irradiation plus hydroxyurea was used [33]. At completion of irradiation, 47% in the control group had complete regression of the primary tumor as compared to 42% in the combined therapy group. Subsequent distant metastases developed in 23% of patients in the combination group as compared to 8% in the control group. With followup of 6 to 33 months, 31% of the control group was alive, free of disease as compared to 22% of the combination group. Half of the patients in the combined therapy group had increased mucositis in the irradiated area of greater intensity and at a lower dose level of irradiation than expected. A white blood count below 2500/mm^3 was noted in 31% of patients on combined therapy. The authors concluded that hydroxyurea as a radiosensitizer resulted in increased toxicity, did not improve the overall results, and may have contributed to increased distant metastases.

Although hydroxyurea showed additive effects *in vivo* and *in vitro* with irradiation and uncontrolled trials suggested enhanced tumor response, three randomized trials have failed to confirm an additive or synergistic effect in patients with head and neck cancer.

3.3. 5-fluorouracil combined with radiation therapy

5-fluorouracil (5-FU) is a fluorinated pyrimidine. Its mechanism of action is inhibition of thymidylate synthetase which results in decreased synthesis of thymidylate and interference with DNA production. 5-FU is also incorporated into RNA to replace uracil. If a cell is deprived of thymidine, it may produce an unstable DNA which would increase its sensitivity to irradiation [34]. However, the exact mechanism of sensitization has not been fully ellucidated. Ehrlich ascites tumor cells to which 5-FU and irradiation had been given showed suppression of uracil incorporation into DNA and increased depolymerization of DNA [34]. 5-FU has caused radiation sensi-

Table 4. Randomized studies of 5-fluorouracil combined with radiotherapy

Author	Howe [38]	Ansfield [39]
# Patients	19	131
Primary sites	Pharynx	All
Stages	III, IV	II, III, IV
Radiation (rad)	6000	6500
Chemotherapy	15 mg/kg × 3	10 mg/kg/d × 3
	7.5 mg/kg × 2	5 mg/kg/d × 4
		5 mg/kg/d bi-weekly
Survival:		
Follow-up	–	60 mo
Radiation	–	15%
Radiation + Chemotherapy	–	36%

tization of transplanted tumors in mice [35]. The major toxicities of 5-FU include leukopenia, stomatitis, nausea, vomiting, and diarrhea.

Initially, several investigators were encouraged by the results of combining 5-FU and irradiation for squamous cancers of the head and neck [36, 37]. Von Essen *et al.* treated 25 patients with T3 or T4 buccal mucosa cancers with 5-FU (15 mg/kg $\times$ 5 days) prior to radiation (6500 rad) [20]. Sixty-seven per cent of patients had total regression of tumor with the combination, but despite these responses, only 25% were tumor free at 2–14 months follow-up.

One of the first randomized trials (Table 4) evaluating the use of 5-FU studied 19 patients with T3 and T4 pharyngeal cancers [38]. 5-FU was given for 5 consecutive days prior to irradiation. Although the combination increased the rate of regression of pharyngeal cancers, there were no differences in survival or long-term control of the primary tumor.

In a second controlled trial, Ansfield *et al.* randomized 134 patients with advanced cancers of the head and neck to receive irradiation alone or irradiation plus 5-FU [39]. 5-FU was given in a schedule in which decremental doses were given during irradiation in an attempt to decrease mucositis (5-FU – 10 mg/kg/day $\times$ 3 days, 5 mg/kg/day $\times$ 4 days, 5 mg/kg/bi-weekly). Five-year survival was 35% for the combination arm and 15% for the radiation therapy alone arm ($p = .006$). Patients with tongue and tonsil primaries had a significant survival advantage with combined therapy. For tongue cancers the 5-year survival for the combination group was 43%, compared to 13% for the control group. For tonsil primaries, the 5-year survival was 59% for the combination group and 10% for the control group. There was no advantage with the addition of 5-FU for patients with hypopharynx, larynx, or nasopharynx primaries. The combination group did experience increased dermatitis, stomatitis and dysphagia.

An update by Gollin *et al.* confirmed these positive results for oral and tonsil cancers [40]. Although control of the primary and regional nodes was better for patients in the combination arm, distant metastases occurred with the same frequency in both groups.

3.4. Bleomycin combined with radiation therapy

Bleomycin (Bleo), a complex of glycopeptides isolated from *streptomyces vertisillus*, causes DNA strand scission. The major toxicities of this drug include pulmonary fibrosis, hypertrophic skin changes, pyrexia, mucositis, alopecia and rare hypotension. The synergy of Bleo and irradiation has been studied *in vitro* and *in vivo* [41, 42], and it has been demonstrated that Bleo interferes with cellular repair following irradiation. The optimal timing of drug administration depends on the cell system used. Jorgenson noted in a transplanted mouse tumor that synergy was obtained when Bleo and irradiation were given simultaneously, but the effect was only additive when Bleo was given intermittently [42].

Early clinical trials were encouraging. Berdal *et al.* combined irradiation (4200 rad) and concurrent Bleo (15 mg daily 1 h prior to irradiation in the first week; 15 mg thrice weekly in the second and third weeks) [43]. Of 46 patients with advanced head and neck cancer, complete responses were noted in 57% and partial responses in 33%. Mucositis did not appear to be greater than from irradiation alone. The authors concluded that the rapid rate of regression was suggestive of synergy, although it would be difficult to distinguish synergistic from additive effect. Following this, multiple non-randomized studies indicated improved response rates with the addition of Bleo to irradiation [44, 45].

Results from randomized trials are conflicting (Table 5). Shanta and Krishnamurthi randomized 145 patients with stage III or IV oral cavity cancers to irradiation alone (6500 rad) versus irradiation plus Bleo (10 or 15 mg thrice weekly IV or by intra-arterial (IA) injection) [46]. The two groups were comparable with respect to patient age, tumor and histologic grade. In the study group, 31% had invasion of the mandible as compared to 23% in the control group. The complete response rate was 77% in the combined therapy group as compared to 21% in the controls. It made no difference whether Bleo was given IV or IA. The disease-free survival at 36 months was 50% in the study group and 20% in the controls. Of patients with mandibular invasion, 75% in the study group responded to therapy and are still free of disease as compared to none in the control group. The

Table 5. Randomized studies of bleomycin combined with radiotherapy

Author	Shanta [46]	Cachin [47
# Patients	145	227
Primary sites	Oral cavity	Oropharynx
Stages	III, IV	
Radiation dose (rad)	6500	6400
Chemotherapy	10–15 mg thrice weekly × 7	15 mg twice weekly × 5
% Complete response:		
Radiation alone	21%	68%-primary 49%-nodes
Radiation + Chemotherapy	27%	67%-primary 62%-nodes
% Survival		
Interval follow-up	36 mo	15 mo
Radiation alone	20%	50%
Radiation + Chemo.	50%	50%

authors noted a marked increase in mucositis which resulted in lowering of total dose of irradiation.

Contrasting data was reported by Cachin et al. in a randomized trial of 227 patients with squamous cell cancer of the oropharynx [47]. Patients were treated with either irradiation alone (6400 rad) or irradiation plus Bleo (15 mg twice weekly × 5). The groups were comparable with regard to important prognostic factors. Mucositis and skin reactions occurred in 71% of patients in the combined therapy group. This resulted in delay of radiotherapy in 22% of patients and discontinuation of therapy in 5%. In contrast, in the control group, 21% had mucositis or skin reactions resulting in a delay of therapy in only 6% of patients. The complete response rate at the primary was 67% in the combined therapy groups, compared to 68% for the control group. Complete regression of lymph nodes was reported in 62% of the combined therapy group, compared to 49% of the control group. At 15 months follow-up, survival was the same in the two groups at 50%. The authors concluded that Bleo does not enhance the efficacy of irradiation in oropharyngeal cancers.

There are several reasons to explain the contrasting results of these two studies. The major difference is that the studies involved two different sites of disease, oral cavity and oropharynx. For recurrent head and neck cancer, response to chemotherapy varies with primary site [48], and so perhaps the additive effect of Bleo to irradiation may also vary with site. Cachin's study took place at 13 different institutions, and time of tumor evaluation varied from less than 1 month to more than 3 months following therapy. Patients in the combined therapy group had significantly more toxicity, resulting in a delay in irradiation. In addition, the total Bleo dose was less in the Cachin study compared to Shanta's study.

The addition of Bleo to preoperative radiation was studied by Kapstad et al. who randomized 29 patients to preoperative irradiation alone (3000 rad) or preoperative irradiation plus Bleo (15 mg thrice weekly on weeks 1, 2, 4 and 5) [49]. There was no difference in the amount of edema, mucosal reaction or skin reaction between the two groups. At two weeks, 60% of patients in the combined therapy group had a least a 50% reduction of tumor as compared to 28% in the radiation alone group. Despite the small numbers, these results were considered encouraging.

A current study of the Northern California Oncology Group randomizes patients with inoperable advanced squamous cell cancers to radiotherapy alone or radiotherapy with concurrent Bleo (5 mg biweekly) followed by maintenance chemotherapy with Bleo and Mtx at completion of radiotherapy [50]. To date, 79 patients have entered the study. No significant hematologic toxicity has been noted in either group. The degree of radiation mucositis, skin reaction, and impairment of swallowing and speech is greater in patients with combined therapy, although this has not resulted in a significant reduction in radiation dose or interruption of radiotherapy. Pulmonary toxicity was moderate in three patients, and severe in one. This study is still coded, and the overall response rate is 62% in arm Y, and 33% in arm X. The median time to failure is 440 days in arm X and has not been reached in arm Y.

In conclusion, *in vivo* and *in vitro* bleomycin has been noted to be a radiation sensitizer. One controlled trial shows a marked improvement with the use of bleomycin, one randomized trial shows no change and a current ongoing trial is encouraging. Thus, further trials need to be done to define the clinical benefit of Bleo in combination with radiation therapy.

3.5. Cisplatin combined with radiation therapy

Cisdiamminedichloroplatinum or cisplatin (CP) is a relatively new chemotherapeutic agent that is efficacious for cancers of the head and neck. CP has as its mechanism of action the following interactions with DNA: monofunctional binding to bases, chelation, and bi-functional cross-linking to bases [51]. Zak *et al.* first noted the interaction of CP and irradiation when survival of mice after single dose whole body irradiation was improved by the addition of CP [52]. Following this Wodinsky *et al.* noted that the survival of mice innoculated with P388 lymphocytic leukemia cells and treated with irradiation was prolonged by the addition of CP compared to either treatment alone [53].

The following mechanisms have been postulated for the CP-irradiation interactions: (1) hypoxic cell sensitizer, (2) inhibition of repair of radiation-induced sublethal or potentially lethal damage, (3) conversion of lesions into chromosomal aberrations, (4) cell cycle perturbations, (5) toxic ligand release, (6) reaction with non-protein SH groups [51, 54, 55].

The effect of drug timing has been studied and was noted to have little effect on survival curves in several tumor systems [54]. Overgaard and Kahn studying C3H mammary carcinoma in mice noted enhanced irradiation response in tumor by a factor of 1.7 when CP was given 30 minutes before irradiation as compared to an enhanced effect of 1.2 when CP was given immediately after or 4 h following radiation [56]. They hypothesized that this was due to radiosensitization of hypoxic tumor cells when the drug was given prior to irradiation.

Cisplatin has been used in human studies as a radiosensitizer in a variety of solid tumors. Utilizing a dose of 40 mg/m^2 weekly during conventional radiation therapy, Reimer *et al.* noted that 91% of patients achieved a partial response [57]. Radiation reactions were only noted in two patients. Creagan *et al.* treated three patients with advanced head and neck cancer with irradiation and CP [68]. They noted significant toxicity including severe nausea and vomiting, malaise, and abscesses. They felt the combination was still not safe for general clinical use.

A study of the Eastern Cooperative Oncology Group evaluated 23 patients with advanced head and neck cancer who received cisplatin – 10 – 30 mg/m^2 per week throughout radiation therapy [59]. Of 18 evaluable patients, 12 were alive without disease at 2 to 16 months following treatment. At a CP dose of 10–20 mg/m^2 only 10% of patients has severe mucositis or myelosuppression. Fifty percent of patients receiving CP at 30 mg/m^2 had severe toxicity. They felt that an acceptable weekly dose of CP was 20 mg/m^2. Based on these results, a randomized study comparing irradiation alone to irradiation plus CP is planned.

3.6. Combination chemotherapy and radiation therapy

Although few randomized trials have shown an advantage for single agent chemotherapy combined with irradiation, several studies of combination chemotherapy with irradiation have been undertaken.

Bitter et al. studied 20 patients with advanced oral cavity cancers utilizing Bleo IA every 4 days followed immediately by Mtx (240 mg/m^2) for 4 courses in combination with irradiation – 6000 rad in 6 weeks [60]. Half of the patients had a complete response, and several patients were rendered disease free following surgery. At one year the survival was 84%. An increase in severity of mucositis was noted, but only 2 patients required delays in radiation therapy.

Smith et al. studied simultaneous radiotherapy, Bleo, adriamycin and 5-FU for patients with stage III & IV head and neck cancer [61]. The chemotherapy regimen was as follows: 5-FU (110 mg/m^2 IV 3 times/week), adriamycin (7.0 mg/m^2 IV weekly), Bleo (4.5 units/m^2 IV or IM twice weekly). The chemotherapy was given 1 hour before irradiation, and irradiation was carried to 5500 to 6500 rads. Following irradiation, patients were evaluated for surgical resection, and surgery was individualized for patients. All patients responded to the initial chemotherapy and irradiation, and 67% had a complete clinical response. Forty-three percent of the patients are surviving without evidence of disease 6 to 8 months following treatment. Although there was impressive tumor shrinkage with combination of these agents and irradiation, the individuality of treatment makes it difficult to drawn any conclusions about long-term control.

Seagren et al. treated 26 patients with a combination of cyclophosphamide, Bleo, and irradiation [62]. They began with in vitro studies in the radiobiology laboratory of Bleo combined with radiotherapy. They noted when combining Bleo with irradiation, that a group of patients with advanced nodal disease did worse than other patients with less advanced nodal status.

They postulated that their poor results in patients with enlarged nodes was because of hypoxic cells. Based on studies that show cyclophosphamide activity against hypoxic cells, they began treating patients with the above combination. They based their drug schedule on studies that indicated that cyclophosphamide given before irradiation gives better cell kill than the same agent given simultaneously or following irradiation. Thus, they gave cyclyphosphamide (1 gm/m^2 every three weeks) 30 min before irradiation. Bleo (15 units) was given twice weekly. The regimen was designed to allow time for recovery from toxicity.

Utilizing this regimen, 13 of 20 patients had a complete response to irradiation and chemotherapy. Following further therapy, 16 of 20 patients were free of disease. However they were disappointed that 11 of 16 patients recurred locally or in regional lymph nodes with a median time to recurrence of only 5 months. The authors felt that the failure of an initial high response rate to be translated into prolonged disease-free survival was in part due to advanced nodal disease. Mucositis was the major dose-limiting toxicity in their study.

In a pilot study, Fu et al. treated 15 patients with advanced squamous cell carcinoma with cyclophosphamide, Bleo, and vincristine during radiation and with cyclophosphamide, Mtx and Bleo following radiation [63]. In this study, cyclophosphamide (750 mg/m^2 IV) was given on day 1, vincristine (1.4 mg/m^2 IV) on day 2, and bleomycin (15 units) on days 3, 4, 5, 8, 10 and then twice weekly during weeks 5 through 9. The mean dose of radiation was 6640 rad. Very few patients were able to complete the chemotherapy because of severe mucositis or appearance of recurrent disease. At the end of radiotherapy 10 of 15 patients were free of disease and 14 of 15 patients had greater than 50% regression. At this of last follow-up, 47% were disease-free with a mean follow-up of 8+ months.

The toxicity from this regimen was considerable, and the mortality rate was 20%. The major toxicities included mucositis and infection. Ten of 15 patients required additional breaks in their irradiation. Late complications occurred in three patients – 2 developed bone necrosis, and one developed an esophageal cutaneous fistula. The authors concluded that although this program may have resulted in enhanced tumor effect, the toxicity was too great to warrant a randomized trial and that alternate treatments should be studied.

4. Radiation therapy followed by chemotherapy

It has been shown in animal models that chemotherapy is most effective when used for the eradication of small tumor volumes [64]. Thus chemotherapy given after definitive radiation therapy to destroy micrometastases may be efficacious. There are no published controlled trials to date investigating post-irradiation chemotherapy but several investigators have noted difficulty delivering chemotherapy to this patient population.

5. Conclusions

The role of chemotherapy in combination with radiation therapy for the treatment of squamous cancers of the head and neck is still controversial. Most of the studies of chemotherapy used prior to radiotherapy are pilot studies lacking long-term follow-up. In these studies, a variety of drug combinations, doses, and schedules have been used. Chemotherapy achieves higher responses when given prior to other modalities than similar regimens used for recurrent disease [2]. The toxicity is acceptable, and pretreatment chemotherapy does not enhance radiation toxocity in the majority of patients. Cisplatin has been included in most of the more effective regimens. Although the effect of drug dose is not yet clear, extrapolations from tumor models suggest that the dose response curve may be steep [65]. It may be that the benefit of pretreatment chemotherapy is related to the ability to achieve a complete response since various investigators have noted a relationship between response to chemotherapy and survival [7]. Although many authors are enthusiastic about their results, it is generally agreed that randomized, controlled trials are necessary before definite conclusions can be drawn.

The majority of combined modality studies are designed to evaluate concurrent chemotherapy and radiotherapy. The ideal radiosensitizer would be one that increases tumor response without an enhanced effect on normal tissues. There are a variety of drugs that have a 'radiosensitizing effect'. *In vitro* and *in vivo* some of these drugs have proven to be synergistic with irradiation, whereas others are merely additive. There are multiple drugs and dose schedules which could be utilized, and the radiobiology laboratory may be helpful in selecting a starting point for clinical studies. Cisplatin, one of the most effective drugs for head and neck cancer, has not yet been tested in many clinical trials and may improve results.

Many of the clinical studies consist of mixtures of patients with different tumor stages, sites, and treatment variables. Numbers of patients in randomized trials must be large enough to balance important prognostic factors. These studies have included mostly patients with stage III and IV disease, and it may be that major improvements will be derived from studies in patients with earlier stages of disease. In particular, the efficacy of a drug as a sensitizer may be negated by large tumor volumes. It may be that selected sites of disease are in fact better suited to radiosensitization than others. For example, those randomized studies that suggested positive results consisted mainly of patients with oral cavity tumors. When Bleo was combined with irradiation, Shanta [46] found an improvement in surgical in patients with oral cavity cancer, whereas Cachin [47] found no improvement in a group with oropharyngeal primaries. Ansfield [39] found improvement of survival with the addition of 5-FU to radiotherapy for patients with cancers of the tongue and tonsil, but not for hypopharyngeal, laryngeal or nasopharyngeal cancers.

Current therapies for advanced cancers of the head and neck are inadequate in the majority of patients. Early results with combined modality therapy are encouraging. Collaborative clinical trials that involve the radiotherapist, otolaryngologist, and medical oncologist should have high priority, and should lead to innovative and improved treatment strategies for these patients.

References

1. Wang CC: General principles of radiation therapy of head and neck tumors. In: Suen JY, Myers EN (eds) Cancer of the Head and Neck. Churchill Livingstone, 1981, pp 123–144.
2. Mead GM, Jacobs C: Changing role of chemotherapy in the treatment of head and neck cancer. Am J Med 73:582–595, 1982.
3. Laster WR, Mayo JG, Simpson-Herren L, et al.: Success and failure in the treatment of solid tumors. II. Kinetic parameters and 'cell cure' of moderately advanced carcinoma 755. Cancer Chemother Rep 53:169–188, 1969.
4. Randolph VL, Vallejo A, Spiro RH, Shah J, Strong EW, Huvos AG, Wittes RE: Combination therapy of advanced head and neck cancer. Cancer 41:460–467, 1978.
5. Glick JH, Marcial V, Richter M, Valez-Garcia E: The adjuvant treatment of inoperable stage III & IV epidermoid carcinoma of the head and neck with platinum and bleomycin infusion prior to definitive radiotherapy. An RTOG Pilot Study. Cancer 46:1919–1924, 1980.
6. Brown AW, Blom J, Butler WM, Garcia-Guerrero G, Richardson MF, Henderson RL: Combination chemotherapy with vinblastine, bleomycin, and Cis-diamminedichloroplatinum (II) in squamous cell carcinoma of the head and neck: Cancer 45:2830–2835, 1980.
7. Al-Sarraf M, Binns P, Vaishampayan G, Loh J, Weaver A: The adjuvant use of cis-platinum, oncovin, and bleomycin (COB) prior to surgery and/or radiotherapy in untreated epidermoid cancer of the head and neck. In: Jones SE, Salmon SE (eds), Adjuvant Therapy of Cancer II. Grune and Stratton, 1979, pp 421–428.
8. Tannock I, Cummings B, Sorrenti V, and the ENT Group: Combination chemotherapy used prior to radiation therapy for locally advanced squamous cell carcinoma of the head and neck. Cancer Treat Rep 66:1421–1424, 1982.
9. Marcial VA, Valez-Garcia E, Figueroa-Valles NR, Cintron J, Vallecillo LA: Multi-drug chemotherapy (Vincristine-bleomycin-methotrexate) followed by radiotherapy in inoperable carcinomas of the head and neck. J Rad Onc Biol Phys 6:717–721, 1980.
10. Petrovich Z, Block J, Kuisk H, MacKintosh R, Casciato D, Jose L, Barton R: A randomized comparison of radiotherapy with a radiotherapy-chemotherapy combination in stage IV carcinoma of the head and neck. Cancer 47:2259–2264, 1981.
11. Bagshaw MA, Doggett RLS: A clinical study of chemical radiosensitization. Front Radiat Ther Oncol 4:164–173, 1969.

284

12. Loken MK, Kim YS, Mosser DG, Marvin JF: The effect of combined irradiation and chemotherapy on cancer growth. Radiology 73:166–174, 1959.

13. Berry RJ: A reduced oxygen enhancement ratio for x-ray survival of hela cells *in vitro* after treatment with methotrexate. Nature 208:1108–1110, 1965.

14. Friedman M: The treatment of squamous cell carcinoma of the head and neck with combined methotrexate and irradiation. Front Radiat Ther Onc 4:106–115, 1969.

15. Kramer S: Use of methotrexate and radiotherapy for advanced cancer of the head and neck. Front Radiat Ther Onc 4:116–125, 1969.

16. Klimo J, Danko T: Methotrexate in combination with radiotherapy in the treatment of squamous carcinomas of the head and neck. Neoplasia 21:451–454, 1974.

17. Taylor SG IV, Bytell DE, DeWys WD, Applebaum E, Sisson GA: Adjuvant methotrexate and leucovorin in head and neck squamous cancer. Arch of Otolaryngol 104:647–651, 1978.

18. Pointon RCS, Askill CS, Hunter RD, Wilkinson PM: Treatment of advanced head and neck carcinoma with synchronous irradiation and methotrexate. Cancer Treat Rep 65 (Suppl 1):145–148, 1981.

19. Kligerman MM, Hellman S, Von Essen CF, Bertino JR: Sequential chemotherapy and radiotherapy. Radiology 86:247–250, 1966.

20. Von Essen C, Joseph L, Simon G, Singh AD: Sesuential chemotherapy and radiation therapy of buccal mucosa carcinoma in South India. AJR 102:530–540, 1968.

21. Knowlton AH, Percarpio B, Bobrow S, Fischer JJ: Methotrexate and radiation therapy in the treatment of advanced head and neck tumors. Radiology 116:709–712, 1975.

22. Richard JM, Sancho H, Lepintre Y, *et al.*: Intra-arterial methotrexate chemotherapy and telecobalt therapy in cancer of the oral cavity and oropharynx. Cancer 34:491–496, 1974.

23. Lustig RA, DeMare PA, Kramer S: Adjuvant methotrexate in the radiotherapeutic management of advanced tumors of the head and neck. Cancer 37:2703–2708, 1976.

24. Faekus JT, Sommer C, Kramer S: Adjuvant intravenous methotrexate or definitive radiotherapy alone for advanced squamous cancers of the oral cavity, oropharynx, supraglottic laynx or hypopharynx. Int J Radiat Oncol Biol Phys 6:533–541, 1980.

25. Sinclair WK: Hydroxyurea: Differential lethal effects on cultured mammalian cells during the cell cycle. Science 150:1729–1731, 1965.

26. Phillips RA, Tolmuch LJ: Repair of potentially lethal damage in x-irradiated hela cells. Radiat Res 29:413–432, 1966.

27. Lerner HJ, Beckloff GL, Lipshutz H, Campbell R, Ritchie D: Hydroxyurea in the management of head and neck cancer. Plast and Reconst Surg 40:233–239, 1967.

28. Richards GJ, Chambers RG: Hydroxyurea: A radiosensitizer in the treatment of neoplasms of the head and neck. Am J Roentgenol 105:555–565, 1969.

29. Richards GJ, Chambers RG: Hydroxyurea in the treatment of neoplasms of the head and neck. Am J Surg 126:513–518, 1973.

30. Lerner HJ: Concomitant hydroxyurea and irradiation. Am J Surg 134:505–509, 1977.

31. Lipshutz H, Lerner HJ: Six year survival in the combined treatment for advanced head and neck cancer under the combined therapy program. Am J Surg 126:519–522, 1973.

32. Hussey DH, Abrams JP: Combined therapy in advanced head and neck cancer: hydroxyurea and radiotherapy. Progress in Clinical Cancer 6:79–86, 1975.

33. Stefani S, Eells RW, Abbate J: Hydroxyurea and radiotherapy in head and neck cancer. Radiology 101:391–396, 1971.

34. Vermund H: Enhancement of radiation effects by chemotherapy. Acta Radiologica Supplementum 311:1–78, 1971.

35. Vermund H, Hodgett J, Ansfield FJ: Effects of combined roentgen irradiation and chemotherapy on transplantal tumors in mice. AJR 85:559–567, 1961.

36. Foye LV Jr, Willett FM, Hall BE, Roth M: The potentiation of radiation effects with 5-fluorouracil. Calif Med 93:288–290, 1960.

37. Hall BE, Foye LVJr, Roth M, Willett FM, Hales DR, Ward JH Jr, Butler HT, Godfrey MH: Treatment of inoperable cancer with 5-fluorouracil and irradiation. Lancet 1:115–116, 1960.

38. Howe CD, Fletcher GH, Suit HD, Samuels ML: Combined 5-fluouracil and cobalt-60 therapy evaluated by double blind technique. Acta Un Int Cancer 20:400–403, 1964.

39. Ansfield FJ, Ramirez G, Davis HL Jr, Korbitz BC, Vermund H, Gollin FF: Treatment of advanced cancer of the head and neck. Cancer 25:78–82, 1970.

40. Gollin FF, Ansfield FJ, Bradenburg JH, Ramirez G, Vermund H: Combined therapy in advanced head and neck cancer: A randomized study. Am J Roentgenol 114:83–88, 1972.

41. Juul Jorgensen SJ: Time-dose relationships in combined bleomycin treatment and radiotherapy. Eur J Cancer 8:531–534, 1972.

42. Bleehen MM: Combination therapy with drugs and radiation. Br Med Bull 29:54–59, 1973.

43. Berdal P, Ekroll T, Iversen OH, Weyde R: Treatment of squamous cell carcinomas in head and neck with bleomycin and with combined bleomycin and x-rays. Acta Otolaryng (Stockh) 75:318–320, 1973.

44. Rygard J, Hansen HS: The place of bleomycin in the treatment of highly differentiated squamous cell cancer either alone or in combination with irradiation. Prog Biochem Pharmacol 11:205–218, 1976.

45. Ichikawa T: Studies of bleomycin: Discovery of its clinical effect, combination treatment with bleomycin and radiotherapy, side effects, and long-term survival, Gann Monograph on Cancer Res 19:99–113, 1976.

46. Shanta V, Krishnamurthi S: Combined therapy of oral cancer bleomycin and radiation: A clinical trial. Clin Radiol 28:427–429, 1977.

47. Cachin Y, Jortay A, Sancho H, Eschwege F, Madelain M, Desaulty A, Gerard P: Preliminary results of a randomized EORTC study comparing radiotherapy and concomitant bleomycin to radiotherapy alone in epidermoid carcinomas of the oropharynx. Eur J Cancer 13:1389–1395, 1977.

48. Goldsmith MA, Carter SK: The integration of chemotherapy into a combined modality approach to cancer therapy. V. Squamous cell cancer of the head and neck. Cancer Treat Rev 2:137–158, 1975.

49. Kapstad B, Bang G, Rennaes S, Dahler A: Combined preoperative treatment with cobalt and bleomycin in patients with head and neck carcinomas- a controlled clinical study. Int J Radiat Oncol Biol Phy 4:85–89, 1978.

50. Fu KK: (Personal Communication)

51. Double EB, Richmond RC: A review of platinum complex biochemistry suggests a rationale for combined platinum-radiotherapy. Int J Radiation Oncology Biol Phys 5:1335–1339, 1979.

52. Zak M, Drobnik J: Effect of cis-dichlorodiammineplastinum (II) on the post-irradiation lethality in mice after irradiation with x-rays. Strahlentherapie 142:112–115, 1971.

53. Wodinsky I, Swiniarski J, Kensler CJ, Venditti JM: Combination radiotherapy and chemotherapy for P388 lymphocytic leukemia in vivo. Cancer Chemother Rep 4:73–97, 1974.

54. Muggia FM, Glatstein E: Summary of investigations on platinum compounds and radiation reactions. Int J Radiol Oncol Biol Phys 5:1407–1409, 1979.

55. Alvarez MV, Cobreros G, Heras A, Zumel Ma CL: Studies on cis-dichlorodiammineplatinum (II) as a radiosensitizer. Br J Cancer 37:68–72, 1978.

56. Overgaard J, Khan AR: Selective enhancement of radiation response in a C3H mammary carcinoma by cisplatin. Cancer Treat Rep 65:501–503, 1981.

57. Reimer RR, Gahbauer R, Bukowski RM, et al.: Simultaneous treatment with cisplatin and radiations therapy for advanced solid tumors. Cancer Treat Rep 65:219–222, 1981.

58. Creagan ET, Fountain KS, Frytak S, DeSanto LW, Earle JD: Concomitant radiation therapy

and cis-diamminedichloroplatinum (II) in patients with advanced head and neck cancer. Med Pediatr Oncol 9:119–120, 1981.

59. Haselow RE, Adams GS, Oken MM, Goudsmit A, Lerner HJ, Marsh JC: Simultaneous cis-platinum (DDP) and radiation therapy (RT) for locally advanced unresectable head and neck cancer. Proc Am Assoc Cancer Res Am Soc Clin Oncol:201, 1982.

60. Bitter K: Bleomycin-methotrexate-chemotherapy in combination with telocobalt-radiation for patients suffering from advanced oral carcinoma. J Maxillofac Surg 5:75–81, 1977.

61. Smith BL, Franz JL, Mira JG, Gates GA, Supp J, Cruz AB: Simultaneous combination radiotherapy and multidrug chemotherapy for stage III and stage IV squamous cell carcinoma of the head and neck. J Surg Oncol 15:91–98, 1980.

62. Seagren SL, Byfield JE, Davidson TM, Sharp JR: Bleomycin, cyclophosphamide and radiotherapy in regionally advanced epidermoid carcinoma of the head and neck. Int J Radiat Oncol Biol Phys 8:127–132, 1982.

63. Fu KK, Silverberg IJ, Phillips TL, Friedman MA: Combined radiotherapy and multidrug chemotherapy for advanced head and neck cancer: results of a radiation therapy oncology group pilot study. Cancer Treat Rep 63:351–357, 1979.

64. Griswold DP Jr: The potential for murine tumor models in surgical adjuvant chemotherapy. Cancer Chemother Rep 5:187–204, 1975.

65. Ervin PJ, Weichselbaum RR, Fabian RL, Karp DD, Posner MR, Miller D: Role of chemotherapy in the multi-disciplinary approach to advanced head and neck cancer: Potentials and problems. Ann Otol 90:506–511, 1981.

13. Preoperative adjuvant induction chemotherapy in head and neck cancer

WAUN KI HONG, JAMES D. POPKIN and STANLEY M.
SHAPSHAY

1. Introduction

Adjuvant chemotherapy for solid tumors has been primarily limited to patients who have attained complete tumor control with surgery and/or radiotherapy [1]. The rationale is based on the use of chemotherapeutic drugs to eradicate residual microscopic disease that persists after local tumor control has been achieved. Unless residual undetectable tumor cells are eliminated, the patient eventually develops local recurrence or distant metastases; and overall survival is not improved [1].

The use of adjuvant chemotherapy for premenopausal breast cancer patients with positive axillary nodes has improved their overall survival [1, 2]. Adjuvant chemotherapy for patients with advanced squamous cell carcinoma of the head and neck who have achieved complete local control after surgery and/or radiotherapy has not been adequately evaluated [3–5].

The enthusiasm of investigators for postoperative adjuvant chemotherapy trials has been minimized by the relative age and poor compliance of the patients with head and neck cancer and by the exigencies of long-term treatment and follow-up [3, 4]. An alternative approach is the recent introduction of induction chemotherapy in previously untreated patients with advanced Stage III and IV tumors prior to definitive surgery and/or radiotherapy [3–5]. The conventional treatment of surgery and/or radiotherapy has not provided adequate tumor control in the majority of patients who present with advanced local/regional disease [4, 5]. Local recurrence occurs in up to 60% of these patients, distant metastases develop in 20 to 30%; and survival remains poor, ranging from 0 to 40% [4–6].

Until recently, chemotherapy was reserved for those patients with recurrence of disease following surgery and/or radiotherapy. Extensive prior therapy, declining performance status, and poor nutritional status of these patients predictably led to poor responses with palliative chemothera-

Gregory T. Wolf (ed), Head and Neck Oncology.
© *1984 Martinus Nijhoff Publishers, Boston. ISBN 0-89838-657-8. Printed in The Netherlands.*

py [3, 7]. However, several recent clinical trials indicate that higher response rates and longer durations of response are achieved with chemotherapy in previously untreated patients compared to patients with recurrent tumors following surgery and/or radiotherapy [8–10]. The rationale and theoretical advantages for preoperative induction chemotherapy are summarized in Table 1. The possible negative effects of using preoperative induction chemotherapy are described in Table 2.

2. Clinical trials

The selection of chemotherapeutic agents for preoperative adjuvant trials has evolved from experience obtained in the treatment of advanced recurrent tumor patients with single-agent treatment or combination regimens. Methotrexate, cisplatin, 5-FU, and bleomycin have been used, either alone or in combination, for preoperative adjuvant chemotherapy.

Table 1. Rationale and potential advantages of preoperative adjuvant chemotherapy in advanced previously untreated head and neck cancer

1. Better performance status and good nutritional status will increase tolerance of chemotherapy.
2. Intact blood supply of previously untreated tumors has the potential advantage of delivering high drug concentrations to the tumor site.
3. Increased tumor cell kill in rapidly growing tumor cells.
4. Potential eradication of subclinical microscopic metastatic disease that is not removed by local treatment.
5. Enhanced efficacy of planned definitive local treatment by cytoreduction of the primary tumor and nodal metastases.
6. Continued use of a chemotherapeutic regimen as a maintenance regimen in patients who initially achieved significant response.

Table 2. Possible adverse effects of preoperative adjuvant chemotherapy in previously untreated advanced head and neck cancer

1. Delay of surgery from complications of chemotherapy.
2. Inaccurate knowledge of tumor margins.
3. Increased immunosuppression.
4. Potential increased risk from postoperative radiation therapy.

2.1. Single agents

2.1.2. Methotrexate (MTX)

MTX has undergone the most investigation and is regarded as standard therapy for recurrent head and neck cancer [3, 7, 10]. MTX is a structural analogue of folic acid, and its antimetabolic action is due to intracellular binding to dihydrofolate reductase. This interferes with the production of thymidine and de novo synthesis of purines required for DNA synthesis. Calcium leucovorin (Citrovorum factor, folinic acid) is capable of reversing this inhibition of DNA synthesis by restoring the end product of the inhibited enzyme, dihydrofolate reductase.

Although MTX has been extensively studied in head and neck cancer, there remains considerable controversy about how best to administer this drug [11, 12]. Recently, MTX has been used in moderate and high doses with leucovorin rescue to enhance the therapeutic index and to rescue normal cells. Three nonrandomized pilot studies of preoperative adjuvant high-dose MTX and leuvorin rescue have been published in the literature.

Tarpley *et al.* used MTX at a dose of 240 mg/m^2 with leucovorin rescue and produced responses in 23 of 30 previously untreated patients. However, the magnitude of response was not defined as other than tumor regression. This cohort of patients was compared to a historical control group and had slightly enhanced disease-free survival [12].

Kirkwood *et al.* evaluated 23 patients with advanced head and neck cancer with high-dose MTX (3.0–7.5 mg/m^2) and leucovorin rescue followed by surgery and/or radiotherapy. Major responses were seen in 52% of patients with prolongation of disease-free survival seen in responders to chemotherapy, compared to nonresponders. These studies emphasized a lack of hematologic toxicity and no apparent increase in the incidence of surgical complications with preoperative chemotherapy [13].

Table 3. Activity of preoperative adjuvant single-agent chemotherapy in previously untreated advanced head and neck cancer

Investigator	Drug schedule	Evaluable patients	Response (%) CR + PR
Tarpley [12]	MTX-LV 240 mg/m^2	30	77
Kirkwood [13]	MTX-LV 3.0–7.5 mg/m^2	23	52
Taylor [14]	MTX-LV 240 mg/m^2	17	75% 2 yrs survival rate
Popkin and Hong [18]	Bleomycin infusion 7 days	21	33
Wittes [23]	Cisplatin 120 mg/m^2 q 3 wks	22	40
Jacobs [24]	Cisplatin 80 mg/m^2 contin. inf.	18	39

PTX: Methotrexate; LV: Leucovorin.

Taylor *et al.* studied 17 patients with Stages III and IV head and neck cancer. MTX at a dose of 240 mg/m^2 with leucovorin rescue was used prior to surgery and/or radiotherapy. A 2-year survival rate of 75% was achieved in 17 patients with advanced cancers, 7 of whom had been previously treated. The authors attributed the encouraging results of this trial to the fact that MTX was escalated in each cycle until mucocutaneous toxicity occurred [14].

As preoperative or adjuvant chemotherapy, MTX has not convincingly shown an improvement in overall outcome or in modification of the natural history of advanced head and neck cancer. Although a fair number of partial responses have been obtained, few if any complete responses have resulted from single agent MTX treatment; therefore, its role as a preoperative adjuvant therapy seems limited. Investigations incorporating this drug in combination with other agents are discussed in Section 2.2.

2.1.3. Bleomycin

Bleomycin is the second most extensively studied chemotherapeutic agent in head and neck cancer [4]. Bleomycin is the generic name for a group of antibiotics isolated in Japan from Streptomyces verticillus. As a single agent, the drug appears generally less effective than methotrexate, although no comparative study has been performed. The initial use of bleomycin was as an intermittent intravenous bolus; however, a compelling amount of indirect evidence has developed favoring the administration of this drug by continuous intravenous infusion. An *in vitro* study suggested the improved therapeutic index of a continuous infusion of bleomycin [15]. Bleomycin has been used as a continuous 24-h infusion in the hope of providing maximum target tissue exposure and cell kill due to its relatively short serum half-life and specific inhibitory effect in the G2-S phase of the cell cycle [15–17].

Due in part to its recent emergence as an active agent, and investigator enthusiasm for combination chemotherapy, there have been few studies evaluating bleomycin alone in a preoperative adjuvant setting. Popkin and Hong *et al.* recently evaluated a 7-day continuous intravenous infusion of bleomycin given prospectively to 21 previously untreated patients with Stage III and IV head and neck cancer prior to surgery and/or radiotherapy. One complete and six partial responses occurred for a 33% response rate [18]. However, there was no apparent benefit derived in this poor prognostic group in terms of increased resectability, or disease-free and overall survival. Furthermore, the response rate was not appreciably different from that reported with intermittent bolus administration in a heterogenous previously treated patient population.

The toxicity of a bleomycin infusion is generally not severe, although fatality from idiosyncratic pulmonary toxicity [19, 20] has been reported to occur at doses well below 300 mg and has occured during continuous infusion. Since this drug rarely causes myelosuppression, its major role in adjuvant chemotherapy in head and neck cancer would seem to be in combination with other agents.

2.1.4. Cisplatin

Of the several platinum compounds tested in experimental tumor systems, cisplatin has been found to have the greatest antitumor activity. The precise mechanism of drug activity is not known but its thought to be similar to that of bifunctional alkylating agents.

Cisplatin rarely causes hematologic toxicity, aside from mild anemia, but major problems seen in early studies were gastro-intestinal toxicity, nephrotoxocity, and ototoxicity. The usefulness of this drug was limited, until it was discovered that prehydration and mannitol diuresis could minimize nephrotoxicity without compromising antitumor activity [21, 22].

Wittes et al. treated 22 previously untreated advanced head and neck cancer patients with cisplatin, 120 mg/m^2 IV, every 3 weeks until maximum response occurred, prior to definitive treatment with surgery and/or radiotherapy. One complete and eight partial responses were obtained for a 40% major response rate [23]. These results were felt to be identical to those of a previous pilot study from the same institution, where a 30% response rate was obtained with single-agent cisplatin in a group of heavily pretreated patients.

Jacobs et al. reported a 39% response rate with single-agent cisplatin, given as a 24-h continuous infusion; however, only 6 of 18 patients studied were previously untreated [24].

2.2. Combination chemotherapy

The experience of combination chemotherapy in the treatment of recurrent or metastatic head and neck cancer has not been encouraging. Recent emphasis has been on the use of chemotherapy as initial treatment before surgery or radiotherapy in patients with locally advanced Stages III and IV head and neck tumors. Cisplatin, bleomycin, methotrexate, 5-FU, and vincristine have been used in combination as induction treatment. The response rate of 60 to 80% observed in induction chemotherapy in previously untreated patients is clearly superior to the rate in patients who have undergone prior surgery, irradiation, or both (Table 4). Cisplatin in conjunction with bleomycin was perhaps the first combination induction regimen for head and neck cancer and has become the most extensively studied.

Randolph et al. used cisplatin, 120 mg/m^2, Days 1 and 22 and continuous bleomycin infusion Days 3–10 for 7 days. A 71% overall response rate with a 19% complete response rate was noted in 21 patients with advanced head and neck cancer. All patients were considered to have unresectable disease and had radiation therapy following the chemotherapy [8].

Hong et al., using a similar regimen, described a 72% response rate with 20% complete responses in 58 patients with advanced head and neck cancer. Twenty-six patients had subsequent surgery, and two had no residual tumor in the surgical specimen. All patients received definitive radiotherapy. Surgery after chemotherapy was accomplished without difficulty. The surgical planes and anatomical landmarks were easily identifiable, except in areas of previous tumor involvement [9].

Glick et al., administered cisplatin by continuous 24-h infusion in combination with bleomycin and noted decreased gastrointestinal and renal toxicity. The overall response rate was 48% with no complete responses. All patients received subsequent radiation therapy, which was well tolerated. Although this regimen was less toxic than the previous two, it did not appear to be as effective, presumably because of reduced drug doses [25].

Elias et al., treated 22 patients with cisplatin, 100 mg/m^2, on Day 1 followed by a 5-day infusion of bleomycin; and on Day 10 methotrexate, 50 mg/m^2, was given, followed by a 36-h infusion of MTX, 1500 mg/m^2 with leucovorin rescue. The overall response rate was 68% with an 18% rate of complete response. Six patients had severe nephrotoxicity, and two died [26].

Al-Sarraf et al., added vincristine to a high-dose cisplatin and bleomycin regimen and reported an impressive 28% incidence of complete response.

Table 4. Induction combination chemotherapy for advanced previously untreated head and neck cancer

Investigator	Drugs used	No. of patients	Major response (%) CR + PR
Randolph [8]	DDP + BLO	21	71
Elias [26]	DDP + BLO + MTX	22	68
Hong [9]	DDP + BLO	58	72
Glick [25]	DDP + BLO	29	48
Spaulding [29]	DDP + BLO + VCR	30	97
Ervin [30]	DDP + BLO + VCR	18	89
Al-Sarraf [28]	DDP + BLO + VCR	77	79
Price [33]	VCR + BLO + MTX + 5-FU + Hydrocortisone	200	67
Perry [31]	DDP + BLO + VCR	64	66
Al-Sarraf [32]	DDP + 5-FU	26	88
Schuller [27]	DDP + BLO + MTX + VCR	58	66

DDP: Cisplatin; 5-FU: 5-Fluorouracil; BLO: Bleomycin; VCR: Vincristine; MTX: Methotrexate.

The complete and partial response rate (CR + PR) was 79% in 77 patients. Chemotherapy was well tolerated, with no fatalities or life-threatening complications [28].

Schuller *et al.*, used a regimen of cisplatin, methotrexate, bleomycin, and vincristine as preoperative chemotherapy in 58 previously untreated patients. Overall major response was 66%. There was no increase in surgical or radiotherapeutic complications as a result of initial chemotherapy [27].

Spaulding *et al.* also administered a cisplatin/vincristine/bleomycin regimen to 29 previously untreated patients. The complete and partial response rate was 95% (11 CRs). No intraoperative or postoperative complications attributable to chemotherapy were noted [29]. Similar results have also been reported by Ervin *et al.* with the addition of high-dose methotrexate/leucovorin to a cisplatin and bleomycin regimen [30].

Perry *et al.* added vinblastine instead of vincristine to a cisplatin and bleomycin regimen and reported a 22% incidence of complete responses. Overall major response (CR + PR) was 66% in 64 patients. All partial responders were rendered disease-free after definitive treatment [31].

Recently, Kish *et al.* used a continuous infusion of 5-FU instead of bleomycin because of the threat of pulmonary complications from bleomycin in patients with poor pulmonary function tests. The 5-Fluorouracil was added to cisplatin, 100 mg/m^2 IV, every three weeks. The initial report was very impressive; major tumor regression was achieved in 88.5% of 26 patients. Although all patients were initially inoperable, six underwent resection following chemotherapy, and another six patients underwent resection after chemotherapy and irradiation. This study concluded that cisplatin and 5-FU infusion was an effective combination with lesser toxicity than bleomycin in patients with previously untreated advanced carcinoma of the head and neck [32].

Price and Hill have explored the use of non-platinum-containing chemotherapy as initial treatment for advanced head and neck carcinoma. Two hundred patients received chemotherapy – consisting of vincristine, bleomycin, methotrexate, 5-FU, and hydrocortisone – given over 24 h as initial therapy on Days 1 and 14, prior to definitive treatment. Of these 200 patients, 195 were assessed for chemotherapy response on Day 28, and 131 had an overall objective response of 67% (8:CR, 123:PR). The complete remission rate following local therapy was significantly greater in chemotherapy responders [33].

None of these induction regimens can be adopted for routine use in advanced head and neck cancer patients as initial treatment until a controlled study can demonstrate that induction chemotherapy increases disease-free and overall survival. These questions are now being addressed in a well-designed clinical trial of operable advanced head and neck cancer patients sponsored by the National Cancer Institute (Table 5). This study is

Table 5. National Cancer Institute Head and Neck Contracts Program operable stages III and IV squamous cell carcinomas of the oral cavity and larynx/hypopharynx [34]

RANDOMIZE:

1. Surgery ⟶ Radiotherapy Follow-up
   4-10 wks postsurgery

2. Induction ⟶ Surgery ⟶ Radiotherapy ⟶ Follow-up
   Day 1   3-7   22-28   4-10 wks postsurgery
   Cisplatin Bleomycin

3. Induction chemotherapy ⟶ Surgery ⟶ Radiotherapy ⟶ Maintenance
   Day 1   3-7   22-28   4-10 wks postsurgery   Chemotherapy Follow-up
   Cisplatin Bleomycin   4 wks after
                                                               radiotherapy and
                                                               every month × 6 mos.

Induction chemotherapy: Cisplatin 100 mg/m² IV push Day 1; Bleomycin 15 U/m² IV push, then 15 U/m²/day × 5 as continuous infusion, Days 3–7.

Maintenance chemotherapy: Cisplatin 80 mg/m² continuous infusion for a 24-h period.

designed to compare standard treatment, consisting of surgery and postoperative radiotherapy; induction chemotherapy using cisplatin and bleomycin, followed by standard treatment; and induction chemotherapy followed by standard treatment with the addition of cisplatin maintenance chemotherapy. The purpose of this study is not only to determine the effect of chemotherapy on local and regional tumor control, but also to assess the impact of induction chemotherapy with and without maintenance chemotherapy on distant metastases and survival. A preliminary report of the NCI trial noted a 50% response rate (8%:CR, 42%:PR) in the first 229 patients receiving induction chemotherapy [34]. The somewhat low response rate to this induction regimen compared to previous pilot studies is presumably due to reduced doses of the chemotherapeutic regimens in this trial. Toxicity was minimal, and no significant differences in operative complicatins were seen. Evaluation of the impact of survival in the induction chemotherapy group has not been reported yet, as this study closed on April 30, 1982.

3. Surgical aspects

3.1. Surgical findings after induction chemotherapy

Surgery after induction chemotherapy has been accomplished without difficulty. Tatoo marking of tumor margins prior to chemotherapy is essential to permanently establish the resection area. Surgical margins should be carefully examined, particularly if induction chemotherapy was effective in reducing tumor bulk. Margins should be designed to extend 1 to 2 cm beyond the tumor, when possible.

If complete response to chemotherapy occurred, areas of fibrosis and induration, similar to the effect of preoperative radiotherapy, are seen at the tumor site. Tumor masses are often somewhat 'sticky' to surrounding tissue; however, resection can proceed without difficulty. Surgical planes and landmarks are for the most part easily identifiable. Areas of fibrosis or edema alert the surgeon to a 'tumorous area' necessitating wider resection margins, when feasible. On occasion, the fibrosis and edema are reminiscent of the heavily irradiated neck. A common surgical finding at the primary site is an area of induration without ulceration of the overlying epithelium [10, 35]. Random biopsies of the primary site after a complete response to induction chemotherapy are often negative for tumor. Complete surgical resection is necessary, because 'nests' of viable tumor cells may be present.

3.2. Histopathologic findings

The most conspicuous findings in tumors treated with cisplatin and bleomycin is a tendency toward increased differentiation of the original cellular structure, if there was a response to chemotherapy. Tumor masses, particularly in the neck, are replaced by a cheesy material identified as keratin on histopathology. There appears to be a direct correlation between the degree of maturation changes and the response to chemotherapy. Necrosis, often noted following radiotherapy of large tumor masses, is conspicuous in its absence. The histopathologic results closely resemble those found after administration of bleomycin alone, although they are considerably accentuated by the addition of cisplatin [10, 35].

3.3. Prognostic factors for initial tumor response with induction chemotherapy

Previous clinical trials indicate that higher response rates and longer durations of response are achieved with chemotherapy in previously untreated patients than in patients with tumors that recur after surgery and radiation therapy. Other factors – e.g., patient performance and nutritional status, the site of tumor, the size of primary tumor, and histologic differentiation – have been suggested as important prognostic factors that influence tumor response to induction chemotherapy [9, 28]. Preliminary reports from the NCI trial indicate that no significant differences were observed in response rates for primary tumors that arose from different anatomical sites [34]. However, there was a trend, based on tumor size, for patients with smaller tumors to have better response rates. Primary tumor response rates (complete and partial) were highest for patients with T1 and T2 primary tumors, compared to T3 and T4 primary tumors, which suggests the valuable impact of induction chemotherapy in the treatment of early stages of head and neck cancer. Response rates for regional lymph nodes with induction chemotherapy were identical among the patients with N1 or N2 adenopathy but were significantly higher than for patients with N3 adenopathy [9, 28, 34].

Previous trials suggest that the histologic differentiation of tumors may predict differences in tumor sensitivity to chemotherapeutic drugs. The conclusions of previous studies regarding histologic differentiation of tumors and chemotherapy response are conflicting. Al-Sarraf [28] suggests that poorly differentiated tumors are associated with the highest complete response rates, while a study from Shapshay and Hong [36] suggests the highest response rates for well-differentiated tumors. The chemotherapy regimens were similar in both of these studies. The recent NCI trial suggests that histologic tumor differentiation is not significantly associated with tumor response.

4. Conclusions

The greatest therapeutic challenge for patients with advanced squamous cell carcinoma of the head and neck is achievement of a complete remission and long-term, disease-free survival. Overall survival has not really improved as a result of the combined therapy program of surgery and radiation therapy. The combined modalities of surgery followed by radiation therapy seem to decrease the local and regional recurrence rate, but the patients subsequently die from distant metastases. The natural course of tumor growth suggests the need for further exploration of some form of systemic chemotherapy.

4.1. Effective induction chemotherapy regimens

Induction chemotherapy prior to surgery or radiotherapy presumably will decrease the volume of tumor at the primary site and will also eradicate subclinical, microscopic, metastases. Methotrexate, cisplatin, bleomycin, and 5-fluorouracil, as single agents or in combination, have been used for induction chemotherapy. Major response rates are significantly higher using combination chemotherapy than those reported in single agent studies in previously untreated patients. The literature indicates a major response rate of 60 to 80%, and complete regression rates of 10 to 20% with induction chemotherapy in previously untreated patients. These results are clearly superior to those achieved in patients with tumors recurrent after surgery and/or radiotherapy. Thus, the relatively common squamous cell carcinoma has become one of the most chemosensitive tumors to induction chemo-therapy in previously untreated patients.

In general, long-term, disease-free survival with initial chemotherapy occurred only in those patients whose tumors completely disappeared prior to surgery and/or radiotherapy. Chemotherapy-induced partial responses predict conversion to complete response by subsequent surgery and/or radiotherapy. Disappointingly, only a small percentage of patients who had less than a partial response will achieve complete response with definitive local treatment. The Goldie and Coldman hypothesis suggests that chemo-therapy should be given in high doses as early as possible and in the shortest interval possible [38]. The development of an effective and powerful induc-tion regimen with acceptable toxicity is the main avenue of current inves-tigation.

4.2. Interrelationship of induction regimen toxicity and subsequent definitive treatment

In general, the toxic effects of induction chemotherapy regimens were mild, as the previous studies indicated. Preliminary results from the NCI Contract Study indicate that there were no delays of surgery or deaths associated with toxic effects from induction chemotherapy. Surgery following induction chemotherapy does not result in increased wound healing complications. Radiation therapy following induction chemotherapy and surgery does not result in enhanced radiotherapy side effects.

4.3. Impact of unresectable tumors

A significant tumor response to induction chemotherapy may allow more aggressive local definitive treatment in patients with unresectable squamous cell carcinoma of the head and neck. Also, cytoreduction of the primary tumor in response to induction chemotherapy possibly allows marginally curable patients to receive more curative local treatment [37]. However, the issue of induction chemotherapy converting unresectable tumor to resectable tumor has not yet been clarified.

4.4. Patterns of relapse

The current on-going clinical trials of induction chemotherapy in head and neck cancer are investigating the adjuvant effect of drugs in conjunction with conventional therapy. If induction chemotherapy reduces the local and distant recurrence rates more than does conventional treatment, then it will provide a rationale for use of chemotherapy in an adjuvant setting in conjunction with conventional treatment.

Several non-randomized clinical trials suggest that induction chemotherapy does not have great impact in reducing distant recurrence rates, compared to historical control groups. This question is vital, particularly because the control of distant metastases is critical to improve the survival rate of head and neck cancer patients. We will have to wait for the results of the NCI trial to know the impact of induction chemotherapy on distant metastases and overall survival.

References

1. Ultmann JE, Kanofsky JR: Adjuvant therapy: Principles and state of the art. In: Salmon S, Jones S (eds) Adjuvant Cancer Therapy II. Adjuvant Cancer Therapy II. New York, Grune ø Stratton, 1979, pp 637–659.
2. Henderson IC, Canellos GP: Cancer of the breast. The past decade. NEJM 302:17–30, 78–90, 1980.

3. Bertino JR, Mosher MB, DeCanti RC: Chemotherapy of cancer of the head and neck. Cancer 31:1141–1149, 1973.

4. Carter SK: The chemotherapy of head and neck cancer. Semin Oncol 4:413–424, 1977.

5. Hong WK, Bromer R: Current concepts: Chemotherapy in head and neck cancer. NEJM 308:75–79, 1983.

6. Probert JC, Thempson RW, Bagshaw MA: Patterns of spread of distant metastases in head and neck cancer. Cancer 33:127–133, 1974.

7. Leone LA, Albala MM, Rege VB: Treatment of carcinoma of the head and neck with intravenous methotrexate. Cancer 21:828–837, 1968.

8. Randolph VL, Vallejo A, Spiro R, et al.: Combination therapy of advanced head and neck cancer. Induction of remissions with diaminedichloroplatinum (II), bleomycin, and radiation therapy. Cancer 41:460–467, 1978.

9. Hong WK, Bhutani R, Shpashay SM, Strong S: Induction chemotherapy of advanced previously untreated squamous cell head and neck cancer with cisplatin and bleomycin. In: Prestayko AW, Crooke ST, Carter SK (eds) Cisplatin: Current Status and New Developments. New York, Academic Press, 1980, pp 431–444.

10. Hong WK, Shapshay SM, Bhutani R, et al.: Induction chemotherapy in advanced squamous head and neck carcinoma with high-dose cis-platinum and bleomycin infusion. Cancer 44:19–25, 1979.

11. DeConti RC, Schoenfeld D: A randomized prospective comparison of intermittent methotrexate, methotrexate with leucovorin, and a methotrexate combination in head and neck cancer 48:1061–1072, 1981.

12. Tarpley Jl, Chretien PB, Alexander AS, et al.: Highdose methotrexate as a preoperative adjuvant in the treatment of epidermoid carcinoma of the head and neck. Am J Surg 130:481–486, 1975.

13. Kirkwood JM, Miller D, Weichselbaum R, Pitman SW: Symposium: Adjuvant cancer therapy of head and neck tumors. Predefinitive and postdefinitive chemotherapy for locally advanced squamous carcinoma of the head and neck. Laryngoscope 89:573–531, 1979.

14. Taylor SG, Bytell DE, DeWys WD, et al.: Adjuvant methotrexate and leucovorin in head and neck squamous cancer. Arch Otolaryngol 104:647–651, 1978.

15. Costanzi JJ, Loukas D, Gagliano RG, et al.: Intravenous bleomycin Infusion as a potential synchronizing agent in human disseminated malignancies. A preliminary report. Cancer 38:1503–1506, 1976.

16. Krakoff IH, Cvitkovic E, Currie V, et al.: Clinical pharmacologic and therepeutic studies of bleomycin given by continuous infusion. Cancer 40:2027–2037, 1977.

17. Sikic BI, Collins JM, Mimnaugh EG, Gram TE: Improved therapeutic index of bleomycin when administered by continuous infusion in mice. Cancer Treat Rep 62:2011–2017, 1978.

18. Popkin JD, Hong WK, Bromer RH, et al.: Induction bleomycin infusion in head and neck cancer. Am J Clin Oncol: Cancer Clin Trials 7:199–204, 1984.

19. Bennett WM, Pastore L, Houghton DC: Fatal pulmonary bleomycin toxicity in cisplatin-induced acute renal failure. Cancer Treat Rep 64:921–924, 1980.

20. Iacovino JR, Leitner J, Abbas AK, et al.: Fatal pulmonary reaction from low doses of bleomycin. An idiosyncratic tissue response. JAMA 235:1253–1255, 1976.

21. Hayes DM, Cvitkovic E, Golbey RB, Krakoff IM: High-dose cisplatinumdiaminedichloride: Amelioration of renal toxicity by mannitol diuresis. Cancer 39:1372–1381, 1977.

22. Wittes RE, Cvitkovic E, Shah J, et al.: Cis-Diaminedichloroplatinum (II) (DDP) in the treatment of epidermoid carcinoma of the head and neck. Cancer Treat Rep 62:359–366, 1977.

23. Wittes R, Heller K, Randolph V, et al.: cis-Dichlorodiamineplatinum (II)-based chemotherapy as initial treatment of advanced head and neck cancer. Cancer Treat Rep 63:1533–1538, 1979.

24. Jacobs C, Bertino JR, Goffinet DR, *et al.*: 24-h infusion of cisplatinum in head and neck cancers. Cancer 42:2135–2140, 1978.
25. Glick JH, Marcial V, Velez-Garcia E: The adjuvant treatment of inoperable Stage III and IV epidermoid carcinoma of the head and neck with platinum and bleomycin infusions prior to definitive radiation therapy: An RTOG pilot study. Cancer 46:1919–1924, 1980.
26. Elias FG, Chetien PB, Monnard E, *et al.*: Chemotherapy prior to local therapy in advanced squamous cell carcinoma of the head and neck. Preliminary assessment of an intensive drug regimen. Cancer 43:1025–1031, 1979.
27. Schuller DG, Wilson HG, Smith RG, *et al.*: Preoperative reductive chemotherapy for locally advanced carcinoma of the oral cavity, oropharynx, and hypopharynx. Cancer 51:15–19, 1983.
28. Al-Sarraf M, Drelichman A, Jacobs J, *et al.*: Adjuvant chemotherapy with cis-platinum, oncovin, and bleomycin followed by surgery and/or radiotherapy in patients with advanced previously untreated head and neck cancerb: Final report. In: Salmon S, Jones S (eds) Adjuvant Cancer Therapy III. New York, Grune & Statton, 1981, pp 145–152.
29. Spaulding MB, Kloach D, Grillo J, *et al.*: adjuvant chemotherapy in the treatment of advanced tumors of the head and neck. Amer J Surg 140:538–542, 1980.
30. Ervin TJ, Karp DD, Weichselbaum RR, Frei III E: Adjuvant chemotherapy for squamous carcinoma of the head and neck. In: Salmon S, Jones S (eds) Adjuvant Cancer Therapy III. New York, Grune & Stratton, 1981, pp 183–189.
31. Perry DJ, Weltz MD, Brown AW, *et al.*: Adjuvant chemotherapy for advanced head and neck cancer. In: Salmon S, Jones S (eds) Adjuvant Cancer Therapy III, New York, Grune & Stratton, 1981, pp 161–168, 1981.
32. Kish J, Drelichman A, Jacobs J, *et al.*: Clinical trial of cisplatin and 5-Fu infusion as initial treatment for advanced squamous cell carcinoma of the head and neck. Cancer Treat Rep 66:471–474, 1982.
33. Price LA, Hill BT: Safe and effective 24-h combination chemotherapy without cisplatin as initial treatment in head and neck cancer: Improved survival at 5 years. Proc Amer Soc Clin Onc 1:202, 1982.
34. Baker SR, Makuch RW, Wolf GT: Preoperative cisplatin and bleomycin in head and neck squamous carcinoma. Arch Otolaryngol 107:683–689, 1981.
35. Shapshay SM, Hong WK, Incze JS, *et al.*: Histopathologic findings of cis-Platinum and bleomycin therapy in advanced previously untreated head and neck carcinoma. Am J Surg 136:534–538, 1978.
36. Shapshay SM, Hong WK, Incze JS, *et al.*: Prognostic indicators in induction cis-platinum and bleomycin chemotherapy for advanced head and neck cancer. Amer J Surg 140:543–547, 1980.
37. Pennacchio JL, Hong WK, Shapshay S, *et al.*: Combination of cis-platinum and bleomycin prior to surgery and/or radiotherapy compared with radiotherapy alone for the treatment of advanced squamous cell carcinoma of the head and neck. Cancer 50:2795–2801, 1982.
38. Goldie JH, Coldman AJ: A mathematical model for relating the drug sensitivity of tumors to their spontaneous mutation rate. Cancer Treat Rep 63:172, 1979.

14. Intra-arterial infusion chemotherapy of head and neck cancer

SHAN R. BAKER and RICHARD WHEELER

1. Introduction

Despite almost three decades of experience, the use of intra-arterial chemotherapy for the treatment of head and neck cancer is not universally accepted [1]. Overall reported response rates are not substantially different from the therapeutic results obtained with systemic therapy. The additional complications associated with establishing and maintaining arterial access have further dampened enthusiasm for this approach. It is clear that considerable improvement in regional therapy techniques and efficacy will be necessary before widespread clinical acceptance of intra-arterial chemotherapy is attained. These improvements must be based on the anatomic and pharmacologic factors that determine the success of regional therapy, and require the development of safe and reliable delivery systems.

The principal objective of regional chemotherapy, as for cancer chemotherapy in general, is tumor cell kill. The rationale for regional delivery is based on the steep dose/response curve exhibited by most antineoplastic agents [2]. Intra-arterial chemotherapy has the potential advantages of (a) increased drug concentration at the tumor site (b) decreased systemic drug levels and toxicity (c) continuous tumor cell exposure to an antineoplastic agent, and (d) the possibility of systemic rescue.

Regional therapy is not applicable to all malignancies or patients. The factors that are necessary for a successful regional approach include (a) a tumor natural history that demonstrates primarily local aggressiveness rather than widespread metastatic dissemination (b) a definable and accessible arterial supply that provides selective access to tumor blood supply with minimal normal tissue distribution (c) antineoplastic agents with favorable pharmacokinetic properties and demonstrable antitumor activity and (d) a delivery system that permits safe continous long-term infusion with minimal patient inconvenience. In this chapter we will review the anatomic and pharmacologic principles that determine the effectiveness of regional thera-

Gregory T. Wolf (ed), Head and Neck Oncology.
© *1984 Martinus Nijhoff Publishers, Boston. ISBN 0-89838-657-8. Printed in The Netherlands.*

py, summarize the clinical studies conducted in head and neck cancer to date, and discuss future directions and alternatives for intra-arterial chemotherapy.

2. Anatomic considerations

The two major anatomic considerations are the extent and location of the malignancy, and the vascular supply of the involved region. The therapeutic advantage of regional therapy, high local drug concentration with a low systemic exposure, becomes a major disadvantage when the tumor extends or metastasizes beyond the infused volume. The maximum impact on patient survival or cure will be achieved only for malignancies that display local aggressiveness with a low or absent propensity for wide-spread metastatic dissemination.

The history of the treatment of head and neck cancer has been one of continual applications of new techniques in the hope of improving cure rates. In the 1930's orthovoltage radiation therapy dominated the management of head and neck cancer, following Coutard's fractionation method, cures were obtained in perhaps 25% of oral, pharyngeal and laryngeal cancers. In the 1940's Dr. Hayes Martin improved the survival statistics by developing new techniques of radical surgery, combining wide resection of the primary tumor in continuity with neck dissection for regional metastases. The philosophy of 'one operation fits all' prevailed, and functional and cosmetic disability was a common trade-off for improved survival rates. In the 1950's improvement in radiation therapy equipment enabled MacComb and Fletcher to introduce the concept of combined therapy consisting of radiotherapy and surgery. Treatment results again improved. The 1960's were marked by the introduction of new surgical concepts such as immediate repair of large defects of the head and neck utilizing regional skin flap repair. Conservative laryngeal surgery emerged as another surgical advancement. In the 1970's the concept of adjuvant chemotherapy was developed and utilized to treat potentially curable head and neck cancer. In the 1980's we can look forward to more multimodality studies searching for improved cure rates in advanced disease, and the development of regional cancer centers for the treatment of head and neck cancer.

Many of the emerging treatment modalities in the 1980's will be directed toward improved local control of head and neck cancer. Approximately 13,000 patients in the United States die yearly of squamous cell cancer of the head and neck [3]. Although the clinical incidence of distant metastases is increased in advanced stage patients who achieve loco- regional control, the majority of patients still die of loco-regional disease [4, 5]. It is this group of patients that will benefit from improved local control rates through

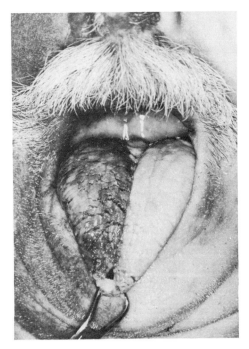

Figure 1 (A). India ink injection of external carotid artery demonstrating ink staining of ipsilateral oral mucosa.

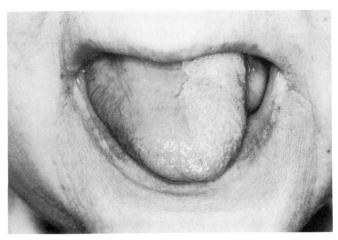

Figure 1 (B). Ipsilateral stomatitis extending only to midline in patient being treated with intraarterial chemotherapy from totally implantable infusion pump. Arch Otolaryngol 108:703–708, 1982. Copyright 1982, AMA.

new therapeutic approaches. Thus, head and neck cancer has an appropriate natural history for the application of a regional approach to therapy.

Vascular anatomu of the head and neck

Most intra-arterial chemotherapy conducted to date has been delivered through catheters placed in the external carotid artery (ECA) by way of the superficial temporal artery, the superior thyroid artery or other accessible branches. Lesions which cross the midline require the insertion of two catheters. In general, long term intra-arterial therapy has been applicable only to lesions supplied by the external carotid artery. The regional lymph nodes in the mid and lower neck, and tumors confined to or extending into the neck beyong the nutrient field of the external carotid artery are excluded from the infused volume. Implantation of a catheter into the thyrocervical trunk can allow infusion of the cervical region, and can be used in conjunction with the standard cranio-facial infusion through the ECA.

The ECA arises from the common carotid artery near the upper border of the thyroid cartilage and passes upward to supply the vast majority of the integument, musculature, skeleton and mucosal lining of the face and upper aerodigestive tract. Unilateral India ink injections of the ECA in fresh cadaver specimens demonstrate ink staining of the mucosal surfaces of the nasal passage, oral cavity, oral pharynx and hypopharynx, as well as the skin of the face, forehead, anterior scalp, and upper neck to the level of the thyrohyoid membrane inferiorly (Fig. 1A). Ink staining extends to the midline of the head and neck. These anatomic studies are confirmed clinically in patients receiving ECA intra-arterial chemotherapy by observing ipsilateral stomatitis and alopeica extending only to the midline (Fig. 1B) [6].

The thyrocervical trunk (TCT) is a short thick vessel arising from the first portion of the subclavian artery close to the medial border of the scalenus anterior (Fig. 2). It divides almost immediately into two constant branches, the inferior thyroid and the suprascapular arteries and a variable third branch, the transverse cervical artery.

The inferior thyroid artery passes upward in front of the vertebral artery and longus colli then turns medialward behind the carotid sheath and the sympathetic trunk. Reaching the lower border of the thyroid gland it divides into two branches, which supply the posterior-inferior part of the gland, portions of the trachea and the upper cervical esophagus. The inferior thyroid artery also supplies the muscles and mucous membrane of the hypopharynx and lower portion of the larynx, and the deep muscles of the neck. Muscular branches supply the infrahyoid strap muscles, longus colli, scalenus anterior, and inferior pharyngeal constrictor muscle.

The suprascapular artery passes downward and lateralward across the scalenus anterior and phrenic nerve deep to the sternocleidomastoideus. It crosses the subclavian artery and the brachial plexus and runs behind and parallel to the clavicle. Distributing branches to the sternocleidomastoideus, subclavius, and neighboring muscles, the suprascapular artery also gives rise

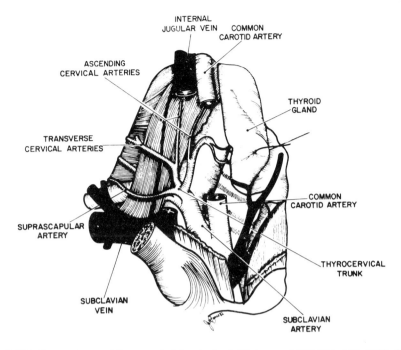

Figure 2. Relative anatomy of thyrocervical trunk. Arch Otolaryngol 108:703–708, 1982. Copyright 1982, AMA.

to a suprasternal branch which supplies the skin of the upper part of the chest, and an acromial branch which pierces the trapezius muscle and supplies the skin over the acromion.

The transverse cervical artery arises from the TCT in 80% of cases. It passes laterally across the posterior cervical triangle in a position somewhat cephalic and dorsal to the suprascapular artery. Medially it crosses superficial to the scalenus anterior muscle and phrenic nerve and lies deep to the sternocleidomastoideus. Laterally it crosses the trunk of the brachial plexus and is covered only by the platysma, investing layer of the deep fascia, and the inferior belly of the omohyoideus. As it reaches the levator scapulae muscle it divides into a superfical and a deep branch supplying much of the trapezius, levator scapulae and neighboring deep cervical muscles. The deep branch, particularly, may arise from the second or third part of the subclavian artery. When this occurs it is called the descending scapular artery, while the superficial branch then receives the name of superficial cervical artery. Infrequently (less than 20%), the entire transverse cervical artery arises from the third part of the subclavian artery [7].

India ink injections of the TCT trunk in fresh cadaver specimens demonstrate excellent staining of the integument and deep structures of the lower neck. Staining of the skin occurs from the clavicle superiorly to the level of

306

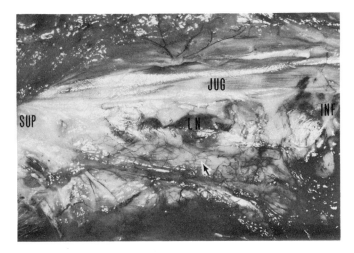

Figure 3. India ink injection of thyrocervical trunk. Note ink staining of fine network of vessels (arrow) surrounding lymph nodes of lower jugular chain. JUG indicates jugular vein; LN, lymph nodes; Sup, superior; and Inf, inferior. Arch Otolaryngol 108:703–708, 1982. Copyright 1982, AMA.

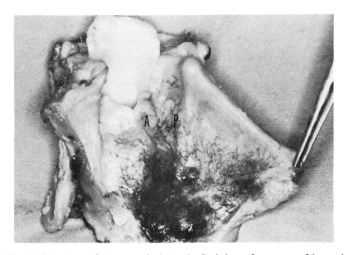

Figure 4. India ink injection of thyrocervical trunk. Staining of mucosa of hypopharynx and pyriform sinus is readily apparent. Dye extends well beyond midline in hypopharyngeal and postcricoid mucosa. A, indicated arytenoid; P, pyriform sinus. Arch Otolaryngol 108:703–708, 1982. Copyright 1982, AMA.

the mid thyroid cartilage. Although skin staining only extends to the level of the mid neck, ink is observed in blood vessels of the subcutaneous tissues of the neck as far superiorly as the level of the body of the mandible. Dissections of the deep structures of the neck in these cadavers demonstrate ink staining of a fine network of vessels surrounding the lymph nodes of the lower jugular chain. Ink extends superiorly to the level of the mid neck (Fig.

3). The lower cervical lymph nodes readily stain with ink. Staining of the mucosa of the hypopharynx, pyriform sinus, and upper cervical esophagus is also apparent. Dye extends well beyond the midline in the hypopharyngeal and postcricoid mucosa (Fig. 4) [6].

3. Pharmacologic considerations

Dose/response and antineoplastic agents

For the vast majority of anticancer drugs, the dose/response curve is steep. In other words, relatively small changes in dose rate have a major impact on the percentage of cells killed. The implication for cancer chemotherapy in general is that maximum tumor regression will be obtained by using the highest dose possible, i.e. the maximum tolerated dose (MTD). Since normal tissue cell kill follows a similar steep curve, the clinical MTD is defined as the highest dose rate that produces an 'acceptable' level of toxicity. The therapeutic advantage of regional therapy is defined by the increase in tumor drug exposure, compared to that achieved by systemic therapy at the MTD.

The steep dose/response curve has been best defined in experimental *in vitro* and animal tumor models. A two fold increase in dose can result in a three to ten fold increase in tumor cell kill [2]. Few clinical trials that examine the effect of dose rate on objective tumor response have been conducted. However, a clear dose effect has been demonstrated in patients with Hodgkin's Disease, Non Hodgkin's lymphoma, testicular cancer and small cell cancer of the lung [2, 8]. Clinical studies have been hampered by the paucity of highly active agents in many solid tumors, and the relatively small dose rate differences employed. In addition many studies have compared low dose, non-toxic therapy with full dose therapy and do not answer the question of extension of the dose response curve beyond the MTD of systemic therapy. Attempts to extend the MTD by use of aggressive supportive care systems, and autologous bone marrow transplantation provide encouraging but not conclusive findings [9, 10]. To the extent that regional therapy can achieve a greater than two to three fold increase in the dose delivered to the tumor it will provide a mechanism to further evaluate the dose response curve. Ultimately a randomized clinical trial comparing maximized regional treatment to aggressive systemic therapy will be necessary to document the value of the regional approach.

The duration of drug exposure is also an important determinant of cytotoxicity. For many agents, particularly phase specific agents (drugs which are cytotoxic only during one phase of the cell cycle), the duration of exposure above a critical concentration is more important than the concentration achieved [11–14]. Non cycle specific agents that are capable of killing resting or cycling cells, (alkylating agents, nitrosoureas) are primarily concentration dependent and are best administered by intermittant bolus with sufficient time between doses to allow normal tissue recovery [12, 15–18]. Cycle specific agents are cytotoxic during more than one phase of the cell cycle, but preferentially kill cycling cells. These agents (many antitumor antibiotics, some antimetabolites) are both concentration and exposure duration dependent. Slowly growing tumor cell populations may be more sensitive to long durations of exposure to cycle specific agents [19]. Effective chemotherapy, systemic or regional, must take into consideration these important variables of dose and duration. Properly designed infusion treatment regimens should be based on the mechanism of action and the cycle specificity of the drugs used, and on the anticipated growth kinetics of the tumor being treated [12, 20].

Factors affecting concentration and exposure duration

The major factors determining drug concentration are the dose rate and the regional blood flow. The higher the dose rate (quantity/unit time) and the lower the regional blood flow (volume/unit time) the greater the drug concentration in the local tumor blood supply [21]. Tumor drug exposure will then be determined by the rate of diffusion or transport of drug across capillary endothelium into the extra cellular fluid [22]. Tumor drug exposure can be maximized by increasing the dose rate, infusing into low blood flow regions (or decreasing the blood flow) and using rapidly diffusing antineoplastic agents [23].

The duration of drug exposure is determined primarily by the infusion system employed. The characteristics of an ideal infusion system includes proper catheter placement and properties that minimize the risks of thromboembolism or hemorrhage, and a pumping mechanism that allows precise long term infusion with minimal intrusion into patients activities. Drug delivery systems are more extensively discussed in a following section.

Therapeutic index

Regional therapy will be potentially beneficial to the extent that tumor exposure to antineoplastic agents can be increased without an increase in drug toxicity. Clinical benefit may occur if the drug exposure is approximately equal to that attained by systemic administration but debilitating systemic toxicity is lessened. In the latter instance, an increase in objective response rate would not be anticipated, and the costs and morbidity of installing and maintaining the infusion system must be considered. Overall evaluation of the efficacy of a particular regional approach must consider the drug exposure attained, the local and systemic toxicity produced, and the monetary, physical and emotional costs of installing and maintaining the system.

The pharmacokinetic principals affecting regional therapy have been extensively reviewed [24, 25]. The therapeutic advantage (R_d) of an intraarterial infusion (assumes the same dose rate is used IA and IV) is defined by the equation:

$$R_d = \frac{(AUC_T)/(AUC_S)\ IA}{(AUC_T/AUC_S)\ IV} + 1$$

where AUC is the area under the concentration × time curve of drug exposure, T refers to the tumor and S to the systemic circulation [21]. For infusion into a body region that does not metabolize drugs (such as the head and neck), equation (1) reduces to:

$$R_d = \frac{Cl_{TB}}{Q} + 1$$

where Cl_{TB} is the total body drug clearance and Q is the regional blood flow [21]. The regional advantage can be increased by using agents with a high total body clearance (which diminishes the systemic drug exposure) and by infusion into regions with a low regional blood flow (which increases regional drug exposure).

Ultimately, the tumor drug exposure attained is limited by the toxicity produced, either local or systemic. The amount of systemic toxicity depends upon the systemic drug level, and varies with the total body clearance of active drug, the first pass extraction of drug as it goes through the regional capillary bed, and the degree of A-V major vessel shunting around the capillary bed. Local toxicity is primarily determined by the drug sensitivity of normal tissues within the infused volume.

Under ideal circumstances an agent infused intraarterially would be entirely removed from the blood during initial transit through the tumor capillary bed. The first pass extraction actually attained depends upon vascular considerations (the capillary surface area and endothelial integrety), the rate of diffusion of the drug across the endothelium into the extracellular space (partition coefficient), drug uptake from the extracellular space into the tumor cell (to maintain the diffusion gradient between the blood and the extracellular space), and cell retention of the drug (determined by drug binding to the intracellular target and/or intracellular metabolism, and the presence or absence of an active transport system extruding the drug) [22, 23].

Even given a high first pass extraction in the capillary bed, substantial systemic toxicity may occur if a high percentage of the drug is shunted from the arterial to the venous circulation via precapillary shunts. The AV shunting that occurs during head and neck infusion has been determined in a small number of patients and varied from less than 10% to over 40% [26]. These studies were performed using radiolabeled macroaggregated albumin that is trapped in the capillary bed, and the first pass extraction in tumor or normal tissue is virtually 100%. These values therefore represent the minimum attainable systemic level. The systemic level of a drug that is not entirely extracted will be higher.

Given some degree of AV shunting and less than complete first pass extraction, the concentration and duration of exposure of systemic tissues will be determined by the rate of active drug clearance. Drug clearance is determined by the rate of drug metabolism (intravascular and/or organ metabolism), drug excretion and, for certain agents, the rate and occurrence of protein binding. Knowledge of the factors that determine the systemic drug level combined with knowledge of the effects of concentration and duration of exposure on the cytotoxicity of a particular agent should allow selection of the optimum schedule of drug administration (bolus vs. long-term infusion).

Potentially systemic toxicity could also be avoided or lessened, in instances where pharmacokinetic manipulations are unsatisfactory, by systemic 'rescue' or administration of an agent that prevents cytotoxicity. The most frequent application of this principle in head and neck intra-arterial therapy is the concommitant use of methotrexate and calcium leucovorin [27]. Despite the wide application of this therapy, clinical studies that establish the superiority of the approach are non-existent. Considerable experimental investigation has shown that the interaction between methotrexate and leucovorin is complex and depends upon the relative concentrations of methotrexate and leucovorin, and the activity of drug uptake mechanisms [28, 29]. Clinical validation of these experimental findings are sorely needed.

Although systemic toxicity can occur with intraarterial therapy, in the majority of instances the dose-limiting side effects are local [30]. The major determinant of local toxicity is the drug sensitivity of the normal tissue within the regional area. Avoidance of agents that characteristically produce toxicity in the infused area would be appropriate. For regional therapy of head and neck cancer this is impractical since the majority of efficacious drugs (methotrexate, bleomycin, fluoropyrimidines) frequently produce mucositis. The investigation and development of regional agents that produce dose-limiting toxicity outside of the head and neck area is necessary.

If precise catheterization that allowed infusion only of the tumor could be accomplished, local toxicity could be avoided. This is not technically feasible and would leave areas adjacent to tumor untreated, providing sanctuaries for tumor spread. Since normal tissue toxicity follows a steep dose/response curve similar to tumor cytotoxicity, physiologic or modulated conditions that would increase drug delivery to the tumor could be advantageous. A low total regional blood flow improves the advantage of intraarterial therapy by increasing the drug concentration at a given dose rate. However, once drug/blood mixing has occurred, drug delivery becomes proportional to the blood flow rate with greater blood flow providing higher drug delivery [23]. Differential drug delivery to tumor and normal tissue is reflected in the blood flow ratio which can vary from 4.2 to 14.1 in favor of tumor flow in head and neck cancer [26]. This favorable blood flow distribution provides some selectivity to intra-arterial therapy. Further augmentation of the ratio by simultaneous infusion of vasoactive agents is currently under exploration [31, 32].

Combination chemotherapy

The use of systemic combination drug chemotherapy is well established in the treatment of malignant disease. Application of combination drug regimens to intraarterial therapy has the potential for similar improvements in the duration and rate of response. Generally accepted principals in systemic combination drug design also apply to regional therapy [18, 33].

Of critical importance is the use of agents active in the disease and avoidance of agents with similar spectrums of toxicity. Although the addition or combination of inactive agents based on a biochemical rationale may provide significant antitumor effect in experimental systems, such combinations have not as yet made an important clinical impact [34, 35].

The use of agents with different toxicities should allow each drug to be given at or close to its individual MTD and exert its maximum antitumor effect. The steep dose/response curve also applies to drugs used in combination. Decreasing dose rates to allow drugs with similar toxicities to be used together will decrease the activity of each agent. The resulting combination may be less active than aggressive use of any of the drugs singly.

4. Drug delivery systems

Catheterization techniques

Early use of intraarterial infusion involved repeated puncture of the selected artery either through direct exposure of the artery or by percutaneous injection. The need for cannulation of the artery to enable longer intervals of infusion soon became evident. Schneierson and Blum [36] described a successful method of continuous arterial infusion using a needle attached to a syringe mounted on a motor-driven cam mechanism which transferred fluid through a one-way intake and output valve assembly into an artery.

Donovan [37] utilized plastic tubing to administer intraarterial heparin. Utilizing the method of Donovan, Klopp et al. [38] developed a suitable technique for repeated intraarterial injection of nitrogen mustard through polyethylene tubing introduced through a proximal arterial branch directly into the artery selected.

Bierman et al. [39] introduced the concept of isolating the major artery leading to a specific organ to the exclusion of other viscera for specific roentgenographic organ visualization. They envisioned the technique could be used for administering chemotherapeutic agents to neoplastic lesions involving an organ. They surgically exposed the common carotid, brachial or femoral artery and were able to pass a catheter into the aorta, and various branches of the aorta. Under fluoroscopic control it was possible to place the catheter in the renal arteries, celiac axis, superior and inferior mesenteric arteries and various small branches of the carotid and subclavian arteries. They injected Diodrast intraarterially and were able to visualize the common and internal carotid artery and the thyrocervical trunk in a patient with a sarcoma of the eye. In two additional patients with head and neck cancer, the external carotid artery was cannulated and fluorescein dye was injected. Three of the 24 patients studied developed hemiplegia following arteriography and one of these patients subsequently died.

Retrograde placement of catheters for the purpose of introducing chemotherapeutic agents was first reported for the treatment of pelvic cancer. Cromer et al. [40] introduced catheters into the deep epigastric or profunda femoral artery and advanced them in a retrograde direction through the external iliac artery into the abdominal aorta. Nitrogen mustard was injected every eight hours in 2-mg quantities. The injections were preceded by application of blood pressure cuffs to both thighs and inflation of the cuffs to a level exceeding systolic pressure. Such a maneuver prevented escape of nitrogen mustard into the circulation of the lower extremities.

The early work of Klopp et al. [38], Bierman et al. [39] and Cromer et al. [40] popularized the use of the catheter method of angiography and intraarterial infusion chemotherapy. The catheter method provided the following advantages over the method of injecting substances by means of single needle: (1) the substance could be injected into a vessel at any level desired; (2) the risk of extravasation of the injected substance was minimized; (3) the patient could be placed in any position required; and (4) the catheter could be left in situ for longer intervals than when a needle was utilized.

The major disadvantage of the catheter technique was the necessity for the direct surgical cannulation of the vessel. However, in 1949 Jonsson [41] performed aortography after puncture of the common carotid artery using a blunt cannula fitted with an inner sharp needle. Peirce [42] in 1951 developed a technique by which polyethylene tubing could be introduced into an artery through a large bore needle. In the same year, Donald *et al.* [43], employing a similar technique, catheterized the common carotid artery. These methods required a large bore needle which limited its usefullness in cannulating smaller arteries. Seldinger [44] used a catheter the same size as the needle thus enabling the use of a smaller needle which could be introduced percutaneously into an artery. A catheter was introduced on a flexible leader through the puncture hole after withdrawal of the puncture needle. He was able to percutaneously cannulate the brachial artery in the antecubital fossa using this method.

The availability of polyethylene tubing and the perfection of equipment and techniques for percutaneous cannulation of arteries allowed for continuous intra-arterial infusion or long term intermittant infusions in contradistinction to periodic intraarterial injections. Payne [45] and Galvin [46] accomplished continuous intraarterial infusions by attaching the infusion catheter to bottles hung approximately 10 feet high from the ceiling of the hospital room. Tandom arrangement of bottles of infusate could be used to safe guard against air emboli. The ever present risk of air emboli prompted Krant *et al.* [47] to develop an air-free closed, disposable infusion system. They maintained a continuous intra-arterial infusion using an externally pressurized collapsible plastic bag connected to a one-way valve. A similar technique was reported by Skinner *et al.* [48]. Sullivan and his associates [49, 50] and Tucker and Talley [51] employed mechanical pumps to administer perfusate intraarterially at a constant rate over prolonged periods.

Ramsden and Duff [52] were the first to cannulate the superficial temporal artery and advance a catheter retrograde for perfusion of the external carotid artery. Duff *et al.* [49] later reported a technique of introducing a catheter into the common or external carotid artery through a purse string suture in the artery. Oettgen, Duff and Clifford [53] also described the purse string technique. In addition they introduced the use of a plastic catheter and needle with the same diameter. The needle with guide was inserted into the artery, and the needle was withdrawn leaving the guide in the lumen of the artery. The catheter was threaded onto the guide and introduced into the artery. The guide was then removed. The catheter was attached to a sleeve with lugs. The lugs were sutured to the arterial wall to secure the catheter. This method was similar to that described by Trussell [54] and Cahill [55] and their colleagues, and was reminiscent of the method introduced by Seldinger [44] and applied by Blaisdell *et al.* [56].

An important concept is the ligation of collateral vessels or vessels arising from the artery being infused but not contributing to the nutrient supply of the neoplasm. Benson *et al.* [57] recommended ligation of collateral vessels to enhance the concentration of infusate in the tumor-bearing area. In a few cases where the external carotid (ECA) was not patent on the tumor bearing side, they utilized the contralateral external carotid artery. To enhance perfusion of tumors extending into the hypopharynx, the thyrocervical trunk was ligated on the involved side.

Complications

Many complications have been associated with intraarterial chemotherapy. Most complications and disadvantages were related to the use of an indwelling catheter. Keeping the catheter in place required accurate surgical technique, good nursing care and a cooperative patient. Clotting of catheters was an ever present complication. Measures used to prevent clotting included continuous infusion, frequent injections with a heparin-saline solution and the use of a wire stylus to clear the catheter of thrombus. When injections were made, considerable care had to be exercised to prevent air embolism and to avoid dislodging small terminal clots formed in the lumen and around the catheter [58].

Arteritis and infection of the skin around the catheter at the skin level eventually develops in all external catheter systems. Arteritis may lead to hemorrhage, leakage of infusate around the catheter and septic embolus. Likewise, unless meticulous care is taken, the lumen of the catheter may become infected and lead to sepsis.

Indwelling arterial catheters may produce vasospasm. Thus catheters near the carotid bulb may cause motor weakness, aphasia, or hemiparesis. Catheters placed in the external carotid artery may sometimes cause neurological sequelae. Retrograde flow of chemotherapy agents may spill into the internal carotid circulation causing seizures and motor weakness. This is most common when partial or complete thrombosis of the external carotid artery has occurred. Catheters located in the distribution of the common or internal carotid circulation are constant sources for thrombus and air emboli to the brain. Convulsions, hemiparesis and death have occurred as a result of embolization.

Neurologic sequelae may also occur from air embolism or inadvertent dislodgement of an atherosclerotic plaque into the internal carotid system. Migration of the infusion catheter from the external carotid artery into the common or internal carotid artery may expose the brain to direct infusion of antimetabolites, resulting in seizures or neurological impairment [59].

Reemtsma [60] reported on the incidence of complications occurring during intra-arterial infusion chemotherapy. The most frequent complications were drug related nausea and vomiting, skin erythema or necrosis. Hanna, Gaisford and Goldwyn [61] reported approximately 100 cases treated with intraarterial nitrogen mustard for palliation and relief of pain in head and neck cancer. The superficial temporal artery was used for catheterization of the external carotid artery in the majority of the patients. Approximately 40% of patients developed some type of complication. The most common was the inadvertent removal of the intra-arterial catheter.

Watkins and Sullivan [62] reviewed much of the work begun by Sullivan. They reported 136 patients treated with intraarterial chemotherapy. As experience was gained with the use of indwelling arterial catheters, the complication rate decreased. The overall complication rate was 40%. Four major embolizations occurred resulting in the death of one patient. Death from hemorrhage occurred in eight patients.

Goldman et al. [58] also reported on the complications of indwelling catheters. Fibrin coating along the catheter was found in 20 patients studied by pull-out arteriography and was associated with clinical symptoms. Major thrombus formation occurred around the catheter tip in 28% of the infused vessels. Systemic heparinization did not reduce the incidence of thrombus formation. Factors that appeared to reduce the incidence of complications were the placement of soft, pliable catheters with small diameters into large arteries.

Newer, soft, flexible silicone elastomer catheters with extremely small lumens (OD 2.5 mm, ID 1.2 mm) have proved to be effective conduits for long term administration of intra-arterial chemotherapy. The small lumen does not readily allow retrograde blood flow into the catheter. The softness and flexibility of the catheter prevents migration or penetration of the catheter through the vessel wall. The extreme flexibility of the catheter requires that it be implanted surgically via an arterotomy since it cannot be easily advanced within an artery. By selecting a branch of the external carotid artery for access, an arterotomy is performed near the origin of the vessel from the external carotid artery. The catheter tip is advanced forward until the tip is just flush with the lumen of the external carotid artery. This technique allows infusate to be delivered directly into the blood stream of the external carotid artery without the need for the catheter to occupy any of the lumen of the vessel. The placement of such a catheter utilizing this technique has allowed the authors to administer intraarterial chemotherapy for many months without thrombosis or obstruction of the catheter system [6].

Drug infusion techniques

Refinements of the infusion apparatus paralleled refinements in the technique of arterial cannulation. Zimmerman and Rand [63] first developed a pressure pump for administering intraarterial fluids when catheterizing the heart. An electrical reciprocating pressure pump that could maintain a constant air pressure over a range of 0 to 400 mm of mercury was used. Instead of a Murphy drip, a safety float valve was used to automatically seal the outflow tubing when the injection fluid was exhausted. Pegg, Trotman and Pierce [64] pointed out the deficiencies of gravity flow especially in controlling the flow rate. Their infusion arrangement consisted of a special drip chamber containing two platinum electrodes; each drop of fluid momentarily connected the electrodes thus providing a signal to operate the monitor. The apparatus was driven by a 6-volt battery and the drip rate was displayed on a meter calibrated from 0 to 50 drops a minute. An alarm sounded if the rate fell below 10 drops a minute for more than $1\frac{1}{2}$ minutes. The device could be used for intraarterial infusion by connecting it to a synchronous motor attached to a driving screw which in turn was attached to a syringe. This automatic syringe was connected to a pressure sensitive switch that was set to operate at 100 mm Hg above the patients measured arterial pressure; this permitted the pump to develop a moderate increase in pressure to overcome variations of flow resistance but stopped it in the event of a complete blockage due to clotting or extravasation. The fluid passed through an air trap and electrodes mounted in the top of this chamber activated a relay if the amount of trapped air increased above a predetermined limit.

The problem of loss of temperature of substances infused intravascularly was solved by Longden [65]. He used polystyrene material to insulate the infusion bottles against the environment. Tests showed that the temperature of fluid within the insulated bottles dropped only 2 degrees F per hour.

Addison and Jennings [66] described a technique for infusion using a vinyl plastic transfusion bag which was made with two separate compartments. One compartment was filled with infusate while the other was connected to a positive pressure oxygen source which progressively caused collapse of the infusate compartment. McDonald [67] described a similar container divided by a partition. The pressure chamber was activated by a sphygmomanometer.

Donaldson and Paletta [68] and others [69, 70] utilized a Barron arterial infusion pump to provide controlled and even infusion pressure. This pump which was originally designed for forced oral alimentation, is of the roller type, and through a series of reciprocal gears provides four speeds, allowing volumes between 400 to 2000 ml per 24 h.

The technique of continuous intraarterial infusion was simplified by a chronometric infusion pump described by Watkins [71]. This spring activated pump was used to dispense 3 to 5 ml of infusate per 24 h. A disposable plastic reservoir within the apparatus contained 25 ml of the infusate, a supply sufficient for several days of treatment. The apparatus was harnessed to the chest and enabled prolonged intraarterial infusion chemotherapy on an ambulatory outpatient basis. Burn and Gains [72] described a similar apparatus. The pump named, the Chemofusor, was powered by a miniature mercury battery. A single roller fixed to a drive plate rotated against the infusion tubing creating the pumping action. The Chemofusor was worn by the patient in a carrying holder and afforded continuous intraarterial infusion chemotherapy in ambulatory patients. More recently, Rutherford and Anderson [73] reported on the management of 152 patients treated on an outpatient basis with continuous infusion cancer chemotherapy using a portable infusion pump system.

Implantable infusion pump

One of the main reasons intraarterial infusion chemotherapy has not been more widely accepted has been the need for prolonged hospitalization and the many complications accompanying the use of external catheters and infusion pumps. To circumvent many of these complications, a percutaneously refillable, totally implantable pump has been designed, built and tested. The pump provides a continuous and uniform rate of infusion. The design, animal trials, and initial experience with this device as a delivery vehicle for heparin in patients with refractory thromboembolic disease have been described in detail [74-78].

The Infusaid pump (Infusaid Corp., Sharon, MA) consists of a hollow titanium disk separated into two chambers by a metal bellows (Figs. 5A and B). The inner chamber contains the infusate, the outer a charging liquid in equilibrium with its vapor phase. At 37°C, the vapor pressure is approximately 450 mm of mercury greater than atmospheric pressure. This vapor pressure provides the power source, exerting pressure on the bellows, and forcing the infusate through a 0.22 micron bacterial filter and a resistance element. The pump is placed beneath the skin and the drug chamber is periodically refilled by percutaneous injections of infusate. The drug chamber is refilled through a self-sealing silicone rubber septum in the top of the pump. The pressure of the refill injection forces the bellows to expand, reducing the volume of the outer chamber, recondensing the volatile-driving vapor. Thus, refilling the drug chamber simultaneously recharges the power source for the next infusion cycle. The resistance element is connected to a silicone rubber delivery catheter which can be inserted into a vein, artery, or body cavity.

The Model 400 Infusaid pump features an auxiliary injection port with a second self-sealing rubber septum. This port connects directly with the infusion catheter and may be used for injection of fluorescein or radioactive

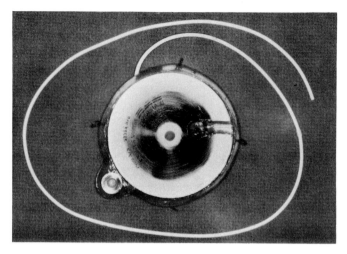

Figure 5(A). Infusaid pump Model 400 attached with silicone rubber infusion catheter.

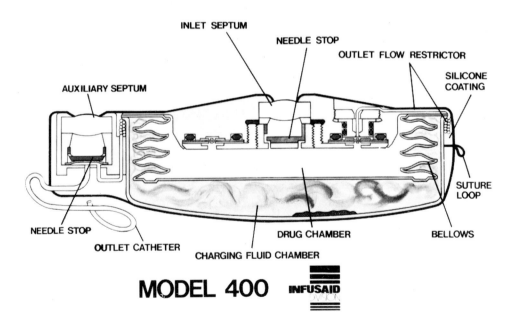

Figure 5(B). Infusaid pump Model 400 schematic (Courtesy of the Infusaid Corporation, Sharon, MA). Arch Otolaryngol 108:703–708, 1982. Copyright 1982, AMA.

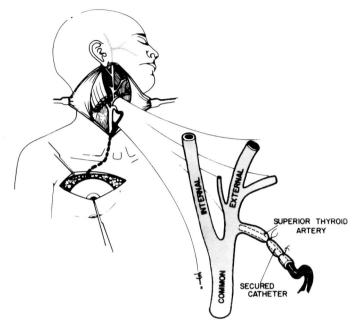

Figure 6. Infusion catheter is advanced until it is flush with the lumen of the external carotid artery. Infusion pump is placed in a subcutaneous pocket superficial to the fascia of the pectoralis major muscle. Head Neck Surg 4:118–124, 1981.

microspheres to confirm the region of infusion. It may also be utilized to bypass the drug chamber for bolus injections of the same or a different drug from that being unfused. The Infusaid pump delivers 45 ml of infusate over a time period of one to five weeks depending on the flow rate selected. For the purpose of intraarterial infusion of head and neck neoplasms, pumps have been utilized which deliver drugs at flow rates of 1 to 5 ml/24 h. A constant flow rate is achieved with this system at constant ambient temperature and pressure conditions. A flow rate variability less than 10% can be expected during a single pump cycle and is described by the performance curve for each pump. The recent development of a dual catheter pump now permits single pump therapy of bilateral or midline head lesions, or unilateral tumors involving the head and neck.

Implantation of the pump and delivery catheter may be accomplished under local or general anesthesia. Neoplasms confined to the head and upper neck are perfused through the external carotid artery. Direct vessel cannulation is accomplished through an incision parallel to the anterior border of the sternocleidomastoid muscle and centered at the level of the hyoid bone. The dissection is carried deep and the external carotid artery is identified and exposed. A branch of the external carotid artery which does not perfuse a region of the neoplasm is selected to receive the catheter (Fig. 6). An arterotomy is performed and the catheter is threaded into the vessel.

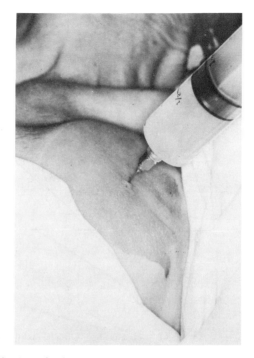

Figure 7 (A). The Infusaid pump is placed beneath the skin of the chest.

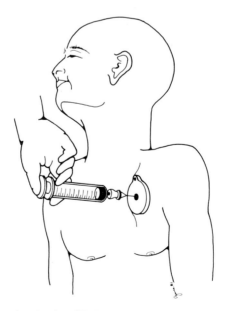

Figure 7 (B). The inner drug chamber is refilled by percutaneous injections through a self-sealing septum. J Surg Oncol 21:125–131, 1982.

The catheter tip is advanced until it is flush with the lumen of the external carotid artery. After the catheter has been inserted, the distal vessel can be ligated and the catheter securely tied in place within the vessel with several separate ligatures.

Additional branches of the external carotid artery that are not directly perfusing the area of the cancer are ligated. For example, when treating carcinoma in the maxillary sinus and pterygopalatine fossa area, the superior thyroid, lingual, occipital, posterior auricular, and superficial temporal arteries should be ligated. Any of the more proximal ligated vessels could act as the recipient artery for the delivery catheter. The proper placement of the catheter and ligation of extraneous vessels should lower the total regional blood flow, provide maximum delivery of chemotherapy to the tumor while sparing as much normal tissue as possible, and lessen the risk of thrombosis of the artery nourishing the neoplasm.

Implantation of the infusion pump requires an incision parallel to and two centimeters below the clavicle. A subcutaneous pocket is made superficial to the fascia of the pectoralis major muscle. The sterile pump is introduced into the pocket and secured to the deep fascia by non-absorbable sutures placed through loops which are attached to the sides of the pump. The arterial catheter is directed toward the subcutaneous pocket created in the subclavicular fossa. The catheter is tunneled through the subcutaneous tissues of the neck and upper chest wall and is connected to the outlet catheter from the pump. The incisions in the neck and chest are closed in layers without drains.

An implanted pump is allowed to infuse sterile saline containing sodium heparin (200 to 500 unit/ml) for the first several postoperative days. The pump is then percutaneously emptied of the heparinized saline, the flow rate is checked, and the pump is refilled with an antineoplastic drug solution (Fig. 7). The drug concentration in the pump is determined by the desired dose rate and the calibrated flow rate. After wound healing is apparent, patients are allowed to return home and are able to continue their regular activities. Therapy thereafter is conducted entirely on an outpatient basis. Patients return for scheduled outpatients visits every one to three weeks, depending on the flow rate of the pump.

During each outpatient visit, patients are assessed for tumor response, pump function, and possible drug toxicity. The pump is emptied by percutaneous needle entry throught the subcutaneous septum, and refilled with antineoplastic drug or sterile heparinized saline. The flow rate is then calculated by subtracting the residual pump infusate volume from the volume used to recharge the pump at the time of previous refill and dividing by the number of infusion days.

At the University of Michigan, 25 pumps have been implanted in 20 patients. Two patients had two pumps implanted to provide bilateral head infusion, three pumps have been replaced. Eight of these patients have received dual catheter infusion systems. There have been no episodes of bleeding. An abrupt decrease in flow rate has occurred in three patients receiving dichloromethotrexate infusions for head and neck cancer. The pump was replaced in two patients, and dichloromethotrexate crystals were noted in the arterial catheter or resistance element. Dichloromethotrexate has subsequently been dissolved in 0.5% sodium bicarbonate to increase drug solubility, and no further infusion malfunctions have occurred. Two patients have developed infections of the pump pocket. One infection occurred while the catheters were externalized for three weeks awaiting pump delivery. The second infection occurred following skin breakdown over the catheter in a patient who had undergone a previous radical neck dissection and neck irradiation. The patient characteristics and pump performance are detailed in Tables 1 and 2.

The infusion pump offers a convenient and versatile mode of access to veins, arteries or body cavities [78–80]. Drug dosage can be altered easily by emptying and refilling the pump with a different concentration of infusate. Similarly, therapy can be intermittently discontinued by replacing the drug infusate with saline. Intraarterial bolus chemotherapy can be accomplished through the auxiliary injection port of the pump.

Table 1. Patient population treated with the unfusaid pump

No. treated	20
Male/Female	13/7
Median age	55
	(18–72)
Prior radiation	16
Prior chemotherapy	6
No prior therapy	4
Cell type	
Squamous	13
Basal cell	2
Undifferentiated	2
Salivary gland	2
Sarcoma	1
Primary site	
Tongue/Tonsil	9
Palate	2
Ethmoid sinus	2
Parotid	2
Skin	2
Larynx	1
Floor of mouth	1
Max. sinus	1

Table 2. Infusaid pump performance

No. implanted	25
Single catheter	(17)
Dual catheter	(8)
No. infusion days	7500+
Median duration of therapy	7+ months
	(3+–31+)
Infections	2
Bleeding	0
Emboli	2
System failure	3

A limiting factor in the use of this implantable pump is related to the infusion drug selected. The chemotherapeutic agents must not react with the titanium pump components, they must be of sufficiently low viscosity to permit infusion, and they must be chemically stable at physiological temperatures over durations of three to four weeks. Therefore drugs must be tested *in vitro* for stability and pump compatibility prior to clinical application.

Distribution of drug delivery

Accurate identification of an artery for cannulation is essential when administering intraarterial chemotherapy to ensure complete infusion of the tumor vasculature. A number of methods have been developed for this purpose, including radiographic visualization and the use of injectable fluorescein or methylene blue dyes. Bierman *et al.* [39] injected diodrast to localize the external carotid in head and neck cancer patients. Duff and his associate [49, 52] injected fluorescein and inspected the head and neck with an ultra violet light to ensure proper identification of the external carotid artery. Engeset, Brennhovd and Stovner [81] introduced the use of patent blue violet dye to test for proper staining of tumors in the head and neck region. Szabo and Kovacs [82] also utilized patent blue staining for precise positioning of the indwelling infusion catheter.

Rapoport *et al.* [83] injected I^{131} labeled albumin macroaggregate followed by scanning of the head and neck to determine infusion patterns and to provide a method of selective catheterization of appropriate branches of the external carotid artery for direct infusion of tumors. Kaplan *et al.* [84] infused radionuclides at low flow rates, approximating those used for drug delivery, to define patterns of intrahepatic infusion. Radiotracer patterns of intra-hepatic infusion are obtained by infusing 4.0 mCi of 99m technetium-macroaggregated albumin via a catheter infusing the hepatic artery and

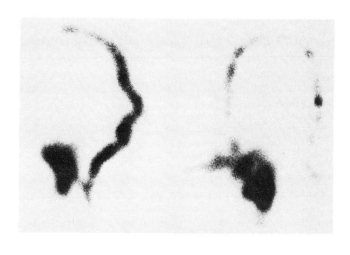

(A)

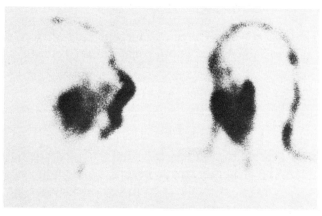

(B)

Figure 8. Radionuclide scan of patient treated with dual-catheter infusion pump. Radioactivity can be demonstrated in lower part of neck from perfusion of thyrocervical trunk (A) as well as upper part of neck from perfusion of external carotid artery (B). A radioactive pen was used to outline the head and neck. Arch Otolaryngol 108:703–708, 1982. Copyright 1982, AMA.

obtaining a radio-nuclide liver scan. The presence or absence of radio-labeled albumin flow to focal tumor defects was compared to a prior technetium-99m-Sulfur colloid liver-spleen scan to assess adequacy of the infusion.

A similar technique has been utilized by the authors of this chapter to assess infusion patterns in head and neck cancer patients treated with intraarterial chemotherapy. We use a slow injection of technitium-99 tagged macroaggregated albumin through the pump auxiliary port, followed by computerized tomographic and static post injection scanning. This allows determination of the infused area, and permits detection of CNS infusion that could result from improper catheter placement or collateral circulation.

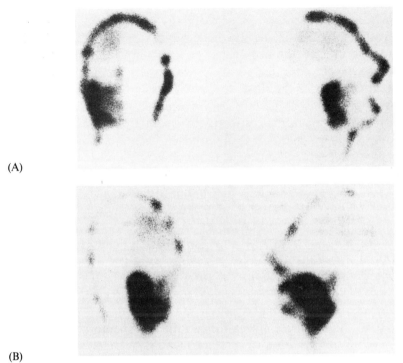

(A)

(B)

Figure 9. Radionuclide scan of patient treated with dual-catheter infusion pump. Catheters were placed in both external carotid arterial (ECA) systems for treatment of extensive tongue cancer. Radioactivity is concentrated in tongue musculature. A. Perfusion of right ECA. B. Perfusion of left ECA. Arch Otolaryngol 108:703–708, 1982. Copyright 1982, AMA.

Figure 8 demonstrates a radionuclide scan of a patient after catheters were placed in the ECA and TCT systems for treatment of an extensive oral pharynx and hypopharyngeal carcinoma and unilateral cervical metastases. Radio-activity can be demonstrated in the lower neck and hypopharynx (Fig. 8A) as well as the upper neck and oral cavity (Fig. 8B). Similarly, Fig. 9 demonstrates a radionuclide scan of a patient treated with a dual catheter pump for an extensive bilateral tongue cancer. No cervical metastases were clinically evident. Radioactivity is concentrated in the tongue musculature suggesting excellent infusion of the tumor.

5. Clinical experience with intra-arterial therapy

Historical developments

The earliest intraarterial injections were for the treatment of infection localized to a specific region. The rationale for intraarterial injection of antiseptic substances was formulated by Parlavecchio [85]. He concluded that the procedure was a feasible method of obtaining a high concentration of a therapeutic agent in a diseased tissue. Ransohoff [86] in 1910 introduced anesthesia in the upper extremities by the intraarterial infusion of 4 to 8 ml of 0.5% cocaine. He utilized a tourniquet to retard venous outflow from the extremity, thus concentrating the cocaine within the extremity while minimizing systemic effects of the drug. In 1925, Hirsch, Myerson and Halloran [87] treated patients with paresis from neurosyphillus with intracarotid infusion of arsenical preparations. Initially, they surgically exposed the carotid artery on repeated occasions to administer chemotherapy. However, repeated incisions became a limiting factor and led them to develop a technique of percutaneous injection.

The accidental administration of nitrogen mustard into the brachial artery of a patient with Hodgkin's disease produced erythema, followed by vesiculation and ulceration of the hand and forearm. Eventually the intense local reaction subsided and no irreversible changes were observed. This suggested that intraarterial injection of nitrogen mustard could produce, within the vascular territory of an artery, an intense reaction from which normal tissue could recover. Thus was born a new method for treating regional carcinoma that had an accessible arterial blood supply. Klopp and his co-workers [38] in 1950 were the first to use intraarterial infusion chemotherapy. They administered nitrogen mustard to several head and neck cancer patients and reported effects not obtained by the intravenous administration of therapeutic amounts of the same drug. In 1951, Barberio et al. [88] administered nitrogen mustard to dogs and showed that the survival times of animals given divided doses of intraarterial nitrogen mustard was increased over those of dogs given the same amount as a single daily injection. Cromer et al. [40] treated 16 patients with carcinoma of the cervix and vagina in 1952 using intraarterial chemotherapy.

Until the late 1950's, the administration of intraarterial chemotherapy agents was largely confined to alkylating agents. Use was limited, however by lack of specificity of nitrogen mustard and the severe toxicity to normal tissue. A number of antimetabolites were studied by the intraarterial route including azaserine, 5-fluorouracil (5-FU) and methotrexate (MTX) [89]. It soon became apparent that single daily arterial administration of these agents resulted in toxic and therapeutic effects similar to those seen with the systemic route of administration. Thus unlike the alkylating agents, the antimetabolites did not demonstrate enhancement of activity by the intraarterial route. Recognition that antimetabolites required a more prolonged duration of drug exposure to achieve maximum antitumor effects directed attention toward prolonging the duration of intraarterial administration.

Clarkson and Lawrence Jr. [90] studied head and neck cancer patients receiving intra-arterial methotrexate or a fluoropyrimidine and confirmed that a 3- to 4-fold higher concentration of methotrexate was present in the distribution of the external carotid artery compared to the concentration in the systemic circulation. Methotrexate (5 mg per day) or 5-fluorodeoxyuridine (5-FUdR) (1.5 mg/kg/24 h) were administered for 5 to 7 days before toxicity developed. The authors recommended treating to the point of development of local or systemic toxicity.

Sullivan, Miller and Sikes [50] treated head and neck cancer, in addition to other tumors, with continuous intraarterial infusion of methotrexate and gave leucovorin intramuscularly every 6 h. Partial or complete responses were observed in 10 of 18 patients treated. In order to evaluate the importance of the intraarterial route of administration, another series of patients received comparable courses of therapy with continuous intravenous methotrexate and intermittent leucovorin factor. The authors concluded that continuous 24-h administration of methotrexate increased toxicity and presumably antitumor effect of a given dose 10-fold or more compared to bolus IV administration.

The methotrexate-leucovorin combination was used by Nahum and Rochlin [27] in 42 advanced head and neck cancer patients. Patients that demonstrated significant regression of tumor were treated with surgical excision and it was in this group that results appeared to be most favorable. Tumor regression was usually noted by the second or third week of intraarterial chemotherapy.

Sullivan et al. [89] reported on the use of several different intraarterial pharmacologic agents. In addition to methotrexate-leucovorin, the authors tested 5-FU (7.5 to 15 mg/kg/24 h) and FUdR (0.5 mg/kg/24 h). Of the 63 patients receiving an adequate course, 38 showed a partial regression of tumor and 15 demonstrated complete regression of neoplasm.

Westbury treated 59 patients and recommended intermittent intraarterial injection of chemotherapeutic agents [91]. Ten of these patients showed complete clinical regression using methotrexate with and without leucovorin or methotrexate in combination with vinblastine. He recommended continuation of intraarterial therapy until the tumor appeared static or complete clinical regression was observed.

The fluoropyrimidines have been used for intraarterial therapy in head and neck cancer for three decades [89, 92]. Johnson and colleagues [93] treated 70 patients with head and neck cancer using 5-FU. Most patients received 15 mg/kg/day for 4-5 days followed by 7.5 mg/kg/day for several more days. Objective response of greater than 50% reduction of tumor size occurred in 15 (36%) of the patients, 12 (17%) demonstrated objective responses of less than 50%. Freckman [94] treated 36 head and neck cancer patients with intraarterial 5-FU (500 mg/24 h for 10–14 days). Results were similar to Johnson et al. with 12 (33%) patients responsing to therapy. The toxicities observed included mucositis and skin erythema in the infused area.

Bleomycin produces a 20%–25% objective response rate in head and neck cancer when given systematically [95]. Bitter [96] using cobalt-57 tagged bleomycin, demonstrated higher tumor concentrations of the drug with intraarterial administration compared to the same dose given systemically. Intraarterial bleomycin used as a single agent or in combination with methotrexate has produced response rates ranging from 18% to 70% [82, 97–101]. Burkhardt and Holtje [97] used 9 to 12 units daily for a median of 32 days and noted 5 of 7 complete remissions. However, Richard and Sancho [98] gave 30 units over 10 to 12 h daily for 6–10 days to 27 patients and obtained responses in only 5 patients. The major toxicity observed has been stomatitis and skin rash in the perfused region. Pulmonary toxicity was observed with high cumulative doses.

Cisplatin is a highly active agent in squamous cell carcinoma of the head and neck. Response rates of 27% to 31% have been achieved in systemic single agent trials [102, 103]. The dose limiting toxicity is renal impairment. Stomatitis and myelosuppression are uncommon. Madajewica et al. [104] examined the organ distribution of intracarotid and extracarotid cisplatin in dogs. Five fold lower renal levels of platinum were found following intracarotid injection. In a phase I study of intracarotid cisplatin, Stewart et al. [105] noted only mild to moderate systemic toxicity, however, severe local-central nervous system (CNS) and retinal toxicity was observed at doses greater than 60 mg/M^2. Calco et al. [106] in a phase I-II trial of percutaneous intra-arterial cisplatin for regionally confined malignancy (excluding the internal carotid artery) documented a safe starting dose of 120 mg/M^2. An overall response rate of 45% was noted with significant responses observed among patients with melanoma, sarcoma, breast carcinoma and neuroblastoma. Side effects included transient renal and bone marrow toxicity as well as neurotoxicity and ototoxicity (6%), the latter usually with residual damage. Lehane et al. [107] treated twenty-six patients with head and neck cancer (19 had no prior therapy) with 100 mg/M^2 of intra-arterial cisplatin infused over one hour and observed responses in 25 patients. No local-regional toxicity was observed. All patients had mild to moderate nausea and vomiting.

Cisplatin may be uniquely active in adenoid cyctic carcinoma of the salivary glands. A multi-institutional survey conducted by Suen and Johns [108] reported on 53 patients with adenoid cystic carcinoma of the head and neck treated with single (45 patients) or multiple drugs (7 patients). The overall response rate to cisplatin (64%) was substantially higher than with other agents. Sessions et al. [109] reported on four patients with adenoid cystic carcinoma treated with intraarterial cisplatin. Responses suggested that this method may be a useful adjunct in the management of this tumor both as a preoperative as well as palliative measure.

Mitomycin-C has not been extensively evaluated in head and neck cancer.

The results from cumulative series suggests a 20% objective response rate with systemic therapy [110]. Intraarterial mitomycin-C has been utilized for head and neck cancer, cancer of the cervix, and for primary or metastatic disease in the liver [111–113]. In a recent study, Tseng et al. [114] found lower systemic blood levels (and less toxicity) when mitomycin-C was given intraarterially in patients with colon cancer. Pelvic as well as intra-hepatic tumors were treated in this study. Andreasson et al. [115] administered mitomycin C (10–20 mg every 2 weeks) by this method to 15 patients with advanced unresectable cancer obtaining a partial response in six patients. Twenty-six of 30 patients (28 previously untreated) responded to the combination of mitomycin-C and bleomycin. Five of these patients had histologically proven complete remissions. Brismar et al. [116] administered intraarterial mitomycin-C to 15 patients with advanced malignant head and neck tumors. Ten to 20 mg of mitomycin-C diluted in saline to a concentration of 1 mg/ml was injected at a rate of approximately 10 ml/min every other week for up to five injections. In 5 patients the tumor decreased significantly in size. A marked decrease in pain was reported by 9 of the 15 patients.

A number of investigators have reported on multiple drug chemotherapy administered intraarterally for the treatment of head and neck cancer. Donegan and Harris [117] combined intraarterial fluorouracil, methotrexate and bleomycin. In all cases, irradiation and/or surgery had previously failed to control the tumor. Tumor regression occurred in 87% of the cases (13/15) and was complete in three (20%) cases. Regressions lasted up to 13 months. Curioni and Quadu [118] treated 47 patients with squamous cell carcinoma of the oral cavity with intraarterial vincristine, methotrexate, bleomycin and adriamycin or mitomycin-C. Regression of tumor occurred in 29 (62%) patients. All patients then received irradiation. Survival after 18 months was 51%.

Szabo and Kovacs [119] administered intraarterial vincristine, bleomycin, methotrexate, and mitolactol to 72 patients as preoperative, postoperative, or palliative management. Used preoperatively, tumor regression occurred in up to 80% of cases. Tumors of the gingiva, parotid gland, maxilla, and tonsil responded very well in contrast to neoplasms in the tongue.

Quadu treated 97 squamous cell carcinomas with intraarterial vincristine, bleomycin, adriamycin and leucovorin factor rescue. A 68% regression rate was observed, however, a high rate of complications and systemic toxicity was seen [120].

A tri-national (Germany, Austria and Switzerland) group, named DO-SAK, is studying intraarterial bleomycin and methotrexate and has observed that complete responses were more prevalent in patients with smaller primary tumors and with minimal or no cervical lymph node involvement [120]. Bier [121] reported on a pilot study conducted by DOSAK in which intraarterial chemotherapy was used to treat 18 patients with Stage I, II or III head and neck cancer without the addition of the standard treatment of radiotherapy or surgery. Bleomycin (total dose 180 mg) and methotrexate (240 mg/M^2) with leucovorin factor were utilized. Clinically, complete remission (CR) was achieved in 2 of 2 T1 tumors, 7 of 8 T2 tumors and 4 of 8 T3 tumors. CR was achieved in 8 of 10 patients with necks classified as NO, 3 of 5 with N1 necks, and 2 of 2 patients with N2 disease. The 5-year survival of 27% was not impressive, and the author concluded that radiation or surgery should be combined with intraarterial chemotherapy.

Chemotherapy delivered through angiographically placed catheters requires patient hospitalization, and is usually limited to short term infusions. Treatment given through surgically placed catheters with external portable infusion pumps permits greater patient freedom and longer infusion durations. However some patient restrictions remain, and thrombotic or infectious complications are common with long term therapy. The Infusaid Pump described above allows long term intra-arterial therapy in an outpatient population. Patient activity is unrestricted and the complication rate has been low. The authors have used this system to deliver single agent and combination drug therapy. The drug regimens, objective responses and toxicity pattern are detailed in Table 3. The majority of patients have

Table 3. Chemotherapy regimens delivered through the infusaid pump

Agent	# Pts.	Median MTD	Spectrum of Toxicity	Response
DCMTX	6	4 mg/M/d × 14 d. (3.4–6.0)	local-5 pts. systemic 1 pt.	2/5
FUDR	6	0.02 mg/kg/d × 14 d (0.15–0.04)	local-6 pts. systemic 0 pt.	1/3
BLM	5	> 4 u/d × 7 d (1–> 4)	local-1 pt. systemic 0 pt.	0/3
CP/FUDR	10	CP-100 m/M FUDR- 0.02 mg/kg/d × 14 (0.015–0.03)	local-8 pts. systemic 8 pts. *	8/10
MTC/BLM	3	MTC 4 mg/M d 1,5 BLM 4 u/d × 7	local-0 pt. systemic 1 pt.	2/2
MTC/BLM/ DCMTX	7	MTC 3 mg/M d 1,5 BLM 4 u/d × 7 DCMTX 3 mg/M/d × 14	local 5 pts systemic 1 pt.	1/5

* Nausea and vomiting only.

responded to at least one drug program. Seven of fourteen patients who had pumps implanted prior to February, 1982 have received therapy for at least one year, and four patients have had functioning systems for over two years. Systemic toxicity (except for nausea and vomiting with cisplatin) has been uncommon. Further clinical experience with these programs will be necessary to fully establish the objective response rate. However the Infusaid Pump has proven safe, effective and has high patient acceptance.

Intraarterial chemotherapy with irradiation or surgery

The rationale for chemotherapy combined with primary therapy for head and neck cancer is based on the fact that large tumors are rarely cured by radiation or surgery alone. Large tumors are less well vascularized, and a greater number of hypoxic cells are present that are less radiosensitive. Induction chemotherapy which converts a large tumor to a small one may allow standard treatment to be more effective. A second concept is that of radiosensitization by a drug, although there is no good clinical evidence that any chemotherapy agent will effect greater radiotherapy sensitization to tumor compared to normal tissue [1]. A third concept is post operative chemotherapy following standard therapy of head and neck cancer. Chemotherapy drugs may be useful in irradicating residual malignant cells in the area of treatment and metastatic microfoci which may have already developed prior to surgery and irradiation but have not become clinically manifest.

The introduction of intra-arterial chemotherapy led quite early to its combination with other modalities in cancer therapy. Reese et al. [122] administered intraarterial triethylenemelamine, an alkylating agent, in combination with radiation therapy to treat three patients with retinoblastomas. Bolman, Holzaepfel and Barnes [123] used intraarterial nitrogen mustard combined with irradiation to treat various gynecologic malignancies. One group of patients received irradiation before nitrogen mustard and another group received intraarterial nitrogen mustard prior to irradiation. They found when nitrogen mustard preceded radiotherapy, complications were more numerous and more severe. However, patients who had received prior irradiation appeared not to be as responsive to intraarterial chemotherapy as the previously untreated patients.

Mallams, Finney and Balla [124], aware of the radiosensitizing effect of oxygen, treated rats with Walker 256 carcinosarcoma implanted into the hind legs with intraarterial hydrogen peroxide followed by a single dose of irradiation. The left control leg received 1250 r in a single dose. The right leg was infused with hydrogen peroxide and immediately following this, 250 r in a single dose was given. Tumors in the right leg disappeared and were biopsy negative while the control left leg showed no change of the tumor in a five week interval. The rationale of potentiating irradiation with oxygenation was applied clinically by Corgill [125]. He treated head and neck cancer patients by daily infusion of 250 cc of a 0.12% solution of hydrogen peroxide in 5% glucose and water. The one hour infusion was concomitant with 200 r of irradiation. The results in some cases were gratifying.

Latourette and Lawton [126] treated 24 patients, most with head and neck cancer using concomitant regional chemotherapy and vigorous radiation therapy. Continuous intraarterial infusion of 5-FU (5 mg/kg/24 h) for up to two weeks was combined with Cobalt 60 irradiation. Satisfactory tumor regression was observed, along with considerable, but acceptable, toxicity.

Balla *et al.* [127] treated 22 head and neck cancer patients with methotrexate (25 mg/24 h) for 12 consecutive days. Following a four week rest period, surgery or radiation therapy was used in most of the patients. They noted several complications in the group of patients undergoing surgery after chemotherapy.

Jesse [128] compared, in a non-randomized study, intraarterial methotrexate to 5-FU in 38 previously untreated patients with head and neck cancer. Both drugs were used in combination with irradiation. Local control of disease for greater than 15 months was obtained in 14% of those patients receiving methotrexate and radiotherapy and 46% of those receiving 5-FU and radiotherapy. Nervi *et al.* [129] employed intraarterial methotrexate plus vinblastine followed by radiotherapy in 129 patients with head and neck cancer. Using historical controls, the results in Stage II and III disease with induction chemotherapy were equivalent but not superior to results with radiation therapy alone.

Cruz, McInnis and Aust [130] treated 44 advanced head and neck patients with triple therapy consisting of intraarterial infusion, followed by radiotherapy, and, when applicable, wide surgical excision and node dissection. Chemotherapy was administered daily to toxicity (5–16 days), and consisted of 5-fluorouracil (15 mg/kg/d), methotrexate (5 mg/d), and vinblastine 0.02 mg/kg/d). Response to chemotherapy alone was 76% (15% CR, 16% PR). Patients completing both chemotherapy and irradiation but not showing complete (100%) regression of the primary tumor usually died of disseminated disease within a year. Patients with lesions not amenable to standard surgical extirpation died usually within two years, of recurrent disease at the primary site even though they had shown complete regression after combined chemotherapy and radiotherapy. Patients undergoing surgical extirpation of the tumor site fared the best of all if their tumor had responded completely to chemotherapy and preoperative radiotherapy.

Bleomycin intravenous infusion (total dose 180–200 mg) plus intra-arterial methotrexate administered immediately after the bleomycin infusion was combined with radiotherapy (6000 rads) for the treatment of 20 patients with advanced oral carcinoma [131]. Survival after one year was 84% and appeared to be superior to historical controls.

A non-randomized study of the efficacy of combined intraarterial chemotherapy preceding standard treatment was performed by Auersperg and associated [132]. Of the 74 patients with locally advanced carcinoma of the oral cavity and oropharynx, 38 were given radiotherapy and 36 received intraarterial chemotherapy followed by radiotherapy. Intraarterial chemotherapy consisted of methotrexate with leucovorin (7 of 36), bleomycin (5 of 36), methotrexate and bleomycin (7 of 36), methotrexate and podophillic acid ethyl hydrazide (4 of 36), or vinblastine with bleomycin and methotrexate (13 of 36). Intraarterial chemotherapy was continued to complete remission (CR) or maximum objective response. Radiotherapy was commenced 10–14 days after completion of intraarterial chemotherapy. Surgical resection was performed when possible. Intraarterial chemotherapy produced an objective response in 28 of 36 patients and a complete response in 13 of 28 responders. All patients were followed for greater than three years or until death. One of 38 radiotherapy treated and 6 of 36 intraarterial chemotherapy treated patients were free of disease at three years. Median survival times were approximately 6 months with radiotherapy and $11\frac{1}{2}$ months for the chemotherapy group. The chemotherapy group had significantly higher survival rates than the radiotherapy group at 5 to 14 months but not at greater than 14 months. Although intraarterial chemotherapy produced good objective responses, lasting results could not be expected unless intraarterial chemotherapy was supplemented by radiotherapy and surgery.

Utilizing intraarterial vincristine and bleomycin, Demard et al. [133] were able to appreciate tumor regression in 30 of 33 head and neck patients treated with sequential chemotherapy before surgery and/or radiotherapy. Similar results were obtained by Danko et al. [134]. Intraarterial methotrexate (total 35–110 mg) and bleomycin (total 5–65 mg) over 6–19 days, was given to 17 patients with orofacial cancer prior to radiotherapy. Some patients also underwent surgery. All patients demonstrated tumor regression of 30–90%. Five resection specimens contained no evidence of malignant cells.

Molinari [135] utilized combined intraarterial chemotherapy to manage 126 patients with locally advanced epidermoid carcinoma of the head and neck. Various single agents and combinations of drugs were administered prior to surgery or irradiation. Methotrexate plus leucovorin, adriamycin, bleomycin, vincristine plus bleomycin and vincristine, bleomycin, plus methotrexate were analyzed. Three successive cycles of vincristine, bleomycin and methotrexate in combination gave the best results with 74% of 24 patients achieving greater than 50% regression and 47% achieving greater than 75% regression. The 3-year survival rates for combined intraarterial chemotherapy and radiotherapy or surgery in patients with greater than 75% tumor regression induced by chemotherapy was 77% compared to 22% for those achieving less than 75% regression.

Hollmann *et al.* [136] treated 69 patients with advanced maxillofacial cancer with combination intraarterial chemotherapy and radiotherapy. Forty of the patients had previous radiotherapy or surgery and 9 of the 40 had also received previous chemotherapy. Most patients received intraarterial infusions of a combination of methotrexate (25 mg per day with leucovorin factor rescue; and bleomycin (15 mg/day) concomitant with radiation therapy (6500 rads to the primary and 4000 rads to the regional nodes). Planned mean total doses of 500 mg of methotrexate and 300 mg of bleomycin were given to most patients. Fifty-three patients were followed for at least one year or until death. Although the one-year survival rate was low (15/53 evaluable patients) it was the authors impression that the potential benefits of intraarterial chemotherapy and simultaneous radiotherapy justified the expense and risk of treatment.

Zielke-Temme *et al.* [101] treated 20 patients with stage III and IV squamous cell carcinoma of the head and neck with bleomycin and methotrexate prior to high dose preoperative radiotherapy and if possible, subsequent resection. The initial clinical evaluation following intraarterial chemotherapy demonstrated tumor regression in 12 of 18 patients. No complete regressions were noted. After the completion of radiotherapy, 6 of 16 patients demonstrated a complete response and 5 demonstrated a partial response. Ten of 18 (56%) were considered free of disease at the end of all three therapy modalities. The initial clinical response after intraarterial chemotherapy combined with radiotherapy correlated well with the findings in the pathological specimen. Five patients who showed a complete response had resected specimens free of tumor. Only 3 of these patients had a partial response to intraarterial chemotherapy alone. Five patients survived 12 or more months free of disease and four of these had tumors of the maxillary antrum. The authors concluded that general use of intraarterial chemotherapy prior to conventional therapy in advanced tumors of the head and neck was not justified. However, intraarterial chemotherapy may be useful in treating patients with operable stage III carcinoma of the maxillary antrum.

The optimism for intraarterial chemotherapy in combination with primary therapy for nasal and paranasal sinus cancer has been supported by other investigators as well. Goepfert *et al.* [137] used intraarterial 5-fluorouracil (6 mg/kg average dose) in 24 of 26 patients with nasal cavity and paranasal sinus cancer, concomitant with radiotherapy (6000–7000 rads in 6–7 weeks). Determinate two and 5-year survival rates were 48% and 26% respectively. They concluded that their results were equal to those which included maxillectomy as part of the treatment. Nervi *et al.* [138] found no statistically significant difference in the four-year survival rate between 12 patients with carcinoma of the maxillary antrum who received intraarterial chemotherapy and irradiation and 13 patients treated by radiation alone even though 8 of 12 patients did show some tumor regression from the chemotherapy. Moseley *et al.* [139] treated 10 patients with Stage III and IV squamous cell carcinoma of the maxillary sinus using intraarterial bleomycin and methotrexate followed by high dose radiotherapy and surgical resection. Seven of the 10 patients had extensive tumor necrosis in the surgical specimen and no evidence of viable residual tumor was found in four of these patients. After a median follow up period of two years there had been only one local recurrence in resected patients, however, three patients had died from pulmonary metastases. The atypical early metastatic spread of head and neck cancer treated with intraarterial induction chemotherapy has been noted by others [140] and may represent a new problem facing the oncologist as better local-regional control of tumor is achieved.

Only two studies have used concurrent randomized controls to evaluate the efficacy of intraarterial chemotherapy combined with radiotherapy. Nervi and colleagues [129] studied 140 patients with advanced squamous cell carcinoma of the oral cavity, oropharynx, or maxillary antrum. Seventy-two patients were randomized to receive intraarterial methotrexate (90–120 mg in 25–40 days according to tolerance), followed by radiotherapy (7000–7500 rads). Both interstitial and external radiotherapy was given to 38 of the methotrexate-treated patients. The other 68 patients were treated with radiotherapy only. All patients were followed for at least four years. In the methotrexate group, the four year determinate survival rates in patients with Stage I, II, III, and IV disease were 93%, 66%, 40% and 10%, respectively. In the radiotherapy only group, four year determinate survival rates were 50% in Stage II, 41% in Stage III and 10% in Stage IV. There was no advantage overall with the addition of chemotherapy. Methotrexate infusion followed by a combination of external and interstitial radiotherapy gave significantly better local tumor control and survival rates as compared with radiotherapy alone in patients with cancer of the oral cavity (82 patients). These improved results were attributed to the increased use of interstitial radiotherapy in this group of patients rather than to a synergism between methotrexate and radiotherapy.

Bagshaw and Doggett [141] reported a controlled study of intraarterial chemotherapy plus irradiation versus irradiation alone. Local control of disease was achieved in 32% (7/22) of patients receiving methotrexate plus radiation therapy versus 38% (6/16) of patients treated with radiotherapy alone.

In the final analysis, most studies utilizing intraarterial chemotherapy preceded by or followed by irradiation or surgery may have yielded some improvement in short term control but randomized studies have not demonstrated a significant increase in long term survival.

6. Future development in intra-arterial therapy

Intraarterial chemo-embolization

Responding to the need for selectivity in cancer chemotherapy, antineoplastic agents have been microencapsulated with ethylcellulose. Administration of the capsule intra-arterially into the vascular bed of tumors causes trapping within the tumor vasculature and subsequent sustained release of the agent. The sustained release properties of microencapsulated mitomycin-C was first studied in animal experiments [142]. Canine kidneys infused with microcapsules retained active mitomycin C for more than 6 h and showed extensive necrosis 5 days after the infusion. the kidneys infused with non-encapsulated mitomycin C rapidly excreted mitomycin C and showed little histological change. The blood level of mitomycin C released from the intrarenal microcapsules was markedly reduced as compared with control levels. The results suggested that selective infusion of microcapsules containing chemotherapy agents into tumor- supplying arteries could facilitate intensive local chemotherapy with minimal systemic side effects.

Intraarterial infusion of ethylcellulose microcapsules containing mitomycin C apparently exerts it therapeutic effects through infarction and sustained drug action. One hundred thirty patients, none with head and neck cancer, have thus far been treated by Kato and his associates [143, 144] with chemoembolization using microcapsules delivered through percutaneous catheterization of arteries as a pre-operative or palliative measure. Substantial tumor reduction of greater than 30% to 50% was achieved in 65% of the patients and pain relief occurred in 80%.

Intraarterial embolization with radioactive seeds has been employed by Lang and Dekernion [145] to treat advanced renal carcinoma. Fourteen patients were treated by embolization of the affected kidney with I^{125} seeds. The total dose delivered ranged from 1600 to 14,000 rads. A similar approach could be utilized in localized head and neck cancer. The approach would provide a low energy emitter allowing selective high dose radiation of the tumor while sparing the adjacent normal tissues.

Other forms of intraarterial embolization have recently been employed. Kuribayashi *et al.* [146] has used gelatin sponge (gelfoam) embolization to reduce gastrointestinal toxicity of patients receiving intraarterial chemotherapy of the liver. Ivalon granules have been used to obtain peripheral occlusion of arteries that range from 25 to 1 mm in diameter [147]. Ivalon granules are easy to use, reach smaller vessels, and cause a more permanent occlusion than Gelfoam particles.

Selective *in vivo* targeting has been studied in animal models using magnetically responsive albumin microspheres containing chemotherapy agents [148, 149]. Magnetic microspheres containing adriamycin and magnetite (Fe 30) as the magnetically responsive material have been injected into the arterial blood supply of sarcoma implanted into the tails of rats. In the experimental group, the microspheres were magnetically targeted by intraarterial injection of the ventral caudal artery while a 5500 oersted magnetic field was placed adjacent to the tumor. In control animals free adriamycin was injected intravenously and intraarterially while other control animals received microspheres without drug. All of the animals receiving the magnetic microspheres containing drug demonstrated marked or total tumor regression. No deaths or metastases occurred. In contrast, control animals failed to show tumor regression and all died of tumor. Using an animal model, Widder *et al.* [148, 149] have also been successful in targeting I^{125} labeled microspheres using a magnetic field. Targeted chemotherapy has not been attempted in man, however, regions of the body such as the extremities and the head and neck where magnetic fields could be readily applied would be ideal sites for application of this methodology.

Intra-arterial immunotherapy

There has been little in the literature concerning intraarterial immunotherapy. The theoretical basis for advocating such therapy is similar to that of regional chemotherapy, i.e. to concentrate the active antitumor agent in the region of the malignancy. The transfer of passive immunity by intraarterial injection of tumor-immune pig lymph node cells has been used to treat bladder cancer in man [150]. Okuda *et al.* [151] treated 24 patients with maxillary sinus carcinoma by topical application of gelatin sponge saturated with phytohemagglutinin combined with intraarterial infusion of 5-FU and concurrent irradiation. Phytohemagglutinin may have immunostimulating properties and has been observed to cause accumulation of immunocytes at the site of infections. Complete clinical regression of tumor occurred in 83% of the cases treated with phytohemagglutinin vs 53% of a control group. On histological examination, 67% of the phytohemagglutinin group of patients showed no signs of tumor vs. 16% of the control group. Unfortunately, there was no signicant difference between the two groups in the three year crude survival rate (68% phytohemagglutinin group and 62% control group).

7. Summary

Despite decades of experience, the place of intraarterial therapy in the treatment of head and neck cancer remains undefined. Published series have reported a wide range of response rates and complications. The recent development of a totally implantable pump system for intraarterial infusion overcomes the majority of technical impediments to regional therapy and makes long-term intraarterial therapy practical in an outpatient population. Further advances in the regional therapy of head and neck cancer will come from the aggressive application of pharmacologically rational drug combinations in primary and recurrent disease. Ultimately, randomized comparisons of systemic and intraarterial therapy must be conducted to establish the efficacy of a regional approach to chemotherapy.

References

1. Carter SK: The chemotherapy of head and neck cancer. Semin Oncol 4:413–424, 1977.
2. Frei E. III, Canellos GP: Dose: a critical factor in cancer chemotherapy. Am J Med 69:583–594, 1980.
3. Silverberg E: Cancer statistics, 1983. Ca 33:9–25, 1983.
4. Probert JC, Thompson RW, Bagshaw MA: Patterns of spread of distant metastases in head and neck cancer. Cancer 33:127–133, 1974.
5. Million RR, Cassisi NJ, Wittes RE: Cancer in the head and neck. In: DeVita VT, Hellman S, Rosenberg SA (eds). Cancer: Principles & Practices of Oncology. J.B. Lippincott Co., Phil, 1982, pp 301–395.
6. Baker SR, Wheeler RH, Medvec BR: Innovative regional therapy for head and neck cancer. Arch Otolaryngol 108:703–708, 1982.
7. Grant JCB, Batsmajian JV: Grants Method of Anatomy, Baltimore, Williams & Wilkins Co., 1965, p 621.
8. Samson MK, Rinkin SE, Jones SE, Costangi JJ, LoBuglio AF, Stephens Rl, Cummings GD: Dose-response and dose-survival advantage for high versus low dose cisplatin combined with vinbalstine and bleomycin in disseminated testicular cancer: A Southwest Oncology Group Study. Cancer (in press).
9. Wheeler RH, Ensminger WD, Thrall JH, Anderson JL: High dose adriamycin: Exploration of dose response in human neoplasia. Cancer Treat Rep 49:493–498, 1982.
10. Thomas ED: The role of marrow transplantation in the eradication of malignant disease. Cancer 49:1963–1969, 1982.
11. Bruce WR, Heeker BE, Powers WE, Valeriote FA: Comparison of the dose- and time-survival curves for normal hematopoietic and lymphoma colony-forming cells exposed to vinblastine, vincristine, arabinosylcytosine and amethopterin. J Nat Cancer Inst 42:1015–1023, 1969.
12. Mellett LB, Considerations in design of optimal therapeutic schedules. In: Pharmacology and the Future of Man. Proc 5th Int Congr Pharmacology, San Francisco, 1972, Vol 3. Karger, Basal, 1973, pp 332–353.
13. Pinedo HM, Chabner BA: Role of drug concentration, duration of exposure, and endogenous metabolites in determining methotrexate cytotoxicity. Cancer Treat Rep 61:708–715, 1977.
14. Chabner BA, Young RC: Threshhold methotrexate concentration for *in vivo* inhibition of DNA synthesis in normal and tumorous target tissues. J Clin Invest 52:1804–1811, 1973.
15. Bruce Hr, Meeder BE, Valeriote FA: Comparison of the sensitivity of normal hematopoietic and transplanted lymphoma colony-forming cells to chemotherapeutic agents administered *in vivo*. J Nat Cancer Inst 37:233–245, 1966.

16. Young RC, Rosenoff SA, Hyers CE, Btereton H, Chabner BA: Alterations in DNA synthesis induced by chemotherapeutic agents *in vivo*: Potential applications to clinical treatment schedules. In: Drewinko B, Humphrey RM, (eds) Growth Kinetics and Biochemical Regulation of Normal and Malignant Cells. Baltimore, Williams & Wilkins Co., 1977, pp 787–809.

17. Skipper HE, Schabd FM: Quantitative and cytokinetic studies in experimental tumor systems. In: Holland JF, Frei E (eds) Cancer Medicine. Philadelphia, Lea and Febiger, 1982, pp 663–685.

18. Blum RH, Frei E, III, Holland JF: Principles of dose, schedule, and combination chemotherapy. In: Holland JF, Frei E III (eds) Philadelphia, Lea and Febiger, 1982, pp 730–752.

19. Ritch PS, Oichipinti SJ, Skramstad KS, Shackney SE: Increased relative effectiveness of doxorubicin against slowly proliferating sarcoma 180 cells after prolonged drug exposure. Cancer Treat Rep 66:1159–1169, 1982.

20. Jusko WJ: A pharmacodynamic model for cell-cycle-specific chemotherapeutic agents. J Pharmacokin Biopharm. 1:175–200, 1973.

21. Collins JM, Dedrick RL: Pharmacokintics of anticancer drugs. In: Chabner B (ed) Pharmacologic Principles of Cancer Treatment. Philadelphia, W.B. Saunders Co., 1982, pp 77–99.

22. Fensmacher J, Gazendam J: Intra-arterial infusions of drugs and hyperosmotic solutions as ways of enhancing CNS chemotherapy. Cancer Treat Rep 65 (Suppl 2):27–38, 1981.

23. Levin VA, Landahl HD, Patlak CS: Drug delivery to CNS tumors. Cancer Treat Rep 65 (Suppl 2):19–26, 1981.

24. Chen HG, Gross JF: Intra-arterial infusion of anticancer drugs: Theoretic aspects of drug delibery and review of responses. Cancer Treat Rep 64:31–40, 1980.

25. Eckman WW, Pallak CS, Fenstermacher JD: A critical evaluation of the principles governing the advantages of intra-arterial infusions. J Pharmacokin Biopharm 2:257–285, 1974.

26. Wheeler RH, Zeissman HA, Medvec BR, Thrall JW, Keyes JW, Baker SR: Pharmacologic basis for intra-arterial (IA) chemotherapy of head and neck cancer (H & N Ca). Proc Amer Assoc Cancer Res 24:1983.

27. Hahum AM, Rochlin DB: Regional arterial chemotherapy of the head and neck. Surg Gynec & Obst 115:478–483, 1962.

28. Goldman ID: Membrane transport considerations in high-dose methotrexate regimens with leucovorin rescue. Cancer Treat Rep 65(Suppl 1):13–18, 1981.

29. Leyva A, Nederlragt H, Lankelma J, Pinedo HM: Methotrexate cytotoxicity: Studies on its reversal by folates and nucleosides. Cancer Treat Rep 65(Suppl 1):45–50, 1981.

30. Baker SR, Wheeler RH: Long-term intra-arterial chemotherapy infusion of ambulatory head and neck cancer patients. J Surg Oncol 21:125–131, 1982.

31. Gyves JW, Ensminger WD, Thrall J, Cho K, Walker S: Dependence of hepatic tumor vascularity on tumor size. Clin Res 30:747A, 1982.

32. Kaelin WG, Shrevastar S, Shand OG, Jirtle RL: Effect of verapamil on malignant tissue blood flow in SMT-2A tumor-bearing rats. Cancer Res 42:3944–3949, 1982.

33. DeVita VT, Schein PS: The use of drugs in combination for the treatment of cancer. Nejm 288:998–1006, 1973.

34. O'Connell MJ, Powis G, Rubin J, Moertel CG: Pilot study of PALA and 5-FU in patients with advanced cancer. Cancer Treat Rep 66:77–80, 1982.

35. Weiss GR, Ervin TJ, Meshad MW, Kufe DW: Phase II trial of combination therapy with continuous-infusion PALA and bolus-injection 5-FU. Cancer Treat Rep 66:299–303, 1982.

36. Schneierson SS, Blum L: A method of continuous arterial infusion bone marrow and blood levels during the administration of penicillin. Surgery 25:30–35, 1949.

37. Donovan TJ: The uses of plastic tubes in the reparative surgery of battle injuries to arteries with and without intraarterial heparin administration. Ann Surg 130:1024–1043, 1949.
38. Klopp CT, Alfordd TC, Bateman J, Berry GN, Winship T: Fractonated intraarterial cancer chemotherapy with methyl bis amine hydrochloride; a preliminary report. Ann Surg 132:811–832, 1950.
39. Bierman HR, Miller ER, Byron RL Jr, Dod KS, Kelly KH, Black DH: Intraarterial catheterization of viscera in man. Am J Roentgenol 66:555–568, 1951.
40. Cromer JK, Bateman JC, Berry GN, Kennelly JM, Klopp CT, Platt LI: Use of intraarterial nitrogen mustard therapy in the treatment of cervical and vaginal cancer. Am J Obst Gynec 63:538–548, 1952.
41. Jonsson G: Thoracic aortography by means of a cannula inserted percutaneously into the common carotid artery. Acta Radio 31:376–386, 1949.
42. Peirce EC: Percutaneous femoral artery catheterization in man with special reference to aortography. SGO 93:56–74, 1951.
43. Donald DC, Kesmodel KF, Rollins Sl, Paddison RM: An improved technique for percutaneous cerebral angiography. Arch Neurol Psych 65:508–510, 1951.
44. Seldinger Si: Catheter replacement of the needle in percutaneous arteriography. Acta Radio 39:368–376, 1953.
45. Payne M: Intraarterial infusion. Nursing Times 57:1356–1357, 1961.
46. Galvin C: Methotrexate in inoperable cancer. Irish J M Sc 449:223–236, 1963.
47. Krant MJ, Hall TC, Lloyd JB, Patterson WB: Utilization of an air free pump for intraarterial infusion. Cancer Chemother Rep 14:39–43, 1961.
48. Skinner DB, Herbst Al, Austen WG, Raker JW: A simplified technique for intraarterial infusion for regional chemotherapy. SGO 115:242–244, 1962.
49. Duff JK, Sullivan RD, Miller E, Ulm AH, Charlson BC, Clifford P: Antimetabolite-metabolite cancer chemotherapy using continuous intraarterial methotrexate with intermittent intramuscular citovorum factor method of therapy. Cancer 14:744–752, 1961.
50. Sullivan RD, Miller E, Sikes MP: Antimetabolite-metabolite combination cancer chemotherapy; effects of intraarterial methotrexate-intramuscular citrovorum factor therapy in human cancer. Cancer 12:1248–1262, 1959.
51. Tucker JL, Talley RH: Prolonged intraarterial chemotherapy for inoperable cancer; a technique. Cancer 14:493–495, 1961.
52. Ramsden CH, Duff JK: Continuous arterial infusion of Head and neck tumors, improvements in technique by retrograde temporal artery catheterization. Cancer 16:133–135, 1963.
53. Oettgen HF, Duff JK, Clifford P: Problems of continuous chemotherapy by arterial catheters. Arch Surg 86:323–330,1963.
54. Trussell RR, Mitford-Barberton G de B: Carcinoma of the cervix treated with continuous intraarterial methotrexaie and intermittent intramuscular leucovorin. Lancet 1:971–972, 1961.
55. Cahill JJ, Zeit PR: Intraarterial infusion of pelvic tumors with amethopteria. Am J Gynec 81:970–977, 1961.
56. Blaisdell FW, Hall AD, Campagna G: An atraumatic needle for percutaneous arterial catheterization. Am J Surg 106:528–530, 1963.
57. Benson JW, Kiehn CL, Holden WD: Cancer chemotherapy by arterial infusion. Arch Surg 87:125–144, 1963.
58. Goldman ML, Bilbao MK, Rosch J, Dotter CT: Complications of indwelling chemotherapy catheters. Cancer 36:1883–1990, 1975.
59. Helsper JT, DeMoss EV: Regional intraarterial infusion of 5-fluorouacil for cancer. Surgery 56:340–348, 1964.
60. Reemtsma K: Complications of regional cancer chemotherapy by perfusion and infusion techniques. Am J Surg 105:645–648, 1963.

61. Hanna DC, Gaisford JC, Goldwyn RM: Intraarterial nitrogen mustard for control of pain in head and neck cancer. Am J Surg 106:783–785, 1963.
62. Wathins E Jr., Sullivan RD: Cancer chemotherapy by prolonged arterial infusion. SGO 118(1):3–19, 1964.
63. Zimmerman HA, Rand JH III: A pressure pump for administering intraarterial or intravenous fluids. J Lab Clin Med 35:993–994, 1950.
64. Pegg DE, Trotman RE, Pierce NH: Apparatus for continuous infusion chemotherapy. Brit M J 1:1207–1208, 1963.
65. Longden N: Insulation of infusion bottles. Lancet 1:1029–1030, 1963.
66. Addison BA, Jennings ER: A simplified technique for cancer infusion chemotherapy. J M A Georgia 52:203–204, 1963.
67. McDonald IR: An assisted infusion apparatus. M J Australia 50(1):661–662, 1963.
68. Donaldson RC, Paletta FX: An improved method of direct cannulation of the carotid artery for infusion. Am J Surg 106:712–715, 1963.
69. Herter FP, Markowitz AM, Feind CR: Cancer chemotherapy by continuous intraarterial infusion of antimetabolites. Am J Surg 105:628–639, 1963.
70. Kisken HA, Johnson RO, currieri AR: A technique of continuous intraarterial infusion. Cancer Chemother Rep 24:27–28, 1962.
71. Watkins E JR: Chronometric infusor – an apparatus for protracted ambulatory infusion therapy. New England J Med 269:850–851, 1963.
72. Burn Jl, Gains E: The chemofusor: a new apparatus for maintaining continuous intraarterial infusion chemotherapy. Brit J Surg 60(5):375–377, 1973.
73. Rutherford WL: H.D. Anderson: treating cancer on an outpatient basis. Tex Hosp 36:10–12, 1980.
74. Blackshear PJ, Dorman FD, Blackshear PL Jr, Varco RL, Buchwald H: A permanently implantable self-recycling low flow constant rate multipurpose infusion pump of simple design. Surg Forum 21:137, 1970.
75. Blackshear PJ, Dorman FD, Blackshear PL Jr, Varco RL, Buchwald H: The design and initial testing of an implantable infusion pump. SGO 134:51–56, 1972.
76. Blackshear PJ, Rohde TD, Varco RL, Buchwald H: One year of continuous heparinization in the dog using a totally implantable infusion pump. SGO 141:176–186, 1975.
77. Rohde TD, Blackshear PJ, Varco RL, Buchwald H: Chronic heparin anticoagulant in dogs by continuous infusion with a totally implantable pump. Trans Am Soc Artif Intern Organs 21:510–514, 1975.
78. Rohde TDD, Blackshear PJ, Varco RL, Buchwald H: Protracted parenteral drug infusion in ambulatory subjects using an implantable infusion pump. Trans Am Soc Artif Intern Organs 23:13–16, 1977.
79. Dakhil S, Ensminger WD, Kindt G, Niederhuber J, Chandler W, Greenburg H, Wheeler R: An implanted system for ventricular drug infusion in central nervous system tumors. Cancer Treat Rep 65:401–411, 1981.
80. Ensminger W, Niederhuber J, Dakhii S. Thrall J, Wheeler R: A totally implanted drug delivery system for hepatic arterial chemotherapy. Cancer Treat Rep 65:393–400, 1981.
81. Engeset A, Brennhovd I, Stovner J: Intraarterial infusions in cancer chemtherapy, a technique for testing drug distribution. Lancet 1:1382–1383, 1962.
82. Szabo G, Kovacs A: Possibilities of enhancing the effectiveness of intraarterial chemotherapy. Int J Oral Surg 9:33–44, 1980.
83. Rapoport A, Sobrinho J de A, Serson D, Nunes JE De O: The value of I 131 labeled albumin macroaggregate in the localization of intraarterial chemotherapy for the treatment of advanced cancer of the head and neck. TUMORI 60:355–359, 1974.
84. Kaplan WD, Ensminger WD, Come SE, Smith EH, D'Orsi CJ, Levin OC, Takvorian RW, Steele GD Jr: Radionuclide angiography to perdict patient response to hepatic artery chemotherapy. Cancer Treat Rep 64(12):1217–1222, 1980.

342

85. Parlavecchio G: Sul lavaggio antisettico interstizaile dei tessut dolla vie arteriosa. Policlinico (sez Prat) 6:667–674, 1899.
86. Ransohoff JL: Terminal arterial anesthesia. Ann Surg 51:453–456, 1910.
87. Hirsch HL, Myerson A, Halloran RD: Intracarotid route in the treatment of general paresis. New England J Med 192:713–717, 1925.
88. Barberio JR, Klopp CT, Ayres WW, Gross HA: Effects of intraarterial administration of nitrogen mustard. Cancer 4:1341–1363, 1951.
89. Sullivan RD, Miller E, Chryssochoos T, Watkins E Jr: The clinical effects of the continuous intravenous and intraarterial infusion of cancer chemotherapeutic compounds. Cancer Chemother Rep 16:449–510, 1962.
90. Clarkson B, Lawrence W Jr: Perfusion and infusion techniques in cancer chemotherapy. M Clin North Amer 45:689–710, 1961.
91. Westbury G: Regional chemotherapy in amignant disease. Ann Roy Coll Surgeons England 32:358–379, 1963.
92. Oettgen HF, Clifford P, Candler P: Continuous intraarterial or intravenous infusion of 5-FU-2′-deoxyuridine: therapeutic and toxic effects. Cancer Chemother Rep 32:35–46, 1963.
93. Johnson RO, Kisken WA, Curreri AR: A report upon arterial infusion with 5-fluorouracil in 100 patients. Surg Gynec obstet 120:530–636, 1965.
94. Freckman HA: Results in 169 patients with cancer of the head and neck treated by intraarterial infusion therapy. Am J Surg 124:501–509, 1972.
95. Hong WK, Bromer R: Chemotherapy in head and neck cancer. N Engl J Med 308:75–79, 1983.
96. Bitter KJ: Pharmacokinetic behavior of bleomycin-cobalt-57 with special regard to intraarterial perfusion of the maxillofacial region. Maxillofac Surg 4:226–231, 1976.
97. Burkhardt A, Holtje WJ: Effects of intra-arterial bleomycin therapy in squamous cell carcinoma of the oral cavity: biopsy and autopsy examinations. Maxillofac Surg 3:217–230, 1975.Richard JM, Sancho H: Intra-arterial chemotherapy of head and neck tumors: Statistical study of 129 cases treated at the Institute Gustave Roussy. Biomedicine 18:429–435, 1973.
98. Inuyama Y: Vleomycin treatment of head and neck carcinoma in Japan. In: Carter SK, Crooke ST, Umeazwa H (eds) Bleomycin: current status and new developments. New York, Academic Press, 1978, pp 267–277.
99. Matras H, Burke K, Watzek G, Kuhbock J, Potzi P, Dimopoulos J: Concept of cytostatic Therapy in advanced canced cancers of the head and neck. Maxillofac Surg 7:150–154, 1979.
100. Zielke-Temme BC, Stevens KR Jr., Everts EC, Moseley HS, Ireland KM: Combined intrearterial chemotherapy rediation therapy and surgery for advanced squamous cell carcinoma of the head and neck. Cancer 45:1527–1532, 1980.
101. Wittes RE, Cvitkovic E, Shah J, Gerold FP, Strong EW: cis-Dichlorodiammineplatinum (II) in the treatment of epidermoid carcinoma of the head and neck. Cancer Treat Rep 61:359–366, 1977.
102. Stephens R, Coltman C, Rossof A, Samson M, Panettiere F, Al-Sarraf M, Albers D, Bonnet J: cisDichlorodiammineplatinum (II) in adult patients: Southwest Oncology Group Studies. Cancer Treat Rep 63:1609–1610, 1979.
103. Madajewica S, Kanter P, West C, Bhargava A, Prajapati R, Caracandos J, Anellanoasa A, Fitzpatrick J: Plasma, spinal fluid and organ distribution of cisplatinum (DDP) following intravenous (IV) and intracarotid (IC) infusion. Proc Amer Amer Assoc Cancer Res and ASCO 22:176, 1981.
104. Stewart DJ, Benjamin RS, Zimmerman S. Caprioli RM. Wallace S, Chuang V, Clavo D, Samuels M, Bonura J, Loo TL: Clinical pharmacology of intraarterial cis-Diamminedichloroplatinum (II). Cancer Res 43:917–920, 1983.

105. Calvo DB III, Patt YZ, Wallace S, Chuand VP, Benjamin RS, Pritchard JD, Hersch EM, Bodey GP Sr., Havligit GM: Phase I–II trial of percutaneous intraarterial cisdiammine-dichloro platinum (II) for regionally confined malignancy. Cancer 45:1278–1283, 1980.

106. Lehane DE, Sessions R, Johnson P, Gomez L, Horowitz B, Bryan RN, DeSantos L, Zubler MA, Durrance FY: Intraarterial cisplatinum administration for advanced squamous cell carcinoma of the head and neck region. International Head and Neck Oncology Research Conference, Rossly, VA, Sept 1980, Abst #2:11.

107. Suen JY, Johns ME: Chemotherapy for salivary gland cancer. Laryngoscope 92(3):235–239, 1982.

108. Sessions RB, Lehane DE, Smith RJH, Bryan RN, Suen JY: Intraarterial cisplatin treatment of adenoid cystic carcinoma. Arch Otolaryngol 108:221–224, 1982.

109. Crooke ST, Bradner WT: Mitomycin-C: a review. Cancer Treat Rev 3:121–139, 1976.

110. Inuyama Y: Mitomycin C Treatment for head and neck cancer in Japan. Carter SK, Crooke ST (eds) Mitomycin C: Current status and new developments. New York, Academic Press, 1979, pp 173–182.

111. Swenerton KD, Evers JA, White GW, Boyes DA: Intermittant Pelvic infusion with vincristine, bleomycin, and mitomycin-C for advanced recurrent carcinoma of the cervix. Cancer Treat Rep 63:1379–1381, 1979.

112. Misra NC, Jaiswal MSD, Singh RV, Das B: Intrahepatic arterial infusion of combination mitomycin-C and 5-fluoroucacil in treatment of primary and metastatic liver carcinoma. Cancer 39:1425–1429, 1977.

113. Tseng MH, Lucj J, Mittleman A, Ledesma EJ, Berjian RA: Chemotherapy of advanced colorectal cancer with regional arterial mitomycin-C infusion and concomitant measurement of serum derug level. Proc Amer Cancer Res and ASCO 22:359, 1981.

114. Andreasson L, Bjorklunk A, Landberg T, Mattson W, Merke C: Combination chemotherapy of advanced melignant head and neck tumors by means of regional intraarterial infusions and systemic treatment. International Head and Neck Research Conference, Rosslyn, VA, sept 1980, Abst #2.10.

115. Brismar J, Bjorklund A, Elner A, Eneroth C-M: Selective intraarterial cytostatic injections in malignat head and neck tumors. Neuroradiol 16:434–437, 1978.

116. Donegan WL, Harris P: Regional chemotherapy with combined drugs in cancer of the head and neck. Cancer 38:1479–1483, 1976.

117. Curioni C, Quadu G: Clinical of intraarterial polychemotherapy in the treament of carcinoma of the oral cavity. J Maxillofac Surg 6:207–216, 1978.

118. Szabo G, Kovacs A: Intraarterial chemotherapy of head and neck Tumors. Acta Chir Acad Sci Hung 20:49–55, 1979.

119. Muggia FM, Wolf Gt: Intraarterial chemotherapy of head and neck cancer: Worth another look? Cancer Clin Trials 3:375–379, 1980.

120. Bier J: Intraarterial chemotherapy in head and neck cancer: clinical and experimental experience of the DOSAK. Rev Sudam Oncol (Argent); 3:35–40, 1979.

121. Reese AB, Hyman GA, Merriam DR Jr, Forrest AW, Kliegerman MM: Treatment of retinoblastoma by radiation and triethylenemelamine. AMA Arch Ophth 53:503–513, 1955.

122. Bolman RE, Holzaepfel JH, Barnes AC: Intraarterial nitrogen mustard in advanced pelvic malignancies. Am J Obst Gynec 72:1319–1325, 1956.

123. Mallams JT, Finney JW, Balla GA: The use of hydrogen peroxide as a source of oxygen in a regional intra-arterial infusion system. South Med 55:230–232, 1962.

124. Corgill DA: Arterial anticancer drug infusion therapy. Laryngoscope 72:1159–1178, 1962.

125. Latourette HB, Lawton RL: Combined radiation and chemotherapy. JAHA 196:1057–1060, 1963.

126. Balla G, Mallams JT, Hutton S, Aronoff BL, Byrd L: The treatment of head and neck

malignancies by continuous intraarterial infusion of methotrexate. Am J Surg 104:699–704, 1962.

127. Jesse R: Combined intraarterial infusion in radiotherapy for treament of advanced cancer of the head and neck. Front Radiat Ther Oncol 4:126–131, 1969.

128. Nervi, Perrino A, Valente V: Protracted intraarterial chemotherapy with sequential courses of antimitotics and radiotherapy in the treatment of extended head and neck cancer. TUMORI 54:199–219, 1968.

129. Cruz AB Jr, McInnis WD, Aust JB: Triple drug intraarterial infusion combined with x-ray therapy and surgery for head and neck cancer. Am J Surg 128:573–579, 1974.

130. Bitter K: Bleomycin-Methotrexate. chemotherapy in combination with Telecobalt-radiation for patients suffering from advanced oral carcinoma. J Maxillofac Surg 5:75–81, 1977.

131. Auersperg M, Furlan L, Marolt F, Jereb B: Intaarterial chemotherapy and radiotherapy in locally advanced cancer of the oral cavity and oropharynx. Int J Radiat Oncol Biol Phys 4:273–277, 1978.

132. Demard F, Colonna d'Istria J, Jausseran M, Vallicioni J, Gaillot M, Scheider M: Intraarterial sequential chemothetapy in Head and neck tumors. Medical Oncology Abstracts of the 4th Annual Meeting of the Medical Oncology sociaty and the Bi-Annual Meeting of the Immunology and immunotherapy Group, Nice, France, December 2–4, 1978. New York, Springer-Verlag, 1978, p 29.

133. Danko J, Satko I, Durkovsky J: Combined regional chemotherapy and radiation therapy in the treatment of epidermoid carcinoma of the oro-facial region. Neoplasma 26(3):345–350, 1979.

134. Molinari R: Experience with intraarterial chemotherapy prior to surgery or adiotherapy for advanced cancer of the oral cavity. Rev Sudam Oncol (Argent) 3:18–25, 1979.

135. Hollman K, Jesch W, Kuehboeck J, Dimopoulos J: Combined intraarterial chemotherapy and radiation therapy of tumours in the maxillofacial region. J Maxillofac Surg 7:191–197, 1979.

136. Goepfert H, Jesse RH, Lindberg RD: Arterial infusion and radiation therapy in the treatment of advanced cancer of the nasal cavity and paranasal sinuses. Am J Surg 126:464–468, 1973.

137. Nervi C, Arcangeli G, Badaracco G, Cortese M, Morelli M, Starace G: The relevance of tumor size and cell kinetics as predictors of radiation response in head and neck cancer: A randomized study on the effect of intraarterial chemotherapy followed by radiotherapy. Cancer 41:900–906, 1978.

138. Moseley HS, Thomas lr, Everts EC, Stevens KR, Ireland KM: Advanced squamous cell carcinoma of the maxillary sinus, results of combined reginal infusion chemotherapy, radiation therapy and surgery. Am j Surg 141(5):522–525, 1981.

139. Dalley VM: Radiotherapy and chemotherapy in treatment of head and neck cancer. Int J Radiat Oncolo Bio Phys 4:173–179, 1979.

140. Bagshaw M, Doggett RLS: A Clinical Study of chemical radiosensitization. Front Rad Ther Oncol 4:164–173, 1969.

141. Kato T, Nemoto R, Mori M, Kumagai I: Sustained-release properties of microencapsulated mitomycin C with ethylcellulose infused into the renal artery of the dog. Cancer 46:14–21, 1980.

142. Kato T, Nemoto R, Mori H, Takahashi M, Tamakawa Y, Harada M: Arterial chemoembolization with microencapsulated anticancer drug. An Approach to selective cancer chemotherapy with sustained effects. JAMA 245:1123–1127, 1981.

143. Kato T, Shindo M, Mori H, Abe R, Tamakawa Y: Early results of chemoembolization with microencapsulated drugs. UICC Conference on Clinical Oncology, October 28–31, 1981. Lausanne, Switzerland. International Union Against Cancer 131, p 181.

144. Lang EK, DeKernion JB: Transcatheter embolization of advanced renal cell carcinoma

with radioactive seeds. J Urol 126:581–586, 1981.

145. Kuribayashi G, Philips DA, Harrington DP, Bettmann MA, Garnic JD, Come SE, Levin DC: Therapeutic embolization of the gastroduodenal artery in hepatic artery infusion chemotherapy. AJR 137:1169–1172, 1981.

146. Chuang VP, Wallace S: Arterial infusion and occlusion in cancer patients. Sem Roentgenol 16(1):13–25, 1981.

147. Widder KJ, Senyei AE, Ranney DF: Magnetically responsive microspheres and other carriers for the biophycical targeting of antitumor agents. Adv Pharmacol Chemother 16:213–217, 1979.

148. Widder KJ, Morris RM, Poore J, Senyei AE: Selective ratgeting of magnetic microspheres containing adriamycin: Total remission in yoshida sarcoma.bearing rats. Proc am Assoc Cancer Res 21:261, 1980.

149. Symes MD, Eckert H, Feneley RCL, Teresa L, Mitchell JP, Roberts JBM, Tribe CR: Transfer of adoptive immunity by intraarterial injectin of tumor.immunepig lymph node cells. Urology 12:399–401, 1978.

150. Okuda M, Sakaguchi K, Tomiyama S, Takahashi M: Use of phytohemagglutinin in the treatment of maxillary cancer. Arch Otolaryngol 229:127–134, 1980.

15. New drug development in head and neck oncology

MARIO EISENBERGER, DANIEL HOTH and JUAN POSADA
Jr.

Introduction

The role of chemotherapy in the treatment of squamous cell carcinomas of
the head and neck remains limited to palliation. Multiple single agents and
combinations have been tested in patients failing initial treatment (surgery
and/or radiation) resulting in an unclear impact on survival. New approaches under extensive evaluation include: (1) development of new drugs,
(2) testing of evolving new concepts of drug interaction and modulation, (3)
testing of different routes of administration particularly the intraarterial
route with the utilization of new techniques and devices such as prolonged
infusion pumps.

1. Single agents

A large number of antitumor drugs have been tested during the past several
years. Among the most active and thoroughly evaluated of the currently
non-investigational agents are Methotrexate (MTX), Cisplatin (CP) and
Bleomycin (BLM). Several other single agents have been tested in broad
phase II trials that usually include numerous malignancies in a single trial.
This approach, commonly utilized in early years of clinical chemotherapy
research, in most instances did not involve standardized criteria for response and rarely included a sufficient number of patients per disease to
allow for a reliable estimation of true response rates in each disease studied.
A common denominator in all these clinical trials is the persistent short
duration of responses (3–4 months) and limited survival. These patients are
generally in a poor nutritional state with a number of associated medical
illnesses caused mostly by excessive alcohol intake and tobacco use [33].
The variability in responses among similar studies may be related to different distribution of elements of prognostic value in each patient population
studied rather than differences in treatment efficacy.

Gregory T. Wolf (ed), Head and Neck Oncology.
© *1984 Martinus Nijhoff Publishers, Boston. ISBN 0-89838-657-8. Printed in The Netherlands.*

Among the drugs that have been tested are cyclophosphamide [1–4], Chlorambucil [5], Nitrogen mustard [6, 7], Nitrosoureas [8–15], Hydroxyurea [6], Vinblastine [17], Actinomycin-D [18], Mitomycin-C [18], Procarbazine [19]. 5-Fluorocuracil [20–28], Adriamycin [29–30], and Cytosine Arabinoside [31]. Table 1 illustrates the activity found with these agents in clinical trials.

Methotrexate (MTX), one of the most extensively investigated drugs in this disease, has been tested in different doses and schedules. Several contributions to a better understanding of the optimal administration of MTX have been made throughout the approximate 25-year period of use in clinical trials. The reversal (rescue) of methotrexate toxicity with different agents with the primary objective of enhancing antitumor effects has also been extensively evaluated. The agent most widely used for this purpose is Calcium Leucovorin (Folinic acid), which will replenish the depleted pool of reduced folates caused by the action of methotrexate [32]. Several clinical trials designed specifically to identify the most effective dose/schedule of this agent have been performed during the past several years (Table 2) [34–39]. As a single agent methotrexate produces regressions in 25–80% of patients with recurrent and/or metastatic disease [33]. Responses are usually partial with less than 10% of patients experiencing complete remissions.

Table 1. Single agent activity

Drug (ref)	Number of studies	Total number of evaluable patients	Response* (%)
Cyclophosphamide [1–4] (in different doses, schedules, and routes)	4	86	2 CR, 3 PR, 45 Improved
Chlorambucil [5]	1	34	1 CR, 4 PR (14%)
Nitrogen Mustard [6, 7]	2	43	5 Improved
Hydroxyurea [16]	1	11	4 Improved
Vinblastine [17]	1	23	4 PR (17%), 7 Improved
Mitomycin-C [18]	1	4	0
Procarbazine [19] (IV or p.o.)	1	31	3 Improved
5-Fluorouracil [20–28] (Different doses, schedules, and routes)	9	115	2 CR, 5 PR, 26 Improved
Adriamycin [29, 30]	2	88	11 PR (12.5%)

* Improved = Less than 50% reduction in tumor mass following the usual criteria for response or otherwise not quantitated.
CR = Complete response.
PR = Partial response.

Table 2. Randomized clinical trials with different doses/schedules of methotrexate in head and neck cancer

Investigators (Ref) MTX dose/schedule	Response Responders/ Evaluable (%) CR + PR	Comments
Levitt *et al.* [34]		
(a) 80–230 mg/m^2 × 30 hrs infusion Q2 weeks	7/16 (44%)	Not statistically significant
(b) 140–1080 mg/m^2 × 36–42 h infusion Q 2 weeks, with LR 36–42 h after MTX	15/25 (60%)	
Woods *et al.* [35]		
(a) 50 mg/m^2 IV push + LR 24 h later	6/23 (26%)	Not statistically significant,
(b) 500 mg/m^2 IV push + LR 24 h later	7/27 (26%)	(c) more toxic
(c) 5 g/m^2 IV push + LR 24 h later	10/22 (45%)	
DeConti & Schoenfeld [36]		
(a) 40 mg/m^2 IV push weekly	21/81 (26%)	Not statistically significant
(b) 240 mg/m^2 IV push + LR 42 h later, Q 2 weeks	19/80 (24%)	
(c) MTX + LR as in (b) + CTX + ARA-C	14/76 (18%)	
Kirkwood *et al.* [37]		
(a) 40–200 mg/m^2 IV push d 1 IM 4 divised doses/day, Q week LR d 2 & 5	12/19 (63%)	No statistically significant differ- ences. Same median duration of response.
(b) 1–7.5 g/m^2 IV push/week LR 24 h later	9/30 (30%)	Arm (b) more toxic
Tejada *et al.* [38]		
(a) 50 mg/m^2 PO weekly	5/21 (24%)	(b) and (c) significantly superior
(b) 25 mg/m^2 PO d 1 & 2 weekly	13/20 (65%)	in response rates than (a), no dif-
(c) 50 mg/m^2 PO d 1 + CP 20 mg/m^2 IV d 1 Q week	13/21 (62%)	ferences in duration of response and survival. Similar toxicity
Vogler *et al.* [39]		
(a) 125 mg/m^2 PO Q 6 h × 4 Q week + LR	11/49 (22%)	Not statistically significant.
(b) 60 mg/m^2 IV push weekly	19/61 (31%)	Arm (b) more toxic
(c) 15 mg/m^2 Q 6 h/4 weekly	12/44 (27%)	

CR   = complete response.
PR   = partial response.
LR   = leukovorin rescue.
MTX   = methotrexate.
CTX   = cytoxan.
ARA-C = cytosine arabinoside.
CP   = cisplatin.

With the exception of one trial by Tejada *et al.* [38] in which a limited number of patients were studied, no statistically significant differences between different doses and schedules of methotrexate could be observed in the studies illustrated on Table 2. However, because many of the trials involved small numbers of patients, only large differences would be detected in these comparisons. Conversely, in the trials where no differences were found between treatment arms, there was insufficient power to support the 'negative' results. Despite these criticisms, clinical experience suggests that it is highly unlikely that doses/schedules other than the commonly used dose of methotrexate of 40–60 mg/m^2/wk intravenously will result in any significant therapeutic advantage.

Bleomycin (BLM) has been extensively evaluated in several solid tumors and has demonstrated activity against a number of squamous cell carcinomas including those of head and neck origin. Few studies with this drug as a

Table 3. Single agent bleomycin (BLM) in head and neck cancer

Investigators BLM dose/schedule	Response responders/ evaluable (%) CR + PR	Comments
Bonnadona *et al.* [41]		
(a) 10, 15 or 30 mg/m^2 IV × 2/weekly	7/24 (29%)	High incidence of pulmonary
(b) 15 mg/m^2/d × 5–8 IV	17/32 (53%)	toxicity with doses higher than
(c) 30 mg/m^2/d × 8 IV	4/6 (67%)	10 mg/m^2 twice weekly
Overall	28/62 (45%)	
Halnan *et al.* [42]		
30 mg IV or IM twice weekly	24/55 (44%)	Mild pulmonary toxicity
Haas *et al.* [43]		
10 mg/m^2 IV or IM twice weekly	12/64 (19%)	Mild pulmonary toxicity
Yagoda *et al.* [44]		
0.25 mg/kg IV daily until cutaneous or mucosal toxicity	6/46 (13%)	Mucosal and cutaneous toxicity
Durkin *et al.* [45]		
10 mg/m^2 IV or IM twice weekly	5/81 (6%)	6 with pulmonary toxicity (1 severe)
EORTC [46]		
10–20 mg/m^2/d × 10–38 days IV or IM (total 150–820) or 20 mg/m^2 IV twice weekly	9/54 (17%)	Mucosal, cutaneous, and pulmonary toxicity
Wasserman *et al.* [47]		
Review of multiple doses/schedules	24/158 (15%)	–

single agent have been reported in the literature. The majority of these trials were broad Phase II trials involving other solid tumors. Response rates with Bleomycin have ranged from 6–45% (Table 3) [41–47]. The most important toxic effects associated with this drug were muco-cutaneous and fever and chills. Pulmonary toxicity has been observed more frequently when total cumulative doses exceeded 300 mg. Because of the relative mild hematological toxicity and lack of overlaping toxic effects with other agents, Bleomycin rapidly advanced into trials of drug combinations [40].

Cis-Dichlorodiamine-Platinum II (CP) has shown significant antitumor activity in a variety of experimental tumors and has been proven, in subsequent clinical trials, to be one of the most active agents currently available for the treatment of several human malignancies [48]. Despite its widespread use in head and neck cancer only a few Phase II trials have been done with this drug as a single agent in this disease. The dose limiting toxicity is primarily renal which may be prevented by vigorous hydration and induced

Table 4. Single agent cisplatin (CP) in head and neck cancer

Investigator CP dose/schedule	Responses responders/ evaluable (%) CR + PR	Comments
Wittes *et al.* [50] 2.5–4.5 mg/kg Q 3 weeks with hydration and mannitol	8/26 (31%)	Mostly reversible mild renal toxicity. Mild myelosuppression
Jacobs *et al.* [51] 80 mg/m^2 24 h-infusion Q 3–4 weeks	9/29 (31%)	Mild myelosuppression, renal toxicity or nausea and vomiting (N & V)
Panetiere *et al.* [52] 50 mg/m^2 d 1 & 8 Q 4 weeks	16/65 (25%)	Moderate reversible renal toxicity, N & V
Creagan *et al.* [53] 90 mg/m^2 24 h-infusion with hydration and mannitol	4/23 (17%)	Moderate/severe N & V. Mild renal and hematological toxicity
Sako *et al.* [54] (a) 120 mg/m^2 IV, Q 3 weeks (b) 20 mg/m^2 IV × 5 days, Q 3 weeks. Hydration and mannitol with both regimens	5/15 (33%) 4/15 (27%)	Significant nephrotoxicity and neurotoxicity with both regimens
Randolph & Wittes [55] 50 mg/m^2/wk no prehydration or induced diuresis	4/13 (30%)	Significant nephrotoxicity in 50%, myelosuppression and N & V

diuresis [49]. Overall responses are observed in approximately 30% of patients with recurrent and/or metastatic disease and, as with other active agents, are mostly of short duration. Table 4 illustrates the trials with this agent alone [50–55]. Since nephrotoxicity can be reasonably prevented, nausea and vomiting, especially with higher doses, became the most significant toxic effect with this drug. Analogs of this compound with a different spectrum of toxicity are under active development (see section on investigational agents).

2. Combination chemotherapy

With the identification of more than one active single agent in this disease and due to the evolving evidence supporting the use of combination chemotherapy in other diseases, such as breast cancer and malignant lymphomas, a large number Phase II clinical trials with two or more drugs have been performed. Table 5 illustrates the results with combinations using the three most extensively investigated agents, Methotrexate, Bleomycin and Cisplatin [56–66]. Despite significant variability in response rates, durations

Table 5. Phase II trials with combinations using CP, BLM and/or MTX in head and neck cancer

Investigators Treatment	Response Responders/ Evaluable (%) CR + PR	Duration of response	Comments
Yagoda *et al.* [56] BLM 15 mg IV MTX 15 mg/m² IV at 4–14 d. intervals	8/15 (53%)	3 + mos (mean)	Mild reversible mucositis
Broquet *et al.* [57] BLM 15 mg IV/weekly MTX 0.6 mg/kg IV/weekly	9/15 (60%)	9 weeks (mean)	Severe hematological and pulmonary toxicity
Medenica *et al.* [58] BLM 15 mg IV/weekly MTX 0.6 mg/kg IV/weekly	13/26 (50%)	35 weeks (mean)	Mild hematological toxicity only
Wittes *et al.* [59] CP 2 mg/kg IV Q 3 weeks BLM 0.25 mg/kg IV daily until toxicity followed by 1–2 mg/day/daily	3/24 (13%)	4 mos (median)	Severe nephrotoxicity

Table 5. Phase II trials with combinations using CP, BLM and/or MTX in head and neck cancer (continued)

Investigators Treatment	Response Responders/ Evaluable (%) CR + PR	Duration of response	Comments

Pitman *et al.* [60]
(a) CP – 80 mg/m² hrs inf.
     Q 2 wks with hydra-
     tion followed by MTX
     3 g/m² IV 1 h Q week
     with LR
	6/9	–	(a) Had more nephrotoxicity,
			myelosuppression and mucositis

(b) MTX followed by CP
     same dose and sche-
     dules
	6/11	–	

Moran *et al.* [61] MTX – 30 mg/m² d 1–5 CP – 50–60 mg/m² IV d 2 repeat Q 22 days	8/23 (35%)	4 mos (median)	Mild stomatitis and leukopenia reversible nephrotoxicity (mild)
Ervin *et al.* [62] CP – 20 mg/m² d 1–5 BLM – 10 mg/m² d 3–7 cont. infusion MTX – 200 mg/m² d 15 & 22 +LR Q 4 weeks × 2	26/26 (100%)	–	Median duration of response for the entire group not available. 15/26 had received no prior treatment (surgery/RT)
Vogl & Kaplan [63] MTX – 40 mg/m² IM d 1 & 15 BLM – 10 mg IM d 1, 8 & 15 CP – 50 mg/m² IV d 4 with hydration & diuresis	19/31 (61%)	PR 3 mos CR 7+mos (median)	Mild myelosuppression and azotemia
Caradonna *et al.* [64] BLM – 15 mg/m² IV d 1 Q 2 wks × 4 MTX – 20 mg/m² IV d 1 Q 2 wks × 4 CP – 120 mg/m² IV d 2 Q 10 wks hydration and diuresis maximum 2 courses	14/19 (74%)	4 mos (median)	Moderate/severe pulmonary, renal and bone marrow toxicity.
Murphy *et al.* [65] CP – 100 mg/m² d 2 hydration and diuresis MTX – 30 mg/m² IV d 1 & 15 BLM – 30 mg d 1 weekly × 6 (max 180 mg)	11/24 (46%)	5 mos (median)	Moderate to severe nephrotoxic- ity, N & V, neuropathy, pulmon- ary fibrosis and myelosuppres- sion

Table 5. Phase II trials with combinations using CP, BLM and/or MTX in head and neck cancer (continued)

Investigators Treatment	Response Responders/ Evaluable (%) CR + PR	Duration of response	Comments
Von Hoff *et al.* [66] CP - 50 mg^2 d 1 hydration BLM - 6 mg/m^2 SQ Q 8 h × 12, d 1-4 MTX - 7.5 mg/m^2 IM d 4-6	9/26 (35%)	3 mos (median)	Significant renal, bone marrow, mucosal toxicity. Severe N & V 2 cases of pulmonary fibrosis

CP = Cisplatin.
BLM — Bleomycin.
MTX = methotrexate.
LR = Leukovorin Rescue.

of response were almost uniformly short throughout most of these studies. The toxicity observed with combination containing Cisplatin and Methotrexate, particularly when the latter agent was used in high doses, suggested a possible higher incidence of nephrotoxicity than with either agent used alone. Pitman's study [60], involving a relatively small number of patients, however, suggests that the timing and order of administration of these drugs may be an important determinant of toxicity. The administration of MTX prior to CP in that trial was followed by less renal and other toxicity than the reverse order. Vogl and Kaplan [55] observed high response rates with minimal toxicity using MTX at smaller doses followed by CP four days later. The introduction of other antifolates with similar mechanisms of action to the parent compound but with a different route of metabolism and excretion, such as Di-Chloromethotrexate (DCM), may reduce the nephrotoxicity and consequently improve the therapeutic index of that combination.

Other trials using multi-drug combinations are illustrated in Table 6 [67–83]. In some cases, combinations were based on specific rationale such as *in vitro* and *in vivo* kinetic interactions of multiple drugs as tested by Price and Hill [68], the partial synchronizing effects of one drug (Bleomycin) to cell cycle specific agent(s) [79–82], or the pharmacological synergism *in vitro* between two drugs such as with sequential methotrexate and 5-Fluoruouracil [73–75]. The encouraging initial results observed by one group of investigators with certain combinations unfortunately have not always been confirmed by others.

Table 6. Phase II trials with multidrug combinations

Investigators Treatment	Response responders/ evalua- ble (%) CR + PR	Duration of response	Comments
Wheeler & Baker [67] VCR – 2 mg IV d 1 & 29 Mito-C – 15 mg/m^2 IV d 1 BLM – 20 u/day × 4 by cont. inf. ± MTX 30 mg/m^2 IV/weekly on day 6	19/26 (73%)	18 weeks (median)	Severe pulmonary toxicity attributed to BLM and Mito-C
Price & Hill [68] every 2–3 weeks VCR – 2 mg IV at 1 h BLM – 60 mg cont. infusion from 12 to 18 h MTX – 100 mg IV at 12, 15 & 18 h Hydrocortisone – 500 mg IV at 12 and 18 h 5-FU – 500 mg IV at 18 h Leucovorin – 15 mg PO or IM Q 6 h × 4 starting at 26 h	20/40 (50%)	NA*	Minimal toxicity
Raafat & Oster [69] Same as Price & Hill	2/15 (13%)	5 wks and 28 wks	Moderate hematological toxicity, substantial mucositis
Creagan *et al.* [70] CTX – 400 mg/m^2 ADM – 40 mg/m^2 CP – 40 mg/m^2 without hydration or induced diuresis every 4 weeks	16/25 (64%)	7 mos (median)	Moderate/severe myelosuppression, N & V and mucositis
Creagan *et al.* [71] CTX – 400 mg/m^2 ADM – 40 mg/m^2 CP – 20 mg/m^2 with hydration only Q 4 wks	0/12	–	As above
Creagan *et al.* [72] CTX – 200 mg/m^2 ADM – 30 mg/m^2 CP – 90 mg/m^2 with hydration and diuresis	7/17 (41%)	4.6 mos (median time to progression)	Severe N & V

Table 6. Phase II trials with multidrug combinations (continued)

Investigators Treatment	Response responders/ evalua- ble (%) CR+PR	Duration of response	Comments

Pitman *et al.* [74]
  MTX – 125–250 mg/m² IV
  5-FU – 600 mg/m² 1 h
  after MTX
	25/35 (71%)	3.6 mos
		(median)
			Moderately severe hematological
			and diarrhea

Jacobs *et al.* [75] same as Pitman *et al.* [74]	5/30 (17%)	4+,5,5,7+, 19+ mos	Severe neutropenia and diarrhea

Brown *et al.* [76[
  VLB – 4 mg/m² IV d 1
  BLM – 15 mg/d IM d 1–7
  BLM – 15 mg/d IM d 1–7
  CP – 60 mg/m² IV 6 h
  inf. on day 8 with induced
  diuresis every 3 wks
	10/22 (45%)	4 mos
		(median)
			Mostly myelosuppression and
			N & V

Amer *et al.* [77]
  VCR – 0.5 mg/m² IV d 1 & 4
  BLM – 30 mg/d cont. infusion
  d 1–4
  CP – 120 mg/m² IV d 6 with
  hydration and diuresis
	13/27 (48%)	NA	1 fatal nephrotoxicity episode

Kish *et al.* [78]
  CP – 100 mg/m² IV with hy-
  dration and diuresis
  5-FU – 1000 mg/m²/day in a
  Q 6 h cont. infusion every 3
  weeks
	23/26 (88%)	NA	Mild/moderate myelosuppression

Eisenberger *et al.* [79]
  BLM – 15 mg/m² IV d 1
  Hydroxyurea – 1000 mg/m²
  d 8–15 every 2 weeks
	9/19 (47%)	130 days
		(median
		time to
		progression)
			Mild to moderate myelosuppres-
			sion, 1 fatal pulmonary fibrosis

Medenica *et al.* [80]
  BLM – 15 mg IV/weekly
  MTX – 0.6 mg/kg/week
  Hydroxyurea – 1000 mg/m²
  PO 3 × week
	21/32 (66%)	Mean
		43 wks CRs
		35 wks PRs
			Mild to moderate myelosuppres-
			sion

Table 6. Phase II trials with multidrug combinations (continued)

Investigators Treatment	Response responders/ evaluable (%) CR + PR	Duration of response	Comments
Constanzi *et al.* [81] BLM – 7.5 mg/m² in 48 h cont. inf. MTX – 30 mg/m² IV d 3 alternating with BLM as above and: Hydroxyurea – 2 g/m² PO d 3	10/17 (59%)	1–8 mos	Mild to moderate myelosuppression
Cortes *et al.* [82] BLM – 15 u/24 h d 1–3 cont. infusion CTX – 500 mg IV d 5 MTX – 50 mg IV d 5 5-FU – 500 mg IV d 5 every 3 weeks × 8	21/39 (54%)	Median CR-11 mos PR-7 mos	Mild myelosuppression
Plasse *et al.* [83] BLM – 8.5 u/m²/day cont. inf. × 3 days (d 1–4, 8–11) followed on days 5 & 12 by: CTX – 300 mg/m² MTX – 30 mg/m² 5-FU – 300 mg/m² every 28 days	5/24 (21%)	3.9 mos (median)	Severe pulmonary toxicity in 2 patients (1 fatal)
Rozencweig *et al.* [83a] MTX – 40 mg/m² IV or IM days 1 and 15 BLM – 10 mg IV or IM days 1, 8, 15 VCR – 2 mg IV days 1, 8, 15 CP – 50 mg/m² day 4 every 28 days	37/76 (49%)	CR-28 wks PR-16 wks (median)	Mild renal and myelotoxicity. 55% stomatitis in previously irradiated patients

* NA – not available.

3. Prospective randomized clinical trials comparing single agents and combination chemotherapy

Although an overall comparison of single agent Phase II trials with combination studies may suggest the superiority of combination programs in relation to single agents, the potential variability of prognostic factors among studies and the higher toxicity observed with combinations compared to single agents are among the reasons cited for the need for prospective randomized comparisons.

Only two trials comparing single agents have been reported in the literature recently. Hong *et al.* [84] compared CP (50 mg/m^2 IV push on days 1 & 8, repeated at 4-week intervals) to MTX (40–60 mg/m^2 IV push weekly), and observed responses in 6/21 (20%) in the CP arm and 4/17 (23%) receiving MTX. Duration of response and survival were quite similar for both treatment programs. A qualitative and quantitative evaluation of toxicity prompted the investigators to conclude that MTX had better overall tolerance. A second trial by Lehane *et al.* [85] compared CP in the same dose and schedule used by Hong *et al.* [84] to MTX (15 mg/m^2 IM, days 1–3, every three weeks), and found that 4/44 (9%) and 11/36 (30%) responded to CP and MTX respectively. These differences, however, were not statistically significant. As with the other trial, methotrexate appeared to be better tolerated, but responses were of short duration. Because of the relatively small number of cases per trial, particularly in Hong's study [84] there is a significant chance for a false negative result (beta error) in these trials.

Table 7 lists trials comparing combinations to single agents. As can be seen, no statistically significant differences were observed between treat-

Table 7. Randomized studies of combinations versus single agents

Investigators Treatment	Responses responders/ evaluable (%) CR + PR	Median duration of response	Median survival	Comments
Lehane *et al.* [86]				
(a) MTX – 15 mg/m^2/day 1–3 IM Q 3 weeks vs.	34/105 (33%)	17 wks	29 wks	(b) Slightly more myelotoxic
(b) MTX – 15 mg/m^2 day 1–3 IM MeCCNU – 200 mg/m^2 PO d 1 BLM – 12, 5 mg/m^2 IM on wks 3, 4, 5 & 6 repeated Q 6 wks	23/91 (26%)	14 wks	25 wks	
Williams *et al.* [87]				
(a) MTX – 45–60 mg/M^2 IV/wkly vs.	11/68 (16%)	21 wks	29 wks	(a) More myelotoxicity & mucositis

Table 7. Randomized studies of combinations versus single agents (continued)

Investigators Treatment	Responses responders/ evaluable (%) CR + PR	Median duration of response	Median survival	Comments
(b) CP – 60 mg/m² d 1 VLB – 0.1 mg/kg d 1 & 15 BLM – 15 u IV weekly	13/66 (20%)	16 wks	23 wks	(b) More renal and GI toxicity
Vogl & Schoenfeld [88] (a) MTX – 40–60 mg/m²/ wks vs.	29/83 (35%)	5 mos	5.6 mos	(b) More toxic
(b) MTX – 40 mg/m² d 1 & 15 BLM – 10 mg IM d 1, 8, 15 CP – 50 mg/m² IV d 4	39/81 (48%)	5.8 mos (median time to progression)	5.6 mos	
Jacobs *et al.* [89] (a) CP – 80 mg/m² Q 3 wks vs.	7/41 (18%)	210 days	370 days	(b) More toxic
(b) CP – 80 mg/m² Q 3 wks MTX – 250 mg/m²+LR	13/39 (33%)	140 days	267 days	
Davis & Kessler [90] (a) CP – 3 mg/kg IV over 4–6 h with induced diuresis vs.	4/30 (13%)	4.2 mos	NA	More myelosuppression on arm (b) (severe), nephrotoxicity, N & V in both (a) & (b)
(b) CP – as above MTX – 50 mg/m² IV d 1 & 15 BLM – 15 mg/m² IV twice/week repeated Q 4 weeks	3/27 (11%)	5.2 mos	NA	
De Conti & Schoenfeld [91] (a) MTX 40 mg/m² IV push/wkly vs.	21/81 (26%)	105 days	154 days	(c) more myelotoxic, (a) more mucositis
(b) MTX – 240 mg/m² IV push+LR Q 2 weeks vs.	19/80 (24%)	42 days	133 days	
(c) MTX+LR as in (b) CTX – 0.5 g/m² IV push ARA-C – 300 mg/m² IV	14/76 (18%)	49 days	98 days	
Tejada *et al.* [92] (a) MTX – 50 mg/m² PO/wkly vs.	5/21 (24%)	NA	NA	No differences in toxicity, duration

Table 7. Randomized studies of combinations versus single agents (continued)

Investigators Treatment	Responses responders/ evaluable (%) CR + PR	Median duration of response	Median survival	Comments
(b) MTX – 25 mg/m² PO d 1,2/wkly vs.	13/20 (65%)	NA	NA	of responses and survival
(c) MTX – 50 mg/m² PO d 1, CP – 20 mg/m² IV d 2 weekly	13/21 (62%)	NA	NA	

ments in any of the studies [86–92]. Although some studies showed differences, they were not statistically significant. Furthermore, these differences usually have not resulted in any impact on duration of response and survival. In one study of Williams *et al.* [87] comparing the combination of CP, BLM and vinblastine to methotrexate alone (Table 7), the overall response rates were similar for each arm. However, when patients with distant metastatic disease (one third of all patients in each arm) were analyzed separately a statistically significant difference favoring the combination was observed (combination 43.5% vs. MTX 9.5% $p \leq 0.01$). This finding has not been confirmed by other investigators [86, 88, 91].

Table 8. Investigational drugs evaluated in advanced head and neck cancer

Agent (Ref)	No. evaluable patients	% response
Methyl G [96–98]	69	25
Amsacrine [101, 102]	43	7
Vindesine [103–105]	56	12
Diaziquone [108]	18	0
Dianhydrogalactitol [109]	28	0
Dibromodulcitol [110, 111]	25	16
Etoposide (VP–16) [114, 115]	31	6
PALA [116, 98]	65	4
Bisantrene [117, 118]	21	4
Ftorafur [119]	14	7
Pyrazofurin [120]	22	9
Maytansine [121]	31	3
Thioprolin [122]	16	0
ICRF 159 [123]	23	9

4. Investigational single agents

There is a good reason to search for effective new drugs in the treatment of these groups of tumors, since the available drugs for treatment of head and neck cancer are limited in number and effectiveness. Many investigational agents [93–134] have been studied in patients with advanced cancer. These trials are described below and summarized in Table 8.

Methyl G

Methylglyoxal-bis (guanylhydrazone), also known as Methyl G, Methyl GAG or mitoguazone, has been in clinical trials for over 20 years [93]. In the early 1960's the drug was administered on a daily schedule and produced substantial antitumor activity but at the cost of severe toxicity [94]. Almost 20 years later, Knight *et al.* [95] designed a weekly infusion schedule that was associated with acceptable toxicity. The findings suggested antitumor activity in a wide variety of solid tumors. Kelsen and co-workers conducted a trial at Memorial Sloan-Kettering Cancer Center [96] with Methyl G that yielded one minor and two partial regressions among 10 evaluable patients with head and neck cancer who were previously treated with cisplatinum, bleomycin or MTX. A study by the Walter Reed Army Medical Center group using weekly infusion of Methyl G showed significant activity in relapsed squamous cell carcinomas of the head and neck [97]. Nine of 22 patients (41%) responded, including 2 complete and 7 partial responses; all of the patients had failed conventional radiotherapy and surgery, and 15 had received prior chemotherapy. The Eastern Cooperative Oncology Group [98] entered 100 patients into a study to assess the activity of Methyl G and PALA. Of 50 patients treated with Methyl G, 37 received and adequate course (more than 4 weeks of therapy at 600 mg IV weekly) and 6 (16%) obtained a PR. The median duration of response and survival was two months and three months respectively. Almost all patients had prior radiation (99%) or chemotherapy (93%). One Methyl G responder had no prior chemotherapy. In summary, in three studies, 17/69 evaluable patients demonstrated a major objective response (PR or CR). Due to the lack of overlaping toxicity with other agents and evidence suggesting drug activity in head and neck cancer, clinical studies with this agent in combination with other active agents are underway.

Amsacrine (m-AMSA)

The drug, 4'-(9-acridinylamine)-methanesulfon-m-anisidine (AMSA), is an acridine derivative synthesized by Cain and Atwell [99] that has activity in a wide spectrum of murine tumors. Although clinical trials have shown definite activity in the treatment of acute leukemia [100], two studies [101, 102] in head and neck cancer showed a combined response rate of 7% (3 PR in 43 patients). These results suggest that this drug is unlikely to play a major role in the treatment of head and neck cancer.

Vindesine

Due to modest activity reported in a single trial of vinblastine in head and neck cancer [17], vindesine, another vinca alkaloid, recently underwent evaluation in three studies [103–105]. Fifty six patients with advanced epidermoid carcinoma of the head and neck were studied. Despite good performace status and no history of prior chemotherapy in a significant number of the patients, only 7 brief partial responses and two minor responses were observed for a combined response rate of 12%. It was concluded that vindesine had limited activity as a single agent in head and neck cancer.

Diaziquone (AZQ)

AZQ is a lypophilic aziridinylbenzoquinone synthesized by Driscoll et al. [106] that produces DNA cross-linking. Substantial activity has been seen only in primary brain tumors [107]. A single phase II trial in 18 heavily pretreated patients with epidermoid cancer of the head and neck produced no objective responses [108]. Another trial with this drug is nearing completion.

Dianhydrogalactitol (DAG)

Although alkylation is not the only mechanism of action of DAG it is regarded primarily as an alkylating agent. Due to its chemically distinct structure and lack of cross resistance with other alkylating agents it was tested in clinical trials. DAG was administered to 28 patients with inoperable advanced carcinomas of the head and neck [109]. All but one of the patients had surgery and/or radiation therapy and 12 had prior chemotherapy. No objective responses were observed. It is unlikely that DAG has substantial activity in this disease.

Dibromodulcitol (DBD)

In a Phase I study of DBD in 96 patients, there were 20 objective remissions, including one of 13 cases of head and neck cancer [110]. A multidisease Phase II trial [111] produced 2 PR and 1 CR in 12 patients with head and neck cancer. The complete responder, with an epidermoid carcinoma of the buccal mucosa, had a response duration of 48 months at the time of the report. The combined response rate in these 2 trials was 16% (4/25 patients). Further single agent studies of this drug in this disease are ongoing.

VP-16 (Etoposide)

This agent is an epipodophyllotoxin derivative that has demonstrated significant activity in the treatment of small cell lung cancer and testicular cancer [112, 113]. In a multidisease Phase II study conducted by the Cancer and Acute Leukemia Group B, 1PR and 3 improvements were observed in 24 patients with head and neck cancer [114]. More recently, a smaller trial [115] reported one PR among seven patients previously treated with radiation and chemotherapy. Further trials with this drug may be indicated in previously untreated patients, particularly in face of the high degree of antitumor activity found in other diseases.

PALA (N-(phosphonoacetyl)-L-Aspartate)

PALA inhibits a key enzyme, aspartate transcarbamylase, necessary for *de novo* pyrimidine nucleotide biosynthesis. Two phase II trials have been reported in head and neck cancer. Creagan, at the Mayo Clinic, observed no objective responses in 19 evaluable patients, including 5 patients with no prior chemotherapy [116]. A second trial [98] by the Eastern Cooperative Oncology Group in 46 evaluable patients, mostly pre-treated with radiation and chemotherapy, reported three partial responses (7%). These two studies failed to support any significant activity of this agent in this disease.

Bisantrene

Bisantrene is an anthraquinone closely related to mitoxantrone [117], an active agent in breast cancer. Forastiere [118] treated 21 evaluable patients including nineteen patients with no prior chemotherapy. One objective response was seen in a patient with previously untreated disease.

Platinum analogs

Although CP is among the most active agents recently introduced in the treatment of head and neck cancer, its activity may be offset by its serious toxicity. The toxicity encountered with platinum administration can be either immediate, consisting of severe nausea, vomiting, renal toxicity, and occasional myelosuppression, or delayed, such as decreased hearing and peripheral neuropathy. The presence of these untoward effects has led to the search for analog compounds that retain a similar spectrum of antitumor activity yet produce less toxicity that the parent compound [124, 125].

A number of platinum analogs have been studied clinically in Phase I studies. These are: CBDCA or Carboplatin (Diamine[1,1 cyclobutanedicarboxylatoplatinum] and CHIP or cis-dichloro-transdihydroxy-bis(isopropylamine) platinum IV, DACCP 1,2-diaminocyclohexane-(4 carboxypthalato) platinum II and TN-06 or Cis 1-1, Di(aminomethyl)-cyclohexane platinum II sulfate. In preclinical models each of the compounds showed less nephrotoxicity than the parent compound [125].

During Phase I trials with carboplatin, several schedules have been tested: single dose, 24 hour infusion weekly and daily $\times$ 5 [126–129]. The dose-limiting toxicity in all studies was thrombocytopenia. Nausea and vomiting were mild and the drug was commonly administered to outpatients without concomitant hydration. Regarding nephrotoxicity, reversible elevations in serum creatinine were seen in two patients [126] with low pretreatment creatinine clearances. Elevations of urinary beta glucoronidase (UBG) at doses greater than 50 mg/m^2 weekly were observed in another trial [127] suggesting subclinical tubular damage. However, no other major renal toxicity was seen. No hepatic, neurologic or oto toxicities have been reported. It appears that cumulative doses of $400-450 \text{ mg/m}^2$ of Carboplatin are safe for Phase II trials.

Two Phase I trials with CHIP showed that hematological toxicities with prominent thrombocytopenia was the dose-limiting side effect [128, 129]. Nephrotoxicity manifest as a drop in creatinine clearance was seen in 1 patient out of 26 treated with 37 courses. The recommended Phase II dose on the single schedule every 4 weeks was 350 mg/m^2 [128]. In the daily $\times$ 5 schedule, decreases in creatinine clearances were observed in 3 patients along with a drug eruption in 1 patient and diarrhea in 2 patients. Thrombocytopenia was the dose-limiting toxicity and was noted at doses ranging from 20 mg/m^2 to 65 mg/m^2 daily for 5 days. The recommended Phase II dose on the daily $\times$ 5 schedule was $45 \text{ mg/m}^2 \times 5$ [129].

Potentially, the platinum analogs may offer an alternative to the parent compound in the treatment of head and neck cancer, either by improving the therapeutic index or substituting another dose limiting toxicity for use in the renal impaired patient. Carefully designed Phase III trials will be required to answer these questions.

5. Combination regimens using investigational drugs

Bleomycin and dibromodulcitol

Based on the initial modest activity seen with the latter agent [111] DBD was added to bleomycin [133]. The activity of the 2 drugs was compared to bleomycin alone. Twelve of 44 patients (27%) treated with the combination achieved a partial regression (PR) compared to 4 of 18 (22%) with bleomycin alone. With the caveat of the small number of patients in this study, it appears that DBD added little to bleomycin.

Cisplatinum and dichloromethotrexate

Methotrexate (MTX) and cisplatin (CP), as discussed in the previous section, are two of the most active single agents in this disease. In combination, however, their nephrotoxic effects may be at least additive. This may delay the renal excretion of MTX, resulting in significant myelosuppression and mucositis. Dichloromethotrexate (DCM) is an analog of MTX, that is metabolized and eliminated entirely by the liver. The different route of excretion of DCM could potentially abrogate the nephrotoxicity seen with MTX and platinum. Based on these principles, a Phase I–II trial of cisplatin and DCM was carried out at the University of Michigan [134]. Patients with advanced measurable head and neck cancer were treated at doses of 100 mg/m^2 of cisplatin and 300 mg/m^2 of DCM for good risk and 70 mg/m^2 of cisplatin and 200 mg/m^2 of DCM for poor risk (PS $\leq$ 70%, creatinine clearance <65 ml/m, Hb<10, albumin <3 grams) patients. Twenty five of thirty patients entered were evaluable for response. The majority had received no prior chemotherapy (25 of the 30 entered). Twelve patients (48%) achieved objective remissions, (3 complete and 12 partial responses). Toxicity was acceptable, with myelosuppression and mucositis emerging as dose limiting. Nephrotoxicity was observed in only two patients. The lack of overlapping toxicity between these two agents and the significant activity in this preliminary trial, indicate that this an attractive combination that deserves further testing.

Conclusions

Despite two decades of research in the systemic chemotherapeutic treatment of patients with recurrent and/or metastatic head and neck cancer, these patients continue to present a major dilemma to oncologists. Survival figures for this group in prospective trials cluster about a median of approxi-

366

mately 6 months and rarely exceed 1 year. These observations strongly support the need for vigorous research and the development of new drugs or other treatment programs. Similarly, these figures do not support the existence of satisfactory treatment for patients failing primary treatment.

In this disease as well as with other tumors, the duration and number of prior chemotherapy drug treatments is a strong determining factor for response and survival. Heavily pretreated patients tolerate chemotherapy poorly and, in general, present with far advanced progressive disease relatively resistant to most forms of treatment.

It is essential that research programs testing new chemotherapeutic agents focus on patient populations in which the new drug is given at the earliest possible time after the patient is incurable by standard therapy.

References

1. Harrison D, Espiner H, Glazebrook G: Cyclophosphamide in head and neck cancer In: Fairley G, Simister J (eds) Cyclophosphamide. Williams and Wilkins Co, Baltimore, 1963, pp 48–55.
2. Foye LV, Chapman CG, Willett FM, Adams WS: Cyclophosphamide, A preliminary study of a new alkylating agent. Arch Int Med 106:365, 1960.
3. Solomon J, Alexander M, Steinfeld JL: Cyclophosphamide, a clinical study. JAMA 183:165–170, 1963.
4. Bergsagel D, Levin W: A prelusive clinical trial of cyclophosphamide. Cancer Chemother Rep 52:120–134, 1968.
5. Moore G, Brass I, Ausman R, Nadler S, Jones Jr R, Slack N, Rimm AA: Effects of chlorambucil (NSC 3088) in 374 patients with advanced cancers. Cancer Chemother Rep 52:661–666, 1968.
6. Karnofsky D, Abelman W, Craver L, Burchenal J: The use of the nitrogen mustards in the palliative treatment of carcinoma. Cancer 1:634–656, 1949.
7. Hurley J, Ellison E, Riesch J, Schulte W: Chemotherapy of solid carcinoma. Jama 174:1696–1700, 1960.
8. Marsh JC, De Conti RC, Hubbard SP: Treatment of Hodgkin's disease and other cancers with 1,3-bis (2-chloroethyl)-nitrosourea (BCNU; NSC-409962). Cancer Chemother Rep 55:599–606, 1971.
9. Ramirez G, Wilson W, Grage T, Hill G: Phase II evaluation of 1,3-bis (2-chloroethyl)-1 nitrosourea (NCNU; NSC-409962) in patients with solid tumors. Cancer Chemother Rep 56:787–790, 1972.
10. Hoogstraten B, Gottlieb J, Caoili E, Tucker WG, Talley RW, Haut A: CCNU I-[2-chloroethyl]-3-cyclohexyl-1-nitrosourea. NSC-079037) in the treatment of cancer. Phase-II Study. Cancer 32:38–43, 1973.
11. Broder LE, Hansen HH: 1-(2-chloroethyl)-3-cyclohexyl-1-nitrosourea (CCNU, NSC-79037): A comparison of drug administration at four-week and six-week intervals. Eur J Cancer 9:147–152, 1973.
12. De Conti RC, Hubbard SP, Pinch P, Bertino J: Treatment of advanced neoplastic disease with 1-(2-chloroethyl)-3-cyclohexylnitrosourea (CCNU, NSC-79037). Cancer Chemother Rep 57:201–207, 1973.
13. Dowell KE, Aemstrong DM, Aust JB, Cruz AB: Systemic chemotherapy of advanced head and neck malignancies. Cancer 35:1116–1120, 1975.

14. Tranun BL, Haut A, Rivkin S, Weber E, Quagliana JM, Shaw M, Tucker WG, Smith FE, Samson M, Gottlieb J: A phase-II study of methyl-CCNU in the treatment of solid tumors and lymphomas. A SWOG study. Cancer 35:1148–1153, 1975.

15. Firat D, Tekuzman G: Treatment of solid tumors and lymphomas with methyl-CCNU (NSC-95441). A Phase II study. Cancer Chemother Rep 59:1021–1023, 1975.

16. Bloedow C: Hydroxyurea (NSC 32065): Results of Phase II studies. Cancer Chemother Rep 40:39–41, 1964.

17. Smart C, Rochlin D, Nahum A, Silva A, Wagner D: Clinical experience with vinblastine sulphate in squamous cell and other malignancies. Cancer Chemother Rep 34:31–45, 1964.

18. Humphrey E, Hymes A: An evaluation of actinomycin D and mitomycin-C in patients with advanced disease. Surgery 50:881–885, 1961.

19. Kenis Y, De Smedt, Tagnon HJ: Action du natulan dans 94 cas de tumeurs solides. Eur J Cancer 2:51–57, 1966.

20. Gold G, Hall T, Shnider B, Selawry O, Colsky J, Owens A, Dederick M, Holland J, Brindley CO, Jones R: A clinical study of 5-fluorouracil. Cancer Res 19:935–939, 1959.

21. Olson K, Geene J: Evaluation of 5-fluorouracil in treatment of cancer. J Nat Cancer Inst 25:133–140, 1960.

22. Weiss A, Jackson L, Carabari R: An evaluation of 5-fluorouracil in malignant disease. Ann Int Med 55:731–741, 1961.

23. Staley C, Kerth J, Cortes N, Preston FW: Treatment of advanced cancer with 5-fluorouracil. Surg Gyn Obstetr 112:185–190, 1961.

24. Ansfield F, Schroeder J, Curreri A: A five year clinical experience with 5-fluorouracil. JAMA 181:295–299, 1962.

25. White J, Ricketts W, Strudwick W: A clinical study of 5-fluorouracil in a variety of far advanced human malignancies. J Nat med Assoc 54:315–317, 1962.

26. Moore G, Bross I, Ausman R, Nadler S, Jones Jr R, Slack N, Rimm AA: Effects of 5-fluorouracil NSC 19893 in 389 patients with cancer. Cancer Chemother Rep 52:641–653, 1968.

27. Young C, Ellison R, Sullivan R, Levick SN, Kaufman R, Miller E, Woldow I, Esher G, Li MC, Karnofsky DA, Burchenal JH: The clinical evaluation of 5-fluorouracil and FUDR in solid tumors in adults. A Progress Report. Cancer Chemother Rep 6:17–20, 1960.

28. Jacobs E, Luce J, Wood D: Treatment of cancer with weekly intravenous 5-fluorouracil. Cancer 22:1233–1238, 1968.

29. Krakoff IH: Adriamycin (NSC-123127) studies in adult patients. Cancer Chemother Rep, Part 3, Vol 6, 2:253–257, October 1975.

30. Blum RH: An overview of studies with adriamycin (NSC-123127) in the United States. Cancer Chemother Rep, Part 3, Vol 6, 2:247–251, October 1975.

31. Papac RJ, Fisher JJ: Cytosine arabinoside (NSC-63878) in the treatment of epidermoid carcinomas of the head and neck cancer. Cancer Chemother Rep 55:193–197, 1971.

32. Goldin A, Vendetti JM, Kline I, et al.: Erradication of leukemic (L1210) cells by methotrexate and methotrexate plus leucovorin factor. Nature 212:1548–1550, 1960.

33. Carter SK: The chemotherapy of head and neck cancer. Seminars in Oncology Vol 4, 4:413–424, December, 1977.

34. Levitt M, Mosher M, De Conti R: Improved therapeutic index of methotrexate with leucovorin recue. Cancer Res 33:1729–1734, July 1973.

35. Woods RL, Fox RM, Tattersall MHN: Methotrexate Treatment of advanced head and neck cancer: A dose response evaluation. Cancer Treat Rep 65 (Suppl 1):155–159, 1981.

36. De Conti R, Schoenfeld D: A randomized prospective comparison of intermitent MTX, MTX+LCV, and a methotrexate combination in head and neck cancer. Cancer 48:1061–1072, 1981.

37. Kirkwood J, Canellos G, Thomas E: Increased therapeutic index using moderate dose

methotrexate and LCU twic weekly vs weekly high dose methotrexate-leucovorin in patients with advanced head and neck cancer. Cancer 47:2414–2421, 1981.

38. Tejada F, Murphy E, Zubrod CG: Time sequential chemotherapy in head and neck cancer: Proceedings, International head and neck oncology research conference, Abstract 214, Rosslyn, Sept 1980.

39. Vogler W, Jacobs J, Moffit S, Velez-Garcia E, Goldsmith A, Johnson L, Mackay S: Methotrexate therapy with or without citrovorum factor in carcinomas of the head and neck, breast and colon. Cancer Clin Trials 2:227–236, 1979.

40. Turrisi A, Rozencweig M, Von Holl U, Muggia F: Current status and new developments. In: Bleomycin. Williams and Wilkins, Baltimore, 1978, pp 151–163.

41. Bonnadona G, Tancini G, Bajetta E: Controlled studies with bleomycin in solid tumors and lymphomas. Prog Biocham Pharmacol 11:172–184, 1976.

42. Halman KE, Bleehen NM, Brewin TB, Deeley TJ, Harrison DFN, Howland C, Kunkler PB, Ritchie GL, Wiltshaw E, Todd IDH: Early experience with bleomycin in the United Kingdom in series of 105 patients. Brit Med J 4:635–638, 1972.

43. Haas Charles, Coltman C: Phase II evaluation of bleomycin. Cancer 38:8–12, 1976.

44. Yagoda A, Mukherji B: Bleomycin, an antitumor antibiotic. Clinical experience in 274 patients. Ann Int Med 77:861–880, 1972.

45. Durkin WJ, Pugh RP, Jacobs E: Bleomycin (NSC-125066) therapy of responsive solid tumors. Oncology 33:260–264, 1976.

46. EORTC, Clinical Screening Group: Study of the clinical efficiency of bleomycin in human cancer. Brit Med J 2:643–645, 1970.

47. Wasserman T, Comis R, Goldsmith M, Handelsman H, Penta JS, Slavik M, soper W, Carter SK: Tabular analysis of the clinical chemotherapy of solid tumors. Cancer Chemother Rep, Part 3, Vol 6, 2:399–419, October, 1975.

48. Durant J: In: Prestayko A, Crooke S, Carter SK (eds) Cisplatin Current Status and New Developments. Academic Press, 1980, pp 317–321.

49. Prestayko A: A preclinical overview. In: Prestayko A, Crroke S, Carter SK (eds) Cisplatin Current Status and New Developments. Academic Press, 1980, pp 1–7.

50. Wittes R, Cvitkovic E et al.: Cis.Platinum in patients with advanced head and neck cancer. Cancer Treat Rep 61:359–366, 1977.

51. Jacobs C: The role of cisplatinum in the treatment of head and neck cancer. In: Prestayko A, Crooke S, Carter SK (eds) Cisplatin Current Status and New Developments. Academic Press, 1980, PP 423–444.

52. Panettiere F, Lehane D, Fletcher WS, Stephens R, Rivkin S, McCracken JD: Cis-platinum outpatient treatment for patients with squamous cell carcinomas. Med Ped Oncol 8:221–226, 1980.

53. Creagan ET, O'Fallon JR, Woods JE, Ingle JN, Schutt AJ, Nichols WC: 24-h continuous infusion cis-platinum in the treatment of advanced head and neckcancer. Cancer 51:2020–2023, 1983.

54. Sako K, Razack M, Kalnins I: Chemotherapy for advanced and recurrent squamous cell carcinoma of the head and neck with high and low dose cis-diammine dichloroplatinum. Amer J Of Surg 136:529–532, 1978.

55. Randolph V, Wittes R: Weekly administration of cis-diammine dichloroplatinum (II) without hydration or osmotic diuresis: Eur J Cancer 14:753–756, 1978.

56. Yagoda A, Lipman AJ, Winn R, Schulman P, Cohen F: combination chemotherapy with bleomycin and methotrexate in patients with advanced epidermoid carcinomas. Proc Amer Assoc Cancer Res 1105:247, 1975.

57. Broquet MA, Jacot-De-Combes E, Montandon A, Alberto P: Traitement des carcinomes epidermoides oro-pharyngo-larynges par combinaison de methotrexate et blemycine. Schweiz Med Wochenshr 104:18–22, 1974.

58. Medenica R, Alberto P, Lehman W: Combined chemotherapy of head and neck squamous

cell carcinomas with methotrexate, bleomycin, and hydroxyurea. Cancer Chemother Pharmacol5:145–149, 1981.

59. Wittes R, Brescia F, Young CW, Magill G, Golbey R, Krakoff I: Combination bleomycin and cisplatinum in head and neck cancer. Oncology 32:202–207, 1975.

60. Pitman SW, Minor DR, Papac R: Sequential methotrexate and cis-platinum in head and neck cancer. Proc Amer Soc Clin Oncol, Abstract C-529, 419, 1979.

61. Moran ME, Goepfert H, Byers RM, Guillamondagui O, Larson D, Medina J: Methotrexate followed by cis-platinum in recurrent head and neck cancer, Proc Amer Soc Clin Oncol. Abstract C-756, 195, 1982.

62. Ervin T, Weishelbaum, Miller D, Meshal M, Posner M, Fabian R: Treatment of advanced squamous cell carcinoma of the head and neck with cis-platinum, bleomycin and methotrexate (PBM). Cancer Treat Rep Vol 65, 9–10:787–789, 1981.

63. Vogl S, Kaplan B: Chemotherapy of advanced head and neck cancer with methotrexate, bleomycin, cis-diammine dichloro-platinum in an effective out-patient schedule. Cancer 44:26–31, 1979.

64. Caradonna R, Paladine W: Methotrexate, bleomycin and high dose cis-dichloro diamine platinum (II) in the treatment of advanced epidermoid carcinoma of the head and neck. Cancer Treat Rep, Vol 63, 3:489–491, 1979.

65. Murphy W, Valdivieso M, Bodey G, Freireich E: Cis-dichloro-diamine platinum II, methotrexate and bleomycin for patients with advanced squamous cell carcinoma of the head and neck. Proc Amer Assoc Cancer Res 21:666, 1980.

66. Von Hoff D, Alberts D, Mattoy D, Coulthard S, Dana B, Manning M, Mvers J, Griffin C: Combination chemotherapy with cis-platinum, bleomycin and methotrexate in patients with advanced head and neck cancer. Cancer Clin Trials 4:215–218, 1981.

67. Wheeler R, Baker S: Combination chemotherapy in head and neck cancer. Proceedings, International head and neck oncology conference, Abstract 2.5, Rosslyn, Sept 1980.

68. Price LA, Hill B: Safe and effective combination chemotherapy without cis-platinum for squamous cell carcinomas of the head and neck: Cancer Treat Rep, Vol 65 (Suppl 1):149–154, 1981.

69. Raafat J, Oster M: Combination chemotherapy for advanced squamous cell carcinomas of the head and neck. Cancer Treat Rep, Vol 64, 1:187–189, 1980.

70. Creagan ET, Fleming TR, Edmonson J, Ingle J, Woods JE: Cyclophosphomide, adriamycin and cis-platinum II in the treatment of patients with advanced head and neck cancers. Cancer 47:240–244, 1981.

71. Creagan ET, Fleming TR, Edmonson J, Ingle J, Woods JE: Chemotherapy for advanced head and neck cancer with the combination adriamycin, cyclophosphamide, and cis-platinum (II): A preliminary assessment for a one day vs three day regimen. Cancer 47:2543–2551, 1981.

72. Creagan ET, O'Fallon JR, Schutt AJ, Rubin J, Richardson R, Woods JE: Cyclophosphamide, adriamycin, and 24 hrs infusion of cis-platinum in advanced head and neck cancer. Proc Amer Soc Clin Oncol, C-770, p 198, 1982.

73. Cadman E, Heimer R, Davis L: Enhanced 5-fluorouracil nucleotide formation after methotrexate administration: Explanation for drug synergism. Science 205:1135–1137, 1979.

74. Pitman S, Fisher D, Kowak C, Sasoki C, Kindiner J, Bertino JR: Sequential methotrexate – 5-fluorouracil in squamous head and neck cancer. Proc Amer Soc Clin Oncol, C-650, 166, 1983.

75. Jacobs C: Use of methotrexate and 5-FU for recurrent head and neck cancer. Cancer Treat Rep 60:1925–1928, 1982.

76. Brown A, Blom J, Butler W, Garcia-querrero G, Richardson M, Henderson R: Combination chemotherapy with vinblastine, bleomycin and cis-platinum in squamous cell carcinoma of the head and neck. Cancer 45:2830–2835, 1980.

370

77. Amer M, Izbicki R, Vaitkevicius V, Al-Sarraf M: Combination chemotherapy with cis-platinum, oncovin and bleomycin in head and neck cancer (COB). Cancer 45:217–223, 1980.

78. Kish A, Drelichman A, Weaver A, Jacobs J, Hoschner J, Kinzie J, Loh J, Al-Sarraf M: Cis-platinum and 5-fluouracil infusion in patients with recurrent and disseminated epidermoid cancer of the head and neck. Proc Amer Clin Oncol, C-750, p 193, 1982.

79. Eisenberger M, Denefrio J, Silverman M, Lessner HE: Combination chemotherapy with bleomycin and hydroxyurea in the treatment of advanced head and neck cancer. Cancer Treat Rep, Vol 66, 6:1439–1440, 1982.

80. Medenica R, Alberto P, Lehman W: Combined chemotherapy of head and neck squamous cell carcinomas with methotrexate, bleomycin and hydroxyurea. Cancer Chemother Pharmacol 5:145–149, 1981.

81. Constanzi J, Loukas D, Gagliano R, Griffiths C, Barranco S: Intravenous bleomycin infusion as a potential synchronizing agent in human disseminated malignancies. Cancer 38:1503–1506, 1976.

82. Cortes EP, Kalra J, Amin VC, Attic J, Eisenloud L, Knafik R, Wolk D, Asal J, Sciubba J, Akbiyik, Heller K: Chemotherapy for head and neck cancer relapsing after radiotherapy. Cancer 47:1966–1970, 1981.

83. Plasse t, Ohnuma T, Goldsmith M, et al.: Bleomycin infusion followed by cyclophosphamide, methotrexate and 5-fluorouracyl in patients with head and neck Cancer. Proc Amer Soc Clin Oncol, C-755, 194, 1982.

83a. Rozencweig M, Dodion P, Bruntsh V, Gallmeyer W, Clavel M, Gignoux B, Cortes Funes H, Cavalli F, Kirkpatrick, Dalesio O, Van Rijmenant M: For the EORTC Head and Neck Cooperative Group. Cancer (Submitted 1983).

84. Hong WK, Schaefer S, Issell B, Cummings, Lvedke D, Bromer R, Fofonoff S, D'Aoust S, Shapshay S, Welsh J, Levin E, Vincent M, Vaughan, Strong S: A prospective randomized trial of methotrexate VS cisplatinum in the treatment of recurrent squamous cell carcinomas of the head and neck. Cancer 52:206–210, 1983.

85. Grose EW, Lehane D, Dixon DO, Fletcher WS, Stuckey WJ: Comparison of methotrexate and cis-platinum in patients with advanced head and neck cancer. Cancer Treat Rep (submitted 1983).

86. Lehane D, Lane M, Gad-el-Mawla N, Thomas LC, O'Bryan RN, Fletcher WS, Dixon DO: A comparison of methotrexate with MeCCNU and bleomycin in patients with advanced squamous cell carcinoma of the head and neck regimen: A SWOG study. Cancer Treat Rep (submitted 1983).

87. Williams SD, Einhorn LH, Velez Garcia E, Essessee I, Ratkin C, Birch R, Garrard J: Chemotherapy of head and neck cancer: Comparison of cis-platinum, velban and bleomycin vs methotrexate. Proc Amer Soc Clin Oncol C-784, 202, 1982.

88. Vogl S, Shoenfeld D: A randomized prospective analysis of methotrexate with a combination of methotrexate, bleomycin and cis-platinum in head and neck cancer. Cancer, in press, 1983.

89. Jacobs C, Meyers F, Hendrickson C, Kohler M, Carter SK: A comparison between cis-platinum and cis-platinum and methotrexate in combination in head and neck cancer. Cancer, in press, 1983.

90. Davis S, Kessler W: Randomized comparison of cis-platinum vs cis-platinum bleomycin and methotrexate in recurrent squamous cell carcinoma of the head and neck. Cancer Chemother Pharmacol 3:57–59, 1979.

91. De Conti R, Schoenfeld D: A randomized prospective comparison of intermittent MTX, MTX with LCV and a methotrexate combination in head and neck cancer. Cancer 48:1061–1072, 1981.

92. Tejada F, Murphy E, Zubrod CG: Time sequential chemotherapy head and neck cancer: Proceedings, International head and neck oncology research conference, Abstract 2.14,

Rosslyn Sept 1980.
93. Mihich E: Current studies with methylglyoxal-bis (guanylhydrazone). Cancer Res 23:1375–1389, 1963.
94. Freireich EJ, Frei E, III, Karen M: Methylglyoxal bis-(guanylhydrazone): A new agent active against acute myelocytic leukemia. Cancer Chemother Rep 16:183–186, 1962.
95. Knight W, Livingston RB, Fabian C, Costanzi J: Methylglyoxal bis-(guanylhydrazone) in advanced human malignancy. Proc Amer Soc Clin Oncol 20:319, 1979.
96. Kelsen DP, Yagoda A, Warrell R, Chapman R, Wittes R. Gralla RJ, Casper E, Young CW: Phase II trials of methylglyoxal-bis (guanylhydrazone) Am J Clin Oncol 5:221–225, 1982.
97. Perry DJ, Crain S, Weltz M, Wilson J, Davis RK, Wolley P, Forastiere A, Taylor HG, Weiss R: Phase II trial of mitoguazone in patients with advanced squamous cell carcinoma of the head and neck. Cancer Treat Rep 67:91–92, 1983.
98. Kaplan BH, Vogl SE, Amato D, Earhart R, Lerner Hb: Single agent chemotherapy of advanced head and neck cancer: methylglyoxal bisguanylhydrazone (MGBG) and N-phosphoacetyl L-aspartate (PALA). Proc Amer Soc Clin Oncol 2:165, 1983.
99. Cain BF, Atwell GJ: The experimental antitumor properties of three congeners of the acridylmethanesulphonanilide (AMSA) series. Eur J Cancer 10:539–549, 1974.
100. Legha SS, Keating MJ, McCredie KB, Bodey GP, Freireich EJ: Evaluation of m-AMSA in preciously treated patients with acute leukemiab: Results of therapy in 109 adults. Blood 60:484–490, 1982.
101. Ratanatharathorn V, Drelichman A, Sexon-Porte M, Al-Sarraf M: Phase II evaluation of 4'-(9-acridinylamino)-methanesulfon-m-anisidine (AMSA) in patients with advanced head and neck cancers. Am J Clin Oncol 5:29–32, 1982.
102. Forastiere AA, Young CW, Wittes RE: A phase II trial of m-AMSA in head and neck cancer. Cancer Chemother Pharmacol 6:145–146, 1981.
103. Cheng E, Young CW, Wittes RE: Phase II trial of vindesine in advanced head and neck cancer. Cancer Treat Rep 64:1141–1142, 1980.
104. Sledge GW, Von Hoff DD, Clark GM, Griffin C, Oines DW: Phase II trial of vindesine in squamous cell cancer of the head and neck and adenocarcinoma of the lung. Proc Amer Soc Clin Oncol C-788, 1:203, 1982.
105. Kaplan BH, Vogl SE, Cinberg J, Berenzweig M, O'Donell M: Phase II trial of vindesine in squamous cancer of the head and neck. Proc Amer Soc Clin Oncol C-775, 1:199, 1982.
106. Chou F, Kahn AH, Driscoll JS: Potential central nervous system antitumor agents. Aziridinylbenzoquinones, 2. J Med Chem 19:1302–1308, 1976.
107. Bender JF, Grillo-Lopez AJ, Posada JG, Jr : Diaziquone (AZQ) Investigational New Drugs 1:071–084, 1983.
108. Forastiere AA, Crain SM, Callahan K, Van Echo D, Mattox D, Thant M, Von Hoff DD, Wiernik PH: Phase II trial of aziridinylbenzoquinone (AZQ) in head and neck cancer. Cancer Treat Rep 66:2097–2098, 1982.
109. Edmonson JH, Frytak S, Letendre L, Kvols LK, Eagan RT: Phase II evaluation of dianhydrogalactitol in advanced head and neck carcinomas. Cancer Treat Rep 63:2081–2083, 1979.
110. Andrews NC, Weiss AJ, Ansfield FJ, Rochlin DB, Mason JH: Phase I study of dibromodulcitol. Cancer Chemother Rep 55:61–65, 1971.
111. Andrews NC, Weiss AJ, Wilson W, Nealon T: Phase II study of dibromodulcitol. Cancer Chemother Rep 58:653–660, 1974.
112. Radice P, Bunn PA, JR, Ihde DC: Therapeutic trials with VP-16-213 and VM-26: Active agents in small cell lung cancer, non-Hodgkin's lymphomas and other malignancies. Cancer Treat Rep 63:1231–1239, 1979.
113. Williams SD, Einhorn LH, Greco FA, Oldham R, Fletcher R: VP-16-213 salvage therapy for refractory germinal neoplasm. Cancer 46:2154–2158, 1980.

114. Nissen NI, Pajak TF, Leone L, Bloomfield CD, Kennedy BJ, Ellison RR, Silver RT, Weiss RB, Cuttner J, Falkson G, Kung F, Bergevin PR, Holland JF: Clinical trial of VP 16-213 (NSC 141540) IV twice weekly in advanced neoplastic disease. Cancer 45:232-235, 1980.

115. Felman IE, Grunberg SM, Gala KV, Owens JC: Phase II trial of Etoposide (VP-16) in squamous cell carcinoma of the head and neck. Proc Amer Soc Clin Oncol 2:162, 1983.

116. Creagan ET, Nochols WC, O'Fallon JR: Phase II evaluation of PALA in patients with advanced head and neck cancer. Cancer Treat Rep 65:827-829, 1981.

117. Von Hoff DD, Myers JW, Kuhn J, et al.: Phase I clinical investigation of 9-10-anthracen-edicarboxaldehyde. Cancer Res 41:3118-3121, 1981.

118. Foesteriere AA, Crane S, Garbino C: A phase II trial of bisantrene in advanced epidermoid carcinoma of the head and neck. Cancer Treat Rep, in press, 1983.

119. Campbell M, Al-Sarraf M: Phase II ftorafur therapy in previously treated squamous cell cancers of the head and neck. Cancer Treat Rep 64:713-715, 1980.

120. Cheng E, Currie V, Wittes RE: Phase II trial of pyrazofurin in advanced head and neck cancer. Cancer Treat Rep 63:2047-2048, 1979.

121. Creagan ET, Fleming TR, Edmonson JH, Ingle JN: Phase II evaluation of maytansine in patients with advanced head and neck cancer. Cancer Treat Rep 63:2061-2062, 1979.

122. Boccardo F, Barbieri A, Canobio L, Guarneri D, Merlano M, Rosso R: Phase II trial of thioproline in advanced eidermoid head and neck tumors. Cancer Treat Rep 66:585-586, 1982.

123. Shah MK, Engstrom PF, Catalano RB, Paul AR, Bellet RE, Creech RH: Phase II trial of razoxane (ICRF-159) in patients with squamous cell carcinoma of the head and neck preciously exposed to systemic chemotherapy. Cancer Treat Rep 66:557-558, 1982.

124. Bradner WT, Rose WC, Huftalen JB: Antitumor activity of platinum analogs In: Prestayko AW, Crooke ST, Carter SK (eds) Cisplatin Current Status and New Developments. Academic Press, 1980, pp 171-182.

125. Schurig JE, Bradner WT, Huftalen JB, et al.: Toxic side effects of platinum analogs. In: Prestayko AW, Crooke ST, Carter SK (eds) Cisplatin Current Status and New Developments. Academic Press, 1980, pp 227-236.

126. Curt GA, Grygiel JJ, Weiss R, Corden B, Ozols R, Tell D, Collins J, Myers CE: A Phase I and pharmacokinetic study of CBDCA (NSC 241240). Proc Amer Soc of Clin Oncol 2:21, 1983.

127. Priego V, Luc V, Bonnem E, Rahman A, Smith F, Schein P, Wolley P: A Phase I study and pharrmaccology of diamine (1,L) cyclobutane dicarboxylato (2-1-0) platinum (CBDCA) administered on a weekly schedule. Proc Amer Soc of Clin Oncol 2:30, 1983.

128. Creaven PJ, Mittleman A, Pendyala L, Tseng M, Pontes E, Spaulding M, Moayeri H, Madajewicz S: Phase I study of a new antineoplastic platinum analog cis-dichloro-trans-dihydrocy-bis-isopropylamine platinum IV (CHIP). Proc Amer Soc of Clin Oncol c-86, 1982.

129. Linsberg S, Lee F, Issel B, Poierz B, et al.: A Phase I study of cisdichloro-trans-hydroxy-bis-(isopropylamine) – Platinum IV (CHIP). Amer Soc Clin Oncol, C-139:35, 1983.

130. Egorin MJ, Van Echo DA, Whitacre MY, Olman EA, Aisner J: Phase I study and clinical pharmacokinetics of carboplatin (CBDCA) (NSA 241240). Proc Amer Soc of Clin Oncol 2:28, 1983.

131. Sternberg CN, Cheng E, Sordillo P, Ochoa M: Preliminary Phase II trial of 1,2-diamino-cyclohexane-(4-carboxyphthalato) platinum (II) [DACCP] in colorectal carcinoma. Proc Amer Soc Clin Oncol 2:36, 1983.

132. Pinedo H, ten Bokkel Huinik W, Gall H, McVie J, Simonetti G, vd Vijgh W, Farber L, Vermorken J: Toxicity of cis-1,1 di(aminomethyl)-cyclohexane platinum (Pt) II sulphate (TNO-6) in relation to method of administration. Proc Amer Soc Clin Oncol 2:33, 1983.

133. Issell BF, Boros G, D'Aoust JC, Banhidy F, Crooke ST, Eckhardt S: Dibromodulcitol plus bleomycin compared with bleomycin alone in head and neck cancer. Cancer Chemother Pharmacol 8:171–173, 1982.
134. Roshon S, Wheeler R, Natale R, Medvec B, Long A: Phase I-II trial of cisplatin (CP) and dichloromethotrexate (DM) in patients with head and neck cancer. Proc Amer Soc of Clin Oncol 2:163, 1983.

16. Tumor immunology, immune surveillance and immunotherapy of head and neck squamous carcinoma

GREGORY T. WOLF

1. Introduction

Overall survival rates for patients with advanced head and neck cancer remain dismal despite intensive combined modality treatment approches using surgery, radiation therapy and chemotherapy. It is well established that single modality treatment strategies employing surgery or radiation therapy for small, locally confined tumors achieve 5-year survival rates of 70–90%. However, in patients with extensive primary tumors or regional metastases, the 5-year survival rates range from 0–60%. These generally poor results have not been significantly improved by intensive combinations of surgery and radiation. This has been attributed to failures in the control or prevention of distant metastases despite occasional reductions in local recurrence rates and prolongation of disease free interval.

Pertinent to our understanding of the reasons for the frequent failure of current conventional treatment regimens to cure patients with advanced head and neck cancer are recent observations related to the diversity of biologic and structural characteristics among cells within spontaneously occurring tumors, the complexity of the immunologic mechanisms involved in tumor rejection *in vivo* and the integrity of the host immune response. Correlations of immune reactivity with tumor extent and prognosis in patients with head and neck cancer suggest that immunocompetence is an important factor in the control of neoplasia in these patients. Furthermore, conventional treatment modalities, particularly radiation therapy, produce significant impairments in immune response that in patients with head and neck cancer may persist even after tumor eradication [1]. Based on these observations, it is increasingly clear that the derivation of treatment strategies that are likely to have a beneficial impact in reducing the causes of failures of current therapy will be those strategies that circumvent either [1] the phenotypic and biologic heterogeneity of large tumors [2] the generation of therapy resistant tumor subpopulations during treatment, or [3] the im-

Gregory T. Wolf (ed), Head and Neck Oncology.
© *1984 Martinus Nijhoff Publishers, Boston. ISBN 0-89838-657-8. Printed in The Netherlands.*

pairments in mechanisms of host immune reactivity consistently demonstrated in patients with head and neck cancer. Of the frontiers of current research, immunologic investigations have provided the largest amount of information likely to be of immediate benefit in the derivation of new treatment strategies. The recent introduction of purified monoclonal antibodies against predefined antigens and the development of methods to characterize subpopulations of immune reactive cells offers the potential of providing new insight into immunologic dysfunction in head and neck cancer. Because of these recent developments, new methods for enhancing nonspecific cellular immune mechanims, restoring immunologic homeostasis and utilizing tumor specific monoclonal antibodies are on the horizon.

In this chapter, traditional concepts of tumor immunology are reviewed in light of new information concerning tumor heterogeneity and cellular immune mechanisms. Where ever possible, this information is extrapolated and discussed in reference to recent studies in head and neck cancer. Detailed descriptions of elaborate animal models are minimized by providing appropriate citations to original work and to comprehensive reviews. Finally, past experiences with and future prospects for the role of immunotherapy in the management of patients with head and neck squamous carcinoma are discussed.

2.   Fundamental concepts

2.1. Tumor specific antigens

The foundations of tumor immunology developed from early studies of immunity in infectious disease and more recently from experimental and clinical observations related to organ transplantation and tissue rejection. A central premise derived from these observations has been that cells foreign to a host's own tissues differ in substantive structural or molecular components that can be recognized by the host's immune system and that this recognition results in systematic cellular and humoral reactions resulting in eradication of the foreign cell. Substances that trigger these immunologic reactions are termed antigens and the ability to do so, termed 'antigenicity'. Antigens are commonly believed to be products of gene expression manifest as proteins on the surface of cells or in the cellular cytoplasm.

A critical assumption in tumor immunology is that unique neo-antigens exist on the surface of cells that have undergone a neoplastic change and that these neo-antigens can be recognized by the host. It is well established that normal human cells possess a variety of well-characterized surface antigens that are representative of genetic blood group type, tissue type or embryologic organ development. Evidence for the existence of specific and unique tumor associated antigens that differed from normal tissue antigens was originally derived from studies using syngeneic animals, i.e. animals repeatedly and closely inbred such that from an immunologic point of view, the animals were genetically identical. Such animals would not reject skin grafts from a similar animal, however, chemical or viral induced tumors able to grow in one animal were readily rejected when transplanted into another syngeneic animal [2]. Such readily recognized antigenicity has not been a notable property however in spontaneously occurring animal tumors. The presence of tumor specific antigens (TSA) in human tumors has been a widely accepted assumption in tumor immunology that until recently has been supported by scant scientific evidence.

The earliest investigations seeking evidence for the existence of human TSA utilized *in vitro* assays of lymphocyte mediated reactions to human tumor cells such as colony growth inhibition [3] and microcytotoxicity [4]. Some of these studies, however, suggested that the targets for these reactions were differentiation antigens shared by tumor cells, normal cells or fetal cells derived from similar tissue. Thus, for many years, the existence of specific TSA was questioned because *in vitro* cytotoxicity studies demonstrated both specific killing of tumor cells by host lymphocytes and non-specific killing of tumor cells by lymphocytes from hosts with unrelated tumors and by lymphocytes from normal subjects. These observations of non-specific cellular cytotoxicity have more recently been attributed to the presence of natural killer cells and macrophages in the population of immune reactive cells in both normal subjects and tumor bearing hosts.

Further indirect evidence for human TSA was provided by studies of leukocyte mediated migration inhibition and adherence inhibition. Leukocytes from patients with breast [5–7], lung [8], colon [6] and pancreatic [9] cancers and melanoma [6, 10] were found to respond to extracts from tumors of similar histologic type but not to extracts from other tumors or normal tissues.

More recently, direct evidence for the existence of TSA has been provided using serologic techniques in which antibodies in a patient's own serum that react with autologous tumor cells are detected by a sensitive hemabsorption assay. Using this technique, Class-1 antigens (restricted to autologous tumor cells) have been demonstrated for melanoma, astrocytoma, renal cell carcinoma and sarcoma [11, 12]. In patients with head and neck squamous carcinoma, direct evidence for the existence of TSA has only recently been reported. Studies using well characterized tissue culture lines have demonstrated that squamous carcinoma cells display surface antigens characteristic of the host's blood group type, B_2-microglobulin, pemphigus antigen, tissue antigens common with normal epidermal cells and other antigens unique to the cell lines [13, 14]. Autologous serum reactivity has been reported in over 50% of patients studied [13]. Using sophisticated hybridoma techniques [14], monoclonal antibodies to squamous carcinoma cell lines have been raised that react specifically with squamous carcinoma cells and not with melanomas, fibrosarcomas or normal fibroblasts [13]. These findings extend the results of prior studies in which indirect evidence for the existence of squamous carcinoma TSA was provided by demonstrations of lymphocyte cytotoxicity [15, 16], colony growth inhibition [17, 18] *in vivo* skin test responsiveness to purified tumor extracts [19] and serum immunodiffusion reactions to antisera prepared against purified tumor extracts [20]. The results of these combined investigations provide strong evidence for the existence of TSA in head and neck squamous carcinomas and demonstrate that in some patients, both cellular and serologic reactivity to these antigens can be detected.

2.2. The immune response

Considerable progress has been made characterizing the components of the immune system that are involved in the control of neoplasia. Using well defined animal models of carcinogenesis and sophisticated *in vitro* techniques for analyzing the function of immune reactive cells in peripheral human blood, quantitative and qualitative aspects of the immune response have been elucidated. Classically, the immune system has been divided into two components, the humoral and the cellular immune system (Fig. 1). In the human humoral system, pluripotent bone marrow stem cells develop under the influence of tissues that are the equivalent of the chicken's Bursa of Fabricius to become committed B lymphocytes (B cells). Under appropriate stimulation these cells differentiate into antibody producing plasma cells. Polymorphonuclear cells and complement also play a role in this system. Although the exact role and overall importance of B lymphocytes and antibody in the immune response to neoplasia is not completely defined, antibody mediated tumor cell destruction, antibody-antigen complex formation and the production of cytophilic antibody are well recognized phenomena that are involved in tumor-host immune reactions.

Traditionally, relatively greater importance has been placed on the role of the cellular immune system in tumor immunology. Observations in animal model systems that tumor immunity could be transferred by lymphocytes but not by serum [21] and that cell mediated cytotoxicity could be demonstrated *in vitro* [22] led to extensive evaluations of *in vitro* cellular tumor immunity in man. Mechanisms of tumor cell cytotoxicity were found to be mediated by thymus dependent lymphocytes (T cells). Multifunctional T lymphocytes comprise the major portion of the circulating lymphocyte pool. Precursor T lymphocytes differentiate under the influence of the thymus into mature T cells that can react directly with antigens via specific mem-

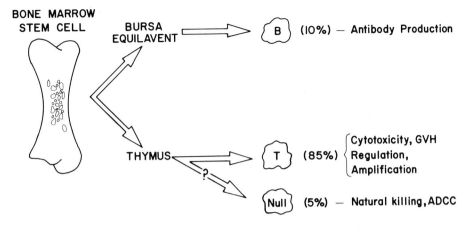

Figure 1. Classical divisions of the lymphocyte immune system into humoral (Bursa equivalent) and cellular (thymus) components. B lymphocytes and T lymphocytes make up approximately 10% and 85% of peripheral blood lymphocytes, respectively. The influence of the thymus on null cell maturation is unknown at present.

brane receptors to become functionally active 'helper' cells, effector cells or immunoregulatory cells. Experimental evidence implicating T cells as the effector cell population in tumor rejection was demonstrated in animal models using murine sarcoma virus induced tumors [23] and certain radiation induced tumors. Further support was provided by studies showing that suppression of the T lymphocyte immune system with antilymphocyte serum or neonatal thymectomy resulted in an increased incidence of tumors induced by RNA or DNA tumor viruses [24]. An important observation from recent studies of ultraviolet (UV) radiation induced tumors in the skin of mice suggest that the T lymphocyte system may also have tumor promoting effects mediated through the generation of T lymphocyte suppressor cells [25]. These cytotoxic effector and suppressor functions of T lymphocytes are facilitated through direct cell contact and the elaboration of soluable factors termed lymphokines. These lymphokines are responsible for modulation and activation of immune reactive cells and the amplification of the inflammatory response.

Because of the complexity and diversity of specific T lymphocyte responses to tumor challenge, reproducible specific cytotoxicity to human tumor cells *in vitro* has not been consistently demonstrated. Discrepancies in results from different laboratories have been attributed to variations in the techniques employed such as length of assay, concentration of tumor and effector cells and compositions of the effector cell population [26]. Moreover, clinically significant correlations of *in vitro* cell mediated cytotoxicity with patient prognosis have not been achieved.

Other cells found to be important in tumor cytotoxicity have included natural killer (NK) cells and monocytes/macrophages. Natural killer cells are large granular lymphocytes that possess non-specific *in vitro* cytolytic effects on tumor cells [27]. Correlations of *in vitro* NK activity and *in vivo* tumor resistence have been provided in experimental animal studies [28]. NK cells may be important in initial tumor development since cytotoxic functions for these cells do not require prior antigen sensitization and in animals bearing progressive tumors, NK activity declines with tumor growth [29]. Furthermore, animals [30] or humans [31] congenitally deficient in NK activity are more susceptible to the development of malignancy.

Monocytes and macrophages are phylogenetically primitive cells of the immune system. When activated by either viral, bacterial, parasitic or tumor stimuli, they respond to produce both antigen-specific and non-specific cytotoxicity. Macrophages play an important role in processing and presenting antigens to T lymphocytes and in regulating leukocyte activities through the secretion of soluable mediators of immune function. Mediators derived from both lymphocytes and macrophages function importantly in creating conditions at the tumor site that encourage accumulation of effector monocytes and lymphocytes that result in amplification of the immune response [32]. Studies of immune regulation and immunosuppression have also demonstrated important suppressive functions of cells of macrophage/monocyte lineage. These functions have been attributed, in part, to monocyte production of prostaglandin E_2, a potent suppressor of T lymphocyte function [33]. Thus, monocytes/macrophages play an important regulatory role that through inappropriate activation of negative feedback mechanisms may contribute to the circumvention of immunologically mediated tumor destruction.

It appears that the intensity and appropriateness of immune response generated during tumor growth and development are critical to the outcome of the tumor-host interaction. Since outcome is the result of both local tumor growth and spread to distant sites, immune recognition and effector mechanisms at both the primary tumor site and in the peripheral blood and lymphatics are involved. A large number of studies of the local immune response to neoplasia have been carried out in animal models in which an initial phase of tumor growth is followed by tumor regression. These studies have implicated involvement of cytotoxic T lymphocytes and macrophages and lymphokines released from antigen-sensitize T cells in the regression phenomenon [23, 24]. In animals manifesting progressive tumor growth, however, cytotoxic activities associated with T lymphocytes [35], NK cells [29] and intratumor macrophages [36] are usually reduced. Although some studies of local tumor immunity in man have demonstrated *in situ* tumor immunity at the primary tumor site [37, 38], most studies demonstrate the presence of suppressor macrophages and suppressor T lymphocytes that are capable of inhibiting cytotoxic and proliferative responses to autologous tumor cells and mitogens [39–42].

The ability of tumors to abrogate local immune reactivity is currently thought to be due in part to the heterogeneity of the tumor cell population that arises by virtue of tumor progression and the selection pressures of the host [43]. This heterogeneity is characterized by differences in growth rate, antigenicity, surface receptors and metastatic capability among cells within the same tumor [44]. The effectiveness of host immune mechanisms to control the dissemination of tumor cells has been found to differ considerably depending on the tumor type, antigenicity, animal species and competence of the immune system. Pertinent to these observations has been evidence from well characterized animal models that the antigenic properties of a tumor influence the effect that an immune response will have on tumor growth [45]. Experimental metastases following intravenous injection of highly antigenic tumor cells are more frequent in immunosuppressed animals than in normal animals. However, injection of a less antigenic tumor of the same type results in fewer metastases in immunosuppressed animals than in immunocompetent animals [45]. Similarly, weakly antigenic fibrosarcomas and melanomas grow and metastasize more readily in immunocompetent animals than in immunologically impaired hosts [46]. Other studies using highly antigenic UV-radiation induced sarcomas demonstrate that enhanced tumor growth and metastasis formation in immunocompetent animals are related to suppressor T lymphocytes specifically induced by the carcinogenic agent [25]. Thus, simply characterizing the type and degree of host immune response may not be sufficient to predict outcome of tumor growth without additional information regarding the antigenic make-up and biologic heterogeneity of the tumor cell population and the degree to which specific local and systemic suppressor cell mechanisms are operative in the local tumor microenvironment. The fact that stimulation of the immune system with exogenous agents results in tumor rejection in some situations and tumor enhancement in others reinforces this conclusion and emphasizes the fact that current generalizations regarding immune response derived from tumor models may be helpful in understanding immune mechanisms but are generally useless in predicting clinical outcome in specific individuals.

2.3. The importance of the immune response

The question posed now is what evidence exists that an immune response is important in the control of human neoplasia? Indirect evidence that immune recognition of tumor antigens and a subsequent appropriate host response is important is provided by several classic observations (Table 1).

Table 1. Indirect evidence for the importance of immune response in neoplasia

---

Increased incidence of malignancy in immunosuppressed patients
Spontaneous regressions of tumors
Increased incidence of malignancy with age
Correlations of immune reactivity with survival

The best illustration of host control of neoplasia is provided by cases of spontaneous regression of malignancies. Although a large number of such cases have been reported [47], the phenomenon of spontaneous regression is exceedingly rare and has been reported most commonly for tumors of melanoma, hypernephroma, choriocarcinoma or neuroblastoma type. However, included in reported spontaneous regressions have been cases of cancers of the larynx [47] and squamous carcinomas of the lung [48]. Spontaneous regressions have frequently followed events that presumably affect host immunologic responses such as blood transfusions, operative trauma and viral or bacterial infections [47]. Furthermore, improved survival rates have been reported in patients developing wound infections following surgery for lung [49] or laryngeal cancers [50].

The importance of the immune system in control of neoplasia is also reflected in the increased incidence of malignancy associated with congenital or acquired immune deficiency disorders [51, 52]. Lymphomas and sarcomas are the most frequent types of malignancy reported in immunodeficiency states, however, epithelial cancers are commonly associated with immune deficiency in Fanconi's syndrome [53, 54] and in immunosuppressed renal transplant patients [55].

It is well known that the risk of cancer development increases with age [56]. Associated with the aging process is a progressive involution of the thymus gland [57] that preceeds a parallel decline in T lymphocyte numbers and function [58–60] and serum thymic hormone levels [61, 62]. These changes along with a concomitant increase in serum levels of immunosuppressive glycoproteins [63] suggests that age related changes in immune reactivity may be related to the increased incidence of spontaneous neoplasms in older individuals.

Further indirect evidence is provided by studies showing correlations of immune reactivity with survival in patients with leukemias [64] and lymphomas [66] and more recently in patients with a variety of solid malignancies [67–69]. In patients with head and neck cancer, similar correlations of immune reactivity and prognosis have been demonstrated using a variety of *in vivo* and *in vitro* assays (see subsequent sections). Of the assays utilized, *in vivo* delayed hypersensitivity skin test response to DNCB has yielded the most consistent correlations with short term prognosis in both patients with limited disease [70–73] and whose with advanced tumors [73]. Skin test reactivity to recall antigens has also correlated with survival in head and neck cancer patients receiving radiation therapy [74]. Results with *in vitro* assays have been less consistent. Some studies have correlated prognosis with *in vitro* lymphocyte responsiveness to mitogens [75, 76], however, most studies have suggested that T lymphocyte numbers and *in vitro* function are more closely related to tumor extent and histology than prognosis [71, 77–79].

The failure of many simple *in vitro* measures of immune reactivity to correlate with patient prognosis cannot be taken as evidence that the immune response is not important in head and neck cancer. The wide variability in specific assay results among individual subjects and the influence of exogenous technical factors on *in vitro* results suggest that such assays are only remotely representative of *in vivo* immune mechanisms. Furthermore, the inability to detect tumor antigenicity or specific T cell responses in many patients with spontaneous tumors reflects the complexity of *in vivo* response patterns involving various effector and suppressor cell subsets and humoral reactions rather than a lack of importance of the immune response.

2.4: Immune surveillance

The concept of immune surveillance as proposed by Ehrlich [80] and expanded on by Burnet [81 postulates that a major function of the immune system is the elimination of developing malignant cells and is based on the premise that TSA exist and can be recognized by host cellular immune mechanisms. Considerable controversy regarding this concept has been generated by difficulties reconciling experimental results in animals models with *in vitro* cellular immune mechanisms and clinical observations of spontaneous tumor development. Previously cited (Section 2.1) experiences with viral and chemically induced tumors in mice supported the existence of TSA and illustrated that the cellular immune system was capable of preventing and eradicating tumor growth. However, the finding that most spontaneously arising tumors did not appear to be antigenic or were only weakly antigenic together with the low incidence of tumor development in immunosuppressive mice congenitally deficient of T lymphocytes (nude mice) [82] argued against the immune surveillance theory. Similarly, in patients with head and neck cancer, tumor antigenicity and specific cellular immunity have been difficult to demonstrate. In many patients, gross deficiencies in T lymphocyte numbers or function have not been identified during early tumor growth [79, 83]. New insights into resolving these apparent inconsistencies with the theory of immune surveillance have been provided by recent studies of effector and regulatory lymphocyte subpopulations and antigen non-specific immune mechanisms mediated by natural killer cells and macrophages.

2.4.1. T lymphocytes

Deficiencies in T lymphocyte numbers and function are consistently demonstrated in patients with advanced head and neck cancers [84–87]. These deficiencies are frequently detected early in the course of disease and are similar to the abnormalities associated with tumor dissemination in cancers of other histologic types [88]. The potential importance of these observations in early tumor recognition is suggested by experimental evidence that T cells control the incidence of certain virus induced tumors [89] and that the development of head and neck cancer is closely associated with viral infections of the herpes type [90–93].

Furthermore, herpes and cytomegalo virus infections are associated with alterations in levels of suppressor lymphocytes [94–96] that are similar to the increase in suppressor lymphocytes assocaited with UV radiation induced tumors in mice [97]. Preliminary studies of suppressor cell function in head and neck cancer patients document elevated levels of suppressor cells bearing receptors for IgG in the peripheral blood [98–101] and draining lymph nodes [102]. Other studies show that levels of cytotoxic/suppressor T lymphocytes as identified by the OKT8 antibody are similar among head and neck cancer patients and normals [103, 104]. Normal levels of T8 cells do not necessarily imply normal suppressor cell function in these patients since the T8 population is made up of differing subsets of cells having either cytotoxic or suppressor function. Overall numbers may not accurately reflect alterations in the function of specific subsets of T8 cells. Furthermore, suppressor cells identified by IgG receptor methods are not identified by the OKT8 antibody [105]. The ratio of inducer/helper cells to suppressor/cytotoxic cells identified by the OKT4 and OKT8 antibodies has recently been reported to be elevated in patients with head and neck cancer [106] and cervical squamous carcinoma [107]. These findings reflect alterations in cellular immune regulation that may be more important than overall T cell numbers in explaining the failure of immune surveillance in these patients.

Experimental models for escape of tumor cells from immunologic destruction have been established with the use of small doses of immunogenic tumors [108] and UV radiation [97]. Results from both models suggest that tumor growth is not due to a failure to generate cytotoxic T cells but rather that growth is facilitated by the induction of suppressor T cells that inhibit the cytotoxic response [25, 97, 109]. Thus, evidence is accumulating that T cell activation occurs and is important in early tumor recognition, but that this response can have positive and negative influences on tumor development. Inappropriate immunostimulation of normal suppressor cell mechanisms may be related to ineffective cytotoxic responses. This conjecture is consistent with preliminary studies of the levels of T cell subpopulations in head and neck cancer patients and prior correlations of suppressor cell levels with impaired lymphocyte response [110–112]. Other factors such as persistent or concomitant viral infection, exogenous environmental factors or tumor antigenicity may also play a role in circumventing T cell cytotoxicity.

It is well established in animal models that tumors are heterogeneous in terms of their cell population [113, 114]. This diversity is best demonstrated by differences in antigenicity and metastatic capability [115, 116] among cells derived from the same tumor. Evidence has been provided for escape of tumor cell lines from susceptibility to cytotoxic T cells based on expression or loss of expression of certain antigens by cells selected from parental tumor lines [117, 118]. Antigenic diversity induced by selection pressures, mutation or unstable genetic differentiation in a progressive tumor may also contribute to failure of host T cell cytotoxic responses to be effective in tumor eradication. There is virtually no available data from patients with head and neck cancer that demonstrate variable cytotoxicity based on tumor cell antigenic differences. However, the successful establishment of cultured cell lines derived from primary and metastatic tumor sites and from previously cultured tumors that have recurred offers the possibility of identifying such differences. Preliminary studies of cell lines from primary tumors and metastatic regional lymph nodes in individual head and neck cancer patients do show variation in growth rates and cell-surface antigen expression [13] that suggest that tumor cell heterogeneity exists in head and neck squamous carcinomas. The role of such heterogeneity in a tumor's escape from immune surveillance remains to be determined.

2.4.2. Natural killer cells

Observations from *in vitro* cytotoxicity studies that non-immune lymphoid cells could produce significant non-specific tumor cell destruction provided the first evidence that immune surveillance might not be solely a T lymphocyte mediated event. Attempts at better characterization of the effector cells in these reactions led to the identification of natural killer (NK) cells and other cytotoxic effector cells that were distinct from specifically immune T lymphocytes. Natural killer cell activity has now been associated with a population of large granular lymphocytes that express receptors for IgG and that also possess some activity in antibody mediated cellular cytotoxicity (ADCC) [119, 120]. These cells differ from macrophages in being non-adherent and non-phagocytic. Studies of surface characteristics and function of NK cells suggest that functional NK cells express surface antigen defined by particular monoclonal antibodies such as Leu 7 (HNK-1) and Leu 11 [121]. Considerable heterogeneity within this population is reflected by variable expression of weak E-rosette receptors [122] and other antigens defined by anti-monocyte [123] and OKT10 antibodies [124].

Although the biologic significance of NK cells remains obscure, evidence from animal studies indicate that these cells play an important role in the surveillance of tumor cells. In particular, nude mice which lack cytotoxic T cells have high levels of NK activity which may explain why the incidence of spontaneous tumors in these animals is no greater than in normal mice [125]. Also, studies using animals congenitally deficient in NK activity (beige mice) or ablated of NK activity show decreased tumor resistance *in vivo* [126–128]. These correlations of *in vitro* NK activity with *in vivo* tumor resistance have been extended to demonstrations of decreased tumor development and increased tumor latency in animals with high NK activity that are exposed to NK suspectible cell lines [129].

NK cells probably do not play an important role in eradication of established tumors. NK cells tend to be decreased in tumor bearing patients and differ morphologically from the population of NK cells in normal subjects [130]. In patients with head and neck cancer, levels of NK cells [130] and NK function [131] are reduced. Most recently, levels of Leu 7 positive NK cells have been found to correlate with impaired lymphokine production [106] in these patients. These findings are in agreement with recent evidence that Leu 7 cells mediate a suppressor cell function in addition to spontaneous cytotoxicity [132].

Current emphasis has been placed on the role of NK cells in control of the hematogenous dissemination of tumor cells. Both spontaneous and experimental metastatic rates in animal models have been shown to be influenced by *in vivo* NK activity [119, 133, 134]. However, it is interesting that in experimental studies of cellular populations associated with the local tumor microenvironment, high levels of suppressor cells and NK cells have been reported [135–137]. Recent studies in man have shown an inverse relationship between peripheral NK activity and local tumor infiltration by lymphocytes [138]. Thus, the respective cytotoxic and regulatory functions of NK cells and their role in the circulation and at the local tumor site need to be clarified before the biologic significance of these cells will be known. This information may be necessary to determine the appropriate clinical use of agents capable of enhancing NK function, such as the interferons, interleukin II, and other lymphokines.

2.4.3. Macrophages

Cells of the reticuloendothelial system, particularly macrophages, are believed to play a primary role in defense against infections and tumor development [139]. Mononuclear phagocytes that arise in the marrow circulate briefly in the blood as monocytes and migrate into the tissues and inflammatory sites where they mature into macrophages. Macrophages, when activated in a specific or non-specific fashion, are characterized by increased size, adherence, content of lysosomes, phagocytosis and secretion of soluble mediators of inflammation and immune function. Specific activation appears to require cooperation of T cells or soluble mediators produced by T cells in response to antigenic challenge [140]. Tumor cell destruction by macrophages can be of the same specificity as the priming T cell or can be non-specific. Activation of macrophage function *in vivo* results in increased resistance to tumors [141], but such resistance may also be due to concomitant enhancement of NK function by the activating stimulus [129]. Studies of the rejection of tumor inocula in mice, however, indicate that macrophage mediated rejection can occur independent of NK cells but is operative only for very small numbers of locally injected tumor cells [142, 143].

A number of studies have examined the influence of macrophage infiltration of local tumors on tumor growth and metastatic rate. In many animal tumors, correlations of macrophage infiltration with loss of the potential for tumors to metastasize have been shown [144, 145], however, these findings have not been consistent in all tumor types studied [146]. Studies of human malignancies including head and neck cancers, indicate that macrophage infiltration of tumors is a frequent occurrence [147, 148], even when lymphoid infiltration is sparse [148]. No significant association of macrophage content with metastatic rate for these tumors has been demonstrated although it has been suggested that locally confined tumors have a greater macrophage content than do primary tumors that have disseminated [149].

The putative role of monocyte mediated cytotoxicity in immune surveillence may be less important than the role macrophages play in processing tumor antigen [150] and regulating lymphocyte responses [151]. Both amplification and suppression of *in vitro* immune responses by monocytes have been reported. An important observation in patients with head and neck cancer has been an association of immunosuppressive adherent monocytes [152] with deficient cell-mediated immunity [87]. In these patients, excessive production of prostaglandin E_2 by monocytes has been implicated in the impaired proliferative response of mononuclear cells to PHA, Con A and in mixed leukocyte cultures [153, 154]. This suppressive effect could be abrogated by prostaglandin synthetase inhibitors (indomethacin) [153–155] suggesting that such agents may be potentially useful as immunomodulators. Supporting this conjecture are preliminary clinical experiences with the use of indomethacin in patients with advanced head and neck cancer in which significant tumor regressions were reported in a small population of patients treated with indomethacin [155, 156].

2.4.4. Escape mechanisms
Abnormalities in immunoregulation due to the presence or function of sup-

388

pressor lymphocytes and monocytes are not the only factors that may contributed to a failure of immune surveillance in patients with head and neck cancer. Elevated serum levels of immunoglobulins [157, 158], antiviral antibodies [90, 93], acute phase proteins [159] and immune complexes [160, 161] have been reported in patients with head and neck cancer and may explain the nonspecific immunosuppressive effects of patient sera on *in vitro* immune function [78, 162, 163]. In particular, elevated levels of IgA [157, 158, 164, 165] have been related to impairments in immune function [157, 166] and to increased levels of immunosuppressive immune complexes in head and neck cancer patients [161, 167]. The biologic function of these serum components is not clear but it has been proposed that they may function as blocking factors in immune mechanisms [168]. This conjecture is consistent with the inhibitory effects of immune complexes *in vitro* [169, 170] and the effects of sera from animals with Maloney virus-induced tumors on lymphocyte mediated cytotoxicity [171, 172]. Similar blocking effects have been reported in man [168] and have been associated with the IgA fraction of the sera in patients with head and neck cancer [166, 173].

Experimental studies suggest that tumors may also escape immune rejection by virtue of their cellular heterogeneity [174] or through mechanisms involving the release of factors that can bind antitumor effector cells and subvert their action [175], or that can mask surface antigens by coating antigenic determinants with sialomucins [176].

Other tumor derived factors that have local and possibly systemic immunosuppressive effects include free tumor antigen [177], acute phase glycoproteins [178] and a variety of factors capable of suppressing macrophage [179, 180] and lymphocyte function [181, 182]. Of these factors, prostaglandins may be of particular importance in head and neck cancer patients because of recent reports of elevated prostaglandin levels [183] and prostaglandin-like material [184] in head and neck tumors, and recent evidence that prostaglandin synthesis inhibitors can improve function *in vitro* [154] and induce tumor regression *in vivo* [155, 156].

3. Immunotherapy

From the preceeding discussion, it is evident that considerable evidence has emerged supporting the existence and importance of an immunologic response to neoplasia in man. Correlation of alterations of *in vivo* and *in vitro* immune reactivity with tumor extent and prognosis suggest that the clinical use of agents that modify the immune response by enhancing or restoring immunologic homeostasis may result in objective benefit in terms of prolonged survival or increased disease free interval. However, the development of appropriate and effective clinical approaches to immunotherapy for patients with head and neck cancer has been limited despite the identification of a large number of agents capable of modifying *in vitro* immune reactivity and the emergence of increasing knowledge of the cellular immune mechanisms involved in immune surveillance and tumor rejection.

Prior approaches to immunotherapy in head and neck cancer utilizing non-specific bacterial immune stimulants have generally failed. This has been attributed to incomplete knowledge of the *in vivo* effects of the agents utilized and the complex cellular and subcellular interactions critical for immunologically mediated tumor eradiation [185]. It is not surprising, therefore, that the results of prior trials that might substantiate the theoretic basis for immunotherapy in head and neck cancer are inconclusive. The recent experimental studies of immune mechanisms that were reviewed in the preceeding sections of this chapter have provided further insight into tumor-host immune interactions. Emerging data suggest that specific immune intervention directed at subpopulations of immunoregulatory cells and enhancement of non-specific mechanisms involving natural killer cells, monocytes, anti-tumor antibodies and lymphokines may lead to more effective immunotherapeutic approaches.

3.1. Immune status and immunotherapy

Agents capable of modulating immune mechanisms have recently been

Table 2. Biologic response modifiers

Immune stimulation
    Bacterial products (BCG, C. parvum, N. rubra)
    Tumor antigens, extracts or vaccines
    Pyran copolymers (MVE-2)
    Interferon
    Muramyldipeptide (MDP)
    Bestatin
    Azimexon

Immune reconstitution
    Thymic hormones
    Levamisole
    Transfer factor
    Prostaglandin inhibitors
    Lymphokines and cytokines
    Anti-tumor antibodies

---

termed biologic response modifiers. They have been broadly classified into categories that discriminate between those agents that act primarily to stimulate or enhance relatively intact immune mechanisms and those that act to reconstitute or restore impaired immune function (Table 2). Because altered immune function in head and neck cancer patients is multifaceted and is also influenced by tumor extent and therapy, such a classification may be clinically useful in the selection of specific biologic response modifiers for specific groups of patients. Factors that may influence the results of immunotherapy, therefore, include not only the type of agent and its effects *in vivo*, but also the relationship of immune competence to existing tumor burden and the effects of conventional therapy on the immune status of the patient.

One of the most consistent and potentially important observations made in patients with cancer of the head and neck is the association of impaired immune reactivity with advanced tumor extent. These observations, in which a variety of *in vivo* and *in vitro* assays were used, indicate that a major portion of the immunologic defect is due to local tumor burden, rather than regional lymphatic or disseminated metastases [78, 186, 187]. Furthermore, immune deficits are frequently detected early in the course of disease when tumor extent is limited [71, 76, 85, 188]. Thus, immunotherapeutic approaches for patients with localized head and neck cancers may differ significantly from those used for patients with other histologic tumor types in which immune reactivity is impaired only with tumor dissemination. A corollary to these observations is evidence from well defined animal models that clinically relevant approaches to immunotherapy have been successful only for tumor prophylaxis or eradication of small tumor burdens that would normally be undetectable in humans. Studies of immune response in head and neck cancer patients following successful tumor eradication frequently demonstrate persistent impairments in parameters of immune reactivity similar to untreated patients [88, 159, 160]. Thus, consideration of immune status both prior to and following conventional therapy (when tumor burden is minimal) may be critical in the appropriate selection of immunotherapeutic approaches.

The relationship of immune reactivity to tumor extent is complicated by the immunosuppressive nature of most conventional therapeutic modalities. Operative intervention and general anesthesia are associated with transient impairments in skin test responsiveness to primary and recall antigens, decreases in levels of circulating T cells, diminished lymphocyte responsiveness to mitogens and loss of leukocyte migration inhibition in response to specific antigens [189]. Immune suppression associated with therapeutic radiation is well-documented [74, 76, 190–192] and may be prolonged in patients with head and neck cancer [1]. Furthermore, alterations in the properties of suppressor and inducer lymphocyte subpopulations have been

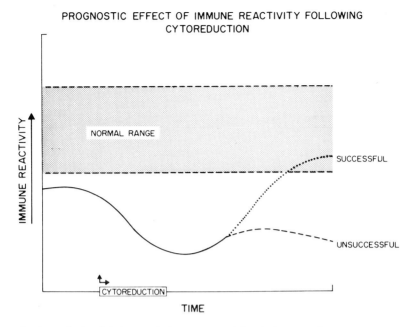

Figure 2. Theoretical serial changes in immune reactivity during and after tumor cytoreductive therapy. Successful cytoreduction is associated with a return of reactivity to normal levels and creates an appropriate setting for immune stimulation. If cytoreduction is unsuccessful, immune reactivity remains at a low level. Immune stimulation in this setting is unlikely to be beneficial and may be detrimental.

associated with radiation therapy [193, 194] and may be related to previously described abnormalities in functional assays [152, 154, 195].

All studies of immune responses in tumor bearing patients demonstrate a range and distribution of immune reactivity that in patients with limited disease overlaps the range of responsiveness in normal subjects. During cytoreductive immune suppressive therapy, immune reactivity declines to levels usually seen in patients with widely disseminated tumors. In general, successful cytoreduction is associated with a rebound in immune reactivity that correlates with prognosis (Fig. 2) [64, 196].

Since effective immune stimulation with bacterial and other non-specific immune adjuvants depends on relatively intact immune mechanisms, an appropriate situation for their use is created after successful cytoreduction. If cytoreduction is not successful, immune reactivity remains at a low level. The lack of effectiveness and inappropriateness of immune stimulation during or immediately following immunosuppressive cytoreduction where regulating immune mechanisms remain impaired has been demonstrated in animal model systems and man [197–199]. These generalizations, derived from experimental and clinical observations, are pertinent to the design of immunotherapy strategies using immune stimulants and may explain in

Table 3. Randomized trials of adjuvant immunostimulants in patients with head and neck squamous carcinoma

Agent	Schedule	Evaluable patients	Results	Investigator
BCG	Monthly post treatment	39	No difference in recurrence rates. Follow-up one year	Taylor *et al.* [209]
BCG	Monthly post treatment	22	No difference in recurrence	Cunningham *et al.* [208]
BCG	Weekly during chemotherapy (BACON)	34	Increased survival, no difference in response rates	Richman *et al.* [210]
BCG	During chemotherapy (MTX), q 3 weeks	23	No difference in response rates or survival	Beuchler *et al.* [206]
BCG	During chemotherapy (MTX), q 3 months	35	No difference in response rates or survival	Papac *et al.* [207]
BCG	Weekly post treatment	127	No difference in survival	Amiel *et al.* [211]
C. parvum	Intralesional preop then subcut. monthly post treatment	99	No difference in recurrence or survival	Beatty [212]
C. parvum	Biweekly post treatment	95	Increased survival for Stage I, II; no overall survival difference	Szpirglas *et al.* [215]
C. parvum	Weekly with MTX	73	No difference in response rates or survival	Vogl *et al.* [213]
C. parvum	Prior to and during RT	57	No difference in survival	Cheng *et al.* [214]

part the failure of early trials with these agents in patients with head and neck cancer. Because of the persistent impairments in immune reactivity demonstrated in head and neck cancer patients after effective cytoreduction, immune stimulation may be inappropriate for many of these patients. Identification of specific alterations in immune mechanisms and restoration of these mechanisms using appropriate agents may be a prerequisite for immune stimulation to be effective.

3.2. Trial results

Of the large number of trials of immunotherapy in man, few have been prospective randomized trials and few have been conducted in patients with head and neck cancer. The majority of trials for head and neck cancer have utilized nonspecific immunostimulants, such as BCG or C.parvum, following surgery or radiation therapy. The results of these trials have been generally disappointing (Table 3). Several preliminary experiences with immune reconstituting agents have suggested more encouraging results and have led to increased interest in reconstituting approaches to immunotherapy in head and neck cancer patients (Table 4).

3.2.1. Bacille Calmette-Guerin
Since Mathe's initial reports of prolonged disease free interval with BCG immunotherapy in acute leukemia [200], non-specific immune stimulation has been studied in a number of solid malignancies including head and neck cancer. Initial encouraging results in ovarian cancer [201], lung cancer [202] and melanoma [203] have not been reproduced in large, carefully done prospective studies [204, 205]. Randomized trials of BCG as an adjuvant to chemotherapy for head and neck cancer patients with either unresectable [206, 207] or potentially curable [208, 209] tumors have failed to demonstrate significant clinical benefit. Other studies have reported modestly increased survival rates when BCG was added to chemotherapy in patients with advanced disease [210] or when BCG was administered following potentially curative local therapy [211]. The interpretation of the results of BCG trials has been difficult due to variability in the BCG preparations used, faulty trial design and lack of standardized regimens in which in vitro tests could be correlated with clinical immunotherapeutic response. Furthermore, extensive investigations of BCG therapy in animal models suggest that the effect of BCG varies with tumor burden and is ineffective when given systemically after a tumor has been established.

3.2.2. Corynebacterium parvum
The results of immunostimulation with C. parvum have been disappointing (Table 3). A variety of trials in which C. parvum was injected intralesionally

Table 4. Randomized trials of adjuvant immunorestorative agents in patients with head and neck squamous carcinoma

Agent	Schedule	Evaluable patients	Results	Investigator
Levamisole	Biweekly post treatment	134	No difference in recurrence or survival at 36 months	Olivari *et al.* [252]
Levamisole	Twice a week with monthly BCG post treatment	57	No difference in immune tests, survival not reported	Olkowski *et al.* [253]
Levamisole	Biweekly post treatment	53	Increased disease free interval ($p < .06$)	Wanebo *et al.* [254]
Levamisole	Biweekly post treatment	24	Decreased recurrence rate at 2 years	Mussche *et al.* [251]
Thymosin Fraction V	Twice weekly During and after RT	75	Early recovery of immune parameters, increased disease free interval ($p < .08$)	Wara *et al.* [236]

or in the region of the draining lymph nodes have failed to document significant clinical benefit [212–214]. In one trial, a decreased recurrence rate was suggested for patients without lymph node metastases who received C. parvum [212]. A similar trial in which C. parvum therapy was compared with postoperative chemotherapy suggested increased survival for patients with limited tumors (Stage I, II) who received either C. parvum or chemotherapy compared to controls receiving standard local therapy [215]. Patients with advanced tumors had earlier and more frequent recurrences with either adjuvant treatment compared with controls. Decreased survival has also been reported in patients with squamous carcinoma of the lung who were treated with C. parvum during immune suppressive chemotherapy [199]. The indication of benefit with C. parvum for patients with limited disease (and a higher likelihood of relatively intact immune mechanisms) and potential detriment for patients with advanced disease (or during immunosuppression) parallels the variable effects of C. parvum immunotherapy in animal models [216, 217] and suggests that results of this therapy may vary depending on host immune function.

3.2.3. Interferons

The interferons consist of a group of antigenically different glycoproteins that share the characteristic biological property of being able to induce a state of resistance to intracellular viral replication [218]. Cellular biosynthesis of interferon can be induced by a variety of viral and chemical stimuli and results in effects that include anti-tumor activity, augmentation of NK activity, enhanced prostaglanding production and other immune regulatory functions. The interferons have been losely grouped into two types: Type I or virally induced interferon, and Type II which is a lymphokine induced by exposing macrophages and leukocytes to mitogens or antigens [219]. The interferons have also been subclassified according to the cell source of the isolated material. Interferons derived from leukocytes are termed alpha, from fibroblasts – beta, and from T lymphocytes – gamma. These various preparations differ in physiochemical characteristics, antigenic properties and immunologic effects [220]. The anticancer properties of the interferons are thought to be related to their ability to enhance natural cytotoxicity, inhibit tumor cell proliferation or regulate immune responsiveness through suppressive effects on antibody and cellular responses [221].

Initial clinical use of interferon in humans has met with variable success and moderate toxicity. Tumor regressions have been reported in nodular lymphomas, multiple myeloma, breast cancer, and squamous carcinoma of the uterine cervix [222–224]. In patients with head and neck cancer, systemic use of interferon has been shown to be of little clinical benefit in nasopharyngeal carcinoma [225]. Intralesional injections of interferon for head and neck cutaneous carcinomas and several oral cavity/oropharynx carcinomas have resulted in histologically complete regressions [226], however, it is unclear whether these regressions were due to an effect of interferon or to an inflammatory reaction incited by the crude, unpurified interferon preparation used.

Because of the postulated role of natural cytotoxicity in immune surveillance and the demonstrated ability of purified interferon to augment NK activity *in vitro* and *in vivo*, the assessment of NK activity has been a major emphasis of most studies of the anticancer potential of interferon. Available data suggest that there is no correlation, however, between the stimulation of NK activity and the occurrence of objective tumor responses [227, 228]. This lack of correlation may be due in part to the fact that most treated patients have had advanced tumors and generally suppressed immune function. Clinical benefit through NK augmentation may be more demonstrable in patients with minimal disease. Although NK activity is decreased in patients with advanced head and neck cancer [130, 131], studies of NK activity in patients with limited tumor extent have not been reported. Future studies of the antitumor effects of interferon in patients with head and neck cancer will have to address these issues in addition to the quantitative and qualitative differences in activities of the many different interferon preparations.

3.2.4. Thymic hormones

Of the natural agents evaluated thus far for their effects on the immune response, the thymic hormones have documented *in vivo* and *in vitro* effectiveness in restoring immune responsiveness in a variety of immune deficiency states including patients with solid malignancies [29]. Evidence that the thymic gland serves a central endocrine function in maintaining cellular immune competence is derived from studies indicating that experimental removal or congenital absence of the thymus gland in animals and humans is associated with impaired cellular immunity and that cellular immune reconstitution can be achieved through administration of soluble thymic extracts. A number of thymic extracts with immunologic activity have been isolated [230], however, the most extensively studied preparation is thymosin fraction V. The results of prior studies of the *in vitro* and *in vivo* effects of thymosin fraction V in cancer patients suggest that the effect of fraction V on impaired cellular immunity is that of restoration of immune reactivity towards normal levels while the effect on levels of cellular immunity higher than normal is modulation towards lower levels [229, 231, 232]. In studies of immunologically impaired patients with disseminated malignancies, thymosin fraction V administration was associated with increases in T cell numbers, mixed lymphocyte culture responses, lymphocyte blastogenesis and the number of positive delayed hypersensitivity skin test responses to recall antigens [229, 233]. Furthermore, in recent controlled trials in patients receiving immunosuppressive chemotherapy [234] or radiation therapy [235], thymosin administration was associated with significantly increased patient survival.

The only randomized clinical trial of thymosin in patients with head and neck cancer suggested early restoration of mixed lymphocyte culture reactivity and mitogen induced blastogenesis in thymosin treated patients receiving immunosuppressive radiation therapy [236]. With a median following of two years, a borderline significant increase in disease-free interval ($p < .08$) was noted. These findings are of importance because of the well documented immunosuppressive effects of radiation therapy. Improvements in local tumor control with postoperative radiation therapy in patients with advanced head and neck cancer have not been accompanied by increased survival rates. This has been attributed to an increased incidence of distant metastases [237-240] that may be related to the immunosuppressive effects of radiation [74, 190, 191, 236]. The results of studies of distant metastases in animal tumor models suggest that immunosuppression following gross tumor eradication is associated with an increased rate of distant metastases [241, 242] and that immunorestorative agents, such as thymosin can decrease this rate of metastases [242-245]. These observations provide rationale for further investigation of immunotherapeutic strategies for preventing or correcting the immunosuppression associated with postoperative radiation in patients with head and neck cancer. The thymic hormones will undoubtedly play an important role in such studies.

3.2.5. Other agents

Levamisole is a synthetic imidazole that has immune reconstituting activity similar to the thymic hormones [246]. Although clinical trials of levamisole in patients with breast and lung cancer have shown encouraging results [247, 248], randomized trials in patients with head and neck cancer have yielded conflicting results (Table 4) [249-252]. Results from two of these trials have suggested, however, that the only groups to benefit from levamisole were those patients with advanced disease who had impaired immune parameters pretreatment [249, 250].

A number of other immunotherapeutic agents are being studied in cancer patients (Table 2) but have not been utilized for trials in patients with head and neck cancer. Provocative preliminary results with prostaglandin synthetase inhibitors [155, 156], intralesional BCG [253], transfer factor [254] and tumor antigen [255] indicate that future approaches could involve a variety of agents with various specific immunologic activities. In particular, the recent emphasis on the importance of non-specific immune mechanisms in tumor control suggests that mediators of immune reactions such as the lymphokines and tumor specific monoclonal antibodies will play an important future role in immunotherapy. The recent discovery of suppressor cells and suppressor mechanisms that interfere with host-mediated immune responses emphasizes the need to better elucidate the role of this phenomenon in tumor control and the specific effects of biologic agents on negative feedback loops present in all immune mechanisms. Indiscriminate use of biologic response modifiers without the necessary insight into these effects and the effects of conventional and immune therapy on immune reactivity and lymphocyte subpopulations will undoubtedly lead to therapeutic failures. The future holds promise for the development of sophisticated quantitative and qualitative indicators of immune reactivity, tumor persistance and tumor recurrence that would be useful in the appropriate selection of patients for immunotherapy, the serial monitoring of the effects of therapy and the early detection of enhanced tumor growth in individual patients.

4. Conclusions

The frontiers of tumor immunology are being pushed forward rapidly through the development and application of new techniques for characterizing tumor cell populations and the immunologic mechanisms of tumor rejection. Concurrent with these developments, laboratory and clinical investigations of agents capable of modifying host biologic responses to malignancy are underway to determine the potential use of these agents in patients with head and neck cancer. Unraveling the complexities of the immune response and identifying mechanisms that permit tumors to escape immunologic destruction remain limiting factors in the development of immunologic approaches to therapy likely to be of use in individual patients. Furthermore, increased knowledge of the effects of traditional therapies on tumor-host interactions and the limitations of such treatments as determined by tumor cell heterogeneity, metastatic behavior and tumor escape mechanisms should permit more rational integration of immune therapy with currently utilized treatment modalities.

Acknowledgement

The author expresses his deepest gratitude to Ms. Rita Brandt for her invaluable support and assistance in the preparation of this manuscript.

References

1. Tarpley JL, Potvin C, Chretien PB: Prolonged depression of cellular immunity in cured laryngopharyngeal cancer patients treated with radiation therapy. Cancer 35:638–644, 1975.

2. Prehn R, Main D: Immunity to methylcholanthrene induced sarcoma. J Natl Cancer Inst 18:768–778, 1957.

3. Hellstrom I: A colony inhibition (CI) technique for demonstration of tumor cell destruction by lymphoid cells in *in vitro*. Int J Cancer 2:65–69, 1967.

4. Hellstrom I, Hellstrom KE, Sjogren HO, Warner GA: Demonstration of cell-mediated immunity to human neoplasms of various histologic types. Int J Cancer 7:1–16, 1971.

5. McCoy JL, Jerome LF, Dean JH, *et al.*: Inhibition of leukocyte migration by tumor-associated antigens in soluable extracts of human breast carcinoma. J Natl Cancer Inst 53:11–17, 1974.

6. Halliday WJ, Koppi TA, Khan JM, Davis NC: Leukocyte adherence inhibition. Tumor specificity of cellular serum-blocking reactions in human melanoma, breast cancer, and colorectal cancer. J Natl Cancer Inst 65:327–335, 1980.

7. Yonomoto RH, Fujisawa T, Waldman SR: Effect of serum blocking factors on leukocyte adherence inhibition in breast cancer patients: specificity and correlation with tumor burden. Cancer 41:1289–1297, 1978.

8. McCoy JL, Jerome LF, Cannon GB, *et al.*: Reactivity of lung cancer patients in leukocyte migration inhibition assays to 3-M potassium chloride extracts of fresh tumor and tissue-cultured cells derived from lung cancer. J Natl Cancer Inst 59:1414–1418, 1977.

9. Goldrosen MH, Russo AJ, Howell JH, *et al.*: Evaluation of mico-leukocyte adherence inhibition as an immunodiagnostic test for pancreatic cancer. Cancer Res 29:633–637, 1978.

10. McCoy JL, Jerome LF, Dean JH, *et al.*: Inhibition of leukocyte migration by tumor-associated antigens in soluable extracts of human malignant melanoma. J Natl Cancer Inst 55:19–24, 1975.

11. Roth JA, Wesley RA: Human tumor-associated antigens detected by serological technique: analysis of autologous humoral immune responses to primary and metastatic human sarcomas by an enzyme-linked immunoabsorbent solid-phase assay. Cancer Res 42:3978–3986, 1982.

12. Ueda R, Shiku H, Pfreundschuh M, *et al.*: Cell surface antigens of human renal cancer defined by autologous typing. J Exp Med 150:564–579, 1979.

13. Carey TE, Kimmel KA, Schwartz DR, *et al.*: Antibodies to human squamous cell carcinoma. Otolaryngology Head Neck Surg 91:482–491, 1983.

14. Sofen H, O'Toole C: Anti-squamous tumor antibodies in patients with squamous cell carcinoma. Cancer Res 38:199–203, 1978.

15. Adelstein EH, Davis WE, Oxenhandler RW, *et al.*: Lymphocyte-tumor cell interaction in patients with and neck cancer: Laryngoscope 88:575–581, 1978.

16. Ariyan S, Krizek TJ, Mitchell MS: Identification of squamous cell carcinoma of the head and neck by tissue culture and immunological testing. Plast Recon Surg 59:386–394, 1977.

17. Aust JC, Rabuzzi D, Reed G: Tissue-cultured head and neck tumors: their use in *in vitro* assays of immune response. Trans Am Aced Ophth Otol 84:603–608, 1977.

18. Kennedy JT: A search for common tumor specific antigen and serum blocking factor in head and neck epidermoid carcinoma. Laryngoscope 85:806–822, 1975.

19. Krause CJ, Nysather J, McCabe BF: Characterization of tumor antigen in epidermoid carcinoma. Ann Otol 84:787–792, 1975.

20. Ibrahim AN, Robinson RA, Marr L, *et al.*: Tumor-associated antigens in cervical cancer tissues and in sera from patients with cervical cancer or with head and neck cancer. J Natl Cancer Inst 63:319–323, 1979.

21. Klein G, Sjogren HO, Klein E, Hellstrom KE: Demonstration of resistance against methylcholanthrene-induced sarcomas in the primary autochthonous host. Cancer Res 20:1561–1572, 1960.

22. Hellstrom I, Sjogren HO: *In vitro* demonstration of humoral and cell-bound immunity

against common specific transplantation antigens of adenovirus 12-induced mouse and hamster tumors. J Exp Med 125:1105–1118, 1967.

23. Gorczyncki RM: Evidence for *in vivo* protection against murine sarcoma virus-induced tumors by T lymphocytes from immune animals. J Immunol 112:533, 1974.

24. Law LW: Studies of the significance of tumor antigens in induction and repression of neoplastic disease: presidential address. Cancer Res 29:1, 1969.

25. Fisher MS, Kripke ML: Further studies on the tumor-specific suppressor cells induced by ultraviolet radiation. J Immunol 121:1139–1144, 1978.

26. Hellstrom I, Hellstrom KE: Cell-mediated reactivity to human tumor-type associated antigens: Does it exist? J Biol Resp Mod 2:310–320, 1983.

27. Rosenberg EB, McCoy JL, Green SS, *et al.*: Destruction of human lymphoid tissue culture cell lines by human peripheral lymphocyte in ^{51}CR-release cellular cytotoxicity assays. J Natl Cancer Inst 52:345, 1974.

28. Riesenfeld I, Orn A, Gidlund M, *et al.*: Positive correlation between *in vitro* NK activity and *in vivo* resistance towards AKR lymphoma cells. Int J Cancer 25:399, 1980.

29. Becker S, Klein E: Decreased 'natural killer' effect in tumor bearing mice and its relation to the immunity against oncorna virus-determined cell surface antigens. Eur J Immunol 6:892, 1976.

30. Karre K, Klein GO, Kiessling R, *et al.*: Low natural *in vivo* resistance to syngeneic leukemias in natural killer deficient mice. Nature 284:624, 1980.

31. Dent PB, Fish LA, White WF, Good RA: Chediak-Higashi syndrome: observations on the nature of the associated malignancy. Lab Invest 15:1634, 1966.

32. North RJ: The concept of the activated macrophage. J Immunol 121:806–809, 1978.

33. Goodwin JS, Webb DR: Regulation of the immune response by prostaglandins. Clin Immunol Immunopath 15:106–122, 1980.

34. Holden HT, Haskill JS, Kirchner H, Herberman RB: Two functionally distinct anti-tumor effector cells isolated from primary murine sarcoma virus-induced tumors. J Immunol 117:440, 1976.

35. Gillespie GY, Hansen CB, Hoskins RG, Russell SW: Inflammation cells in solid murine neoplasms. IV. Cytolytic T lymphocytes isolated from regressing or progressing Moloney sarcomas. J Immunol 119:564, 1977.

36. Russell SW, McIntosh AT: Macrophages isolated from regressing Moloney sarcomas are more cytotoxic than those recovered from progressing sarcomas. Nature 268:69, 1977.

37. Jondal M, Svedmyr E, Klein E, Singh S: Killer T-cells in a Burkitt's lymphoma biopsy. Nature 255:405, 1975.

38. The TH, Eibergen R, Lamberts HB, *et al.*: Immune phagocytosis *in vivo* of human malignant melanoma cells. Acta Med Scand 192:141, 1972.

39. Vose BM, Moore ML: Suppressor cell activity of lymphocytes infiltrating human lung and breast tumors. Int J Cancer 24:579, 1979.

40. Houck JF, McCormick KJ, Panje WR, *et al.*: Modulation of mitogenic response by cells from regional lymph nodes of head and neck cancer patients. Proc Am Assoc Cancer Res 24:202, 1983.

41. Yu A, Watts H, Jaffe N, Parkman R: Concomitant presence of tumor specific cytotoxic and inhibitor lymphocytes in patients with osteogenic sarcoma. N Engl J Med 297:121, 1977.

42. Uchida A, Micksche M: Suppressor cells for natural killer activity in carcinomatous pleural effusions of cancer patients. Cancer Immunol Immunother 11:255, 1981.

43. Fidler IJ, Hart IR: Biologic diversity in metastatic neoplasms: origins and implications. Science 217:998, 1982.

44. Fidler IJ, Kripke ML: Tumor cell antigenicity, host immunity and cancer metastasis. Cancer Immunol Immunother 7:201–205, 1980.

45. Fidler IJ, Gersten DM, Kripke ML: The influence of immune status on the metastases of

three murine fiborsarcomas of different immunogenicities. Cancer Res 39:3816, 1979.

46. Fidler IJ, Gersten DM, Hart IR: The biology of cancer invasion and metastasis. Adv Cancer Res 28:149, 1978.

47. Cole WH: Spontaneous regression of cancer and the importance of finding its cause. Natl Cancer Inst Monogr 44:5–9, 1976.

48. Baker RR: Spontaneous regression of bronchogenic carcinoma. Natl Cancer Inst Monogr 44:31–33, 1976.

49. Ruckdeschel JC, et al.: Postoperative empyema improves survival in lung cancer: documentation and analysis of a natural experiment. N Engl J Med 287:1013–1017, 1972.

50. Schantz SP, Skolnik EM, O'Neill JV: Improved survival associated with postoperative wound infection in laryngeal cancer: an analysis of its therapeutic implications. (Abstract), Research Forum, American Academy of Otolaryngology, October 1979.

51. Harris JP, Penn I: Immunosuppression and the development of malignancies of the upper airway and related structures. Laryngoscope 91:520–528, 1981.

52. Good RA, Finstad J: Essential relationship between the lymphoid system, immunity and malignancy. Natl Cancer Inst Monogr 31:41–58, 1969.

53. Kennedy AW, Hart WR: Multiple squamous-cell carcinomas in Fanconi's anemia. Cancer 50:811–814, 1982.

54. Reed K, Ravikumar TS, Gifford RRM, Grage TB: The association of Fanconi's anemia and squamous cell carcinoma. Cancer 52:926–928, 1983.

55. Birkeland SA: Malignant tumors in renal transplant patients. Cancer 51:1571–1575, 1983.

56. Burbank F: Patterns in cancer mortality in the United States: 1950–1967. Natl Cancer Inst Monogr 33:1–594, 1972.

57. Henry L: Involution of the human thymus. J Path Bact 93:661, 1967.

58. Weksler ME, Hutteroth TH: Impaired lymphocyte function in aged humans. J Clin Invest 53:99–104, 1974.

59. Carosella ED, Mochanko K, Braun M: Rosette forming T cells in human peripheral blood at different ages. Cell Immunol 12:323–325, 1974.

60. Waldorf DS, Willkens RF, Decker JL: Impaired delayed hypersensitivity in an aging population. J Am Med Assoc 203:111, 1968.

61. Bach JF, Papiernick M, Lavasseur P, et al.: Evidence for a serum-factor secreted by the human thymus. Lancet 2:1056–1058, 1972.

62. McClure JE, Lameris N, Wara DM, Goldstein AL: Immunochemical studies on thymosin: radioimmunoassay of thymosin a_1. J Immunol 128:368–375, 1981.

63. Wolf GT, Chretien PB, Weiss JF, et al.: Effects of smoking and age on serum levels of immune reactive proteins. Otolaryngol Head Neck Surg 90:319–326, 1982.

64. Hersh EM, Whitecare JP, McCredie KB, et al.: Chemotherapy, immunocompetence, immunosuppression and prognosis in acute leukemia. N Engl J Med 285:1211–1216, 1971.

65. Leventhal BG, Halterman RH, Rosenberg EB, Herberman RB: Immune reactivity of leukemia patients to autologous blast cells. Cancer Res 32:1820–1825, 1972.

66. Sokal JE, Aungst CW: Cellular responses and prognosis in malignant lymphomas. Natl Cancer Inst Monogr 34:109–112, 1971.

67. Eilber FR, Morton DL: Impaired immunologic reactivity and recurrence following cancer surgery, Cancer 25:362–367, 1970.

68. Israel L, Mugica J, Chahinian P: Prognosis of early bronchogenic carcinoma. Survival cures of 451 patients after resection of lung cancer in relation to the results of pre-operative tuberculin skin tests. Biomedicine 19:68–72, 1973.

69. Pinsky CM, Wanebo HJ, Mike V, et al.: Delayed cutaneous hypersensitivity reactions and prognosis in patients with cancer. Ann NY Acad Sci 276:407–410, 1976.

70. Maisel RH, Ogura JH, Dinitrochlorobenzene skin sensitization and peripheral lymphocyte

count: predictors of survival in head and neck cancer. Ann Otol Rhinol Laryngol 85:517–522, 1976.

71. Hilal EY, Wanebo HJ, Pinsky CM, et al.: Immunological evaluation and prognosis in patients with head and neck cancer. Am J Surg 134:469–473, 1977.

72. Mandel MA: Skin testing for prognosis or therapy formulation in cancer patients: caveat emptor. Plast reconstr Surg 57:64–66, 1976.

73. Bosworth JL, Thaler S, Ghossein NA: Delayed hypersensitivity and local control of patients treated by radiotherapy for head and neck cancer. Am J Surg 132:46–48, 1976.

74. Stefani S, Kerman R, Abbate J: Serial studies of immunocompetence in head and neck cancer patients undergoing radiation therapy. Am J Roentgenol Radium Ther Nucl Med 126:880–886, 1976.

75. Rayn RE, Neel HB: Correlation of preoperative immunologic test results with recurrence in patients with head and neck cancer. Otolaryngol Head Neck Surg 88:58–63, 1980.

76. Jenkins VK, Griffiths CM, Ray P, et al.: Radiotherapy and head and neck cancer. Role of lymphocyte response and clinical stage. Arch Otolaryngol 106:414–418, 1980.

77. Eastham RJ, Mason JM, Jennings BR, et al.: T-cell rosette test in squamous cell carcinoma. Arch Otolaryngol 102:171–175, 1976.

78. Catalona WJ, Sample WF, Chretien PB: Lymphocyte reactivity in cancer patients: correlation with tumor histology and clinical stage. Cancer 31:65–71, 1973.

79. Mason JM, Kitchens GG, Eastham RJ, Jennings BR: T-lymphocytes and survival of head and neck squamous cell carcinoma. Arch Otolaryngol 103:223–227, 1977.

80. Ehrlich P: Uber den jetzigen Stand der Karzinoforschung. In: Himmelweit H (ed) The Collected Papers of Paul Ehrlich, Vol 11. London, Pergamon, 1957, p 550.

81. Burnett MF: Immunological surveillance in neoplasia. Transplant Rev 7:3–25, 1971.

82. Rygaard J, Povlsen CO: The nude mouse vs. the hypothesis of immunological surveillance. Transplant Rev 28:42, 1976.

83. Deegan MJ, Coulthard SW: Spontaneous rosette formation and rosette inhibition assays in patients with squamous cell carcinoma of the head and neck. Cancer 39:2137–2141, 1977.

84. Olkowski ZL, Wilkins SA: T-lymphocyte levels in the peripheral blood of patients with cancer of the head and neck. Am J Surg 130:440–444, 1975.

85. Deegan MJ, Coulthard SW, Qualman SJ, Schork MA: A correlative analysis of in vitro parameters of cellular immunity in patients with squamous cell carcinoma of the head and neck. Cancer Res 37:4475–4481, 1977.

86. Wanebo HJ, Jun MX, Strong EW, et al.: T-cell deficiency in patients with squamous cell carcinoma of the head and neck. Am J Surg 130:445–451, 1975.

87. Zighelboim J, Dorey F, Parker NH, et al.: Immunologic evaluation of patients with advanced head and neck cancer receiving weekly chemoimmunotherapy. Cancer 44:117–123, 1979.

88. Chretien PB: Unique immunobiological aspects of head and neck squamous carcinoma. Can J Otolaryngol 4:225–235, 1975.

89. Allison AC: Interactions of antibodies, complement components and various cell types in immunity against viruses and pyogenic bacteria. Transplant Rev 19:3, 1974.

90. Hollingshead AC, Lee O, Chretien PB, et al.: Antibodies to herpes virus nonvirion antigens in squamous carcinoma. Science 182:713–715, 1973.

91. Shillitoe EJ, Greenspan D, Greenspan JS, et al.: Neutralizing antibody to herpes simplex virus type[1] in patients with oral cancer. Cancer 49:2315–2320, 1982.

92. Sheinin R: Viruses: Causative agents of cancer. Laryngoscope 185:468–486, 1975.

93. Smith HG, Chretien PB, Henson DE, et al.: Viral-specific humoral immunity to herpes simplex-induced antigens in patients with squamous carcinoma of the head and neck. Am J Surg 132:541–548, 1976.

94. Arneborn P, Biberfeld G: T-lymphocyte subpopulations in relation to immunosuppression

in measles and varicella. Infection and Immunity 29:29–37, 1983.

95. Waele MD, Thielmans C, VanCamp BKG: Chracterization of immunoregulatory T cells in EBV-induced infectious mononucleosis by monoclonal antibodies. N Engl J Med 304:460–462, 1981.

96. Carney WP, Rubin RH, Hoffman RA, et al.:Analysis of T-lymphocyte subsets in cytomegalovirus mononucleosis. J Immunol 126:2114–2116, 1981.

97. Kripke ML: Immunobiology of photocarcinogenesis. In: Parrish JA (ed) The Effect of Ultraviolet Radiation on the Immune System. Johnson and Johnson, 1983, pp 87–100.

98. Yata J, Shimbo T, Sawaki S: Changes in T-cell subsets and their clinical significance in cancer patients. In: De-The G, Ito Y (eds) Nasopharyngeal Carcinoma: Etiology and Control. Lyon, IARC Scientific Publication No. 20, 1978, pp 511–521.

99. Vena GA, Angelini G, D'Ovidio R, et al.: Cell-mediated immunity in squamous cell and basal cell carcinomas. G Ital Dermatol Venereol 117:263–267, 1982.

100. Vena GA, Angelini G, D'Ovidio R, et al.: T-lymphocytes with Fc-IgG receptors in skin cancers. Acta Dermatovener (Stockholm) 61:555–577, 1981.

101. Balaram P, Vasudeven DM: Quantitation of Fc receptor-bearing T-lymphocytes (T_G and T_M) in oral cancer. Cancer 52:1837–1840, 1983.

102. Saxon A, Portis J: Lymphoid subpopulation changes in regional lymph nodes in squamous head and neck cancer. Cancer Res 37:1154–1158, 1977.

103. Camacho ES, Schecter P, Graham R, Camacho SA: Immune competence evaluation including T-cell subsets in patients with lung or head and neck carcinomas and smokers. Proc Am Soc Clin Oncol 1:40, 1982.

104. Johnson JT, Rabin BS, Hersch B, Tharel PB: T-lymphocyte subpopulations in head and neck carcinoma. (Accepted for publication), Otolaryngol Head Neck Surg, June 1983.

105. Reinherz EL, Moretta L, Roper M, et al.: Human lymphocyte subpopulations defined by Fc receptors and monoclonal antibodies. J Exp Med 151:969–974, 1980.

106. Wolf GT, Lovett EF, McClatchey K, et al.: Impaired lymphokine production in patients with head and neck cancer correlates with alterations in lymphocyte subpopulations. (unpublished).

107. Lipscomb H, Jacobs AJ, Bechtold T, et al.: Lymphocyte subpopulations in patients with cervical carcinoma. (Abstract), Eleventh Midwest Autumn Immunology Conference Workshops, Chicago. Illinois, November 1, 1982.

108. Moller G, Moller E: Immunological surveillance against neoplasia. In: Castro JE (eds) Immunologic Aspects of Cancer. Baltimore, University Park Press, 1978, p 206.

109. Gatenby PA, Basten A, Creswick P: 'Sneaking through', a T-cell dependent phenomenon. Br J Cancer 44:753, 1981.

110. Broder S, Waldmann TA: The suppressor-cell network in cancer. New Engl J Med 299:1335–1341, 1978.

111. Kapp JA, Pierce CW, Theze J, Benacerraf B: Modulation of immune responses by suppressor T cells. Fed Proc 37:2361–2364, 1978.

112. Hersh EM, Patt YZ, Murphy SG, et al.: Radiosensitive, thymic hormone sensitive peripheral blood suppressor cell activity in cancer patients. Cancer Res 40:3134–3140, 1980.

113. Hart IR, Fidler IJ: The implications of tumor heterogeneity for studies on the biology and therapy of cancer metastases. Biochem Biophys Acta 651:37–50, 1981.

114. Poste G: Experimental systems for analysis of the malignant phenotype. Cancer Metastasis Rev 1:141–199, 1982.

115. Kripke ML, Gruys E, Fidler IJ: Metastatic heterogeneity of cells from an ultraviolet light-induced murine fibrosarcoma of recent origin. Cancer Res 38:2962–2967, 1978.

116. Fidler IJ, Kripke ML: Metastasis results from pre-existing variant cells within a malignant tumor. Science 197:893–895, 1977.

117. Gooding LR: Characterization of a progressive tumor from C3H fibroblasts transformed in

404

vitro with SV-40 virus: immunoresistance *in vivo* correlates with phenotypic loss of H-2K. J Immunol 129:1306, 1982.

118. Urban JL, Burton RC, Holland JM, *et al.*: Mechanisms of syngeneic tumor rejection, susceptibility of host-selected progressor variants to various immunological effector cells. J Exp Med 155:557, 1982.

119. Timonen T, Ortaldo JR, Herberman RB: Characterization of human large granular lymphocytes and the relationship to natural killer and K cells. J Exp Med 153:569–582, 1981.

120. Landazuri MO, Silva A, Alvarez J, Herberman RB: Evidence that natural cytotoxic and antibody dependent cellular cytoxicity are mediated in humans by the same effector cell populations. J Immunol 123:252–258, 1979.

121. Lanier LL, Le AM, Phillips JH: Subpopulations of human natural killer cells defined by expression of the Leu-7 (HNK-1) and Leu-11 (NK-15) antigens. J Immunol 131:1789–1796, 1983.

122. West WH, Boozer RB, Herberman RB: Low affinity E-rosette formation by the human K cell. J Immunol 120:90, 1978.

123. Kay HD, Horwitz DA: Evidence by reactivity with hybridoma antibodies for a probable myeloid origin of peripheral blood cells active in natural cytotoxicity and antibody-dependent cell-mediated cytotoxicity. J Clin Invest 66:847, 1980.

124. Ortaldo JR, Sharrow SO, Timonen T, Herberman RBb: Determination of surface antigens on highly purified human NK cells by flow cytometry with monoclonal antibodies. J Immunol 127:2401, 1981.

125. Stutman O: Delayed tumor appearance and absence of regression in nude mice infected with murine sarcoma virus. Nature 253:142, 1975.

126. Roder JC, Halistes T: Do NK cells play a role in anti-tumor surveillance? Immunol Today 1:96, 1980.

127. Habu S, Fukui H, Shimamura K, Kasai M, *et al.*: *In vivo* effects of anti-asialo GMI, reduction of NK activity and enhancement of transplanted tumor growth in nude mice. J Immunol 127:34–36, 1981.

128. Talmadge JE, Meyers KM, Prieur DJ, Starkey JR: Role of NK cells in tumor growth and metastasis in beige mice. Nature 284:622–624, 1980.

129. Hanna N: Role of natural killer cells in control of cancer metastases. Cancer Metastasis Rev 1:45, 1982.

130. Balch CM, Tilden AB, Dougherty PA, Cloud G, Abo T: Depressed levels of granular lymphocyte with natural killer cell function in 247 cancer patients. Proc Am Assoc Cancer Res 23:905, 1983.

131. Ching CY, Hokama Y, Jim E, *et al.*: Evaluation of natural killer function and interferon *in vitro* in patients with selected malignancies. Proc Am Assoc Cancer Res 23:909, 1983.

132. Tilden AB, Abo T, Balch CM: Suppressor cell function of human granular lymphocytes identified by the HNK-1 (Leu 7) monoclonal antibody. J Immunol 130:1171–1175, 1983.

133. Gorelik E, Wiltrout R, Okumura K, *et al.*: Acceleration of metastatic growth in anti-asialo GM-1-treated mice. In: Herberman RB (ed) NK Cells and Other Natural Effector Cells. New York, Academic Press, 1982, pp 1331–1337.

134. Hanna N, Fidler IJ: Relationship between metastatic potential and resistance to natural killer cell-mediated cytotoxicity in three murine tumor systems. J Natl Cancer Inst 66:1183–1190, 1981.

135. Brodt P, Lala PK: Changes in T cell subsets in mice during the growth of spontaneous mammary tumors. Proc Am Assoc Cancer Res 23:236, 1983.

136. Buessow SC, Paul RD, Lopez DM: The isolation and characterization of lymphocytes infiltrating a mammary adenocarcinoma. Proc Am Assoc Cancer Res 23:238, 1983.

137. Flannery GR, Robins RA, Baldwin RW: Natural killer cells infiltrate chemically induced

sarcoma. Cell Immunol 61:1–10, 1981.

138. Hersey P, Hobbs A, Edwards A, *et al.*: Relationship between natural killer cell activity and histological features of lymphocyte infiltration and partial regression of the primary tumor in melanoma patients. Cancer Res 42:363–368, 1982.

139. Levy MH, Wheelock EF: The role of macrophages in defense against neoplastic disease. Adv Cancer Res 20:131, 1974.

140. Evans R, Alexander P: The role of macrophages in tumor immunity, I. Cooperation between macrophages and lymphoid cells in syngeneic tumor immunity. Immunology 23:615, 1972.

141. Gelboin HV, Levy HB: Polyinosinic-polycytidylic acid inhibits chemically induced tumorigenesis in mouse skin. Science 167:205, 1970.

142. Chow DA, Greene MI, Greenberg AH: Macrophage-dependent NK-cell-independent 'natural' surveillance of tumors in syngeneic mice. Int J Cancer 23:788, 1979.

143. Chow DA, Miller VE, Carlson GA, *et al.*: Natural resistance to tumors is a heterogeneous immunological phenomenon: Evidence for non-NK cell mechanisms. Invas Metas 1:205, 1981.

144. Birbeck MSC, Carter RL: Observations on the ultrastructure of two hamster lymphomas with particular reference to infiltrating macrophages. Int J Cancer 9:249–257, 1972.

145. Eccles SA, Alexander P: Macrophage content of tumors in relation to metastatic spread and host immune reaction. Nature 250:667–669, 1974.

146. Talmadge JE, Key M, Fidler IJ: Macrophage content of metastatic and nonmetastatic rodent neoplasms. J Immunol 126:2245–2248, 1981.

147. Gauci CL: The significance of the macrophage content of human tumors. In: Mathe G (ed) Recent Results in Cancer Research, Vol 56. Berlin, Spinger-Verlag, 1976, pp 122–130.

148. Wood GW, Gollahon KA: Detection and quantitation of macrophage infiltration into primary human tumors with the use of cell-surface markers. J Natl Cancer Inst 59:1081–1087, 1977.

149. Alexander P, Eccles SA, Gauci CLL: The significance of macrophages in human and experimental tumors. Ann NY Acad SCi 276:124–133, 1976.

150. Brunda MJ, Raffel S: Macrophage processing of antigen for induction of tumor immunity. Cancer Res 37:1838–1844, 1977.

151. Shen HH, Talle MA, Goldstein G, Chess L: Functional subsets of human monocytes defined by monoclonal antibodies: a distinct subset of monocytes contains the cells capable of inducing the autogous mixed lymphocyte culture. J Immunol 130:698–705, 1983.

152. Berlinger NT, Hilal EY, Oettgen HF, Good RA: Deficient cell-mediated immunity in head and neck cancer patients secondary to autologous suppressive immune cells. Laryngoscope 88:470–482, 1978.

153. Balch CM, Dougherty PA, Tilden AB: Excessive prostaglandin E$_2$ production by suppressor monocytes in head and neck cancer patients. Ann Surg 196:645–650, 1982.

154. Maca RD, Panje W: Indomethacin sensitive suppressor cell activity in head and neck cancer patients pre and postirradiation therapy. Cancer 50:484–489, 1982.

155. Panje WR: Regression of head and neck carcinoma with a prostaglandin-synthesis inhibitor. Arch Otolaryngol 107:658–663, 1981.

156. Hirsch B, Johnson JT, Rabin BS, Thearle PB: Immunostimulation of patients with head and neck cancer. Arch Otolaryngol 109:298–301, 1983.

157. Wara WM, Wara DW, Phillips TL, Amman AJ: Elevated IgA in carcinoma of the nasopharynx. Cancer 35:1313–1315, 1975.

158. Katz AE, Yoo TJ, Harker LA: Serum immunoglobulin A (IgA) levels in carcinoma of the head and neck. Trans Am Acad Ophthalmol Otolaryngol 82:131–137, 1876.

159. Wolf GT, Chretien PB, Elias EG, *et al.*: Serum glycoproteins in head and neck squamous carcinoma: correlations with tumor extent, clinical tumor stage and T cell levels during chemotherapy. Am J Surg 138:489–500, 1979.

406

160. Baskies AM, Chretien PB, Maxim PE, *et al.*: Circulating immune complexes correlate with levels of seum immune reactive proteins and clinical tumor stage in head and neck squamous carcinoma. Surg Forum 30:516–518, 1979.
161. Wolf GT, Wolfe RA, Chretien PB: Circulating immune complexes in patients with nasopharyngeal carcinoma (manuscripts submitted to Otolaryngol Head Neck Surg).
162. Sample WF, Gertner HR, Chretien PB: Inhibition of phytohemagglutinin induced *in vitro* lymphocyte transformation by serum from patients with carcinoma. J Natl Cancer Inst 46:1291–1297, 1971.
163. Sample WF, Gertner HR, Futrell JW, Chretien PB: Suppression of in vitro reactivity of lymphocytes from normal persons by serum from carcinoma patients. Surg Forum 21:116–118, 1970.
164. Watanabe T, Iglehart JD, Bolognesi DP: Secretroy immune response in patients with oropharyngeal carcinoma. Ann Otol Rhinol Laryngol 92:295–299, 1983.
165. Brown AM, Lally ET, Frankel A, *et al.*: The association of the IgA levels of serum and whole saliva with the progression of oral cancer. Cancer 35:1154–1162, 1975.
166. Sundar SK, Ablashi DV, Kamaraju LS, *et al.*: Sera from patients with undifferentiated nasopharyngeal carcinoma contain a factor which abrogates specific Epstein-Barr virus antigen-induced lymphocyte response. Int J Cancer 29:407–412, 1982.
167. Veltri RW, Sprinkle PM, Maxim PE, *et al.*: Immune monitoring protocol for patients with carcinoma of the head and neck. Ann Otol 87:692–700, 1978.
168. Hellstrom I, Sjogren HO, Warner GA, *et al.*: Blocking of cell-mediated tumour immunity by sera from patients with growing neoplasms. Int J Cancer 7:226–237, 1971.
169. Veltri RW, Radman SM, Sprinkle PM, Quick C: Circulating soluable immune complexes and immunodepression in patients with squamous cell carcinoma of the head and neck. Proc Am Assoc Cancer Res 21:235, 1980.
170. Theofilopoulos An, Andrews BS, Urist MM, *et al.*: The nature of immune complexes in human cancer sera. J Immunol 119:657–663, 1977.
171. Hellstrom I, Hellstrom KE: Studies on the cellular immunity and its serum mediated inhibitors in Maloney-virus induced tumors. Int J Cancer 4:587–600, 1969.
172. Sjogren HO, Hellstrom I, Bansal SC, Hellstrom KE: Suggestive evidence that the blocking antibodies of tumor bearing individuals may be antigen- antibody complex. Proc Natl Acad Sci 68:1372–1375, 1971.
173. Mathew GD, Qualtiere LF, Neel HB, Pearson GR: IgA antibody, antibody-dependent cellular cytotoxicity and prognosis in patients with nasopharyngeal carcinoma. Int J Cancer 27:175–180, 1981.
174. Wheelock EF, Robinson ML: Endogenous control of the neoplastic process. Lab Invest 48:120–139, 1983.
175. Dvorak HF, Orenstein NS, Carvalho AC, *et al.*: Induction of a fibrin-gel investment: an early event in line 10 hepatocarcinoma growth mediated by tumor secreted products. J Immunol 122:166, 1979.
176. Sanford BH: An alteration in tumor histocompatability induced by neuraminidase. Transplant 5:1273–1279, 1967.
177. Black PH: Shedding from the cell surface of normal and cancer cells. Adv Cancer Res 32:75–199, 1980.
178. Yoshimura S, Tamaoki N, Ueyama Y, Hata J: Plasma protein production by human tumors xenotransplanted in nude mice. Cancer Res 38:3474–3476, 1978.
179. Pike MC, Snyderman R: Depression of macrophage function by a factor produced by neoplasms: a mechanism for abrogation of immune surveillance. J Immunol 117:1243–1249, 1976.
180. Cheung HT, Cantarow WD, Sundharadas G: Characteristics of a low molecular weight factor extracted from mouse tumors that affects *in vitro* properties of macrophages. Int J Cancer 23:344–352, 1979.

181. Wong A, Mankovitz R, Kennedy JC: Immunosuppressive and immunostimulating factors produced by malignant cells *in vitro*. Int J Cancer 13:530–542, 1974.

182. Plescia OJ, Smith AH, Grinwich K: Subversion of immune system by tumor cells and role of prostaglandin. Proc Natl Acad Sci 72:1848–1851, 1975.

183. Johnson JT, Rabin BS, Wagner RL: Prostaglandin E_2 of the upper aerodigestive tract. (Abstract), Eastern Society, Triological Society, January 1984.

184. Bennett A, Carter RL, Stamford IF, Tanner NSB: Prostaglandin-like material extracted from squamous carcinoma of the head and neck. Br J Cancer 41:204–208, 1980.

185. Wolf GT, Chretien PB: The chemotherapy and immunotherapy of head and neck cancer. In: Suen JY, Myers EN (eds) Cancer of the Head and Neck. New York, Churchill Livingstone, 1981, pp 782–820.

186. Olivari A, Pradier R, Feierstein J, *et al.*: Cell mediated immunity in head and neck cancer patients. J Surg Oncol 8:287–290, 1976.

187. Wanebo HJ: Immunobiology of head and neck cancer: Basic concepts. Head Neck Surg 2:42–55, 1979.

188. Eilber FR, Morton DL, Ketcham AS: Immunologic abnormalities in head and neck cancer. Am J Surg 128:534–538, 1974.

189. Browder JP, Chretien PB: Immune reactivity in head and neck squamous carcinoma and relevance to the design of immunotherapy trials. Sem Oncol 4:431–439, 1977.

190. Stewart CC, Perez CA: Effect of irradiation of immune responses. Radiology 118:201–210, 1976.

191. Order SE: The effects of therapeutic irradiation on lymphocytes and immunity. Cancer 39:737–743, 1977.

192. Hoppe RT, Fuk ZY, Strober S, Kaplan HS: The long term effects of radiation on T and B lymphocytes in the peripheral blood after regional irradiation. Cancer 40:2071–2078, 1977.

193. Rabou M, Heise ER, Kucera LS, *et al.*: Effects of irradiation on lymphocyte subpopulations. In: Dubois JB, Serrou B, Rosenfeld C (eds) Immunologic Effects of Radiation Therapy. New York, Raven Press, 1981, pp 321–328.

194. Wasserman J, Baral E, Biberfeld G, *et al.*: Effects of *in vitro* irradiation on lymphocyte subpopulations and cytoxicity. In: Dubois JB, Serrou B, Rosenfeld C (eds) Immunologic Effects of Radiation Therapy. New York, Raven Press, 1981, pp 123–135.

195. Baskies AM, Chretien PB, Baer SB: Radiation therapy: its effects on immune reactivity. Prog Clin Cancer 8:215–226, 1982.

196. Cheema AR, Hersh EM: Patient survival after chemotherapy and its relationship to *in vitro* lymphocyte blastogenesis. Cancer 28:851–855, 1971.

197. Colmerauer ME, Koziol JA, Pilch YH: Enhancement of metastasis development by BCG immunotherapy. J Surg Oncol 15:235–241, 1980.

198. Mathe G, Florentin I, Olsson L, *et al.*: Pharmacologic factors and manipulation of immunity systemic adjuvants in cancer therapy. Cancer Treatment Rep 62:1613, 1978.

199. Blomberg BME, Glerum J, Croles JJ, *et al.*: Harmful effects of I.V. Corynebacterium parvum given at the same time as cyclophosphamide in patients with squamous-cell carcinoma of the bronchus. Br J Cancer 41:609–617, 1980.

200. Mathe G, Amiel JL, Schwarzenberg L, *et al.*: Followup of the first (1962) pilot study on active immunotherapy of acute lymphoid leukemia: A critical discussion. Biomed 24:29, 1977.

201. Alberts DS: Adjuvant immunotherapy with BCG of advanced ovarian cancer: A preliminary report. In: Salmon SI, Jones SE (eds) Adjuvant Therapy of Cancer. Amsterdam, Elsevier/North-Holland Biomedical Press, 1977, p 327.

202. McKneally MF, Maver C, Kause HW: Regional immunotherapy of lung cancer with intrapleural BCG. Lancet 1:337, 1976.

203. Morton DL, Eilber FR, Holmes EC: Present status of BCG immunotherapy of malignant

408

melanoma. Cancer Immunol Immunother 1:93–98, 1976.
204. Veronesi U, Adamus J, Aubert C, *et al.*: A randomized trial of adjuvant chemotherapy and immunotherapy in cutaneous melanoma. New Engl J Med 307:913–916, 1982.
205. Mountain CF, Gail MH: Surgical adjuvant intrapleural BCG treatment for Stage I non-small cell lung cancer. J Thor Cardiovasc Surg 82:649–657, 1981.
206. Beuchler M, Mukherji B, Chasin W, Nathanson L: High dose methotrexate with and without BCG therapy in advanced head and neck malignancy. Cancer 43:1095, 1979.
207. Papac R, Minor DR, Rudnick S, *et al.*: Controlled trial of methotrexate and bacillus Calmette-Guerin therapy for advanced head and neck cancer. Cancer Res 38:3150, 1978.
208. Cunningham TJ, Antemann R, Paonessa D, *et al.*: Adjuvant immuno and/or chemotherapy with neuraminidase-treated autogenous tumor vaccine and bacillus Calmette-Guerin for head and neck cancer. Ann NY Acad Sci 277:339, 1976.
209. Taylor SG, Sisson GA, Bytell DE: Adjuvant chemo immunotherapy of head and neck cancer. Recent Results Cancer Res 68:297, 1979.
210. Richman SP, Livingston RB, Gutterman JU, *et al.*: Chemotherapy versus chemo immunotherapy of head and neck cancer: Reports of a randomized study. Cancer Treat Rep 60:535–537, 1976.
211. Amiel JL, Sancho-Garnier H, Vandenbrouck G, *et al.*: First results of a randomized trial on immunotherapy of head and neck tumors. Recent Results Cancer Res 68:318, 1979.
212. Beatty DJ, Terz JJ, Brown PW, *et al.*: Adjuvant intralesional and systemic Corynebacterium parvum immunotherapy for surgically treated head and neck cancer. Surg Forum 31:155–156, 1980.
213. Vogl SE, Schoenfeld DA, Kaplan BH, *et al.*: Methotrexate alone or with regional subcutaneous Corynebacterium parvum in the treatment of recurrent and metastatic squamous cancer of the head and neck. Cancer 50:2295–2300, 1982.
214. Cheng VST, Suit HD, Wang CC, *et al.*: Clinical trial of Cornybacterium parvum (intralymph node and intravenous) and radiation therapy in the treatment of head and neck carcinoma. Cancer 49:239–244, 1982.
215. Szpirglas H, Chastang C, Bertrand JC: Adjuvant treatment of tongue and floor of the mouth cancers. Recent Results cancer Res 68:309–315, 1979.
216. Cruse JP, Lewin MR, Clark CG: Corynebacterium parvum enhances colonic cancer in dimethydrazine-treated rats. Br J Cancer 37:639–643, 1978.
217. Fisher B, Gebhardt M, Linta J, Saffer E: Comparison of the inhibition of tumor growth following local or systemic administration of Corynebacterium parvum or other immunostimulating agents with or without cyclophosphamide. Cancer Res 38:2679–2687, 1978.
218. Isaacs A, Lindenmann J: Virus interference: The interferon. Proc Royal Soc 147:258–267, 1957.
219. Sonnenfeld G, Merigan TC: A regulatory role for interferon in immunity. Ann NY Acad Sci 332:345–355, 1979.
220. Pang RHL, Yip YK, Vilcek J: Immune interferon induction by a monoclonal antibody specific for human T cells. Cellular Immunol 64:304–311, 1981.
221. Friedman RM: Interferons and cancer. J Natl Cancer Inst 60:1191–1194, 1978.
222. Gutterman JU, Blumenschein GR, Alexanian R, *et al.*: Leukocyte interferon-induced tumor regression in human metastatic breast cancer, multiple myeloma and malignant lymphoma. Ann Intern Med 93:399–406, 1980.
223. Horning SJ, Levine JF, Miller RA, *et al.*: Clinical and immunologic effects of recombinant leukocyte A interferon in eight patients with advanced cancer. J Am Med Assoc 247:1718–1722, 1982.
224. Krusic J, Kirhmajer V, Knezevic M, *et al.*: Influence of human leukocyte interferon on squamous cell carcinoma of uterine cervix: clinical, histological and histochemical observations. J Cancer Res Clin Oncol 101:309–315, 1981.
225. Connors JM, Andiman WA, Merigan TC, *et al.*: Treatment of nasopharyngeal carcinoma

with interferon: Epstein-Barr virus serology and clinical results of a pilot study. Proc Am Soc Clin Oncol 1:198, 1982.

226. Padovan I, Brodarec I, Ikic D, et al.: Effect of interferon in therapy of skin and head and neck tumors. J Cancer Res Clin Oncol 100:295–310, 1981.

227. Krown SE, Real FX, Cunningham-Rundles S, et al.: Recombinant leukocyte A interferon in homosexual men with Kaposi's sarcoma. N Engl J Med 308:1071–1074, 1983.

228. Einhorn S, Ahre A, Blomgren H, et al.: Interferon and natural killer activity in multiple myeloma. Lack of correlation between interferon-induced enhancement of natural killer activity and clinical response to human interferon-alpha. Int J Cancer 30:167–172, 1982.

229. Schafer LA, Goldstein AL, Gutterman JN, Hersh EM: In vitro and in vivo studies with thymosin in cancer patients. Ann NY Acad Sci 277:609–612, 1976.

230. Schulof RS, Goldstein AL: Clinical application of thymosin and other thymic hormones. Recent Adv Clin Immunol 3:243–286, 1983.

231. Kenady DE, Chretien PB, Potvin C, Simon RM: Thymosin reconstitution of T cell deficits in vitro in cancer patients. Cancer 39:575–580, 1977.

232. Wolf GT, Kerney SE, Chretien PB: Improvement of impaired leukocyte migration inhibition by thymosin in patients with head and neck squamous carcinoma. Am J Surg 140:531–537, 1980.

233. Constanzi JJ, Gaghano RG, Delaney R, et al.: The effect of thymosin on patients with disseminated malignancies. Cancer 40:14–19, 1977.

234. Lipson SD, Chretien PB, Makuch R, et al: Thymosin immunotherapy in patients with small cell carcinoma of the lung. Cancer 43:863–870, 1979.

235. Schulof RS, Lloyd M, Cox J, Goldstein AL: Synthetic thymosin alpha 1 following mediastinal irradiation: a randomized trial in patients with locally advanced non-small cell lung cancer. Proc Am Soc Clin Oncol 2:185, 1983.

236. Wara WM, Neely MH, Amann AJ, Wara DW: Biologic modifications of immunologic parameters in head and neck cancer patients with thymosin fraction V. In: Goldstein AL, Chirigos MA (eds) Lymphokines and Thymic Hormones: Their Potential Utilization in Cancer Therapeutics. New York, Raven Press, 1981, pp 257–262.

237. Fletcher GH: Place of radiation modulation in the management of head and neck cancer. Sem Oncol 4:375–385, 1977.

238. Jesse RH, Lindberg RD: The efficacy of combining radiation therapy with a surgical procedure in patients with cervical metastasis from squamous cancer of the oropharynx and hypopharynx. Cancer 35:1163–1166, 1975.

239. Schuller DE, McGuirt WF, Krause CF, et al.: Increased survival with surgery alone versus combined therapy. Laryngoscope 89:582–594, 1979.

240. Strong MS, Vaughn CW, Kayna NL, et al.: A randomized trial of preoperative radiotherapy in cancer of the oropharynx and hypopharynx. Am J Surg 136:494–500, 1978.

241. Baker D, Elkan D, Lim M, et al.: Does local x-irradiation of a tumor increase the incidence of metastases? Cancer 48:2394–2398, 1981.

242. Lundy J, Lovett EJ, Wolinsky SM, Conran P: Immune impairment and metastatic tumor growth. Cancer 43:945–951, 1979.

243. Serrou B, Rosenfeld C, Caraux J, et al.: Thymosin modulation of suppressor function in mice and man. Ann NY Acad Sci 332:95–100, 1979.

244. Klein AS, Shoham J: Effect of the thymic factor, thymostimulin (TP-1) on the survival rate of tumor-bearing mice. Cancer Res 41:3217–3221, 1981.

245. Cupissol D, Touraine JL, Serrou B: Ability of lymphocytes treated with thymic factor to decrease lung metastases in tumor-bearing mice. Thymus 3:9–16, 1981.

246. Goldstein G: Made of action of levamisole. J Rheumatol 5:143, 1978.

247. Amery WK: Final results of a multicenter placebo-controlled levamisole study of resectable lung cancer. Cancer Treat Rep 62:1677–1680, 1978.

410

248. Rojas AF, Feierstein JH, Glait HM, Olivari AJ: Levamisole action in breast cancer Stage III. In: Terry WD, Windhorst D (eds) Immunotherapy of Cancer: Present Status of Trials in Man. New York, Raven Press, 1977, p 635.
249. Mussche RA, Kluyskens P: Prognosis of primarily treated localized laryngeal carcinoma ameliorated through levamisole treatment. Oncology 35:329–335, 1980.
250. Olivari AJ, Glait HM, Guardo A, et al.: Levamisole in squamous cell carcinoma of the head and neck. Cancer Treat Rep 63:983, 1979.
251. Olkowski Z, McLaren J, Skeen M: Effects of combined immunotherapy with levamisole and bacillus Calmette-Guerin on immuno-competence of patients with squamous cell carcinoma of the cervix, head and neck and lung undergoing radiation therapy. Cancer Treat Rep 62:1651, 1978.
252. Wanebo HJ, Hilal EY, Pinsky CM, et al.: Randomized trial of levamisole in patients with squamous cancer of the head and neck: A preliminary report. Cancer Treat Rep 62:1663–1669, 1978.
253. Bier J, Rapp HJ, Borsos T, et al.: Randomized clinical study on intratumoral BCG-cell wall preparation (CWP) therapy in patients with squamous cell carcinoma on he head and neck region. Cancer Immunol Immunother 12:71–79, 1981.
254. Goldenberg GJ, Brandes LJ: In vivo and in vitro studies of immunotherapy of nasopharyngeal carcinoma with transfer factor. Cancer Res 36:720–723, 1976.
255. Nair PNM, Gangal SG, Agashe SS, Rao RS: Immunologic studies on human oral cancer. Ind J Cancer 13:64–69, 1976.

17. Tumor immunity and tumor markers in head and neck cancer

ROBERT W. VELTRI and PETER E. MAXIM

1. Introduction

Any review of Head and Neck (H & N) cancer today, irrespective of the organ site, must consider the host, his environment, personal habits, as well as the biology of the tumor of interest [1–6]. The rapidly advancing fields within biotechnology such as genetic engineering, cell cloning, monoclonal antibodies, nonisotopic immunoassay and the allied instrumentation for rapid automated data processing have provided the basis for improved understanding of the etiology, pathogenesis, diagnosis, and treatment of human malignancies.

Another factor which has contributed to our improved knowledge for the management of cancer was derived from the commitment to cancer research with respect to diagnosis and prevention made under the National Cancer Act pased in 1971. This program provided the foundation for major breakthroughs in the isolation and identification of biochemical as well as immunological markers produced during the malignant process. In addition new imaging techniques and reagents combined with development of new hardware and software further improved prospects for diagnosis and treatment of cancer in the 1980's [7, 8].

The National Cancer Institute's forecast for new cases of cancer of the H & N region in the USA for 1982 was approximately 52 000, with a prediction of 16 000 deaths in that forecast. The breakdown according to site was:

Site	No. cases	No. deaths
Buccal cavity and oropharynx	26 600	9 150
Laryngeal	10 700	3 700
Thyroid	9 900	1 050
Nose paranasal sinuses nasopharynx	3 800	2 100

Gregory T. Wolf (ed), Head and Neck Oncology.
© *1984 Martinus Nijhoff Publishers, Boston. ISBN 0-89838-657-8. Printed in The Netherlands.*

Cancers of the H & N region account for only about 5% of all the cancers in the USA. However, internationally the contribution of incidence of cancers for this region is significantly greater. For example, Nasopharyngeal carcinoma in the Chinese occurs twenty-five times more often than in the Caucasian population. Another illustration of this difference is observed in the statistics, for instance, of H & N cancer in Bombay, India where these tumors account for 50% of all diagnosed malignancies.

The leading etiological factors which are known to be involved in H & N cancer invariably direct our attention to tobacco and alcohol consumption [9–12]. The most potent offending agents consist of a long list of chemical irritants and carcinogens produced during pyrolosis, as well as the chronic irritation resulting from radiant and thermal heating and the mechanical insults [11]. The purported role of viruses as causative agents of H and N cancer range from the better defined correlation between Epstein-Barr Virus (EBV) [13–17] and Nasopharyngeal Carcinoma (NPC) and the enigma of a possible role of Herpes Simplex Virus (HSV) [18–23] in the etiology of H and N cancer.

The high degree of variability in regards to susceptibility to this form of cancer appears to be related to genetic, demographic, as well as ecologic factors. In addition it is evident that alcohol serves as a potent promoter while the by products of smoking tobacco generate both initiators and promoters of the carcinogenic process.

Another factor important to the etiopathogenesis of H and N cancer is the nutritional status of the host [6, 24–26]. Protein and calorie intake play a significant role in sustaining the immunological tonus of the host [25, 26]. Several authors have documented that protein-calorie malnutrition (PCM) is a frequent cause of acquired immune deficiency in man. The data to support this conclusion use the same *in vivo* and *in vitro* immunological parameters as have been used previously for immunological monitoring of cancer patients.

2. Tumor immunity in head and neck cancer

2.1. Overview of immunity in cancer

Several excellent reviews of the immune status of cancer patients as well as the immune response to their tumors have been published [27–31]. In general there is a large amount of data to support the importance of the immune system in regulation of tumor growth and metastases. For example, the incidence of cancer in patients undergoing immunosuppressive therapy for purposes of transplantation has been demonstrated to exceed, by several times, the expected values [30, 31]. Also, patients with diseases having a constituent component that includes naturally occurring immunodeficiency, such as the Wiskott-Aldrich Syndrome, demonstrate an abnormally high incidence of De Novo tumors. As a correlate to these observations one must consider the relevance and origin of the universal data bank of literature which documents the immunodepressed status of the cancer patient both at diagnosis and often well into the post-therapy period [27–29]. This review will present immunity in H and N cancer and will address not only the immune status of the tumor-bearing patient but will also evaluate the factors which may contribute to a persistent immunodepressed state.

2.2. Humoral factors in H & N cancer

In an analysis of the humoral immune system and factors produced during the development of H and N cancer it is appropriate to assess both the local and systemic compartments. Several early reports on the local salivary IgA response to infectious agents, such as viruses [32, 33] provided a basis for investigations of the specific IgA local immune response to EBV coded antigens in nasopharyngeal carcinoma patients [13–17, 34]. The results were most encouraging and led to other studies of the local IgA response which proved relevant to H and N cancer. For example, a study in smokers revealed elevated levels in this important control group [35]. A more direct relationship to H and N cancer was provided in a study by Brown et al. [36] that demonstrated an association between salivary and serum IgA levels and status of 102 patients with squamous cell carcinoma of the H and N. These authors found the highest levels of salivary IgA in patients with advanced or recurrent disease. Even if the patients were cured, the IgA levels were well above levels in the controls. In the event new H and N TAA are eventually identified, it will be most appropriate to assess the local IgA immune response to such antigens.

The serum immunoglobulin response in H and N cancer was thoroughly assessed in patients with squamous cell carcinoma by Katz et al. [37]. This prospective analysis demonstrated a significant elevation of serum IgA levels both pre- and post-therapy. Later in a larger patient sample he extended and confirmed these observations [38] and developed an index to determine patient prognosis. This method is described in detail below (Section 3.3). Our laboratories at West Virginia University conducted similar prospective serum immunoglobulin studies of H and N cancer patients [39].

A brief summary of immunoglobulin levels of our patient sample is provided in Table 1. The IgA levels were persistently elevated throughout the course of our study. A more recent analysis by Ockhuizen et al. [40] utilizing part of The West Virginia University serum panel, confirmed the elevated IgA levels and in addition demonstrated for the first time a significantly increased incidence of the Km(l) IgA phenotype marker ($p<0.001$). Additional data on elevated IgA levels has been reported for NPC in both the American and Chinese populations [13–17, 34]. However, the majority of these studies were correlated with specific antibody responses to the EBV coded antigens, which is a unique opportunity since this virus is very closely related to the cause of this type of cancer. These types of data would indicate the possible existence of H and N cancer TAA and may have a broader application to understanding H and N cancer etiology if applied to both virion and non-virion antigens of Herpes simplex virus [5–10]. In this case it will be necessary to discriminate between whether or not the relationship is a primary or co-factorial one or if the virus is serving as a passenger virus and has been reactivated from a latent state [41]. Additional support for an immune response to TAA in H and N cancer is derived from observations of immunoglobulin secreting plasma cells within or bordering the tumor. In a small group of squamous cell tumors studied by Koneval *et al.* [42] most IgG positive cells were noted in both the tumors and their margins and IgA was observed on one occasion. In a more expanded study of 202 patients by Loning and Burkhardt [43], high number of both IgA and IgG secreting plasma cells were observed in cases of leukoplakia with dysplasia and much fewer of such cells were seen in well differentiated tumors. The relationship

Table 1. Immunoglobulin levels in pre- and post-therapy head and neck cancer sera

	Cancer patients (mg %)			Normal donors (mg %)			
	Visit	Mean	CI_{95}	Visit	Mean	CI_{95}	Alpha*
IgG	1[a]	1107	(955–1258)	1	1022	(880–1163)	n.s.
	3[b]	1078	(1065–1091)	3	975	(834–1115)	0.01
	5[c]	0899	(729–1066)	5	981	(871–1090)	n.s.
IgA	1	319	(266–371)	1	0214	(168–259)	0.001
	3	325	(263–386)	3	0223	(159–286)	0.01
	5	296	(234–357)	5	0215	(172–257)	0.01
IgM	1	286	(234–336)	1	0253	(202–301)	n.s.
	3	294	(238–348)	3	0200	(155–244)	n.s.
	5	253	(194–310)	5	0225	(173–274)	n.s.
IgD	1	4.07	(2.50–5.63)	1	2.83	(1.14–4.51)	n.s.
	3	2.99	(1.80–4.12)	3	2.00	(1.23–2.76)	n.s.
	5	2.90	(1.65–4.14)	5	2.08	(0.825–3.33)	n.s.

* Student's *t*-test for independent samples.
[a] Pre-therapy sample.
[b] 3–5 months post-therapy.
[c] 5–7 months post-therapy.

of elevated serum and salivary immunoglobulins, specific antiviral antibodies, local antibody producing cell infiltrates at the tumor site and related studies to be presented below focus attention on the possible existence of specific tumor antigens and immune responses in H and N cancer.

The analysis of immunoglobulins and specific antibodies in H and N cancer sets the stage for presenting new and interesting studies of soluble circulating immune complexes (CIC) in cancer of the H and N. Our laboratory reported the existence of such CIC in a high percentage of these patients (at least 75)) using both the Raji cell assay [44, 45] and later employing the PEG precipitation method [47]. Another collaborative effort with Baskies *et al.* [46] in patients with NPC also showed a similar universal elevation of CIC in these cancer patients.

Table 2 summarizes data on these patient samples using the PEG method of Digeon [47] combined with the measurement of total precipitable protein by the Lowry method. Statistically significant increases in PEG-CIC levels were demonstrated both pre- and post-therapy. As a followup to the historical data gathered on H and N cancer which demonstrated elevations in serum IgA and CIC, Dr. Michael Baseler working in our laboratories developed an IgA-specific immune complex enzyme immunoassay (IgA-IC.)

Table 2. Immune complex in head and neck cancer sera

Cancer patients (μg/ml PEG-Protein)			Normal donors (μg/ml PEG-Protein)			
Visit	Mean	CI_{95}	Visit	Mean	CI_{95}	Alpha*
1 [a]	1107	(387–729)	1	223	(152–293)	.001
3 [b]	1078	(295–478)	3	226	(147–302)	.01
5 [c]	0899	(296–482)	5	182	(126–236)	.001

* Student's *t*-test for independent samples.
[a] Pre-therapy sample.
[b] 3–5 months post-therapy.
[c] 5–7 months post-therapy.

Table 3. Serum-IGA immune complex levels in head and neck cancer

	Sample size	Serum IgA-IC* (μg/ml)	Alpha*
Normals	57	5.12± 4.07	–
H & N cancer (WVU study)	42	11.38±12.54	<.0025
Nasopharyngeal cancer (NCI study)	37	13.36±17.56	<.0025

* IgA-specific ELISA developed by Dr. Michael Baseler.

These data from our laboratory are summarized in Table 3 and illustrate the significant increases in this unique category of CIC. A complete manuscript on this subject is now in preparation. Recent evidence in support of the importance of IgA-IC to the pathogenesis of H and N cancer comes from an investigation which has revealed an IgA-like substance in cancer sera capable of abrogating the *in vitro* lymphocyte mitogenic response to EBV [48]. At this time knowledge and technology are available to more completely assess the role of such CIC in immunoregulation as well as to delineate the types of cancer associated antigens contained in these unique IgA-IC materials.

2.3. Cell-mediated immunity in H & N cancer

The analysis of cell-mediated immunity (CMI) in carcinoma of the H and N has been much more extensive and at least one review that covers methodology and results has been published [47]. In general, during the last ten years authors have assessed one or more of the following *in vivo* and *in vitro* correlates of CMI in H and N cancer patients:

1. *In vivo* DNCB sensitization.
2. *In vivo* specific recall antigen testing.
3. Total small lymphocyte count.
4. Surface lymphocyte marker analysis for lymphocytes T and B.
5. *In vitro* CMI correlates:
   polyclonal mitogenesis;
   specific recall antigen mitogenesis;
   leukocyte adherence inhibition;
   leukocyte migration inhibition.

The most consistent and reproducible results have been produced using *in vivo* DNCB sensitization. The earliest report was by Maisel and Ogura [49] who tested 55 patients with H and N cancer and found 88% of the positive reactors to be alive and tumor free one year after diagnosis and treatment. Of interest, however, was the fact that 53% of nonresponders were also disease free. This provided the first evidence that CMI defects could persist in successfully treated H and N cancer patients. Twomey and Chretien [50] and Eilber *et al.* [51] in 1974 extended and verified these observations in a similar patient sample. In 1976 Maisel and Ogura [52] published a follow-up of their previous patient sample that included some new patients. The results extended the positive correlation of the value of DNCB testing in assessing and the CMI system and showed that 85% of patients with recurrent tumors fell into the nonresponder group of patients. Other clinical investigators attempted to used DNCB to determine patient prognosis and found its value to be limited to early Stage I and II carcinoma of the H and

N [49, 53–55]. In advanced H and N cancer (Stage III and IV) in addition to depressed delayed cutaneous hypersensitivity responsiveness to DNCB, other investigators used *in vitro* CMI correlates to substantiate a persistent state of immunodepression [53–57]. These studies employed one or more of the following assays: total small lymphocyte count, polyclonal mitogenesis, T-lymphocyte count and, more recently, suppressor T-lymphocyte subset counts determined with monoclonal OKT8+ [58].

An apparent relationship between circulating humoral factors and depressed CMI surfaced during studies of circulating immune complexes and cell mediated immunity in H and N cancer patients [39, 59]. The results indicated a consistent relationship between elevated CIC and depressed CMI functions when analyzed by *in vitro* CMI methods. Alternatively, extensive prospective longitudinal studies by Wolf *et al.* [60] have demonstrated that selected serum glycoproteins elevated during H and N carcinogenesis correlate to the depressed immune state of these patients. Also, as mentioned previously, an IgA-CMI blocking factor has been demonstrated in NPC patients' sera [48]. It therefore becomes apparent that circulating humoral as well as cellular factors may combine to collectively-like exert a negative control over the immune response in H and N cancer.

The only additional data to support the existence of immunity to H and N cancer associated antigens has resulted from the application of some rather controversial, yet acceptable, *in vitro* assays. Using the leukocyte adherence-inhibition (LAI) method several investigators have reported positive reactions to crude H and N cancer antigen preparations [61–64]. The very best results were obtained using a homogeneous laryngeal carcinoma patient sample and the homologous extract where the results were 86% positive for the test population [63]. Also, the existence of Laryngeal cancer associated antigens are suggested by data obtained using the leukocyte inhibition factor (LIF) release assay with 3M KCL extracts of homologous tumors in the presence and absence of adherent cells [64].

The above review on humoral and cell-mediated immunity in H and N cancer summarizes current knowledge regarding specific and nonspecific immunity in this patient population. It is apparent that ample opportunities exist to test new ideas on the etiology and pathogenesis of H and N cancer. The following material deals with a closely related area of H and N cancer immunology, that is 'tumor markers'.

3. Tumor markers in head and neck cancer

3.1. Overview of cancer markers

During the course of tumor development, qualitative and quantitative changes occur in levels of a variety of substances in serum [7, 65–69]. Such substances are referred to as tumor markers or biochemical serum markers. The source of these markers may be from the tumor as with the ectopic production of hormones by tumors not generally associated with hormone production such as in lung cancer [68]. Alternatively, some tumors release an excess of metabolic growth products or may overproduce oncofetal antigens. In addition, selected serum markers may be produced by the host in response to the developing tumor. This is probably the case when highly elevated levels of serum glycoproteins are seen in cancer patients.

Many of the different substances that have been previously described as tumor markers are presented in Table 4. The list is not comprehensive and only intended to demonstrate the variety and extent of tumor markers that

Table 4. Classification of substances used as tumor markers

1. Oncofetal antigens
    Carcinoembryonic antigen (CEA)
    Alpha fetoprotein (AFP)
    Ferritin
    Placental proteins

2. Enzymes

Alkaline phosphatases	Lysozyme
Acid phosphatases	Glutamyltranspeptidase
Lactic dehydrogenases	t-Deoxynucleotidyl transferase
Glycosyl transferases	

3. Hormones/Receptors

Calcitonin	Prolactin	Estrogen receptors
ACTH	MSH	
HCG	vasopressin	

4. Immunological parameters
    Immunoglobulin levels
    Lymphokines
    Immune complexes

5. Serum proteins

Alpha-1 antitrypsin	Haptoglobin
Beta-2 microglobulin	Prealbumin
Alpha-1 acid glycoprotein	Ceruloplasmin

6. Metabolic products

Polyamines	Nonhistone proteins
t-RNA	Protamine

7. Candidate tumor associated antigens of head and neck cancer
    Herpes simplex nonvirion antigens
    Epstein Barr virus-associated antigens
    AG-4
    CaCx

have been described. Patients may also present with a highly variable profile when examined for the presence of tumor markers. A patient with squamous cell carcinoma of the head and neck may have abnormal levels of several such markers or none of these. A patient with a relatively small tumor may have high serum levels of a particular marker, whereas a patient with a large tumor may have only slightly elevated or normal levels of a markers. It is therefore advantageous to utilize a panel or battery of tests to measure multiple markers or to select markers based on initial levels when the patient first presents.

Much diversity exists among the types and levels of markers seen not only between patients with different types of tumors, but also among patients with a particular type of cancer. Just as these patients are highly diversified in their response to tumor growth, we now recognize that tumors are highly heterogeneous in many of their biological properties [4, 29, 70, 71]. For example, within a population of B-16 melanoma cells a subpopulation of cells can be cloned that has the capacity to produce a pigment. If these cells are recloned, there will develop subpopulations of cells that are no longer able to produce pigment [70]. In addition, colon cancer cells grown *in vitro* vary considerably in the amount of carcinoembryonic antigen produced per million cells [72]. Lung tumor cells have also been shown to produce various hormones ectopically [70]. Also within a tumor, certain cells exist that have the potential to metastasize and will do so as the result of many different host-tumor interactions [72]. The diversity or heterogeneity therefore that exists with respect to tumor markers is probably a function of both the host and the tumor.

Table 5 outlines some potential uses of tumor markers. Probably the most familiar use is in monitoring the outcome of therapy through the use of longitudinal sampling [34, 39, 45, 60]. If a serum or plasma sample is obtained at the time of diagnosis, baseline (pretreatment) values of one or more markers can be established for the patient. Serial samples are obtained following treatment at preselected intervals. If therapy has been successful and if there has been a reduction of tumor mass, the serum level of the

Table 5. Potential uses of tumor markers

1. Monitoring outcome of therapy
   a. reduction of tumor mass
   b. detecting recurrence or metastases
2. Determination of prognosis
3. Targeting of therapeutic agents
4. Localization of tumor foci (*in vivo* imaging)
5. Screening for early diagnosis/risk assessment

marker should decrease. In the absence of any recurrence, or if there were no distant metastases, the serum level would be expected to remain low. If, however, there is a persistent rise in the level of the marker, this would be evidence to suggest recurrence of the primary tumor, unsuccessful treatment, or growth of unexpected metastatic lesions. All of this, of course, assumes that the serum level of the tumor marker is related to tumor burden.

Because marker level is often associated with tumor burden, an upper limit can be assigned such that patients with serum concentration of the marker higher than the upper limit will have a poorer prognosis than those patients with lower levels. For example, after extensive sampling, a poorer prognosis may be expected from individuals with a pretreatment CEA level greater than 20 ng/ml [74]. Because of the variation and diversity in levels of such markers single determinations are not as accurate as the sequential monitoring of a patient.

Two other potential uses of tumor markers involve the use of antibodies raised to these markers. These antibodies can be radiolabeled, injected into the patient and allowed to concentrate at areas of high antigen (marker) concentrations. Thereafter, through imaging techniques small primary tumor foci, metastatic lesions, or extent of tumor spread from the primary site can be visualized. Radioimmunodetection and localization was the subject of a recent UICC workshop; the results of which have been reported in detail [74]. Similarly, highly radioactive antibodies to ferritin have been used by Order et al. [75] for the treatment of various tumors. The radiolabel in this case is used as a therapeutic agent once it is concentrated at the tumor site.

A potential diagnostic use for tumor markers might relate to their ability to screen large groups of individuals at risk of developing a particular type of tumor. All of the tumor markers tested to date are inadequate for this purpose because of a lack of specificity and sensitivity. They lack specificity because these substances are often elevated in a variety of non-neoplastic diseases as well as during tumor development. CEA for example is elevated not only in colon cancer but in breast and lung cancer, chronic diseases and in cigarette smokers. Furthermore, because almost all of these markers are present in low levels in the non-tumor bearing host, differences in serum concentrations are generally not seen until tumors have reached a significant size. These difficulties could be alleviated by identification and isolation of tumor associated or tumor specific antigens associated with a definite histologic type of tumor and possibly with the use of monoclonal antibody technology for measurement.

In spite of these shortcomings, evidence has accumulated that there are several different tumor markers that may be of some value to the head and neck oncologist in evaluating or monitoring his patients.

3.2. Enzymes

Enzymes have been used as disease biomarkers for many years [77, 78]. Quantitation of serum or tissue levels was usually accomplished using catalytic assays but, more recently, immunoassays have been developed for many of these enzymes [79]. Because many of these enzymes exist as isoenzymes it may be more important to measure a particular isoenzyme rather than total serum enzyme levels. For example, with lactic dehydrogenase, the LDH 5 isoenzyme has been found to be predominant in cancer tissue. In a group of patients with colorectal cancer 52% had elevated levels of LDH5, whereas the total serum LDH was elevated in only 24% [80].

In patients with head and neck cancer Katz et al. [81] measured serum alkaline phosphatase (AP) levels prior to induction chemotherapy. Of the 55 patients studied 40 exhibited a favorable response which was defined as a 50% reduction in tumor mass. In those patients with an AP level greater than 80 mU/ml, 21/24 (88%) were found to respond to chemotherapy. In those patients with levels below 80 mU/ml 19/31 (62%) responded to therapy with cis-platinum and bleomycin. The source of the AP has not been determined although the most likely sources are the liver or the tumor itself. The preliminary evidence presented in this paper indicates that AP levels may offer some predictive value concerning responsiveness to therapy although more detailed studies will be needed. These authors [81] also examined serum glutamic oxaloacetic transaminase levels but found no difference in pretreatment levels between responders (mean 24 mU/ml and nonresponders (mean 21 mU/ml). One other report on a small group of patients (N = 25) has shown significant elevations of salivary beta-glucuronidase activity, but no such elevation of enzyme activity was seen in patients' serum or urine [82].

3.3. Immunoglobulins

Many investigators have used changes in host immunoglobulin levels to monitor response to therapy. The major differences in circulating serum immunoglobulin levels reside with the IgA and IgE classes [37, 38]. An evaluation of 245 patients with carcinomas of the head and neck and 111 controls showed no significant difference between the two groups, when IgG, IgM or IgD levels were compared. With IgE, however, 26.2% of the patients had values in excess of 200 IU/ml, whereas only 7.2% of the controls had similar levels [38]. With IgA, 41.6% of the head and neck patients but only 14.1% of the controls had IgA levels greater than 325 mg/dl. Both of these values were significant at $p<0.0001$ by the Chi square test.

Katz compared the above immunoglobulin data with the success or failure of treatment in these patients (personal communication). He found the treatment failure rate was inversely proportional to the serum IgE level and directly proportional to the serum IgA level. Of the 13 patients in this study with IgE values greater than 1000 IU/ml only 2 were treatment failures. Seven patients had IgE levels less than 100 IU/ml. Six of these were treatment failures. In those patients with IgE less than 1000 IU/ml, a more favorable prognosis was associated with a higher IgE value. However, the IgA level impacted on the rate of treatment failures in that the number of failures increased as the IgA level increased.

A serum immunoglobulin prognostic index (SIPI) using multiple immunoglobulin markers was formulated based on the patient IgE, IgA and IgD levels. A positive SIPI indicated a relative excess of IgA over IgE and IgD and was associated with increased failure rates. When this formula was applied to the test groups it was found to be accurate in predicting treatment failures and successes when the SIPI score was either highly positive or negative. However, the overall accuracy of the SIPI was 60.5%. The accuracy of using these markers was increased when combined with patients' clinical information such as stage, age and lymphocyte count.

In head and neck cancer patients circulating immune complexes (CIC) have been shown to be elevated [44–46, 59]. Immune complexes have been described in many different disease states as well as cancer. Baskies *et al.* [34] working in collaboration with our laboratories, examined polyethyleneglycol precipitated CIC in untreated head and neck cancer patients, cured patients (tumor-free after five years) healthy smokers and healthy nonsmokers. CIC levels were lowest in nonsmokers, higher in smokers and highest in untreated patients. Stage III and IV individuals had higher CIC levels than patients with Stage I and II tumors. In the cured patients, CIC levels were still greater than smoker controls and did not differ from levels found in untreated patients. These findings are consistent with previous observations showing that head and neck cancer patients remain immunosuppressed for years following successful treatment. The presence of elevated levels of CIC in a high risk group (smokers) as well as their persistence in the cured group (at high risk for a second tumor) offers some interesting potential for monitoring these groups.

3.4. Nonimmunoglobulin serum proteins

Wolf *et al.* [60] examined changes in concentration of several different serum proteins. They examined both nonsmoker and smoker controls as well as untreated head and neck cancer patients. Since chronic cigarette smoking is a universal finding in head and neck cancer patients, the control groups were first evaluated. Of the six proteins studied, two (alpha-1 antitrypsin and prealbumin) were found to be significantly different in the smokers when compared to nonsmokers. Serum haptoglobin levels were found to be increased in all tumor stages. Alpha-1 acid glycoprotein (AAG) and alpha-1 antitrypsin (AAT) were also found to be elevated in all tumor stages and increased progressively with tumor stage and extent. Serum albumin, prealbumin and alpha-2 HS glycoprotein levels were decreased, but only alpha-2 HS glycoprotein decreased progressively with increasing stage of tumor.

In cured patients, haptoglobin and alpha-1 acid glycoprotein levels were lower than untreated or recurrent patients indicating that reduced levels correlate with reduction of tumor burden. Similarly alpha-2 HS glycoprotein and prealbumin levels were elevated above untreated groups. During preoperative chemotherapy, alpha-2 HS glycoprotein levels as well as T-cell levels declined during therapy and returned to pretreatment levels after completion of therapy. The authors state that their findings show that alpha-1 antiyrypsin and alpha-1 acid glycoprotein are good indicators of tumor stage and local/regional extent and alpha-2 HS glycoprotein can be used as an indicator of the patients' cellular immune status.

Baskies *et al.* [34] in a study similar to the one described above reported findings in Chinese patients with nasopharyngeal carcinoma. Increased antibody titers to Epstein-Barr Virus (EBV) associated antigens were related to tumor presence but not to tumor stage. Levels of immunoglobulins, haptoglobin, alpha-1 acid glycoprotein, and alpha-1 antitrypsin were increased significantly over normal controls. In contrast to Wolf's study, haptoglobin was the protein most directly related to tumor stage. Haptolobin levels also directly correlated with anti-EBNA antibody titers (Epstein Barr Nuclear Antigen). Again, alpha-2 HS glycoprotein levels were reduced in the NPC patients and in this study were found to correlated with titers of IgA antibodies to EBV early antigen.

Al-Sarraf *et al.* [83] and Carey *et al.* (personal communication) examined alpha-1 acid glycoprotein levels in 47 patients with advanced (Stage III and IV) squamous cell carcinoma of the head and neck and in patients with recurrent disease. They found this marker to be elevated in 52% of untreated patients and 70% of patients with recurrent disease. The levels of this marker correlated well with the size of the tumor mass but not with tumor site or histological differentiation. This marker was also found to be a sensitive indicator of tumor remission.

3.5. Oncofetal antigens

Oncofetal antigens are substances produced by fetal tissues and tumors but usually found in very low quantities in normal adults. Carcinoembryonic antigen (CEA) is a 180,000 MW glycoprotein found in nanogram quantities in normal serum. It was originally described by Gold and Freedman [84] as a new tumor specific antigen for colorectal cancer. This was found not to be the case as the protein was detected in normal serum and in patients with tumors other than colon. In colorectal cancer, CEA is a very good tumor marker and in many instances a good indicator of response to therapy. This marker has also been used with some success in breast and lung cancer [85, 86]. In head and neck cancer, Silverman [87] compared CEA levels in 439 patients with squamous cell carcinoma of the head and neck, 154 healthy smokers and 122 nonsmokers. Among nonsmokers 5 ng/ml served as a cutoff for 95% of the population. This was increased to 7 ng/ml for the smokers. In the cancer population, 36% had CEA levels greater than 5 ng/ml but only 17% had values greater than 7 ng/ml. Based on these data the authors concluded that CEA levels alone were not likely to serve as a prognostic indicator but because of declines in CEA levels seen during therapy, serial determinations could be of value in monitoring tumor response.

Carey et al. (personal communication) in a more recent study, used CEA levels in conjunction with alpha-1 acid glycoprotein levels to monitor head and neck cancer patients. In patients with untreated disease CEA levels exceeded 2.5 ng/ml in 81% and exceeded 5 ng/ml in 37%. In patients with recurrent disease 85% and 55% of the patients exceed the above limits. When used in conjunction with AAG levels, both markers were elevated in 44% of untreated patients and 59% of those with recurrence. The value of selecting more than one marker whenever possible was shown in this study when 88% of the untreated and 94% of the recurrent patients were positive for at least one marker. In serial testing, the AAG was a more sensitive indicator of tumor remission, whereas CEA was more indicative of tumor progression.

Ferritin is another oncofetal protein that is produced during fetal development and also by tumor cells [88]. Ferritin exists in normal serum at concentrations between 30–320 ng/ml. Ferritin also exists as an array of isoferritins with pIs between 4.6 and 5.7. Each characteristic array depends upon the subunit composition of the isoferritin. The subunits are either H or L chains and can be assembled in any combination of H and L to equal 24. The liver and spleen (basic) ferritins are primarily composed of the L subunit whereas the heart and tumor ferritins (acidic) are composed primarily of the H type. In addition to the biochemical differences there are also immunological differences among the basic and acidic isoferritins which become important in the choice of assay system to measure these ferritins [89, 90].

Serum ferritin has been shown to be elevated in many different types of cancer [89, 91, 92]. Representative values obtained in our laboratory (unpublished data) using a double antibody enzyme immunoassay capable of measuring a broad range of isoferritins are presented in Table 6. Note that significantly elevated levels are present in patients with head and neck cancer. When the head and neck cancer patients were evaluated on the basis of stage of disease, ferritin levels did not directly correlate with increasing stage of disease, but were significantly higher in patients with Stage III and IV tumors versus patients with Stage I and II tumors (Table 7). Serum ferritin levels were increased in patients with regional disease as opposed to those with only local disease. In those patients considered cured (tumor free five years) the ferritin level had declined but remained at levels comparable to Stage I and II patients.

The usefulness of serum ferritin levels in head and neck cancer was dependent on serial serum determinations. Twenty five patients were evaluated monthly for serum ferritin levels. At visit 1, which was the time of diagnosis, the mean ferritin value for this group was 172.4 ± 35.9 ng/ml. The

Table 6. Serum ferritin levels in patients with tumors

Population	Sample size	Serum ferritin (ng/ml)
Normal control	118	32.2 ± 2.8
Lung cancer	43	232.0 ± 55.3
Breast cancer	20	289.6 ± 75.6
Colon cancer	9	202.2 ± 68.1
Head and neck cancer	113	242.0 ± 30.6

Each cancer group differed significantly from normals ($p < 0.001$) according to Student's t-test for unpaired data.

Table 7. Serum ferritin in treated and untreated head and neck cancer patients

Population	Sample size	Serum ferritin (ng/ml)
Untreated		
Total	113	242.0 ± 30.6
Stage 1	19	129.1 ± 16.7
Stage 2	19	130.9 ± 18.6
Stage 3	26	230.3 ± 70.3
Stage 4	35	247.3 ± 46.9
Treated		
Cured	28	114.1 ± 18.4

1. Cured indicates clinically free of disease for five years.
2. Student's t-test for independent samples showed all groups significantly higher than normal controls ($p < 0.05$); stage 3 and 4 higher than stage 1 and 2 ($p < 0.05$), and cured lower than total head and neck cancer group ($p < 0.05$).

patients were then treated by surgery, x-irradiation or a combination. By three months following therapy there had been no significant change in the serum ferritin level of this group (157.6 ± 32.2). By 5-6 months post diagnosis the mean serum ferritin level had declined to 96.5 ± 22.7 ng/ml ($p < 0.01$) in the 20 patients that remained in this group.

Appropriate isoferritin determinations are a good monitor of a head and neck cancer patient's response to therapy. When examined individually, those patients with an unfavorable outcome to therapy had high ferritin levels which remained high or increased following therapy. In those patients with a favorable outcome, the ferritin value decreased or remained low with respect to time following therapy [92].

The above information supports the concept that several different substances can be used as markers for head and neck cancer. The appropriate selection of one or more of these substances can assist the clinician in monitoring response to therapy, assessing the host's immune status and possibly predicting prognosis. Future studies should be designed to utilize and expand the markers that are of value in head and neck cancer and to assess whether increased sensitivity and specificity can be achieved by using multiple markers. It might also be appropriate to include in such new prospective studies some of the candidate tumor associated antigens listed in Table 4.

References

1. Strong LC: Genetic and environmental interactions. Cancer 1:1861–1866, 1977.
2. Krontiris TG: The emerging genetics of human cancer. NEJM 309:404–409. 1983.
3. Oppenheimer SB: Causes of cancer: Gene alteration versus gene activation. American Laboratory 40:40–46, 1982.
4. Fidler IJ, Hart IR: Biological diversity in metastatic neoplasms: Origins and implications. Science 217:998–1003, 1982.
5. Correa P, Cuello C, Fajardo LF, Haenskel W, Bolanos O, deRamirez B: Diet and gastric cancer: Nutrition survey in a high-risk area. JNCI 70:673–678, 1983.
6. Ames BN: Dietary carcinogens and anti-carcinogens: Oxygen radicals and degenerative diseases. Science 221:1256–1264, 1983.
7. Sell S: Cancer markers: Diagnostic and developmental significance. Clifton, NJ, The Humana Press, 1980.
8. Rosenberg SA: Serologic analysis of human cancer antigens. New York, Academic Press, 1980.
9. Fraumeni JF: Respiratory carcinogenesis: An epidemiological appraisal, JNCI 55:1039–1046, 1975.
10. Binnie WH, Rankin KV, Machenzie IC: Etiology of squamous cell carcinoma. J Oral Pathology 12:11–29, 1983.
11. Decker J, Goldstein JC: Risk factors in head and neck cancer. NEJM 306:1151–1155, 1982.
12. Miller AB: Trends in cancer mortality and epidemiology. Cancer 51:2413–2418, 1983.

13. Ho HC, Ng MH, Kwan HC, Chau JCW: Epstein-Barr virus specific IgA and IgG-specific antibodies in nasopharyngeal carcinoma. Br J Cancer 34:656–659.
14. Ho HC, Ng MH, Kwan HC: IgA antibodies to Epstein-Barr viral capsid antigen in saliva of nasopharyngeal carcinoma patients. Br J Cancer 34:656–659, 1976.
15. Coates HL, Pearson Gr, Bryan N, Weiland LH, Devine KD: An immunologic basis for the detection of occult primary malignancies of the head and neck. Cancer 41:912–918, 1978.
16. Ho HC, Kwan HC, NG MH: Immunohistochemistry of local immunoglobulin production in nasopharyngeal carcinoma. Br J Cancer 37:514–519, 1978.
17. Ho HC, NgMH, Kwan HC: Factors affecting serum IgA antibody to Epstein-Barr virus capsid antigens in nasopharyngeal carcinoma. Br J Cancer 37:356–362, 1978.
18. Hollinshead A: DHR-ST, LMIT and CF tests to identify herpes simplex tumor associated antigens and antibody. In: Herberman RB (ed), Compendium of Assays for Immunodiagnosis of Human Cancer. New York/Amsterdam/Oxford, Elsevier-North Holland, 1979, pp 489–497.
19. Hollinshead A, Tarro G, Foster WA, Siegel LJ, Jaffurs W: Studies of tumor-specific and herpes non-biron antigens. Cancer Research 34:1122–1125, 1974.
20. Tarro G: Analysis and description of procedures used in the study of the relationship of Herpes simplex virus 'non-virian' antigens to certain cancers. In: de-The G, Epstein MA, zur Hausen H (eds) Oncogenesis and Herpesviruses II. Lyon, IARC Publications, 1975, pp 291–297.
21. Accini R, Terrara R, Tarro G, Sisillo E, Privitera L, Biancardi C, Bartorelli A: Preliminary studies of non-virion antigens associated with herpes simplex 1 and 2 (HSV-1 and HSV-2). Boll Ist Steroter Milanese 55:122–128, 1976.
22. Shillitoe EJ, Greenspan D, Greenspan JS, Silverman S: Immunoglobulin class of antibody to HSV in patients with oral cancer. Cancer 51:65–71, 1983.
23. Shillitoe EJ, Greenspan D, Greenspan JS, Hansen LS, Silverman S: Neutralizing antibody to herpes simplex virus type 1 in patients with oral cancer. Cancer 49:2315–2320, 1982.
24. Weisburger JH, Horn C: Nutrition and cancer: Mechanisms of genotoxic and epigenetic carcinogens in nutritional carcinogenesis. Bull New York Acad Med 58:296–312, 1982.
25. Cunningham-Rundles S: Effects of nutritional status on immunological function. Am J Clin Nutrition 35:1202–1210, 1982.
26. Chandra RK, Tejpar S: Diet and immunocompetence. Int J Immunopharmacology 5:175–180, 1983.
27. Wanebo H: Immunobiology of head and neck cancer: Basic concepts. Head and Neck Surgery 2:42–55, 1979.
28. Richards V: Cancer immunology – An overview. Prog Exp Tumor Research 25:1–60, 1980.
29. Nelson DS, Nelson M, Tarram E, Inoue Y: Cancer and subversion of host defences. JEBAK 59:229–262, 1981.
30. Penn I: Depressed immunity and the development of cancer. Clin Exp Immunol 46:459–474, 1981.
31. Thomas L: On immunosurveillance in human cancer. Yale J Biol and Med 55:329–333, 1982.
32. Tokumaru T: A possible role of Gamma A immunoglobulin in herpes simplex virus infection in man. J Immunol 97:248–259, 1966.
33. Douglas GR, Couch RB: A prospective study of chronic herpes simples virus infection and recurrent herpes labialis in humans. J Immunol 104:289–295, 1970.
34. Baskies AM, Chretien PB, Yang CS, Wolf G, Makuch RW, Tu SM, Hsu MM, Lynn TC, Yang HM, Weiss JF, Spiegel HE: Serum glycoproteins and immunoglobulins in nasopharyngeal carcinoma. Correlations with Epstein-Barr virus associated antibodies and clinical tumor stage. Am J Surgery 138:478–488, 1979.

428

35. Lewis DM, Lapp NL, Burrell RG: Quantification of secretory immunoglobulin A in chronic pulmonary disease. Am Rev Resp Dis 101:55–59, 1970.
36. Brown AM, Lally ET, Frankel A, Harwick R, Davis LW, Rominger CJ: The association of IgA levels of serum and whole saliva with the progression of oral cancer. Cancer 35:1154–1162, 1975.
37. Katz AE, Nysather JO, Harker LA: Major immunoglobulin ratios in carcinoma of the head and neck. Ann Otol Rhinol and Larynol 87:412–416, 1978.
38. Katz AE, Yoo TJ, Nysather JO, Harker LA, krause CJ: Serum immunoglobulin concentrations in carcinoma of the head and neck. In: Neiburgs HE (ed) Prevention and Detection of Cancer. New York, Marcel-Dekker, 1980, pp 1335–1349.
39. Veltri RW, Rodman SM, Sprinkle PM, Quick C: Circulating soluble immune complexes and immunodepression in patients with squamous cell carcinoma of the head and neck. Proc Am Assoc Cancer Res 21:235.
40. Ockhuizen T, Pandey JP, Veltri RW, Arlen M, Fudenberg HH: Immunoglobulin allotypes in patients with squamous cell carcinoma of the head and neck. Cancer 49:2021–2024, 1982.
41. Klein RJ: The pathogenesis of acute, latent and recurrent herpes simplex virus infections. Arch Virology 72:143–168, 1982.
42. Koneval T, Applebaum E, Popovic D, Gill L, Sisson G, Wood GW, Anderson B: Demonstration of immunoglobulin in tumor and marginal tissues of squamous cell carcinomas of the head and neck. JNCI 59:1089–1097, 1977.
43. Loning T, Burkhardt A: Plasma cells and immunoglobulin-synthesis in oral pre-cancer and cancer. Virchows Arch Path Anat Histol 384:109–120, 1979.
44. Maxim PE, Veltri RW, Sprinkle PM, Puseteri RJ: Soluble immune complexes in sera from head and neck cancer patients: A preliminary repart. Ann Otol Rhinol Laryngol 86:428–432, 1978.
45. Veltri RW, Sprinkle PM, Maxim PE, Theophilopoulos AN, Rodman SM, Kinney CL: Immune monitoring protocol for patients with carcinoma of the head and neck: Preliminary report. Ann Otol Rhinol Laryngol 87:692–701, 1978.
46. Baskies AM, Chretien PB, Maxim PE, Veltri RW, Wolf GT: Circulating immune complexes correlate with levels of serum immune reactive proteins and clinical tumor stage in head and neck squamous carcinoma. Surg Forum 31:526–527, 1980.
47. Digeon M, Laver M, Riza J, Bach JF: Detection of circulating immune complexes by simplified assays with polyethylene glycol. J Immunological Methods 16:165–183, 1977.
48. Sundar SK, Ablashi DV, Kamaraju L, Levine PH, Faggione A, Armstrong GR, Pearson GR, Krueger GRF, Hewetson JF, Bertram G, Sesterhenn K, Menezes J: Sera from patients with nasopharyngeal carcinoma contain a factor which abrogates specific Epstein-Barr virus antigen-induced lymphocyte response. Int J Cancer 29:407–412, 1982.
49. Maisel RH, Ogura JH: Abnormal dinitrochlorobenzene skinsensitization as a prognostic sign of survival in head and neck squamous cell carcinoma. The Laryngoscope 83:2012–2019, 1973.
50. Twomey PL, Catalona WJ, Chretien PB: Cellular immunity in cured cancer patients. Cancer 33:435–440, 1974.
51. Eilber FR, Morten DL, Ketcham AS: Immunologic abnormalities in head and neck cancer. Am J Surgery 128:534–538, 1974.
52. Maisel RH, Ogura JH: Dinitrochlorobenzene sensitization and peripheral lymphocyte count: Predictors of survival in head and neck cancer. Ann Otol Rhinol Laryngol 84:517–522, 1976.
53. Zighelboim J, Dorey F, Parker NH, Calcaterra T, Ward P, Fahey L: Immunologic evaluation of patients with advanced head and neck cancer receiving weekly chemotherapy. Cancer 44:117–123, 1979.
54. Hilal EY, Wanebo HJ, Pinsky CM, Middleman P, Strong EW, Oettgen HF: Immunologic

evaluation and prognosis in patients with head and neck cancer. Am J Surgery 134:469–473, 1977.

55. Papenhausen PR, Kukwa PR, Croft CB, Borowiecki B, Silver C, Emerson EE: Cellular immunity in patients with epidermoid cancer of the head and neck. The Laryngoscope 86:538–549, 1979.

56. Jenkins VK, Ray P, Ellis HN, Griffiths CM, Perry RR, Olsen MH: Lymphocyte response in patients with head and neck cancer. Arch Otolaryngol 102:596–600, 1976.

57. Eastham RJ, Mason JM, Jennings BR, Belew PW, Maguda TA: T-cell rosette test in squamous cell carcinoma of the head and neck. Arch Otolaryngol 102:171–175, 1976.

58. Camacho ES, Schechter P, Graham R, Camacho SA: Immune competence evaluation including T-cell subsets in patients with lung or head and neck carcinomas and smokers. Proc Am Soc Clin Oncology 1:156, 1982.

59. Maxim PE, Veltri RW, Davis M: Occurrence of ferritin-bound immune complexes in the sera of cancer patients and controls. Proc Am Assoc Cancer Res 23:1982.

60. Wolf G, Chretien PB, Elias EG, Makuch RW, Baskies AM, Spiegel HE, Weirs JF: Serum glycoproteins in head and neck squamous carcinoma: Correlations with tumor extent, clinical tumor stage, and T-cell levels during chemotherapy. Am J Surgery 128:489–500, 1979.

61. Vetto RM, Burger DR, Vandenbark AA, Jenke PE: Changes in tumor immunity during therapy determined by leukocyte adherence-inhibition and dermal testing. Cancer 41:1034–1039, 1978.

62. Holan V, Sibl O, Hasek M: Monitoring of antitumor immunity in patients with larynx cancer by tube leukocyte adherence-inhibition assay. Cancer Research 39:651–653, 1979.

63. Yetto RJ, Sako K, Dasmahapatra K, Raina S, Rajack S, Holojoke ED, Goldrosen MH: Detection of tumor immunity by the computerized tube leukocyte adherence-inhibition assay in patients with squamous cell carcinoma of the head and neck. Tumor Diagnostik 2:74–78, 1981.

64. Cortesina G, Bussi M, Morra B, Cavallo GP, Beatrice F, Fortunato V Di, Poggio E, Orecchia R, Gabriele P, Rendine S, Sartoris A: Specific LIF production in laryngeal cancer patients: Evidence of suppressor activity exerted by adherent cells. IARC Med Sci 10:243–244, 1982.

65. Lehman F-G (ed): Carcinoembryonic Proteins. Amsterdam, Elsevier/North Holland, 1979.

66. Herberman RB, McIntire KR (eds): Immunodiagnosis of Cancer, Vols 1–2. New York, Marcel Dekker Inc., 1979.

67. Herberman RB (ed): Compendium of Assays for Immunodiagnosis of Human Cancer. Developments in cancer research, Vol. 1. New York, Elsevier/North Holland Inc., 1979.

68. Ruddon RW (ed): Biological Markers of Neoplasia. New York, Elsevier/North Holland, 1978.

69. Klavins JV: Advances in Biological Markers for Cancer. Annals Clin Lab Sci 13:275–280, 1983.

70. Primack A: The production of markers by bronchogenic carcinoma: A review. Sem Oncol 1:235–244, 1974.

71. Hart I, Fidler IJ: The implications of tumor heterogeneity for studies on the biology and therapy of cancer metastases. Biochim Biophys Acta 651:37–50, 1981.

72. Fidler IJ, Hart IR: The development of biological diversity and metastatic potential in malignant neoplasms. Oncodevel Biol Med 4:161–176, 1982.

73. Shi ZR, Tsao D, Kim YS: Subcellular distribution synthesis and release of carcinoembryonic antigen in cultures human colon adenocarcinoma cell lines. Cancer Research 43:4045–4049, 1983.

74. Ewing HP, Newsom BD, Hardy JD: Tumor markers. Current Problems in Surgery 19:57–94, 1982.

430

75. Goldenberg DM (ed): Radioimmunodetection of cancer: A UICC workshop. Cancer Research 40:2953–3087, 1980.
76. Order SE, Klein JL, Leichner PK: Antiferritin IgG antibody for isotopic cancer chemotherapy. Oncology 38:154–160, 1981.
77. Schwartz MK: Enzymes as tumor markers. In: Chu TM (ed) Biochemical Markers for Cancer. New York, Marcel Dekker, 1982, PP 81–92.
78. Schwartz MK, Fleisher M: Enzymes in cancer. J Clin Immunoassay 6:247–252, 1983.
79. Mahan DE: Immunologic methods for the quantitation of prostatic acid phosphatase. J Clin Immunoassay 6:221–227, 1983.
80. Wood DC, Vasela V, Palmquist M: Serum lactic dehydrogenase and isoenzymes in clinical cancer. J Surg Oncol 5:251, 1977.
81. Katz AE, Hong WK, Bhutani R, Berman LD, Blanchard GJ, Koff RS, Shapshay SM, Strong MS: Prognostic indicators in chemotherapy for head and neck carcinoma: Alkaline phosphatase levels. Laryngoscope 90:924–929, 1980.
82. Kothary PM, Mehts AR, Bapat CV: β-glucuronidase activity in oropharyngeal cancers and its value as a tumor marker. Proc Internat Head and Neck Oncol Res Conf, Rosslyn, VA, 1980.
83. Al-Sarraf M, Chu C Y-T, Lai L, Carey MK, Drelichman A: Multiple tumor markers in monitoring patients with epidermoid cancer of the head and neck. Proc Am Assoc Cancer Res 22:285, 1981.
84. Gold P, Freedman SO: Demonstration of tumor specific antigens in human colonic carcinomata by immunological tolerance and absorption techniques. J Exp Med 121:439–462, 1965.
85. Goslin RH, Skarin AT, Zamcheck N: Carcinoembryonic antigen: a useful monitor of therapy of small cell lung cancer. JAMA 246:2173–2176, 1981.
86. Woo KB, Waalkes TP, Ahmann DL, Tormey DC, Gehrke CW, Oliverio VT: A quantitative approach to determing disease response during therapy using multiple biologic markers: Application to carcinoma of the breast. Cancer 41:1685–1703, 1978.
87. Silverman NA, Alexander JC, Chretien PB:CEA levels in head and neck caner. Cancer 37:2204–2211, 1976.
88. Arosio P, Adelman TG, Drysdale JW: On ferritin heterogeneity: further evidence of heteropolymers. J Biol Chem 253:4451–4458, 1978.
89. Drysdale JWb: Ferritin as a tumor marker. J Clin Immunoassay 6:234–240, 1983.
90. Hazard JT, Yokota M, Arosio P, Drysdale JW: Immunologic differences in human isoferritins: Implications for immunological quantitation of serum ferritin. Blood 49:139–146, 1977.
91. Maxim PE, Veltri RW, Prather JR: Serum ferritin as a tumor marker for patients with carcinoma of the head and neck. Proc Amer Assoc Cancer Res 21:233, 1980.
92. Maxim PE, Prather JR, Veltri RW: Ferritin levels in tissue extracts and serum of patients with cacinoma of the lung. Fed Proc 39:23, 1980.

18. Local immunotherapy – Experimental and clinical research

JÜRGEN BIER, STEPHEN J. KLEINSCHUSTER and JOOST RUITENBERG

1. Introduction

Numerous immunostimulants are able to influence the growth of transplanted syngeneic or autochthonous malignant tumors. This also includes living and dead bacterial components.

The possible influence of acute bacterial infections on 'spontaneous remissions' of malignant tumors has been conjectured for over 200 years [1, 2] and led to the clinical therapy measures that were carried out by Coley in the 1890's [3, 4]. If different neoplasias were treated with bacterial toxins, extensive regressions could be observed when an acute infection was provoked in or at the tumor site by direct tumor contact of the toxin. For a number of years, this therapeutic principle of Coley's has determined a therapeutic approach that deals empirically and by experimental analysis with the treatment of malignant tumors and has led to local immunotherapy with Bacillus Calmette-Guerin (BCG).

1.1. BCG and the immune system

BCG was obtained in 1920 by Calmette and Guerin at the Pasteur Institute in Paris from the virulent 'Nocard' strain of mycobacterium tuberculosis of the bovine variety [5, 6]. Animals that were immunized with bacteria of this attenuated strain developed an increased resistance to virulent tuberculosis bacteria. In humans, BCG was first administered to newborns in 1920. Up to the present time, more than 100 million immunizations have been performed by scarification or intradermal injection [7]. Very early, Hirayama (1930) observed 'paraspecific' mechanisms in BCG against heterologous infections, which were later confirmed by various authors for different infective agents [8, 9]. This non-specific BCG activity was soon correlated with a stimulation of cellular immunity [10–12]. In humans and in various

Gregory T. Wolf (ed), Head and Neck Oncology.
© *1984 Martinus Nijhoff Publishers, Boston. ISBN 0-89838-657-8. Printed in The Netherlands.*

animal species, BCG is able to produce an immunity against virulent tuberculosis organisms. Transmission of immunity was possible in animal experiments by the transfer of lymphoid cells [13–16], while this effect was not detectable with antimycobacterial sera [16]. An analysis of BCG antigenicity and an explanation for its protection against tuberculosis has not yet been provided, a situation which can be explained by the complex chemical structure of mycobacterial cell walls [17]. Among other things, however, reports have been presented on cross-reactivities with various strains of bacteria [18], human [19], and experimental tumor cells [20].

Immunological mechanisms induced in the host organism by BCG are extremely complex. They are mediated by manifold interactions of T cells, such as cytotoxic T cells, helper and suppressor T cells, B cells, macrophages, NK (natural killer) cells, and various mediator substances.

1.2. BCG, carcinogenesis and tumor protection

A possible concordance between tubercle bacteria and malignant tumors has been conjectured in the past by clinical and epidemiological observations, which permitted the assumption of an antagonism between tuberculosis and neoplasia [21, 22]. As early of 1929, Pearl reported that patients with florid tuberculosis only showed a malignant tumor in exceptional cases. Furthermore, the inhibiting influence of BCG on carcinogenesis has been investigated experimentally. Tumor development could be delayed and the frequency reduced for chemically [23–30], virally [31–40], and radioactively induced [41] tumors. With BCG, the development of various tumors (carcinomas: [25, 42, 26]; sarcomas: [23, 28, 29, 43]) could also be inhibited in different animal species. Of course, this protective effect was usually only temporary. On the other hand, a permanent protective effect of BCG and MER (methanol extraction residue) was observed for the carcinogenic activity of some oncogenic viruses [32, 33, 38–40].

A direct antitumorigenic activity of BCG was first demonstrated by the inhibition of tumor growth in animals that had been infected with live tubercle bacteria [11, 23, 44–47] or with mycobacterial components [12, 48] before tumor cell inoculation. In order to prevent tumor growth, it was necessary for the experimental animals to be systemically infected with BCG at least seven days prior to tumor cell transplantation [46, 23]. Further investigations in various BCG-infected animal species (mice, rats, hamsters, guinea pigs) showed different results for transplantable spontaneous, viral or chemically induced tumors. In spite of successfull experimental results with BCG in the reduction of carcinogenesis and the protection of BCG immunized animals, established tumors are resistant to a systemic immunotherapy with BCG.

Following Coley's observations (see above), it became known that intra-tumoral injection of bacteria or bacterial products could lead to tumor regressions. Observations by Klein [49–51] have shown that delayed hyper-sensitivity (DTH) reactions in the area of cutaneous tumors can cause a tumor regression. In the early 1970's, these observations led to the concept of local immunotherapy of experimental tumors with BCG. Investigations in different animal tumor models (guinea pig: [52–55]; mice: [56–58]; rat: [59, 60]) showed a complete suppression of tumor growth if tumor cells were mixed with BCG before injection into syngeneic receiver animals. However, simultaneous injection of tumor cells and BCG in different body regions of the animals led to progressive tumor growth.

1.3. Intratumoral BCG therapy

Subsequent to these observations, Zbar [61–64] successfully treated estab-lished tumors with live BCG. Inbred guinea pigs (strain 2) received an intradermal transplantation of 10^6 syngeneic tumor cells obtained from an ascitic variant of a diethylnitrosamine-induced hepatocellular carcinoma (line 10). One week after tumor cell inoculation, a skin tumor developed that measured 1 cm in diameter and weighed about 100 mg. At this time, metastases were already detectable in the draining lymph nodes, and a sur-gical exicision of the primary tumor was no longer a therapeutic success. Untreated tumor-bearing animals died of generalized metastases within 2–3 months. A single intratumoral injection on the eighth day after tumor cell transplantation of 10^7 live BCG organisms led to complete tumor regression and elimination of the metastases in 80% of the animals. In addition, the cured animals developed a tumor-specific immunity that was proven by repeated introduction of homologous tumor cells into the animals. Using the same animal tumor model, Hanna and Peters [65] demonstrated that intratumoral BCG therapy in combination with radical surgery (primary tumor and regional metastatic lymph nodes) only led to a successful antitu-mor therapy if the animals additionally received intravenous application of a limited number of tumor cells. This systemic effect of intratumoral BCG application was also described by Morton et al. [66] for patients with recur-rent cutaneous melanoma metastases. In addition to metastases directly injected with BCG, the regression of non-BCG-injected cutaneous melano-ma metastases was also reported, a phenomenon that has been observed by other study groups [67]. These findings strongly indicated that, in addition to local tumor regressions, intratumoral BCG therapy also produced a gen-eral immunoreaction that could lead to the destruction of disseminated tumor cells. In the experiment of Hanna and Peters [65], however, addition-al radical surgery was absolutely necessary for a therapeutic success.

In the meantime, successful local tumor immunotherapy has been described using a number of viruses, bacteria, and agents (vaccina virus: [68, 69]; mycobacterium: [56, 63, 70, 71]; Coryne-bacterium: [72–75]; Listeria monocytogenes: [76–78]; Bordetella pertussis: [79]; dinitrochlorobenzene: [49]). Since the most information is available on the use of the attenuated form of mycobacterium, BCG, it is useful to describe the limiting factors of intratumoral immunotherapy for this system.

Successful intratumoral immunotherapy with BCG is only possible when a sufficient number of live organisms with satisfactory antitumor activity are used. There is even a clear dose effect relationship between the number of tumor cells to be destroyed and the number of BCG organisms to be injected in order to cure tumor-bearing animals [62]. If strain 2 guinea pigs with 8-day-old carcinomas are treated with an increasing BCG dose, up to 100% of the animals can be cured. On the other hand, the therapeutic success is dependent on the antitumor activity of the applied BCG preparation.

Tumor size is a limiting factor for the success of intratumoral BCG therapy. While 8-day-old line 10 tumors in strain 2 guinea pigs with a tumor weight of 100 mg are cured at an average rate of 80%, therapy of a tumor weighing 425 mg is successful in less than 20% of animals. Of course, when the tumor weight is higher, the greater potential for metastases must also be taken into consideration [62]. The ability of the tumor host to generate a cellular immunoresponse and to respond to mycobacterial antigens with a DTH reaction is codeterminative for the therapeutic success of an intratumoral BCG treatment. Tumor-bearing experimental animals that can no longer develop a DTH reaction to PPD (purified protein derivate of tuberculin) because of treatment with antilymphocyte serum, corticosteroids, sublethal whole-body irradiation or perinatal thymectomy, can not be cured by intratumoral BCG administration [80, 58]. Treatment also fails in tumor animals that have developed a tolerance for mycobacterial antigens by intravenous BCG application and no longer evidence a DTH reaction to PPD [53].

It is possible that the antigenicity of the experimental tumors used also determines the success or failure of intratumoral BCG immunotherapy. For line 10 tumors in strain 2 guinea pigs [62], and for the masto-adenocarcinoma no. 13762 in rats [81] and other rat tumors [82–84] with proven antigenicity, immunotherapeutic successes are reproducible with great regularity. But if tumors with and without detectable immunogenicity are tested for their reactivity to BCG, complete remissions are shown in non-immunogenic tumors only in exceptional cases and in immunogenic tumors frequently. In addition, a direct correlation between antigenicity and the number of tumor cells able to be eradicated by local BCG treatment can be detected for tumors with different antigenicity. When the same therapeutic amount of

BCG is applied, more tumor cells with high than with low antigenicity are destroyed [85].

Only direct contact between tumor cells and BCG can cure tumor-bearing animals. BCG injection before tumor cell transplantation, or at the same time but without direct contact with the tumor cells, has no curative effect. All animals die of progressive tumor growth [59, 62, 84, 86]. Of course, progressive tumor growth can still occur in spite of the close proximity of tumor cells and BCG. In the above described guinea pig tumor model, tumor transplants in the peritoneal cavity, muscle tissue [87], lungs or lymph nodes [86] showed resistance to local immunotherapy with BCG, while intradermal tumors were destroyed. For other syngeneic and autochthonous tumors, tumor regressions have also been described in the colon [88], eye [89], breast [26, 90] and lung [82, 83].

2. Experimental and clinical investigations

2.1. Intratumoral BCG therapy in the syngeneic guinea pig tumor model

The impaired non-specific immunoreactivity [91] and the generally unfavourable prognosis [92] of patients with squamous cell carcinomas in the head and neck region led to the consideration of immunotherapeutic measures to influence the course of the disease. As a result of increasing knowledge about cellular immunomechanisms and experimental experience with bacterial vaccines for tumor therapy, suitable animal experiments were performed to examine whether a rational basis could be found for immunotherapy in the head and neck region.

Intratumoral injection with BCG as an immunotherapeutic treatment has already led to remarkable experimental findings [62] and early clinical experiences [66]. A possible application of this therapeutic approach in the head and neck region of humans was first dealt with experimentally. Care was taken that the experimental tumors were localized in the head and neck region and could be regarded as epithelial tumors with primarily lymphogenous formation of metastases. Because of the known toxicity to live BCG on the human organism [93], animal investigations were done to compare the therapeutic effect of live BCG with that of BCG cell wall preparations (CWP).

In a syngeneic, lymphogenously metastasizing guinea pig tumor model, it was possible to transplant tumors normally growing intradermally into the planum buccale of the animals. The tumors grew there locally with all signs of malignancy and metastasized into the draining submandibular and cervical lymph nodes of the neck. After approximately 60 days, untreated animals died of the tumor. This experimental system was used to test the effect of a simultaneous injection of tumor cells and BCG and CWP on locally established and already lymphogenously metastasized tumors. Animals treated by local and radical surgery were observed for comparison.

Injection of tumor cells and live BCG or BCG-CWP

After anesthesia strain 2 guinea pigs in two groups of six animals each were injected in the right upper planum buccale with line 10 tumor cells ($1 \times 10^6 \cong 0.1$ ml) mixed with live BCG (1×10^6 pfu 0.2 ml) (Group 1) or BCG-CWP (225 μg CW$\cong$0.8 ml) (Group 2). A control group (Group 3) received only line 10 tumor cells ($1 \times 10^6 \cong 0.1$ ml). The local reaction, the tumor growth at the site of injection and the draining lymph nodes were measured at weekly intervals over a period of 30 days. Animals that were clinically tumor-free after 30 days were injected again with 1×10^6 line 10 tumor cells in the upper left planum buccale and observed for another 30 days. After this period of time, animals still tumor-free were injected with 1×10^6 line 10 tumor cells in the left lower planum buccale and again observed (30 days).

Intratumoral injection of live BCG or BCG-CWP

Three groups of strain 2 guinea pigs were injected with 1×10^6 line 10 tumor cells in the right upper planum buccale after anesthesia. Six days after the transplantation, Group 1 (10 animals) was intratumorally injected with $1 \times 10^8 \cong$pfu 0.3 ml of BCG organisms and Group 2 (20 animals) with 675 μg of CW$\cong$0.3 ml BCG-CWP. Group 3 (6 animals) remained untreated. Clinically tumor-free animals were again given 1×10^6 line 10 tumor cells 60 days after transplantation and 1×10^6 line 1 tumor cells on day 90 in the left upper and lower planum buccale. The animals were examined for tumor and regional lymph node size at weekly intervals over a period of 4 months.

Operations

Strain 2 guinea pigs in 3 groups of 6 animals each were injected with 1×10^6 line 10 tumor cells in the right upper planum buccale. Six days after the transplantation, Groups 1 and 2 were operated under anesthesia; Group 3 remained untreated. In the animals of Group 1, the primary tumor and the submandibular and cervical lymph nodes on the tumor side were resected as a block. In the animals of Group 2, only the tumor was locally excised. The application of line 10 and 1 tumor cells in tumor-free animals and the continuous control of the animals was done in the same sequence as described above.

Results

Injections of tumor cells and live BCG or BCG-CWP. After 30 days, strain 2 guinea pigs that were injected in the oral mucosa with line 10 tumor cells and live BCG (Group 1) or BCG-CWP (Group 2) showed no clinical evidence of a primary tumor in the planum buccale or in lymph nodes draining the injection site. In contrast, animals in Group 3, in which exclusively line 10 tumors had been transplanted, showed progressive tumor growth at the injection site and in the draining lymph nodes. Tumor-free animals (Group 1, 2) were again injected with line 10 tumor cells on day 30. After 60 days, no tumor was clinically detectable in any living animal of Group 1 or 2. One animal of Group 2 died on day 43 without a tumor. The surviving animals were injected with line 1 tumor cells on day 60, after which all animals showed increasing tumor growth (Table 1).

Intratumoral injection of live BCG or BCG-CWP. Six days after injection of line 10 cells into the planum buccale, a tumor was palpable at the site of injection, and metastatic draining lymph nodes were palpable around day 21. Untreated animals died between the 50th and 60th day after tumor cell transplantation. The single intratumoral injection of live BCG led to tumor regression and prevented the manifestation of metastatic lymph nodes in 10 out of 10 treated animals. Twenty out of 20 animals were cured by intratumoral injection of BCG-CWP. All living and tumor-free animals were again subjected to the application of line 10 tumor cells on day 60. No tumor growth was evidenced by 9 out of 10 animals treated with live BCG and by 19 out of 20 that had received therapy with BCG-CWP. One animal injected with BCG-CWP died tumor-free on day 79. No animal survived the application of line 1 tumor cells on day 90 (Table 2, Figs. 1, 2).

Operations
The possibilities of surgical measures on the 6th day after tumor cell trans-

---

Table 1. Injection of tumor cells and live BCG or BCG-CWP into the oral mucosa of strain 2 guinea pigs [1]

Animals tumor-free	Tumor cells plus live BCG (Group I)	Tumor cells plus BCG-CWP (Group II)	Untreated control (Group III)		
Day 30	6/6	6/6	0/6 [2]		
Day 60	6/6	5/6 [3]	–	0/6 [2]	
Day 90	0/6	0/5	–	–	0/6

[1] Day 0: Gr. I 1×10^6 line 10 tumor cells with 1×10^6 pfu BCG
 Gr. II 1×10^6 line 10 tumor cells with 100 µg BCG-CW as BCG-CWP
 Gr. III 1×10^6 line 10 tumor cells
 Day 30: Gr. I, II, III 1×10^6 line 10 tumor cells
 Day 60: Gr. I, II, III 1×10^6 line 1 tumor cells
[2] Significant ($p < 0.01$) vs. Gr. I, II (Chi-Square-Test).
[3] Death of one animal on day 43 without tumor.

438

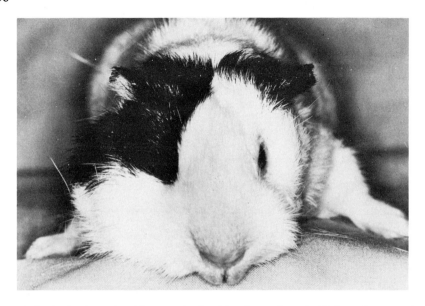

Figure 1. Strain 2 guinea pig with tumor in the right planum buccale 30 days after transplantation of line 10 tumor cells.

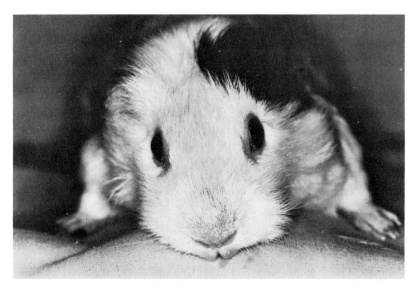

Figure 2. Strain 2 guinea pig without tumor in the right planum buccale after intralesional injection of BCG-CWP 30 days after transplantation of line 10 tumor cells.

plantation were tested by tumor excision and removal of the first lymph node stations (Group 1) or by local tumor excision (Group 2). The 3rd Group remained untreated for control purposes. Radically operated animals (tumor and lymph nodes) survived tumor-free the entire 60 days. In one out of six of these animals, a second application of line 10 tumor cells did not result in any tumor growth. A re-injection of the surviving animal with line 1 cells led to a progressively growing tumor. In all locally operated animals (primary tumor), there was increasing tumor growth in the submandibular lymph nodes. All control animals died of the tumor (Table 3).

Table 2. Intratumoral injection of line 10 tumors with live BCG or BCG-CWP in the oral mucosa of strain 2 guinea pigs.[1]

Animals tumor-free	Live BCG (Group I)	BCG-CWP (Group II)	Controls (Group III)		
Day 60	10/10	20/20	0/6[2]		
Day 90	9/10	18/20[3]	–	0/6[2]	
Day 120	0/9	0/18	–	–	0/6

[1] Day 0: Gr. I, II, III 1×10^6 line 10 tumor cells
  Day 6: Gr. I 1×10^8 pfu BCG
    Gr. II 675 µBCG-CW as BCG-CWP
  Day 60: Gr. I, II, III 1×10^6 line 10 tumor cells
  Day 90: Gr. I, II, III 1×10^6 line 1 tumor cells
[2] Significant ($p < 0,01$) vs. Gr. I, II (Chi-Square-Test).
[3] Death of one animal on day 79 without tumor.

Table 3. Operation on line 10 tumors of the oral mucosa of strain 2 guinea pigs[1].

Animals tumor-free	Radical operation (Group I)	Local operation (Group II)	Controls (Group III)		
Day 60	6/6[2]	0/6	0/6		
Day 90	1/6	–	–	0/6	
Day 120	0/1	–	–	–	0/6

[1] Day 0: Gr. I, II, III 1×10^6 line 10 tumor cells
  Day 6: Gr. I Excision of the primary tumor and the draining lymph nodes
    Gr. II Excision of the primary tumor
  Day 60: Gr. I, III 1×10^6 line 10 tumor cells
  Day 90: Gr. I, III 1×10^6 line 1 tumor cells
[2] Significant ($p < 0,01$) vs. Gr. II, III (Chi-Square-Test).

2.2. Intratumoral BCG therapy in cows with spontaneous squamous cell carcinomas in the head and neck region

Despite the numerous advantages in experimental procedure, syngeneic tumor-animal models with artificially induced tumors have disadvantages in comparison to human neoplasias. In experimental systems, inbred animals are used, while humans represent an 'outbred' population. Experimental tumors are artificial, e.g. virally or chemically induced tumors, and not, as in humans, spontaneously developing tumors. Also, the behavior pattern of metastatic development in almost all syngeneic tumor-animal models does not correspond to the situation with epithelial human tumors. No murine-tumor model, the most frequently used system in experimental tumor therapy, is characterized by local growth combined with predominantly lymphogenous formation of metastases. Murine tumors either do not metastasize at all or only hematogenously or hematogenously and lymphogenously. In addition, other syngeneic tumor-animal models in various inbred animal species do not demonstrate purely lymphogenous metastases of epithelial, induced tumors. One exception to this is the inbred guinea pig model described above. Because of these considerations, the clinical application of tumor therapy derived in experimental animals is limited. An ideal experimental animal tumor model for human epithelial tumors would have to potentially metastasize lymphogenously and develop spontaneously in a large, outbred animal population. A tumor occurring in the eyes of cows – called 'cancer eye' – fulfills these prerequisites. It is a keratinizing squamous cell carcinoma with all the characteristics of a malignant tumor, such as invasive-destructive growth and lymphogenic metastases [94]. The etiology of the tumor is unknown, ultraviolet light [95], non-pigmented periorbital skin [96], insects [97], chemicals [98], viruses [99] and genetic disposition [94] are implied as concomitant causal factors of the disease. Hereford cows, followed by black-and-white Holsteins, appear to be the breeds most frequently affected in the USA and Australia [94]. The tumors occur in the third year of life at the earliest and most frequently around the eighth year [99]. Tumors can occur on all parts of the outer eye and/or its adnexa. They develop, in order of decreasing frequency, at the lateral corneoscleral junctions (limbus), medial corneoscleral junction, lower eyelid, third eyelid (plica semilunaris conjunctivae) and lacrimal lake (lacus lacrimalis). By invasive growth, the tumor can infiltrate into the orbital cavity and destroy the conjunctival sac, the eye musculature, the orbital fat and the optic nerve. In addition, progressive growth of the carcinoma can also affect periorbital tissue, such as periorbital skin, muscles, bones, sinuses and brain (Fig. 3). Progressive growth of this tumor leads to metastases in the draining lymph nodes. The metastatic stations are shown in Fig. 4 and drain via the parotid lymph node and the retropharyngeal lymph node into the truncus trachealis and ductus thoracicus.

Tumor bearing animals of this outbred species with spontaneous, invasive, metastatic tumors of epithelial origin that are localized in the head and neck region appear to provide a suitable therapy model for the treatment of human epithelial tumors. This may be particularly valid for squamous cell carcinomas in the head and neck region that also show histological characteristics identical to those of 'cancer eye' (Fig. 5).

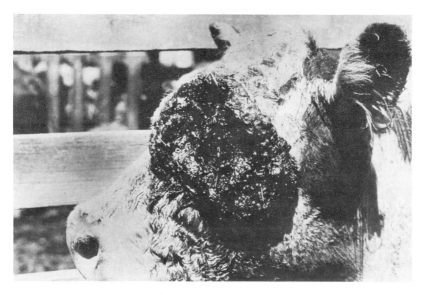

Figure 3. Bovine ocular squamous cell carcinoma.

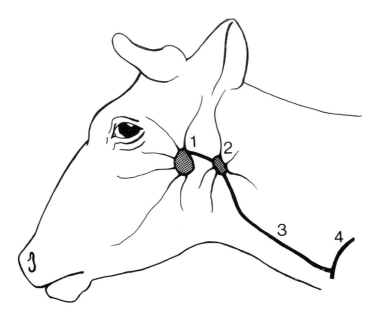

Figure 4. Metastatic regions of bovine ocular squamous cell carcinoma. 1 = parotid lymph node; 2 = retropharyngeal lymph node; 3 = truncus trachealis; 4 = ductus thoracicus.

To test whether intratumoral BCG therapy leads to tumor regression and cure of animals bearing 'cancer eye', surgical treatment methods were carried out and the results compared to untreated animals and animals injected with live BCG or BCG-CWP.

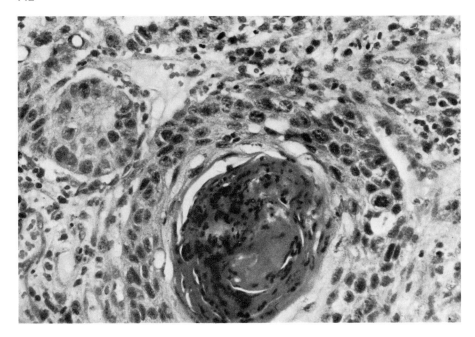

Figure 5. Histology of bovine ocular squamous cell carcinoma. Hematoxylin and eosin, ×296.

Experimental procedure

In a period of four years, 49 tumor-bearing cows were included in the experiments. The animals were divided into 5 groups that were homogeneous with regard to tumor size. Group 1 (10 animals) was intratumorally injected with BCG-CWP and Group 2 (9 animals) with live BCG. Group 3 (10 animals) underwent local (primary tumor) and Group 4 (10 animals) radical (primary tumor and draining lymph nodes) tumor excision. Group 5 (10 animals) remained untreated.

The animals were observed at weekly intervals. The following criteria were used to assess therapy after BCG injection:

(a) complete regression without clinical evidence of a still existent tumor;
(b) partial regression with a measurable decrease in tumor size compared to pretreatment measurements;
(c) progressive growth with measurable increase in the size of the tumor and increasing involvement of surrounding tissue and/or lymphatic metastases.

The following were used to assess therapy for the operated animals:

(a) clinically free of the tumor and metastases;
(b) local tumor recurrence and/or formation of tumor metastases.

In all test groups, animals that developed advanced tumor size, recurrence and/or formation of metastases were killed. Primary tumor, recurrent tumor, draining lymph nodes and other organ regions in which metastases were suspected were examined macroscopically and histologically. The preparations were fixed in 10% buffered formalin, sectioned, stained with hematoxylin-phloxine saffron and assessed.

Intratumoral injection of BCG-CWP
Ten animals were intratumorally injected with BCG-CWP. The preparations contained 1.5 mg CW/ml. Approximately 0.25 ml was intratumorally infiltrated per 1 cm^3 of the tumor. If necessary, a local anesthesia (Lidocaine) was applied in the tumor area before the BCG-CWP injection in order to prevent pain from the injection. Paratumoral injections of BCG-CWP at the time of intratumoral administration could not always be avoided, since some of the preparation escaped because of the partly porous tumor structure. Single injections were performed, sometimes with several punctures in the tumor. Care was taken to infiltrate the entire tumor with the preparation.

Intratumoral injection of live BCG
Nine animals were given single intratumoral injections of live BCG. Approximately 0.25 ml per cm^3 of tumor was applied using the prepared suspension (1×10^8 pfu/ml). The injections were performed in the same way as for BCG-CWP.

Local operation
In 10 animals, local surgical excision of the primary tumor was performed within a suitable margin of safety; the draining lymph nodes were not removed. Independent of the tumor localization and size, a partial excision of the lower eyelid and enuclatio bulbi was performed in two cases each. In six animals, an orbital exteneration was carried out without any or with only partial maintenance of the eyelid skin. No bone resections were done. The operations were performed under local anesthesia using aseptic technique.

Radical operation
Ten animals underwent radical tumor resection. A method was developed for this based on the technique of neck dissection used for human tumors in the head and neck region. Draining lateral retropharyngeal and parotid lymph nodes were removed as a block with the primary tumor.

Untreated controls
Ten animals remained untreated. Progressive growth of the tumor and metastases was observed.

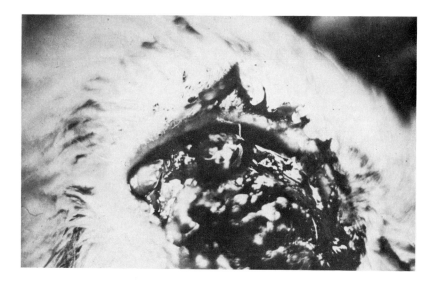

Fig. 6

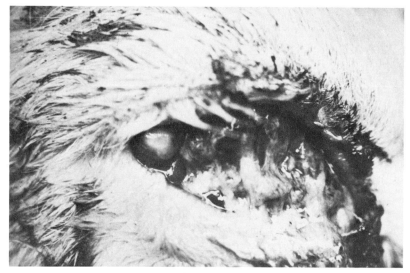

Fig. 7

Results

In all surviving animals [37], the results were based on findings made one year after therapy. Fifteen animals with advanced tumor growth were killed before the observation year had passed (between the 6th and 12th month). The therapy results are presented in Table 4.

Intratumoral injection of BCG-CWP

Only half (5/10) of the animals that had been treated intratumorally with BCG-CWP were clinically tumor-free (Figs. 6–9) after one year. Two animals

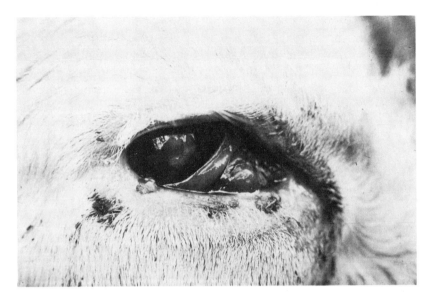

Fig. 8

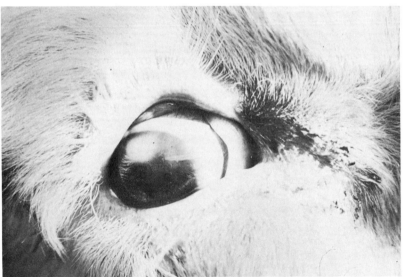

Fig. 9

Figures 6-9. Bovine ocular squamous cell carcinoma before (6) and after (7-9) intratumoral injection.

showed a partial remission, and three showed progressive tumor growth. Two of the three animals with progressive tumor were killed after 6 and 11 months. In both animals, tumor was found in the parotid lymph node, while the lateral retropharyngeal lymph nodes and all other organs were tumor free.

Intratumoral injection of live BCG

Two thirds (6/9) of the animals that had been treated intratumorally with live BCG were clinically tumor-free after one year. In one animal, there was partial remission of the tumor with subsequent arrest of tumor growth. Enlarged lymph nodes suspected of containing metastases were not palpable after a year. Two animals showed progressive tumor growth; one of them was killed seven months after therapy because of a generally deteriorating state of health and progressive formation of lymph node metastases. Distant metastases could not be detected in this animal.

Complete tumor regression after intratumoral BCG therapy occurred within the same period of time for both BCG treated groups. Complete healing was attained with 10–25 weeks subsequent to a short-term (4–5) day inflammatory tumor enlargement after injection of live BCG or BCG-CWP. Tumors in animals manifesting progressive tumor growth after BCG administration showed a slight decrease in growth rate compared to those of untreated control animals. A significant therapeutic difference could not be detected between treatment groups 1 and 2.

Table 4. Treatment of 'cancer eye'

Treatment	it. BCG-CWP (Group I)	it. live BCG (Group II)	Local operation (Group III)	Radical operation (Group IV)	Controls (Group V)
Complete regression	5/10	6/9			1/10
Partial regression	2/10	1/9			0/10
Progressive growth	3/10	2/9			9/10
Tumor-free			5/10	10/10	
Local recurrence and/or metastasis			5/10	0/10	

Local operation

Over a period of one year, local surgical tumor therapy was successful in half of the operated animals (5/10); the other half (5/10) developed local recurrence or metastases. Two of the animals developed local recurrence after 4 and 7 months, and 3 developed parotid lymph node metastases after 6, 8 and 12 months. Four of these 5 animals with local or regional recurrence were killed between the 7th and 12th postoperative month. Tumor tissue was found in the draining parotid lymph nodes of all 4 animals and also in the lateral retropharyngeal lymph nodes and in the lung of one animal each.

Radical operation

Radically operated animals were all clinically free of local recurrence or metastases one year after the operation (Fig. 10).

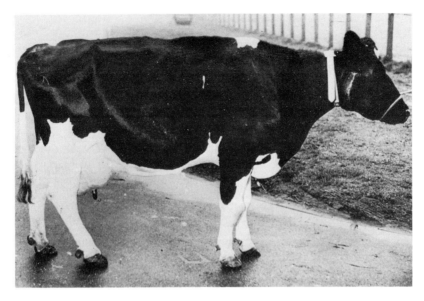

Figure 10. Cow one year after radical surgery.

Untreated control

In the untreated control group, there was a spontaneous total regression of tumor in one animal between the 4th and the 6th month, while the other 9 control animals showed progressive tumor growth. Eight of them were killed between the 6th and 9th month of observation. Metastatic tumor in parotid lymph nodes was found in 6 of the sacrificed animals. Tumor was evident in the lateral retropharyngeal cervical lymph nodes of 3 of the animals, and pulmonary metastases were detected in 2 of them. One animal was free of metastases.

2.3. Discussion of experimental findings

The considerations that led to these experiments were based on clinical observations. Patients with malignant tumors can be successfully treated by radical surgery. Some of the patients treated in this way, however, develop either local recurrences and/or metastases that form from tumor-cell nests already present before the surgical intervention. Current surgical techniques do not always render it possible to completely remove these tumor cells in the vicinity of the primary tumor and the micrometastases in the draining lymphatic vessels. For this reason, conventional treatment methods frequently utilize combination therapies. Either radiotherapy or chemotherapy is given before or after surgery with the aim of destroying these tumor foci. Up to now, however, even these treatment methods in conjunction with surgical measures have only led to limited success.

Considerations derived from the concept of tumor 'immuno-surveillance' could be applied within the framework of these combination-therapy protocols in the following manner: if one assumes that, in the process of their development, malignant tumors give off characteristic neoantigens, it would be conceivable for these tumor-specific determinants to be recognized as foreign antigens and tumor cells destroyed by a neoantigen-induced immunoreaction. The obvious dilemma involved in this consideration, however, is the question of how the primary development of a clinically manifest tumor could occur at all. Independent of this problem, it seems important to prove that it may be possible to induce antitumor reactivity against autochthonous tumors and/or their neoantigens. If this were true, it would be conceivable to remove the primary tumor mass by local or radical surgery and activate the potential immunoreactivity against micrometastases in such a way that cellular immunoreactions destroy the remaining local tumor cell nests and micrometastases in the lymphatic drainage area.

The purpose of the present study was to confirm experimental findings from the literature indicating that the cellular immunoreactivity against syngeneic tumors can be increased by BCG or BCG-CWP to such an extent that tumor-bearing animals can be cured in the experimental system. These observations were confirmed first in the guinea pig system with line 10 tumor cells. Since experimentally induced tumors are not directly comparable to autochthonous tumors, a second step was taken to determine the effect of BCG on the tumor growth of spontaneously developing squamous cell carcinomas in cows. The goal of the animal experiments was to derive experiences gained with intratumoral BCG immunotherapy in the guinea pig and cow models that would be clinically applicable in the human system.

The findings in literature that led to the application of the experimental approaches described here were reported by Zbar et al. [53, 62]. Concisely stated, Zbar succeeded in showing that progressive growth of line 10 tumors from strain 2 guinea pigs could be arrested when, either at the time of tumor inoculation or several days after tumor transplantation, live BCG was directly applied to the tumor. A significant observation in this connection was that the BCG-dependent antitumor effect was not limited to the primary tumor. Control experiments showed that there was not only regression of the primary tumor but also elimination of metastases that had already formed in the regional lymph nodes. In addition, Zbar reported that treated animals developed a tumor-specific immunity, i.e., reintroduction of the same tumor did not lead to any tumor growth, while antigenetically different tumors were not rejected by the animals. It is important in this connection that the BCG effect described by Zbar appears to be largely limited to intradermally growing tumors and does not apply to all tumor types. For example, tumor transplants in the peritoneal cavity [100], musculature [87], lung and lymph nodes [86] could not be effectively treated with this therapeutic protocol. Only Harmel [88] observed the regression of a colonic tumor in the guinea pig after intratumoral BCG therapy. In addition, Simova and Bubnik [101] showed that virus-induced mouse and rat sarcomas were resistant to intratumoral BCG therapy. Sparks and Breeding [102] described similar observations for chemically induced sarcomas. At present, it is still unclear whether these failures were determined by the tumor type or were related to the BCG strain used.

At the center of oncological activity in the field of head and neck surgery is the treatment of squamous cell carcinomas of the oral cavity, which largely metastasize into the regional submandibular and cervical lymph nodes. Since the BCG effect described by Zbar is almost exclusively restricted to epidermally growing tumors, it was our primary aim to test the principles described by Zbar on experimental tumors in the head and neck region. Line 10 tumor cells were thus transplanted into the planum buccale of strain 2 guinea pigs, and the influence of BCG was defined in this model.

If live BCG and BCG-CWP were injected into the planum buccale together with line 10 tumor cells, no growth of the tumor could be observed. Animals treated in this manner developed immunity to the injected tumor, while an antigenetically different tumor cell line (line 1) led to progressive tumor growth (Table 1). In a second experimental assay, line 10 tumor cells were first transplanted into the planum buccale. Six days after transplantation of the tumor cells, live BCG or BCG-CWP was injected intratumorally. As can be seen from Table 2, this experimental protocol led to regression of the primary tumor and prevented the development of lymph node metastases. In addition, animals treated in this manner showed a specific immunity to line 10 tumor cells. In the third experimental assay, tumors were resected six days after tumor inoculation. Animals remained tumor-free after removal of the primary tumor and the draining submandibular and cervical lymph nodes (radical operation). Although these guinea pigs were cured, they did not have any tumor-specific immunity, i.e. progressive tumor growth developed after reapplication of the same tumor. In contrast to the radical operation, locally operated animals developed lymph node metastases after removal of the primary tumor (Table 3).

On the basis of these findings, it can be concluded that in the guinea pig model, the curative effect of an intratumoral therapy with live BCG or BCG-CWP is comparable to that of radical surgery, while local excision of the primary tumor does not represent sufficient treatment. Cured animals in both treatment groups differed since BCG-treated animals developed a tumor-specific immunity, while animals that had undergone radical surgery did not (Table 2).

It seems interesting to compare the experimental results from animals treated by local surgery (6 days after tumor transplantation) and animals that had been treated intratumorally at the same time with live BCG or BCG-CWP. All locally operated animals developed progressive metastatic tumor growth, while the animals that had received intratumoral treatment with BCG showed no tumor growth. Since animals treated by local surgery developed metastases, it can be assumed that at the time of therapy the group of animals that received intratumoral BCG had also already developed metastases in the draining lymph nodes. Thus, the BCG-induced antitumor effect in the planum buccale does not appear to be locally limited to the primary tumor, but includes a systemic antitumor effect on metastases. This argument is supported by investigations of Zbar et al. [62]. At the time of successful intratumoral BCG therapy of intradermal tumors, tumor cells were histologically detectable in the draining lymph nodes, and transplantation of these lymph nodes into tumor-free animals led to the growth of solid tumors. The development of a tumor-specific immunity provides indirect evidence for the systemic effect of intratumoral BCG therapy. The trigger mechanism of this cellular immunity is as yet unknown, and it should be tested whether tumor-specific T-cells are carriers of this specific immunity.

Because of the toxicity of live BCG, BCG-CWP was also tested for its antitumor effect in the planum buccale. An injection of live BCG frequently induces a systemic BCG infection in addition to a massive, chronically proliferating local inflammation. It has been reported, however, that BCG-CWP gives rise to a similar local inflammatory effect but does not cause any side effects in the sense of a BCG-osis or BCG-itis. In addition, Zbar has shown [103] that BCG-CWP has a lower toxicity and a comparable antitumor effect as live BCG. The latter finding was confirmed by our results. Table 2 shows that, in the planum buccale, the antitumor effect of live BCG and BCG-CWP is comparable.

The mechanism of BCG-induced tumor regression at the primary tumor site and the draining lymph nodes has not as yet been entirely clarified. *In vitro*, BCG in co-cultivation with tumor cells shows no cytotoxic effect [104, 105] which suggests a participation of the host organism in local, *in vivo*, tumor regression. Evidence for a T-cell dependent mechanism was first provided by Bartlett et al. [104] and Chung et al. [58]. Mice that had been immunosuppressed by thymectomy, whole body irradiation and treatment with antilymphocyte serum or cortisone did not show any BCG-mediated antitumor effect. For line 10 tumors in the guinea pig, the curative effect of an intratumoral BCG injection could be prevented by antilymphocyte serum [80]. Similar findings have also been reported with antilymphocyte serum in other animal-tumor models [106, 107].

In addition to T-cells, however, the findings of Chassox and Salomon [108] suggest that a decisive role must also be ascribed to macrophages. After application of fine silicon dioxide particles that are especially toxic for macrophages, no BCG-mediated tumor regression occurred in tumor-bearing animals. Similar results were reported by Tanaka *et al.* [107] after blockage of phagocytic cells by fine latex particles.

There is a controversy over the question of whether BCG intensifies a cellular immunoresponse of the organism to tumor antigen [62, 104] or possibly represents a reaction affecting only BCG antigen. Zbar [85] described an apparent dose-effect relationship for tumors of different antigenicity that suggested that BCG treatment of strongly immunogenic tumor cells led to high tumor regression rates while treatment of slightly immunogenic tumors resulted in low regression rates. Moore *et al.* [105, 109, 110] could not confirm this dose-effect relationship.

Studies of the cellular immunoresponse of BCG-treated mice by Mackaness [111] and Blanden *et al.* [112] suggest a theoretical sequence of cellular mechanisms in BCG-determined tumor regression. After the application of BCG in the tumors, the bacteria drain into the regional lymph nodes and induce a proliferation of BCG-specific lymphocytes by their antigenicity. These sensitized lymphocytes are released into the periphery with a latency of a few days and accumulate at the site of the bacterial antigen, in the tumor and in the draining lymph nodes. The reaction between BCG and specifically sensitized lymphocytes leads to the release of lymphocyte-produced mediator substances with recruiting [113, 114], arresting [115, 114] and activating [116, 117] activity. Activated macrophages either have a direct cytotoxic effect on syngeneic tumor cells [118–121] or act by the secretion of tumoricidal substance [122–125]. In addition, they produce a lymphocyte-activating substance (LAF) which may possibly be necessary for the proliferation of T-lymphocytes with subsequent formation of specifically cytotoxic T-cells [126–128].

The development of tumor-specific immunity was tested by subjecting the animals to a reintroduction of line 10 tumor cells and a first application of line 1 tumor cells. Tumor specific immunity was demonstrated in animals that had been simultaneously injected with tumor cells and live BCG or BCG-CWP and for animals with established tumors that had been cured by intratumoral BCG treatment. The development of tumor-specific immunity was dependent on BCG and was possibly related to mechanisms that are triggered by BCG and tumor cells. For tumors treated intradermally with BCG, the development of tumor-specific immunity was reported by Zbar *et al.* [62], who proved that this phenomenon can be observed $2\frac{1}{2}$–12 months after intratumoral treatment, while simultaneous inoculation of the animals with a second application of tumor cells on the day of BCG therapy did not lead to the development of immunity. These findings of immunity against syngeneic tumor cells in animals that had previously received injections of tumor cell and BCG led to concepts of active immunization. For live line 10 tumor cells and live BCG organisms, this effect was described in 1972 by Zbar for intradermal tumors. Changes in tumor cell activity after irradiation or mitomycin-C treatment of the cells [54, 129] lead to development of immunity in combination with BCG in the same way as did lyophilized tumor cells and BCG [130]. Live BCG organisms were interchangeable with heat-destroyed bacteria, BCG extracts, and CWP without loss of activity of these tumor cell BCG vaccines [62, 129]. In all experiments, however, the simultaneous administration of BCG and tumor cells at the same site was always necessary. Spatially and temporally separated injections or the exclusive injection of BCG or attenuated tumor cells did not lead to immunization. The same or similar findings have also been made in other syngeneic animal tumor models [60, 131–133]. In addition, attempts have been made to isolate tumor antigen either directly from tumor cells [134, 135] or from the serum of tumor-bearing animals [136] and to use it for immunization [137].

Currently, knowledge is incomplete on the specific role of BCG in the augmentation of tumor-specific immunity. However, it seems more complex than simply an intensification of the immunoreaction against tumor-specific or associated antigens. Various studies of cellular immunomechanisms suggest T-cell involvement is important for the regression of BCG-injected tumors. No tumor-specific immunity could develop in animals exposed to whole-body irradiation [138], in athymic mice [139] and in thymectomized animals that had undergone bone marrow reconstitution [140]. In addition, Hawrylko [133] demonstrated higher cytotoxicity of spleen and lymph node cells from immunized animals than of cells from non-immunized tumor-bearing animals. Cytotoxicity was observed after cell transfer of the lymphocytes into untreated tumor-bearing animals. An increased cytotoxicity of cells from immune animals compared to those from non-immune animals has also recently been reported using an *in vitro* assay [141].

Despite insufficiently clarified mechanisms of the induction and effect of intratumoral BCG therapy, the following observations have been made:

1. a tumor experimentally placed in the planum buccale is eliminated;
2. regionally manifest metastases do not fully develop; and
3. tumor-specific immunity can be demonstrated in successfully treated animals.

Compared to radical surgery that has the same curative effect, intratumoral BCG treatment has the obvious advantage of inducing a tumor-specific immunity. It must be emphasized that these conclusions apply only to the experimental system, i.e. to line to 10 tumor cells in the planum buccale of strain 2 guinea pigs.

Immunotherapy in experimental systems with inbred animals and experimentally induced tumors has often been successful. At the same time it is apparent that there is a relative lack of positive data for autologous systems. It is at present unclear why spontaneously developing tumors in inbred and outbred animals were not very successfully influenced by immunotherapeutic measures. It is possible that the postulated neoantigens of spontaneously occurring tumors are so slightly immunogenic that no effective antitumor immunoreactivity is developed. But if suitable 'conditioning' made it possible to optimize the immune system for a regular immunoreactivity, an effective inducible immunoreactivity against autochthonously growing tumors would be conceivable. This consideration led us to use an outbred animal population with autochthonous epithelial tumors in the head and neck region. The purpose of the study was to examine the influence of live BCG and BCG-CWP on the growth of squamous cell carcinomas in cows. Forty-nine tumor-bearing cows were divided into five groups analogous to the above mentioned guinea pig model (Table 4). There was progressive tumor growth in the untreated control group except for one spontaneous regression. In the groups receiving a single intratumoral injection of live BCG and BCG-CWP, over 70% of the animals reacted with a tumor regression, and 11 of 19 cows were tumor-free after one year. Half of the locally operated animals were free of recurrence and metastases, while all the animals in the radically operated group were tumor-free after one year. If one compares the results from the cows (Table 4) with those from the guinea pigs (Tables 2 and 3), there is an obvious discrepancy in the experimental findings. While, with the guinea pig model, all locally operated animals developed lymph node metastases, the local operation in cows led to a clinical cure in 50% of the cases. Radically operated animals in both species remained tumor-free. In contrast to the guinea pig model, in which an intratumoral BCG injection led to an outcome similar to that for radically operated animals, the success of an intratumoral BCG injection in cows was only comparable to a local operation. With the present state of experimental knowledge, proof is still lacking in the cow model that clinical cure by intratumoral injection of BCG is accompanied by a tumor-specific immunity. Supporting evidence cannot be provided, since genetically homogeneous bovine animal material is not yet available.

There have been occasional reports of spontaneous remissions of bovine carcinomas in the literature [142]. In our study, a spontaneous regression of this kind occurred in one animal in the untreated control group. Although the cause and mechanisms of spontaneous remissions are largely unknown, they have been associated with cytotoxic cells in recent case descriptions of human neoplasias [143–145]. The therapeutic success of intratumoral BCG therapy in tumor-bearing cows can possibly be attributed to the fact that the tumor in this experimental system is one with relatively marked TSTA. Before experiences based on the bovine model can be generalized, however, additional studies must be carried out with different autochthonously growing tumors in various animal species. Nevertheless, on the basis of the present animal material, we feel it is justified to conclude that intratumoral BCG application in squamous cell carcinomas of cows has an effectiveness similar to that of a local operation.

The following observations must be considered in order to obtain an overall view of the effect of BCG on the growth of malignant tumors in animals: (1) In cases of limited tumor size, intratumoral live BCG or BCG-CWP injection leads in a clear dose-effect relationship to tumor regression in certain experimental systems. (2) BCG is ineffective when it is not applied in the tumor. (3) A tumor regression is accompanied by the development of a tumor-specific immunity that appears to be cell-mediated, i.e. it is not transmissible by antibodies. (4) The activation of macrophages or macrophage-like cells appears to be necessary for the induction of tumor regression. Since the immunity is tumor-specific, macrophages do not appear to be likely effector cells. A postulated sequence of events that incorporates these observations is as follows: by the intratumoral injection of BCG, a DTH reaction of the tuberculin type is induced at the application site, that place in the organism where there are tumor-specific antigens in concentrated form. In the tumor, this reaction leads to an accumulation of cells of both the RES (macrophages) and the lymphocytic system (T-cells). Since it is known that the activation of T helper cells against foreign antigens (tumor-specific neoantigens) requires the cooperation of syngeneic macrophages, and that for this activation a macrophage-produced factor (LAF) is necessary, the requisites for an optimal activation of T helper cells is created by the intratumoral DTH-reaction. Activated T helper cells are likewise a prerequisite for the induction of antigen-specific T killer cells. Activated T killer cells are then able to eliminate tumor cells in cases where the tumor mass is limited.

3. Intratumoral BCG-cell wall preparation therapy in patients with squamous cell carcinoma in the head and neck region

Based on the animal experiments, a clinical study with BCG cell wall preparation (CWP) was undertaken. Patients with head and neck carcinomas stage $T_{1-2}N_{0-2}M_0$ were randomized. One group received surgical treatment only and a second group received preoperative intralesional (i.t.) BCG-CWP. Twenty-four untreated patients (10 female, 14 male) with a histologically confirmed diagnosis of squamous cell carcinoma and clinical tumor stage $T_{1-2}N_{0-2}M_0$ were included in the study. The age of the patients ranged from 52 to 86 years. The average age was 68 years. The tumor patients are listed in Table 5 according to age, sex, TNM classification (UICC 1976), and tumor localization.

3.1. Recurrence and survival

The results of the recurrence and survival observation are summarized in Table 6. Twenty-four patients were included in the study over a period of three years. Twelve patients received i.t. injections of BCG-CWP and were subsequently subjected to radical surgery (Group 1). Twelve patients were treated by surgery only (Group 2). The average observation period for patients in Group 1 was 380 days, and that for patients in Group 2, 365 days.

Recurrence of the tumor became manifest during the observation period in 3 patients in Group 1 and 5 patients in Group 2. The recurrences in Group 1 were local and occurred after an average of 167 days. There was a

Table 5. Listing of the carcinoma patients according to age, TNM classification (UICC 1976), and tumor localization

Patient no.	Sex	Age	TNM	Localization
1	Male	72	$T_2N_2M_0$	Middle lower lip
2	Female	68	$T_2N_2M_0$	Alveolar process UJ, right
3	Male	85	$T_2N_2M_0$	Sulcus gloss-alveolaris, Lingus, left
4	Male	74	$T_2N_2M_0$	Alveolar process LJ, Sulcus buccomandibularis, left
5	Female	65	$T_1N_2M_0$	Lingua, left
6	Male	62	$T_2N_0M_0$	Lingua, left
7	Male	67	$T_2N_1M_0$	Alveolar process LJ, Sulcus glosso-alveolaris, left
8	Female	74	$T_2N_1M_0$	Alveolar process LJ, right
9	Male	71	$T_1N_2M_0$	Sulcus glosso-alveolaris, right and left
10	Female	58	$T_2N_1M_0$	Lower lip, left
11	Female	64	$T_2N_1M_0$	Alveolar process LJ, right
12	Male	52	$T_2N_0M_0$	Alveolar process UJ, Sulcus buccomandibularis, Planum buccale, left
13	Female	67	$T_2N_1M_0$	Alveolar process LJ, Sulcus buccomandibularis, right
14	Male	74	$T_2N_0M_0$	Lower lip, right
15	Male	72	$T_2N_2M_0$	Sulcus glosso-alveolaris, left
16	Female	70	$T_2N_2M_0$	Alveolar process LJ, Sulcus glosso-alveolaris, right
17	Male	80	$T_2N_0M_0$	Alveolar process LJ, Trigonum retromolare, right
18	Female	61	$T_2N_1M_0$	Alveolar process LJ, Trigonum retromolare, right
19	Male	69	$T_1N_1M_0$	Lower lip, left
20	Male	57	$T_2N_1M_0$	Alveolar process LJ, Trigonum retromolare, right
21	Male	68	$T_2N_2M_0$	Alveolar process LJ, Sulcus glosso-alveolaris, right and left
22	Female	67	$T_2N_2M_0$	Alveolar process LJ, left
23	Male	60	$T_2N_2M_0$	Sulcus glosso-alveolaris, left
24	Female	86	$T_2N_1M_0$	Planum buccale, left

local recurrence in one case in Group 2. There were metastases in the lymph drainage area in the neck region of the primary tumor in three patients with a pretreatment classification of N_0. In one case, a metastasis occurred on the contralateral side of the neck following primary en bloc tumor removal. The average recurrence-free interval for these patients was 116 days.

Two of the 3 recurrence patients in Group 1 died after radiation therapy. The third patient received surgical salvage treatment and was free of tumor recurrence during the last examination period. Three of the 5 recurrence patients in Group 2 who were given surgical and chemotherapy salvage treatment died. Two patients were clinically free of any tumor growth during the last follow-up examination after repeated therapy.

The life-table calculations for both treatment groups are shown in Figs. 11 and 12. The cumulative proportion of living patients for the entire study was 61% (SD 41%) and for the patients in primary complete tumor remission, 52% (SD 13%). After the study group had been subclassified into

Table 6. Listing of the tumor patients according to type of therapy an observation period

Patient no.	Therapy type	Observation period in days			
		Total	Without recurrence	With recurrence	To death
1	BCG-CWP, OP	922	922		
2	BCG-CWP, OP	832	832		
3	BCG-CWP, OP	210	186	24	210
4	OP	451	201	250	451
5	OP	762	762		
6	OP	397	127	270	397
7	BCG-CWP, OP	293	203	90	293
8	OP	673	135	538	
9	OP	603	603		
10	BCG-CWP, OP	603	603		
11	BCG-CWP, OP	588	588		
12	OP	466	54	412	466
13	OP	372	372		
14	OP	288	61	227	
15	BCG-CWP, OP	288	288		
16	BCG-CWP, OP	265	265		
17	BCG-CWP, OP	202	202		
18	BCG-CWP, OP	197	110	87	
19	OP	106	106		
20	OP	106	106		
21	BCG-CWP, OP	98	98		
22	BCG-CWP, OP	69	69		
23	OP	67	67		
24	OP	61	61		

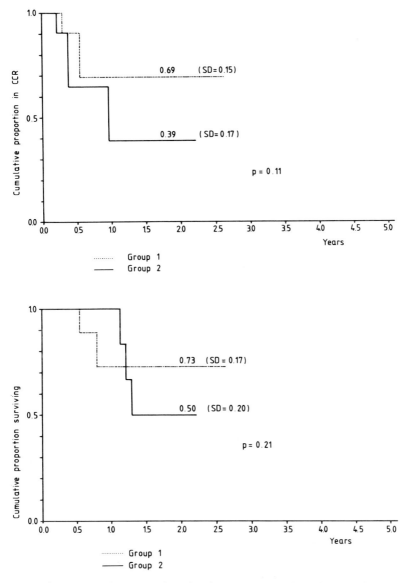

Figures 11 and 12. Cumulative proportion of patients pretreated with BCG-CWP i.t. (. . . . .) and patients not pretreated (———) surviving.

BCG-CW-pretreated and non-pretreated patients, a cumulative proportion of living patients in Group 1 was 73% (SD 17%) (Fig. 11). This value was 23% higher than that for patients in Group 2 (50%, SD 20%). The cumulative proportion of patients who were in complete clinical tumor remission was 69% (SD 15%) for Group 1 and 39% (SD 17%) for Group 2 (Fig. 12).

3.2. Toxicity

An average temperature increase of 2 °C over the pretreatment values was observed in Group 1 at 3–24 h after the injection of BCG-CWP. An average temperature increase of 1 °C was recorded on the first post-operative day for patients in Group 2. The values in Group 1 were increased on day 1 in comparison to those in Group 2. In both therapy groups the body temperature normalized for ten (Group 1) and nine (Group 2) patients by the second or third day after treatment.

Two patients in Group 1 and three in Group 2 were conspicuous in that the increased temperatures persisted up to day 14. The values in Group 1 were increased over the pretreatment initial values on days 1, 2 and 5. In Group 2, they were increased over the pretreatment values on day 1. Comparison of the groups with one another indicated that the temperatures in Group 1 were increased over those in Group 2 on day 1.

The pulse rate on the first day after the BCG-CWP injection (Group 1) increased by an average of 25 beats/minute from $\tilde{x} = 75$ to $\tilde{x} = 100$. Normal values were again registered on day 2. There was a slight increase in pulse rate in the surgical group up to the third postoperative day. Normalization occurred in intervals up to the seventh postoperative day.

Slight to moderately severe chills developed in five patients in Group 1. This symptom disappeared in three patients after 24 h, and in two patients by the fourth day after the i.t. injection. Gastrointestinal complaints including nausea and vomiting were reported by two patients in this group. Anaphylactic or general allergic reactions were not observed and hypotention or hypertension did not occur in either of the therapy groups.

Laboratory examinations before and after therapy indicated no significant changes in the erythropoietic system (Ery, Hb, HbE, HT, Reti) for either group. The leukocyte values in Groups 1 and 2 increased above the norm on the first day after treatment (Group 1 $\tilde{x} = 8$, 200 cells/mm^3, Group 2 $\tilde{x} = 11,400$ cells/mm^3) although these values did not differ significantly from pretreatment values. The leukocyte count for the BCG-pretreated patients was lower on the first day in comparison to that in Group 2. There was also a fall in the values on day three in comparison to day one for Group 1. In both treatment groups the relative lymphocyte count was significantly decreased on day 1 after therapy and back to normal values on day 3.

A slight post-therapeutic drop in platelet counts by a maximum of 30,000 cell/mm^3 was significant in both groups with similar limited changes in PTT and the Quick value. All of the values were within the normal range. There was no proof that the therapy influenced levels of electrolytes, creatinine, glucose, alkaline phosphatase, transaminases, total protein, albumin, globulins, or cardiovascular or urine status. The changes in clinical and laboratory examinations after surgical procedures on the BCG-CWP-pretreated patients corresponded to those observed in the group treated with surgery alone. There was no indication that the i.t. injection had any influence on the parameters tested.

3.3. Local reaction to BCG-CWP

Tumor and draining lymph nodes in patient Group 1 were examined for local changes following the injection of BCG-CWP. Similar infiltrates of varying intensity developed in all patients. No correlation was observed between the tumor and lymph node reactivity and the appearance of a recurrence. Surgical complications did not occur following the BCG-CWP injections, however, postoperatively there were disturbances in the healing of the wound in three instances. Such phenomena, however, were observed to the same extent in the group which received only surgical treatment.

An infiltration which varied in intensity formed at the primary tumor of all patients 6–12 h after the injection. The maximum intensity was reached after 24–48 h. Over a period of several days, ulcerations with exudate developed. These conditions regressed as the infiltrate decreased. There was clinical regression of the infiltrate and partial healing of the ulcerations over a period of 2–6 weeks. During this period the patients did not indicate that they suffered from any pain. In seven patients there was a measurable change in the size of the primary tumor after the injection of BCG-CWP.

Table 7. Listing of the tumor patients according to reaction to BCG-CWP injection on the tumor and in the draining lymph node and according to size change in the tumor

Patient no.	BCG-CWP reaction		Size change in tumor
	On tumor	In lymph node	
1	Severe	Severe	Smaller
2	Moderate	None	None
3	Clear	Moderate	None
7	Severe	Severe	None
10	Severe	Severe	Smaller
11	Clear	Moderate	Smaller
15	Clear	Clear	Smaller
16	Severe	Clear	Smaller
17	Severe	Severe	Smaller
18	Severe	Clear	None
21	Clear	Clear	Smaller
22	Clear	Moderate	None

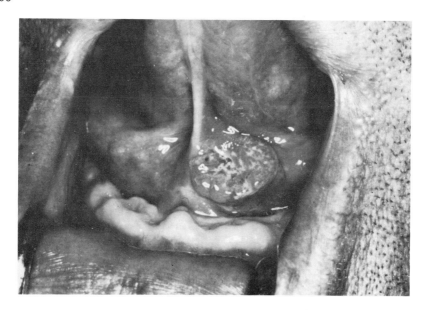

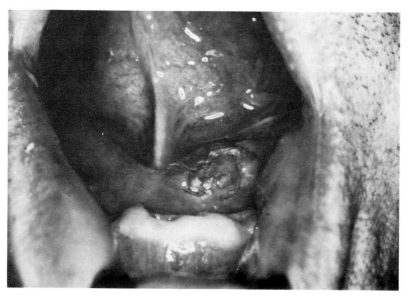

Figures 13 and 14. Squamous cell carcinoma of the oral cavity before (13) and 3 weeks after (14) a single injection of BCG-CWP.

Tumor regressions were up to 50% of the original tumor size (Figs. 13 and 14). Two patients reacted with a partial demarcation of the tumor. In five cases there was no change. Progressive tumor growth was not observed in any patient during the interval between injection and surgery. Of the three patients who recurred, none showed a reduction in the size of the tumor following the injection of BCG-CWP (Table 7).

With the exception of one patient, there was always a reaction in the region of the draining neck lymph nodes. In comparison to inflammation of the primary tumor, lymph node reactions were delayed by 1-2 days and were manifest by swelling of the submandibular and cervical neck nodes and partial reddening of the skin. No reaction occurred in the only patient in this group suffering from a carcinoma of the upper jaw (Table 7).

3.4. Skin tests

Pretreatment dinitrochlorobenzene (DNCB) reactivity of patients in Group 1 was slightly higher for the concentrations 10, 50, and 12.5 µg than for patients in Group 2. The values for 25 µg were identical. Three to 24 months after the BCG-CWP therapy, DNCB reactivity was unchanged in 5 patients in Group 1, positive in 4 patients and negative in 1 patient. In comparison to initial values, quantitative DNCB reactivity after therapy increased for 6 patients in this group and decreased for 1 patient. In the surgical group, a decrease in DNCB skin reactions after therapy was noted in 4 patients. Three patients remained unchanged and positive and 2 patients, negative. Two patients in this group showed a post-therapy quantitative increase in reactivity.

All pretherapy skin tests for PPD were negative. Four patients in Group 1 and 1 patient in Group 2 changed from negative to weakly positive up to three months after the therapy. All patients (10 in Group 1, 8 in Group 2) who were tested after 6 months with increasing concentrations of PPD up to a maximum of 10 IU had markedly positive skin reactions. There were no observed differences between Group 1 and Group 2.

3.5. Conclusions and future prospects

The patients given preoperative i.t. BCG-CWP therapy had more favorable values for the cumulative proportion of patients in clinical complete remission and proportion of living patients according to the analysis of the life-table calculations compared to the group that was treated exclusively by surgery. Clinically there was an increase in the body temperature and pulse rate following i.t. BCG-CWP treatment in comparison to the surgical group. Nausea and vomiting were observed in some of the patients. The laboratory values indicated changes in white blood counts. The local reaction following BCG-CWP injection produced an inflammatory infiltrate at the primary tumor and in the region of the draining lymph nodes. In some patients, there was a significant increase in the infiltrate cells for the BCG-CWP-pretreatment group and the formation of granulomas and proliferates.

After a three-year observation period, results for the BCG-CWP-pre-treated patients are better than for the surgically treated patients with respect to both complete tumor remission and survival expectancy. The differences between the two groups for the cumulative patient proportion in complete tumor remission are not yet statistically significant ($P = 0.11$). However, it appears that the addition of i.t. BCG-CWP therapy has not adversely affected the survival chances of the patients treated. A classification of the patients according to tumor localization, tumor differentiation, age or sex does not appear indicated on the basis of the limited number of cases now available.

Comparable reports concerning BCG-CWP therapy are not yet available. However, the beginning of a similar study with living BCG for patients with malignant melanoma Clark level IV and V has been indicated by Rosenberg and Rapp [146]. Results are available from a similar study of melanoma patients pretreated with Vaccina virus i.t. [69]. Forty-eight previously un-treated patients were randomized to receive either preoperative i.t. therapy with a minimum of 1×10^8 Vaccina virus for 14 days or surgical treatment only. The life-table analysis 48 months after the beginning of the study indicated a higher rate of recurrence-free patients in the patient group that received i.t. pretreatment.

Prior reports of i.t. BCG therapy have overwhelmingly dealt with patients having very advanced stages of malignant melanoma. Partial or total regressions of small skin metastases following i.t. live BCG injections were described for the first time in 1970 by Morton et al. [147]. Four years later another report from the same group [66] reported regression of 90% of the injected skin metastases and 17% of the uninjected metastases in immuno-competent patients. The total number of patients studied was 151. Of these patients, 25% had remained tumor-free for 1–6 years. Several working groups have in the meantime confirmed the original observation made by Morton et al. [81, 146, 148–160]. In almost all of these studies, advanced disease stages, visceral metastases, and lack of reactivity of PPD were limiting factors for success of i.t. BCG therapy. Some authors have also reported instances of tumor enhancement following BCG injection [142, 152, 161].

In addition to living BCG, the clinical use of mycobacterial components has also been reported recently. Seven patients with pulmonary carcinomas were injected intraoperatively with skeletized BCG cell walls [162]. No pre-liminary information is yet available on these patients. Richman et al. [163] reported 18 melanoma and five carcinoma patients with recurrences who had been treated with skeletized cell walls and P_3 i.t. Tumors that were less than 1 cm in diameter reacted up to 58%, while larger tumors responded only up to 33%. Total regressions were not described. The same substances have been used by Vosika et al. [164] for the therapy of malignant melanomas, hypernephromas, and pulmonary and mammary carcinomas. Although 7 of 17 melanoma patients demonstrated partial regressions, no effect was observed for the remaining types of tumors.

In our clinical study, side effects following the i.t. injection of BCG-CWP were limited. Clinically, moderate increases in temperature and pulse rate were noted and in some instances slight chills and nausea with vomiting. The laboratory values indicated no changes other than a short term alteration in the white blood cell count with leukopenia and lymphopenia.

Although our observations of temperature increases, nausea, vomiting, slight chills, lymphopenia, and leukopenia are in agreement with the observation of others [81, 148, 165–173] following the injection of living BCG-CWP, a large number of additional side effects, in some instances with fatal consequences, have been reported which we did not observe in our study with BCG-CWP. Following i.t. treatment with living BCG, McKhann et al. [174] observed two cases with fatal complications. A possible cause was hyperreactivity to BCG which led to high fever, pronounced coagulation disturbances, hypertension and anuria. Clifford [175] also reported two cases with a fatal outcome. Following a single injection of living BCG and subsequent surgical procedures after an interval of three days in patients with head and neck tumors, coagulation disturbances developed that could not be controlled. Hyperreactivity reactions with anaphylactic symptoms in some instances have been described by Morton [168], McKhann et al. [174], Pinsky et al. [157], Sparks et al. [176], and Robinson [177]. Thrombocytopenias with values as low as 3,000 cells/mm^3 have been described by Norton et al. [178]. Hepatomegaly and liver dysfunction with markedly increased alkaline phosphatase levels [165, 167, 157, 173, 169, 81] have been reported as have generalized infections with BCG [81, 179–182].

The large number of severe side effects in some instances can probably be attributed to two factors in all of these studies. Living BCG has been used and this produces a general septicemia. Secondly, multiple injection procedures have also been primarily used, which can lead to local and in some instances generalized hyperergic reactions.

No total regressions were observed in our patients with head and neck tumors. This is possibly due to the fact that the period between BCG-CWP injection and radical surgery was too short. This assumption is supported by the observations recorded in BCG-treated cows with tumors, which only indicated a total tumor regression after several weeks to months [89]. In addition, the only goal of this study was to determine whether the prognosis of patients who undergo radical surgery could be improved by means of additional preoperative BCG-CWP therapy.

Immunological investigations were limited to tests of delayed-type skin reactions. Although the group of BCG-CWP-treated patients showed a general increase in reactivity to DNCB in comparison to patients treated only surgically, no clear changes could be determined for PPD. All patients in both groups developed positive skin reactions as the PPD dose was increased.

At the present, the prognostic effect of combination therapy (BCG-CWP and surgery) is still unclear for patients with squamous cell carcinomas in the head and neck region. The patient numbers in this trial were too limited to permit statistically significant statements. On the basis of the information presented, however, it is possible to state that the extent of side effects described for living BCG can be drastically reduced and partially avoided by using BCG-CWP. Furthermore, the cumulative proportion of patients presently in complete tumor remission is 69% for the combination therapy (BCG-CWP and surgery) group and 39% for patients who only underwent radical surgery. If the available data are carefully interpreted, a trend favoring combination therapy is evident. However, it should be emphasized here that this trend is not yet statistically significant. In the sense of a negative exclusion, the combination therapy has not yet led to complications which would make it necessary to discontinue the study. The outlook for intratumoral BCG-CWP that was used for the first time in the human system is therefore favorable and the study will be continued until sufficient patients have been examined to allow a statistically significant statement concerning the influence of i.t. BCG-CWP on the clinical course of treated patients with head and neck squamous cell carcinoma.

References

1. Nauts HC: The apparently beneficial effects of bacterial infection on host resistance to cancer. NY Cancer Res Inst Monogr 1:1, 1969.
2. Nauts HC: The apparently beneficial effects of bacterial infection on host resistance to cancer. NY Cancer Res Inst Monogr 2:373, 1969.
3. Coley WB: Further observations upon the treatment of malignant tumors with the toxin of erysipelas and Bacillus prodigiosus, with a report of 160 cases. Bull Johns Hopkins Hosp 65:157, 1896.
4. Nauts HC, Fowler GA, Bogatka F: A review of the influence of bacterial infection and of bacterial products (Coley's toxins) on malignant tumors in man. Acta Med Scand 276:5, 1953.
5. Guérin C: In: Rosenthal SR (ed) The History of BCG. BCG Vaccination Against Tuberculosis. Boston, Little, Brown and Company 1957, p 48.
6. Crispen RG: Immunoprophylaxis with BCG. In: Crispen RG (ed) Neoplasm Immunity: BCG vaccination. Chicago, Ill., Schori Press, 1974.
7. Eickhoff TC: The current status of BCG immunization against tuberculosis. Annu Rev Med 28:411, 1977.
8. Dubos RJ, Shaedler RW: Effects of cellular constituents of mycobacteria on resistance of mice to heterologous infections. I. Protective effect. J Exp Med 106:703, 1957.
9. Brown JAK, Stone MM, Sutherland J: BCG vaccination of children against leprosy in Uganda: results at end of second follow-up. Br Med J 1:24, 1968.

10. Biozzi G, Benacerraf B, Grumbach F: Étude de l'activité granulopexique du système réticulo-endo thélial au cours de l'infection tuberculeuse expérimentale de la souris. Ann Inst Pasteur 87:291, 1954.

11. Old, LJ, Clarke DA, Benacerraf B: Effect of Bacillus Calmette-Guérin infection on transplanted tumours in the mouse. Nature (Lond) 184:291, 1959.

12. Weiss, DW, Bonhag RS, De Que, KB: Protective activity of fractions of tubercle bacilli against isologous tumours in mice. Nature (Lond) 190:889, 1961.

13. Suter E: Passive transfer of acquired resistance to infection with mycobacterium tuberculosis by means of cells. Am Rev Respir Dis 83:535, 1961.

14. Millmann I: Passive transfer of resistance to tuberculosis. Am Rev Respir Dis 85:30, 1962.

15. Fong J, Chin D, Elberg SS: Studies on tubercle bacillus-histiocyt relationship. V. Passive transfer of cellular resistance. J Exp Med 115:475, 1962.

16. Lefford MJ, McGregor DD, MacKaness GB: Immune response to Mycobacterium tuberculosis in rats. Infect Immun 8:182, 1973.

17. Lederer E, Adam A, Ciorbaru R, Petit JF, Wietzerbin J: Cell walls of Mycobacteria and related organisms; chemistry and immunostimulant properties. Moll Cell Biochem 7:87, 1975.

18. Minden P, McClatchy JK, Cooper R, Bardane EJ, Farr RS: Shared antigens between Mycobacterium bovis (BCG) and other bacterial species. Science 176:57, 1972.

19. Minden P, Sharpton TR, McClatchy JK: Shared antigens between bacteria and guinea pig line 10 hepatocarcinoma cells. Cancer Res 36:1680, 1976.

20. Borsos T, Rapp HJ: Antigenic relationship between Myobacterium bovis (BCG) and guinea pig hepatoma. J Natl Cancer Inst 51:1085, 1973.

21. v. Rokitansky C (ed): A manual of pathological anatomy. Blanchard u. Lea, Philadelphia, 1855.

22. Pearl R: Cancer and tuberculosis. Am J Hyg 9:97, 1929.

23. Old LJ, Benacerraf B, Clarke DA, et al.: The role of the veticuloendothelial system in the host reaction to neoplasia. Cancer Res 21:1281, 1961.

24. Hattori S, Matsuda M: Relationship between cancer and tuberculosis II. A retarding effect of BCG inoculation for tumor induction in mice with INH or urethane-4NQO injections. Kekkaku 39:449, 1964.

25. Inooka SJ: Relation between tumor growth and host resistance. Sci Rep Res Inst Tohoku Univ (Med) 12:240, 1965.

26. Piessens WF, Heimann R, Legros N, et al.: Effect of Bacillus Calmette-Guérin on mammary tumor formation and cellular immunity in dimethylbenz-(a)anthracene-treated rats. Cancer Res 31:1061, 1971.

27. Weiss DW: Nonspecific stimulation and modulation of the immune response and of states of resistance by the methanol-extraction residue fraction of tubercle bacilli. Natl Cancer Inst Monogr 35:157, 1972.

28. Kataoka T, Nakamura RM, Yamamoto S, et al.: Effect of BCG on carcinogen-induced tumor development in mice. Jap J Med Sci Biol 25:377, 1972.

29. Vollegov AI: Local intensification of cellular immunological reaction and resistance to the development of neoplasms. Vestn Akad Med Nauk SSSR 27(2):91, 1972.

30. Lavrin DH, Rosenberg SA, Conner RJ: Immunoprophylaxis of methylcholanthrene-induced tumors in mice with Bacillus Calmette-Guérin an methanol-extracted residue. Cancer Res 33:472, 1973.

31. Lemonde P, Clode M: Effect of BCG infection on leukemia and polyoma in mice and hamsters. Proc Soc Exp Bid Med 111:739, 1962.

32. Lemonde P, Clode-Hyde M: Influence of Bacille Calmette-Guérin infection on polyoma in hamsters and mice. Cancer Res 26:585, 1966.

33. Sjögren HO, Ankerst J: Effect of BCG and allogeneic tumor cells on adenovirus typ 12

tumorigenesis in mice. Nature (Lond) 221:863, 1969.

34. Lemonde P: Protective effects of BCG and other bacteria against neoplasia in mice and hamsters. Natl Cancer Inst Monogr 39:21, 1973.

35. Schwartz DB, Zbar B, Gibson WT, et al.: Inhibition of murine sarcom virus oncogenesis with living BCG. Int J Cancer 8:320, 1971.

36. Larson CL, Ushijima RN, Florey MJ, et al.: Effect of BCG on Friend disease virus in mice. Nature (New Biol) 229:243, 1971.

37. Larson CL, Baker RE, Ushijima RN, et al.: Immunotherapy of Friend disease in mice employing viable BCG vaccine. Proc Soc Exp Bid Med 140:700, 1972..

38. Ankerst J, Jonsson N: Inhibitory effects of BCG on adenovirus tumorigenesis: dependence on administration schedule. Int J Cancer 10:351, 1972.

39. Houchens DP, Goldberg AI, Gaston MR, et al.: Studies of the effect of Bacillus Calmette-Guérin on Moloney sarcoma virus-induced tumors in normal and immuno-suppressed mice. Cancer Res 33:685, 1973.

40. Haran-Ghera N, Weiss BW: Effect of treatment of C57BL?6 mice with the methanol extraction residue fraction of BCG on leukemogenesis induced by the radiation leukemia virus. J Natl Cancer Inst 50:229, 1973.

41. Nilson A, Révész L, Stjernswärd J: Suppression of Strontium-90-induced development of bone tumors by infection with Bacillus Calmette-Buérin (BCG). Radiat Res 26:378, 1965.

42. Weiss DW, Lavrin DH, Dezfulian M, et al.: Studies on the immunology of spontaneous mammary carcinomas of mise. In: Burdette WJ (ed) Viruses Inducing Cancer. Salt Lake City, University of Utah Press, 1968, p 138.

43. Lavrin DH, Rosenberg SA, Conner RJ: Immunoprophylaxis of methylcholanthrene-induced tumors in mice with Bacillus Calmette-Guérin and methanol-extracted residue. Cancer Res 33:472, 1973.

44. Helpern Bn, Biozzi G, Stiffel C, et al.: Effet de la stimulation du système réticulo-endo-thélial par l'inoculation du bacille Calmette-Guérin sur le développement de l'épithélioma atypique T-8 de Guérin chez le rat. C R Soc Biol (Paris) 153:919, 1959.

45. Biozzi G, Stiffel C, Halpern BN, et al: Effet de l'inoculation du bacille de Calmette-Guérin sur le développement de la tumeur asclique d'Ehrlich chez la souris. C R Soc Bid (Paris) 153:987, 1959.

46. Old LJ, Clarke DA, Benacerraf B, et al.: The reticuloendothelial system and the neoplastic process. Ann N Y Acad Sci 88:264, 1960.

47. Old LJ, Clarke DA, Benacerraf B: Effect of prior splenectomy on the growth of sarcoma 180 in normal and Bacillus Calmette-Guérin infected mice. Experientia 18:335, 1962.

48. Weiss DW, Bonhag RS, Leslie P: Studies on the heterologous immunogenicity of a methanol-insoluble fraction of attenuated tubercle bacilli (BCG). II. Protection against tumor isografts. J Exp Med 124:1039, 1966.

49. Klein E: Hypersensitivity reactions at tumor site. Cancer Res 29:2351, 1969.

50. Klein E, Holtermann OA, Papermaster B, Milgrom H, Rosner D, Klein L, et al.: Immunologic approaches to various types of cancer with the use of BCG and purified protein derivates. Natl Cancer Inst Monogr 39:229, 1973.

51. Klein E, Holtermann OA, Heim F, Rosner D, Milgram H, Adler S, et al.: Immunologic approaches to the management of primary and secondary tumors involving the skin and soft tissues: Review of ten Year program. In: Cancer and Transplantation. NY, Grune and Stratton, 1975.

52. Zbar B, Bernstein I, Tanaka T, et al.: Tumor immunity produced by the intradermal inoculation of living tumor cells and living Mycobacterium bovis (strain BCG). Science 170:1217, 1970.

53. Zbar B, Bernstein I, Rapp HJ: Suppression of tumor growth at the site of infection with living Bacillus Calmette-Guérin. J Natl Cancer Inst 46:831, 1971.

54. Bartlett GL, Zbar B: Tumor-specific vaccine containing mycobacterium bovis and tumor cells: safety and efficacy. J Natl Cancer Inst 48:1709, 1972.

55. Littmann BH, Meltzer MS, Cleveland RP: Tumor-specific, cell-mediated immunity in guinea pigs with tumors. J Natl Cancer Inst 51:1627, 1973.

56. Tanaka T, Tokunaga T: Suppression of tumor growth an induction of specific tumor immunity by intradermal inoculation of a mixture of living tumor cells and life Mycobacterium bovis in syngenic mice. Gann 62:433, 1971.

57. Tokunaga T, Kataoka T, Nakamura RM, et al.: Tumor immunity induced by BCG-tumor cell mixtures in syngenic mice. Jap J Med Sci Bid 26:71, 1973.

58. Chung EB, Zbar B, Rapp HJ: Tumor regression mediated by Mycobacterium bovis (strain BCG): effects of isonicotinic acid hydrazide, cortisone acetate, and antithymocyte serum. J Natl Cancer Inst 51:241, 1973.

59. Baldwin RW, Pimm MV: Influence of BCG infection on growth of 3-methyl-cholanthrene-induced rat sarcomas. Rev Eur Etud Clin Biol 16:875, 1971.

60. Baldwin RW, Pimm MV: BCG immunotherapy of local subcutaneous growth and post-surgical pulmonary metastases of a transplanted rat epithelioma of spontaneous origin. Int J Cancer 12:420, 1973.

61. Zbar B, Tanaka T: Immunotherapy of cancer: regression of tumors after intralesional injection of living Mycobacterium bovis. Science 172:271, 1971.

62. Zbar B, Rapp HJ, Ribi E: Tumor suppression by cell walls of Mycobacterium bovis attached to oil droplets. J Natl Cancer Inst 48:831, 1972.

63. Zbar B: Tumor regression mediated by Mycobacterium bovis (strain BCG). Natl Cancer Inst Monogr 35:341, 1972.

64. Zbar B, Ribi E, Rapp HJ: An experimental model for immunotherapy of cancer. Natl Cancer Inst Monogr 39:3, 1973.

65. Hanna MG Jr, Peters LC: Efficacy of intralesional BCG therapy in guinea pigs with disseminated tumor. Cancer 36:1298, 1975.

66. Morton DL, Eibler FR, Homes EC, et al.: BCG immunotherapy of malignant melanoma: Summary of a seven year experience. Annal Surg 180(4):635, 1974.

67. Bast RC Jr, Zbar B, Borsos T, Rapp HJ: BCG and cancer. New Engl J Med 290:1413, 1974.

68. Hunter-Craig I, Newton KA, Westbury G, Lacey BW: Use of vaccina virus in the treatment of metastatic malignant melanoma. Brit Med J 2:512, 1970.

69. Everall JD, Wand J, O'Doherty CJ, Dowd PM: Treatment of primary melanoma by intralesional vaccina before excision. Lancet 2:583, 1975.

70. Tokunaga T, Kataoka T, Nakamura RM, et al.: Tumor immunity induced by BCG-tumor cell mixtures in syngenic mice. Jap J Med Sci Bid 26:71, 1973.

71. Yamamura Y, Azuma I, Tariyama T, Ribi E, Zbar B: Suppression of tumor growth and regression of established tumor with oil attached Mycobacterial fractions. Gaun 65:179, 1974.

72. Scott MT: Corynebacterium parvum as an immuno therapeutic anticancer agent. Sem Oncol 1:367, 1974.

73. Scott MT: Corynebacterium parvum as a therapeutic antitumor agent in mice: I. Systemic effects from intravenous injection. J Natl Cancer Inst 53:855, 1974.

74. Scott MT: Corynebacterium parvum as a therapeutic antitumor agent in mice: II. Local injection. J Natl Cancer Inst 53:861, 1974.

75. Likhite VV, Halpern BN: Lasting rejection of mammary adeno carcinoma cell tumors in DBA/2 mice with intratumor injection of killed Corynebacterium parvum. Cancer Res 34:341, 1974.

76. Youdim S, Moser M, Stutman O: Non-specific suppression of tumor growth by an immune reaction to Listeria monocytogenes. J Natl Cancer Inst 52:193, 1974.

77. Bast RC Jr, Zbar B, MacKanness GB, Rapp HJ: Antitumor activity of bacterial infection.

I. Effect of Listeria monocytogenes on growth of a murine fibrosarcoma. J Natl Cancer Inst 54:749, 1975.

78. Bast RC Jr, Zbar B, Miller TE, MacKaness GB, Rapp HJ: Antitumor activity of bacterial infection. II. Effect of Listeria monocytogenes on growth of a guinea pig hepatoma. J Natl Cancer Inst 54:757, 1975.

79. Likhite VV: Rejection of mammary adenocarcinoma cell tumors and prevention of progressive growth of incipient metastases following intratumor permeation with killed Bordatella pertussis. Cancer Res 34:2790, 1974.

80. Hanna MG, Snodgrass MJ, Zbar B, Rapp HJ: Histopathology of tumor regression after intralesional injection of mycobacterium bovis. IV. Development of immunity to tumor cells and BCG. J Natl Cancer Inst 51:1897, 1973.

81. Sparks FC, O'Connell TX, Lee YT: Adjuvant preoperative and postoperative immunochemotherapy for mammary adenocarcinoma in rats. Surg Forum 24:118, 1973.

82. Baldwin RW, Pimm MV: BCG immunotherapy of rat tumors of defined immunogenicity. Natl Cancer Inst Monogr 39:11, 1973.

83. Baldwin RW, Pimm MV: BCG immunotherapy of pulmonary growth from intravenously transferred rat tumor cells. Brit J Cancer 27:48, 1973.

84. Baldwin RW, Pimm MV: BCG immunotherapy of local subcutaneous growth and postsurgical pulmonary metastases of a transplanted rat epithelioma of spontaneous origin. Int J Cancer 12:420, 1973.

85. Zbar B, Ribi E, Kelly M, Granger D, Evans C, Rapp HJ: Immunologic approaches to the treatment of human cancer based on a guinea pig model. Cancer immunol Immunother 1:127, 1976.

86. Smith HJ, Bast RC Jr, Zbar B, Rapp HJ: Eradication of microscopic lymph node metastases after injection of living BCG adjacent to the primary tumor. J Natl Cancer Inst 55:1345, 1975.

87. Littman B, Zbar B, Rapp HJ: Effects of Mycobacterium bovis (BCG) on tumor cell growth in muscle. Proc Am Ass Cancer Res 13:96, 1972.

88. Harmel RP Jr, Zbar B, Rapp HJ: Suppression and regression of a transplanted tumor in the guinea pig colon mediated by Mycobacterium bovis, strain BCG. J Natl Cancer Inst 54:515, 1975.

89. Kleinschuster SJ, Rapp HJ, Lueker DC, Kainer R: Regression of bovine ocular carcinoma by treatment with a mycobacterial vaccine. J Natl Cancer Inst 58:1807, 1977.

90. Simmons RL, Rios A, Kersey JH: Regression of spontaneous mammary carcinomas using direct injections of neuramidase and BCG. J Surg Res 12:57, 1972.

91. Bier J, Bitter K, Nicklisch U: Immundefekte bei Patienten mit Plattenepithelkarzinomen der Mundhöhle. Dtsch Z Mund-Kiefer-Gesichts-Chir 1:210, 1977.

92. Fries R, Platz H, Wagner R Stickler A, et al.: Karzinome der Mundhöhle. Zur Frage der Abhängigkeit der Prognose von der Lokalisation (Etagen und Bezirke) des Primärtumors. Dtsch Z Mund-Kiefer-Gesichts-Chir 1:127, 1977.

93. Aungst CW, Sokal JE, Jager BV: Complications of BCG vaccination. Proc Am Assoc Cancer Res 14:108, 1973.

94. Russel WO, Wynne ES, Loguvam GS: Studies on bovine ocular squamous carcinoma ('cancer eye'). I. Pathological anatomy and historical review. Cancer 9:1, 1956.

95. Lush JL: Red-eyed Herefords preferred; sunlight shown to be hard on white-eyed and white-skinned animals in southern latitudes. Breed Gaz 88:489, 1925.

96. Guilbert HR, Wahid A, Wagnon KA, Gregory PW: Observations on pigmentation of eyelids of Hereford cattle in relation to occurrence of ocular epitheliomas. J Animal Sc 7:426, 1948.

97. Craig J: Disease of dairy cattle: Warts and eye cancer. J Deps Agri West Australia 1:861, 1952.

98. Kinsley AT: Ocular tumors with case reports. Am Vet Rev 43:291, 1913.

99. Nair KP, Sastry GA: A survey of animal neoplasms in the Madras State. I. Bovines, Indian Vet J 30:325, 1954.

100. Hunter (personal communication).

101. Simova J, Bubenik J: Failure of Bacillus Calmette-Guérin (BCG) infection to suppress the growth of transplanted mouse and rat sarcomas. Folia Bid (Prague) 19:296, 1973.

102. Sparks FC, Breeding JH: Tumor regression and enhancement resulting from immunotherapy with Bacillus Calmette-Guérin and neuramidase. Cancer Res 34:3262, 1974.

103. Zbar (personal communications).

104. Bartlett GL, Zbar B, Rapp HJ: Suppression of murine tumor growth by immune reaction to the Bacillus Calmette-Guérin strain of Mycobacterium bovis. J Natl Cancer Inst 48:245, 1972.

105. Moore M, Lawrence N, Witherow PJ: Suppression of transplanted rat sarcomata mediated by Bacillus Calmette Guérin (BCG). Eur J Cancer 10:673, 1974.

106. Ray PK, Poduval TB, Sundaram K: Antitumor immunity. V. BCG-induced growth inhibition of murine tumors. Effect of hydrocortisone, antiserum against theta antigen, and gamma-irradiated BCG. J Natl Cancer Inst 58:763, 1977.

107. Tanaka T, Nakawaga H, Kato A, et al.: Effect of anti-thymocyte serum, anti-macrophage serum, and latex particles on the therapeutic efficacy of BCG or Corynebacterium liquefaciens in syngeneic mice. Gann 68:45, 1977.

108. Chassoux D, Salomon JC: Therapeutic effect of intratumoral injection of BCG and other substances in rats and mice. Int J Cancer 16:515, 1975.

109. Moore M, Lawrence N, Nisbet NW: Tumor inhibition mediated by BCG in immunsuppressed rats. Int J Cancer 15:897, 1975.

110. Moore M, Lawrence N, Nisbet NW: Inhibition of transplanted sarcomas mediated by BCG in rats with a defined immunological deficit. Biomedicine 24:26, 1976.

111. MacKaness GB: The influence of immunologically committed lymphocytes on macrophage activity in vivo. J Exp Med 129:973, 1969.

112. Blanden RV, Lefford MJ, MacKaness: The host response to Calmette-Guérin bacillus in mice. J Exp Med 129:1079, 1969.

113. Snyderman R, Altmann LC, Hausmann MS, Mergenhagen SE: Human mononuclear leucocyte chemotaxis: A quantitative assay for mediators of humoral and cellular chemotaxis factors. J Immunol 108:857, 1972.

114. David JR: Lymphocyte mediators and cellular hypersensitivity. N Engl J Med 288:143, 1973.

115. David JR, Lawrence HS, Thomas L: Delayed hypersensitivity in vitro: II. Effect of sensitive cells on normal cells in the presence of antigen. J Immunol 93:274, 1964.

116. David JR: Delayed hypersensitivity in vitro: Its mediation by cell-free substance formed by lymphoid cell-antigen interaction. Proc Nat Acad Sci Wash 56:72, 1966.

117. David JR, Piessens WF, Churchill WH Jr: Macrophage activation by lymphocyte mediators and tumor immunity: a brief review. In: Fink MA (ed) The Macrophage in Neoplasia. New York, Academic Press, 1976, p 67.

118. Holtermann OA, Casale GP, Klein E: Tumor cell destruction by macrophages. J Med 3:305, 1972.

119. Hibbs JB Jr: Macrophage nonimmunologic recognition: Target cell factors related to contact inhibition. cience 180:868, 1973.

120. Alexander P: Activated macrophages and the antitumor action of BCG. Natl Cancer Inst Monogr 39:127, 1973.

121. Keller R: Cytostatic elimination of syngeneic rat tumor cells in vitro by nonspecifically activated macrophages. J Exp Med 138:625, 1973.

122. Heise ER, Weiser RS: Factors in delayed hypersensitivity: Lymphocyte and macrophage cytotoxins in the tuberculin reaction. J Immunol 103:570, 1969.

123. Pinous WB: Tissue injury and delayed hypersensibility. Ann Allergy 28:93, 1970.

470

124. Kramer JJ, Granger GA: The *in vitro* induction and release of a cell toxin by immune C57BL/6 mouse peretoneal macrophages. Cell Immunol 3:88, 1972.
125. Ferluga J: Increased cytolytic activity of a subcellular fraction from mouse liver after BCG infection. Lancet 2:1476, 1973.
126. Gery I, Waksman BH: Potentation of the T-lymphozyte response to mitogens. II. The cellular source of potentating mediator(s). J Exp Med 136:143, 1972.
127. Mitchell M, Kirkpatrick D, Mohys M, Gery I: On mode of action of BCG. Nature (New Biol) 243:216, 1973.
128. Calderon JJ, Kiely M, Lefko JL, Unanue ER: The modulation of lymphocyte function by molecules secreted by macrophages. I. Description and partial biochemical analysis. J Exp Med 142:151, 1975.
129. Bekierkonst A: Immunotherapy and vaccination against cancer with non-living BCG and cord factor (trehalose-6,6'-dimycdate). Int J Cancer 16:442, 1975.
130. Yarkoni E, Rapp HJ, Zbar B: Immunotherapy of a guinea pig hepatoma with ultrasonically prepared mycobacterial vaccines. Cancer Immunol Immunother 2:143, 1977.
131. Tanaka T, Saito T: Immunotherapy of cancer: induction of tumor immunity with a mixture of tumor cell-BCG,and the effect of intratumor injection of BCG and of nonliving BCG-preparations. Gann 66:631, 1975.
132. Embleton MJ: Influence of cell-free tumor-associated antigen preparations on the developement of immunity to chemically induced rat tumors. Int J Cancer 18:622, 1976.
133. Hawrylko E: Influence of BCG potentatiated immunotherapy in tumor bearing mice. J Natl Cancer Inst 59:359, 1977.
134. Pellis NR, Kahan BD: Specific tumor immunity induced with soluble materials: restricted range of antigen dose and of challenge tumor load for immunoprotection. J Immunol 115:1717, 1976.
135. Price MR, Baldwin RW: Tumor-specific, complement dependant serum cytotoxicity against a chemically induced rat sarcoma. Int J Cancer 20:284, 1977.
136. Rao VS, Bonavida B: Detection of soluble tumor-associated antigens in serum of tumor-bearing rats and their immunological role *in vivo*. Cancer Res 37:3385, 1977.
137. Price MR, Preston VE, Robins RA, Zollner M, Baldwin RW: Induction or immunity to chemically-induced rat tumors by cellular or soluble antigens. Cancer Immunol Immunother 3:247, 1978.
138. Pimm MV, Baldwin RW: Influence of whole body irradiation on BCG contact suppression of a rat sarcoma and tumor-specific immunity. Br J Cancer 34:453, 1976.
139. Hopper DG, Pimm MV, Baldwin RW: Silica abrogation of mycobacterial adjuvant contact suppression of tumor growth in rats and athymic mice. Cancer Immunol Immunoth 1:143, 1976.
140. Bomford R: Active specific immunotherapy of mouse methylcholanthrene induced tumors. Br J Cancer 32:551, 1975.
141. Rella W, Chaput B: Immunotherapy with tumor cells and BCG in the guinea pig, studied by immunological *in vitro* and *in vivo* experiments. Oncology 35:136, 1978.
142. Spredbrow PB, Wilson BE, Hoffmann D, Kelly WR, Francis J: Immunotherapy of bovine ocular squamous cell carcinomas. Vet Record 100:376, 1977.
143. Maurer L, McIntyre O, Rueckert F: Spontaneous regression of malignant Melanoma. Pathologic and Immunologic study in a ten year survivor. Am J Surg 127:286, 1974.
144. Bulkley GB, Cohen MH, Banks PM, *et al.*: Long-term spontaneous regression of malignant melanoma with visceral metastases. Cancer 36:485, 1975.
145. Bodurtha AJ, Berkelhammer J, Kim YH, Laucius JF, Mastrangelo MJ: A clinical, histologic, and immunologic study of a case of metastatic malignant melanoma undergoing spontaneous remission. Cancer 37:735, 1976.
146. Rosenberg SA, Rapp HJ: Intralesional immnotherapy of melanoma with BCG. Med Clin N Amer 60:419, 1976.

147. Morton DL, Gilber FR, Malmgren RA, Wood WC: Immunological factors which influence response to immunotherapy in malignant melanoma. Surgery 68:159, 1970.
148. Bornstein RS, Mastrangelo MJ, Sulit H, et al.: Immunotherapy of melanoma with intralesional BCG. Natl Cancer Inst Monogr 39:213, 1973.
149. Cohen MH, Jessup JM, Felix El, et al.: Intralesional treatment of recurrent metastatic cutaneous malignant melanoma. Cancer 41:2456, 1978.
150. Grant RM, Cochran AJ, MacKie R, et al.: Results of administering BCG to patients with melanoma. Lancet 2:1096, 1974.
151. Krementz ET, Samuels MS, Wallace JH, et al.: Clinical experiences in immunotherapy of cancer. Surg Gynecol Obstet 133:209, 1971.
152. Levy NL, Mahaley MS, Day ED: Serum-mediated blocking of cell-mediated anti-tumor immunity in a melanoma patients: Assocation with BCG immunotherapy and clinical deterioration. Int J Cancer 10:244, 1972.
153. Lieberman R, Wybran J, Epstein W: The immunologic and histopathologic changes of BCG-mediated tumor regression in patients. with malignant melanoma. Cancer 35:756, 1975.
154. Mastrangelo M, Bornstein RS, Sulit H, et al.: Immunotherapy of malignant melanoma. Ann Intern Med 76:877, 1972.
155. Mastrangelo MJ, Kim YH, NBornstein RS, et al.: Clinical and histologic correlation of melanoma regression after intralesional bCG therapy. J Natl Cancer Inst 52:19, 1974.
156. Nathanson L: Regression of intradermal malignant melanoma following intralesional injection of Mycobacterium bovis strain BCG. Cancer Chemother Rep 56:659, 1972.
157. Pinsky MC, Hirshaut Y, Oettgen HF: Treatment of malignant melanoma by intratumoral injection of BCG. Natl Cancer Inst Monogr 39:225, 1973.
158. Rosenberg E, Powell R: Active tumor immunotherapy with BCG. South Med J 66:1359, 1973.
159. Seigler HF, Shingleton WW, Metzgar RS, et al.: Immunotherapy in patients with melanoma. Ann Surg 178:352, 1973.
160. Smith GV, Morse PA Jr, Derlaps DG: Immunotherapy of patient with cancer. Surgery 74:59, 1973.
161. Mastrangelo MJ, Berd D, Bellet RE: Critical review of previously reported clinical trials of cancer immunotherapy with nonspecific immunostimulants. Ann NY Acad Sci 277:94, 1976.
162. Yamamura Y, Azuma I, Taniyama T, et al.: Immunotherapy of cancer with cell wall skeleton of Mycobacterium bovis-Bacillus-Calmette-Guérin. Ann NY Acad Sci 277:209, 1976.
163. Richman SP, Gutterman JU, Hersh EM, Ribi EE: Phase I-II study of intratumor immunotherapy with BCG cell wall skeleton plus P_3. Cancer Immunol Immunother 5:41, 1978.
164. Vosika G, Schmidtke J, Goldman A, et al.: Phase I-II study of intralesional immunotherapy with oil-attached mycobacterium smegmatis call wall skeleton and trehalose dimycolate. Cancer Immunol Immunother 6:135, 1979.
165. Mastrangelo M, Bellet RE, Berkelhammer J, et al.: Regressions of pulmonary metastatic disease associated with intralesional BCG therapy of intracutaneous melanoma metastases. Cancer 36:1305, 1975.
166. Hunt JS, Silverstein MJ, Sparks F, et al.: Granulomatous hepatitis: A complication of BCG immunotherapy. Lancet 2:820, 1973.
167. McKneally MF, Maver C, Kausel HW: Regional immunotherapy of lung cancer with intrapleural BCG. Lancet 1:377, 1976.
168. Morton DL: Immunological studies with human neoplasms. J Reticuloendothel Soc 10:137, 1971.
169. Rosenberg Sa, Seipp C, Sears HF: Clinical and immunologic studies of dissemenated BCG

infection. Cancer 41:1771, 1978.

170. Morton DL, Holmes EC, Eibler FR, *et al.*: Immunological aspects of neoplasia: A rational basis for immunotherapy. Ann Int Med 74:587, 1971.

171. Sparks FC: Hazards and complications of BCG immunotherapy. Med Clin N Am 60:499, 1976.

172. Krown Se, Hilal EY, Pinsky CM, *et al.*: Intralesional injection of the methanol extraction residue or Bacillus Calmette-Guérin (MER) into cutaneous metastases of malignant melanoma. Cancer 42:2648, 1978.

173. Richman SP, Mavligit GM, Wolk R: Epilesional scarification. JAMA 234:1233, 1975.

174. McKhann CF, Hendrickson CG, Spilter LE, *et al.*: Immunotherapy of melanoma with BCG: Two fatalities following intralesional injection. Cancer 35:514, 1975.

175. Clifford (personal communication).

176. Sparks FC, Highton A, Hunt JS: Generalized reaction associated with the intratumor injection of BCG. Chest 68:725, 1975.

177. Robinson JC: Risks of BCG intralesional therapy: An experience with melanoma. J Surg Oncol 9:587, 1977.

178. Norton JA, Shulman NR, Corash L, *et al.*: Severe thrombozytopenia following intralesional BCG therapy. Cancer 41:820, 1978.

179. Augnst CW, Sokal JE, Jager BV: Complications of BCG vaccination in neoplastic disease. Ann Intern Med 82:666, 1975.

180. Hanna MG Jr, Zbar B, Rapp HJ: Histopathology of tumor regression after intralesional injection of Mycobacterium bovis: I. Tumor growth and metastasis. J Natl Cancer Inst 48:1441, 1972.

181. Mansell PWA, Krementz ET: Reactions to BCG. JAMA 226:1570, 1973.

182. Bodurtha A, Kim YH, Laucius JF, *et al.*: Hepatic granulomas and other hepatic lesions associated with BCG immunotherapy for cancer. Am J Clin Path 61:747, 1974.

19. Biostatistical considerations for head and neck cancer research

ROBERT MAKUCH and MARY JOHNSON

Introduction

The proper application of statistical principles to research in clinical oncology can have a tremendous impact on the validity and persuasiveness of results. The biomedical literature contains some very comprehensive discussions of design considerations for clinical studies in cancer and guidelines for collecting and evaluating data from such trials (e.g., see [1, 2]). These references provide a statistical rationale for the main features of a clinical trial, which include:

(1) A clear, unambiguous protocol.
(2) Detailed description of the experimental design.
(3) Justification for the sample size and expected duration of the trial.
(4) Well-defined eligibility criteria.
(5) Clear description of treatment regimens.
(6) Explicit definition of the end-points for evaluation.
(7) Patient record forms and data management procedures.
(8) Proposed statistical analysis and data monitoring procedures, including methods for handling drop-outs and protocol violations.

All of these aspects are important, although the way in which they are implemented will vary depending on the goal of the particular trial and the nature of the disease and treatment under study.

The purpose of this chapter is to relate some of these general principles to Phase III comparative clinical trials designed for the study of therapies for head and neck cancer. In the process, some recent developments in biostatistical methodology in the context of this specific cancer research setting will be critically examined. In particular, various approaches to study design, sample size determination, patient allocation procedures, and methods of statistical analysis will be explored. Also highlighted are the statistical difficulties posed by multiplicities arising in the analysis of head and neck

Gregory T. Wolf (ed), Head and Neck Oncology.
© *1984 Martinus Nijhoff Publishers, Boston. ISBN 0-89838-657-8. Printed in The Netherlands.*

cancer trials (e.g., repeated significance tests for the purpose of terminating an on-going trial or addressing a large number of previously unanticipated hypotheses) and current methods to accommodate these situations are described. Emphasis has therefore been placed on selected biostatistical principles as well as methodologic alternatives for applying these principles. While the methods discussed are broadly applicable, they have particular relevance to the planning and evaluation of clinical trials in head and neck cancer.

Study design

One of the most critical stages in the evaluation of new therapies for head and neck cancer involves the planning of Phase III comparative clinical trials. Proper planning is essential to help insure that a clinical trial has a high probability of identifying the better treatment (if there is one) and producing results that are statistically valid and convincing to others. Inherent in the interpretation of Phase III studies is the comparison of results against some type of 'control'. To this end, the concurrent randomized controlled clinical trial is generally the favored technique since it guards against systematic selection bias in the assignment of treatment. Thus one can likely attribute any observed treatment differences to the treatment, rather that some other factor introduced consciously or unconsciously. Also, the treatment groups will tend to be comparable in regard to both known and unknown prognostic factors. This is important since, although statistical adjustment procedures can be used to adjust for any known differences among treatment groups, one cannot account for imbalances in currently unknown yet important factors. A third advantage of randomization is that it guarantees the validity of the statistical significance tests used to evaluate comparative treatment efficacy [3].

The search for new and innovative approaches to the design of clinical trials in cancer has recently been spurred on by certain practical as well as ethical limitations of the randomized clinical trial. For any particular trial, a randomized design may appear to be optimal and, theoretically, yield unbiased estimates of treatment efficacy with a certain degree of precision. However, this design may be difficult to implement successfully in the face of: (1) low or variable patient accrual rates at some or all participating institutions, (2) lack of acceptance of the trial plan on the part of some investigators who wish to participate, (3) limited financial resources and research facilities, and (4) ethical considerations. Alternatives to the randomized, controlled trial have been proposed to help solve or circumvent these and other problems encountered in studies of new cancer therapies. Since good experimental design is a *sine qua non* of ethical research in humans, the advantages and disadvantages of a number of alternative experimental designs are reviewed in terms of their operational feasibility as well as their biostatistical features.

Historical controls

In spite of the benefits of randomization, some clinical investigators prefer to treat all eligible patients with an experimental therapy and compare these patients to a set of controls who previously received standard therapy. The quality of data and degree of documentation for such historial control groups often depend on their source, ranging from fairly scant descriptions of 'literature controls' to more extensive and verifiable information from recently completed studies conducted by the same investigator or group of investigators.

Many reasons have been put forth to support the use of historical controls [4]. Among the most frequently mentioned reasons are that (1) all patients receive the new treatment, thereby shortening the overall completion time and accrual objectives relative to those required for a randomized study, (2) the control and experimental groups can be guaranteed to be comparable in regard to those characteristics used as a basis for selecting the control patients, and (3) such studies are more ethical since all new patients are given the experimental (and often thought to be the better) treatment. Although the first two points are uncontestable, the ethical argument is more controversial. Byar states that 'We may reasonably ask, if we do a study that convinces us but convinces no one else and is then either ignored or requires confirmation by yet another study, whether we have really acted in the most ethical fashion in the long run' [5]. Shaw and Chalmers state that 'random allocation of patients in a scientific trial is more ethical than the customary procedure, that of trying out a new therapy in an unscientific manner by relying on clinical impression and comparison with past experience' [6].

Another proposed justification for historical controls is based on the development of statistical procedures which allow adjustment for differences in known prognostic factors among the treatment groups. Examples of such procedures include the linear logistic model for binary response [7] and the life-table regression method of Cox [8]. However, such retrospective adjustment has important limitations. These include: (1) historical data which may contain many errors and missing values in factors required for adjustment, (2) inability to account for imbalances in important, but currently unrecognized, prognostic factors, and (3) complex statistical techniques which entail certain statistical assumptions about the data that may or may not be tenable for the particular study being analyzed. Another drawback of historical controls is that no protection exists from potential biases introduced by changes over time in diagnostic methods, staging criteria, supportive care, referral patterns, and effects of unmeasured or unknown prognostic factors [3]. Farewell and D'Angio [9] illustrate this point using data from two consecutive randomized studies conducted by the same research group, each employing the same control treatment arm. They found that conclusions of the second study differed materially if the control group from the first study has been used rather than the concurrent randomized controls. A review by Pocock [10] of the cancer clinical trial literature also revealed the instability of results with the same treatment in consecutive clinical trials. Pocock reported that, in 19 instances where collaborative groups used the same treatment in two consecutive trials, the results when one arm was compared with the supposedly identical arm in a subsequent trial were substantially dissimilar, with 4 of the 19 differences in death rates significant at the 2% level. If historical comparisons of this type were reliable, one would not expect such a notable difference in survival for two groups receiving the same treatment. Thus, the notion of Gehan and Freireich [4] that historical controls are acceptable, particularly when they arise from the most recent in a sequence of previous studies in which similar kinds of patients are admitted and similar evaluation criteria are used, should not be accepted automatically.

Although the issues mentioned above indicate that historical controls are rarely an adequate substitute for concurrently randomized controlled clinical trials in head and neck cancer, they can be useful in the study of diseases so rare that sufficient patient accrual over a reasonable period of time is impossible in a prospective randomized clinical trial. Another valid reason for using historical controls as a comparison group is if one can identify a subset of patients for which death (or any other well-defined outcome event) is inevitable within a relatively short and predictable period of time. Then any new treatment that prolongs survival beyond that point can be recognized quickly as a therapeutic advance. This holds since any dramatic change in the endpoint can reasonably be attributed to the new therapy by virture of the fact that the outcome is inevitable and not subject to much variability, selection bias or other unknown patient features. However, this situation is generally inapplicable for patients with head and neck cancer, given that the disease course is highly variable and influenced by many treatment-related and non-treatment-related factors.

Randomized consent designs

Zelen recently introduced a class of alternatives to conventional randomized trials known as pre-randomized or randomized consent designs in an effort

DOUBLE RANDOMIZED CONSENT DESIGN

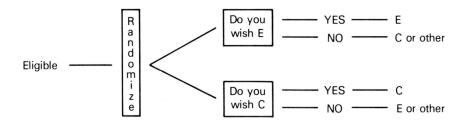

E = New experimental treatment
C = Best standard treatment

Figure 1

to increase participation by both patients and physicians [11]. He believes that some physicians are unwilling to participate in studies where they must inform the patient that treatment is chosen by a chance mechanism. Perhaps the most widely used of his pre-randomized designs is the double randomized consent design, displayed in Fig. 1. Patients who are eligible for the study are randomized to either one of two treatment groups and are asked if they wish to receive the assigned treatment. Patients in one group are assigned to receive the control therapy (C) while the other group of patients is assigned to receive the new experimental therapy (E). All patients are informed of their involvement in the study. If the patient agrees to participate, an informed consent is obtained. If the patient refuses the assigned therapy then he will receive the alternate treatment, or perhaps some other therapy not under investigation in this study.

According to Zelen, this design should increase patient accrual since the physician approaches the patient only to discuss a single therapy, and the patient knows which treatment will be given before providing consent. Thus, the design does not threaten or compromise the physician's role as a competent decision-maker or the patient's right to make an informed choice. On the other hand, there are some potentially significant scientific and ethical concerns associated with the use of the prerandomized consent design.

One problem is that a bias can be introduced into the study since the physician knows the next treatment assignment prior to approaching the patient for consent. To illustrate what the bias is, and how it can affect the interpretation of results, assume that a well-defined group of Stage III and IV head and neck cancer patients could be split into good and poor prognostic categories. During the consent process, the physician (consciously or unconsciously) presents the more aggressive experimental therapy E (relative to the control therapy C) in a less favorable light to the poor prognosis patients than to the good prognosis patients with the consequence that most of the poor prognosis patients refuse E and elect instead to receive C. Assume that E is in fact the superior treatment for both the good and poor prognosis patients. Since Zelen states that 'all patients must be analyzed in the group to which they were randomized, regardless of the treatment in fact received' [11], the true treatment difference will be diluted since most of the poor prognosis patients assigned to E in fact received the inferior treatment. Thus the true overall beneficial effect of E is masked, and one would conclude falsely that no significant treatment difference exists. It is less likely that such a faulty interpretation would arise in a classical randomized trial since the physician is unaware of the treatment assignment until consent has been obtained, and patients who are fully informed about the study and consent to be randomized are much less likely to refuse the assigned treatment.

Zelen is aware of this possible dilution effect resulting from the probability of rejecting the designated treatment [12]. He indicates that, if 10% of the patients refuse the assigned treatment, 1.6 times as many patients are required to obtain the same sensitivity in this design as in a conventional randomized design. If there is a 20% refusal rate, then 2.8 times as many patients are required. This dilution effect has been observed to be even greater in some clinical trials. Thus, one of the proposed advantages of increased accrual with Zelen's design can be markedly compromised. In addition, as the refusal rate to the assigned therapy increases, it may become increasingly attractive to compare the treatment groups according to the treatment actually received by each patient, rather than the treatment assigned. The results from an analysis based on the former approach are subject to severe bias, and the value of a randomized clinical trial is totally neglected.

From an ethical standpoint, difficulties with this design arise if the patient is given a biased presentation of the relative merits of the assigned treatment during the consent process. In the interest of obtaining consent, potential benefits of the assigned treatment may be overemphasized while the risks are inadequately stressed. Since one can reasonably expect the best standard treatment to have a very low refusal rate, pressure may grow more acute to recruit patients into the experimental group, particularly if the clinical investigator is conscious of a moderately high refusal rate. This runs counter to the informed consent process which, as Fleming points out, should provide the patient with 'a discussion of the risks and benefits of the various therapeutic options in order to facilitate and guarantee informed decisions' [13].

Potential drawbacks of the randomized consent design should be carefully considered in the context of any particular application. The true treatment

Factor 1: Type of Neck Dissection	Factor 2: Induction Chemotherapy Received? Yes No
Radical Modified	

Figure 2. A 2 × 2 factorial design: treatments consist of all combinations that can be formed from the two factors.

difference will be diluted in a randomized consent design unless essentially all randomized patients agree to receive the treatments as assigned. Since the design is insensitive to small treatment differences when the consent rate is less than 100%, its use should clearly be discouraged in the comparative evaluation of conservative therapies, i.e., studies which are intended to show some degree of 'equivalence' between a new therapy and a standard. In multi-clinic studies, variability of consent rates among investigators could produce significant treatment-by-clinic interactions which make the combined data more difficult to interpret. Nevertheless, some studies may not be possible using a classical randomized design, and in these instances the idea of pre-randomization certainly should be entertained.

Factorial designs

Peto [14] recommended that 2 × 2 factorial designs be considered for wider use in cancer clinical trials. In these designs there are two factors, each of which represents a controllable treatment option offered at two levels, and all the combinations of levels of each factor are randomly allocated to the patients. The design can thus be used to evaluate the comparative therapeutic efficacy of several treatment strategies in the same clinical trial.

To illustrate how this design is used, suppose we wish to examine the survival impact of induction chemotherapy and type of neck dissection (radical vs. modified) in patients with advanced, operable head and neck cancer. In the 2 × 2 factorial design seen in Fig. 2, patients are assigned to one of four groups: (1) radical neck dissection (RND) + induction chemotherapy (IC), (2) RND + no IC, (3) modified neck dissection (MND) + IC, and (4) MND + no IC. To evaluate the difference between radical and modified neck dissection, patients in groups (1) and (2) combined are compared to patients in groups (3) and (4) combined. Likewise, to evaluate the efficacy of induction chemotherapy, patients are compared in each of two induction groups, regardless of the type of neck dissection performed. Thus, by using this design, Peto claims that two independent treatment questions are answered for the price of one since only one clinical trial has been performed. Strictly speaking, this is only approximately true since the 2×2 factorial trial should be somewhat larger to take into account the multiple treatment comparisons to be made when analyzing the data. Reasons for this will become clearer when we return to discuss the multiple comparisons issue in more detail later in this chapter.

In addition to analyzing the main effects of each treatment factor individually, one can examine whether the survival difference between patients receiving a modified or radical neck dissection is the same for those who received induction chemotherapy as for those who did not receive induction chemotherapy. Conversely, one can examine whether the survival difference between patients receiving and those not receiving chemotherapy is the same independent of the type of neck dissection performed. If it is found that the response to one treatment is not altered by the level of the other treatment, then the treatment effects are said to be independent. On the contrary, if one type of neck dissection is superior in patients not receiving induction chemotherapy, and the other type of neck dissection is superior in patients receiving induction chemotherapy, then it is said that an interaction exists between the type of dissection and induction chemotherapy.

If treatment effects are independent, the factorial design is very useful since it (1) provides a broader picture of the effects of the various therapeutic options, and (2) can result in a considerable savings in time and material when compared to carrying out two single-factor clinical trials. If treatments are *not* independent, then the effects of a treatment vary according to the particular level of the other treatment factor. In this case, '2×2 designs will point unbiasedly to the complicated truth, while misleading conclusions could well emerge from other designs' [14]. Although this is true for large clinical trials, one is often not sure whether or not an interaction exists between treatments in smaller studies since the small sample sizes do not provide adequate power to detect interaction. Thus if the effects of the treatments are not independent, results from a clinical trial which used this design will not necessarily point to the complicated truth, and misleading conclusions could emerge from the design.

As an example, assume the survival duration among patients who received no induction chemotherapy is significantly different according to the type of neck dissection received, while the survival difference based on type of neck dissection is negligible among patients who underwent induction chemotherapy. Then the overall comparison of radical versus modified neck dissection will not show a significant difference unless the overall difference is large relative to the degree of variability. Significance tests could be performed separately within each subset of patients receiving or not receiving induction chemotherapy. However, our experience suggests that sample size requirements for factorial studies usually are calculated as if they were designed as single-factor experiments. Thus the limited number of patients within each combination of treatment levels usually makes the practice of subset analysis undesirable because the sensitivity of the statistical test to detect treatment differences is low.

If one is planning to do a clinical trial utilizing this design, we recommend that sample sizes be large enough to provide adequate ability to detect not only differences between the levels of each treatment factor, but also some clinically important degree of interaction between treatment effects. Then, even if it is not possible to reduce results of the trial to simple overall treatment effects, the experiment will yield more definitive information about treatment interrelationships.

Institutional choice design

Another design which has been used in several recent multi-center cancer clinical trials allows participating institutions to randomize patients to only a subset of the treatments under study. This design, referred to as the 'institutional choice' design [15], may involve the evaluation of three treatments, two experimental treatments (E1 and E2) and one control treatment (C). Each institution selects to compare in a randomized prospective fashion either E1 versus C or E2 versus C. Thus, each institution uses only one of the two experimental treatments. The motivation for such a nonstandard design is based on the frequently encountered difficulty of obtaining agreement among investigators with varied orientations and patient support facilities to utilize a common set of treatment regimens at all institutions. Although the design appears to be attractive at first glance, the analysis and interpretation of data can be problematic. The deficiencies of the design have been thoroughly described by Makuch and Simon [16], and are reviewed here. Suppose the trial is viewed as two separate randomized studies. Then the efficacy of treatment E1 can only be evaluated with respect to control patients in institutions that chose treatment E1; likewise, patients on treatment E2 should be compared only to control patients randomized at the same institutions. As a consequence, more patients are needed to compare E1 and E2 to a control arm than for a randomized 3-arm study in which all institutions use equal 3-way randomization.

The advocates of this design cite the fact that the two substudies have a 'common control arm'. It is argued that, if the two control groups are comparable, the design allows a comparison of each experimental therapy with the pooled control groups and a valid direct comparison of the two experimental treatments. However, such optimism regarding the analysis may be unrealistic. If the two control groups do respond differently, statistical adjustment procedures may be needed to adjust for group imbalances when comparing each experimental group to pooled controls or when comparing experimental treatments to each other. This procedure may not be adequate to salvage the study since the comparison of treatments E1 and E2 will suffer from some of the same limitations as the use of historical controls. That is, the comparison will depend on the validity of the statistical model and no adjustment can be made in the model for unknown prognostic factors. Second, it takes very large numbers of patients to demonstrate approximate comparability of the control groups, as we will show later in this chapter. However, even if the comparability of control groups is demonstrated convincingly, one cannot rule out the possibility of bias in the comparison of treatments E1 and E2. Some institutions may have greater competence than others in administering certain experimental treatments, which may explain the preference for some institutions to select E1 and others to select E2. This preference alone could explain any observed differences between groups, and may invalidate any comparison between E1 and E2 patients since it is impossible to discriminate between the impact of treatment and hospital on the endpoint of interest.

In summary, the study designs mentioned above represent just a few alternatives to the traditional randomized trial. From our discussion it is clear that a variety of factors must be considered before selecting a particular experimental design for a clinical trial. These factors include anticipating patient and investigator willingness to participate in the study, issues of statistical validity and bias, and other practical, ethical and financial constraints. While innovative approaches in study design will continue to be developed to meet changing research needs, their limitations as well as their advantages should be similarly appraised. Our general recommendation is that standard, randomized prospective clinical trial designs be used for the evaluation of comparative treatment efficacy unless their disadvantages significantly outweigh the advantages of some alternative study design.

Size of the study

An important aspect of study planning is the calculation of sample sizes. Appropriate determination of the required number of patients leads one to evaluate critically whether sufficient number of patients can be accrued over a reasonable time while the primary study objectives remain of interest. With this information, the modification of eligibility criteria or other design parameters required to attain accrual goals can be made prior to the start of the study. Zelen indicates that the patient accrual period should not exceed three years in most instances [17]. Accrual often drops measurably after this time, especially if medical advances render the existing study obsolete. All too frequently, studies are commenced without such careful consideration, and there are insufficient patient numbers upon completion of the study to detect moderate, but clinically important, differences. Freiman *et al.* have highlighted this problem in a review of 71 'negative' trials in major medical journals, pointing out that 50 of these trials carried a 10% risk of missing a 50% therapeutic improvement [18].

The usual approach for sample size estimation in comparing two treatments requires that one specify a true treatment difference, D, which is considered important to detect together with the Type-I and Type-II error rates associated with the statistical test to be used. A Type-I error represents the event of falsely rejecting the null hypothesis that the treatments are equivalent. The probability of making this error is denoted by α. The other type of decision-making error occurs when the null hypothesis is not rejected although the alternative hypothesis that a difference exists between the treatments is in fact true. This is called Type-II error, and the probability of making this error is specified as β. The power of the test, i.e., the probability of detecting a true treatment difference, is $(1-\beta)$. Underlying this hypothesis-testing framework is the notion that a statistical test is performed at the end of the trial on a major endpoint of interest, and one wishes to test the null hypothesis of no difference in treatment efficacy. This is done by calculating a p-value based on the value of the test statistic calculated for the observed data. The conventionally accepted p-value to reject the null hypothesis is 0.05. This implies that, assuming that there is no true difference in treatment efficacy, the probability of obtaining a difference in the data as extreme as that observed is 0.05. Thus the p-value does not describe the probability that the null hypothesis is true, but the probability of an observed difference assuming that the null hypothesis is true.

Commonly-used endpoints for sample-size planning in clinical trials for head and neck cancer are either dichotomous (e.g., success versus failure, where 'success' may be defined as tumor response or survival for two years) or the time to some critical event (e.g., tumor recurrence or death). For the first type of endpoint in which two treatments are compared, assume that p_T is the proportion of 'success' patients in the experimental treatment group and p_C is the proportion of 'success' patients in the control treatment group. Suppose we wish to have a total of N patients in each group so that, with high probability, we can detect a true difference of absolute magnitude $D = |p_T - p_C|$. This probability is the power of the test, and is usually specified for planning purposes between 0.80 and 0.95. One must also specify the significance level α of the test; it is usually chosen to be 0.05 or 0.01.

Table 1 indicates the number of patients required per group in order to achieve a specified power and significance level as a function of the true success rates. These values were obtained using the approximation formula of Casagrande, Pike, and Smith [19], and the table is used in the following way. Suppose we wish to detect an increase in the complete response rate from 40% to 70% between a standard and new induction chemotherapy regimen for patients with Stage III or Stage IV head-and-neck squamous carcinoma. Although one expects the new regimen to provide a higher response rate, unexpected morbidity or mortality could arise in this group and the response rate could be lower than that for the standard group. A two-sided significance level is therefore selected. Two-sided significance levels should be used for planning purposes unless a strong justification exists for expecting a difference in only one direction between the two treatments.

Table 1. Number of patients in each of two treatment groups (two-sided test)

Smaller success rate	Larger minus smaller success rate									
	.05	.10	.15	.20	.25	.30	.35	.40	.45	.50
.05	620*	206	113	74	54	42	33	27	23	19
	473†	159	88	58	43	33	27	22	18	16
.10	956	285	146	92	64	48	38	30	25	21
	724	218	112	71	50	38	30	24	20	17
.15	1250	354	174	106	73	53	41	33	26	22
	944	269	133	82	57	42	32	26	21	18
.20	1502	411	197	118	79	57	44	34	27	22
	1132	313	151	91	62	45	34	27	22	18
.25	1712	459	216	127	84	60	45	35	28	23
	1289	348	165	98	65	47	36	28	22	18
.30	1880	495	230	134	88	62	46	36	28	22
	1414	375	175	103	68	48	36	28	22	18
.35	2006	522	239	138	89	63	46	35	27	22
	1509	395	182	106	69	49	36	28	22	18
.40	2089	537	244	139	89	62	45	34	26	21
	1571	407	186	107	69	48	36	27	21	17
.45	2132	543	244	138	88	60	44	33	25	19
	1603	411	186	106	68	47	34	26	20	16
.50	2132	537	239	134	84	57	41	30	23	17
	1603	407	182	103	65	45	32	24	18	14

* Upper figure: significance level 0.05, power 0.90.
† Lower figure: significance level 0.05, power 0.80.

Table 1 shows that 62 patients are needed in each group to detect a difference, $D = 0.30$ ($= 0.70 - 0.40$) with probability (power $= 1 - \beta$) 0.90 for $\alpha = 0.05$. Forty-eight patients are required per group if one is willing to have probability 0.80 (rather than 0.90) of detecting a difference in the response rates, keeping all other parameters unchanged. When the success rate exceeds 0.50, the table is used by considering the failure rate and entering the table with 1-(success rate).

This table illustrates that the number of patients increases as the expected magnitude of the true treatment difference decreases between the two treatment groups. Thus, some investigators may specify a larger treatment difference for planning purposes than may be realistic in order to justify that the study can be completed within a reasonable period of time and the hypotheses adequately tested. One must guard against such optimism during the planning stages of a clinical trial, since the power of the study may be very low for detecting differences of moderate, but still clinically important, magnitude. With such experimental design characteristics, it is possible that a new experimental treatment will be found not to differ significantly from the standard therapy. As a consequence, other investigators may lose interest in testing the new treatment any further and it will be passed over for further evaluation although it represents a true therapeutic advance. Furthermore, since limited patient, monetary, and clinical resources could have been redirected towards a more definitive study, one must also weigh the 'opportunity' costs associated with embarking on a study which has little chance of providing convincing results.

A recent phenomenon in cancer clinical trials is the use of 'conservative' or less intensive treatments in which the primary objective is to determine if the two treatments yield similar therapeutic results. For instance, in the treatment of Stage II head and neck cancer patients with oral cavity sites of primary disease, the hypothesis that radiotherapy produces as good a survival result as surgery may be of interest. Makuch and Simon describe a method to calculate the number of patients required for such trials [20]. The anticipated overall proportion of successes P (e.g., proportion alive at three years) is specified, along with a value d such that if the two treatments are truly equally effective the upper $100 \cdot (1 - \alpha)$ percentage confidence level for the true difference in proportion of successes on the two treatments does not exceed d with probability $(1 - \beta)$. Then the required number of patients, N, per treatment group is $2 \cdot P \cdot (100 - P) \cdot (z_{\alpha/2} + z_\beta)^2 / d^2$, where z_α is the upper α tail point of the standard normal distribution (e.g., for $\alpha = 0.05$ and $\beta = 0.20$, $z_{\alpha/2} = 1.96$ and $z_\beta = 0.84$).

To demonstrate the required calculations, assume that the proportion of Stage II patients who receive either radiotherapy or surgery alone and are alive at three years is $P = 0.75$. We wish the sample to be large enough so that with a high degree of confidence $(1 - \beta = 0.80)$, one can conclude that the treatments differ in regard to three-year survival by no more than $d = 0.10$. For $\alpha = 0.05$, we calculate the number of patients required in each group to be $2 \cdot (.75) \cdot (.25) \cdot (1.96 + .84)^2 / .1^2 = 294$. As many trial planners fail to appreciate, this example demonstrates that large sample size are often needed in 'conservative' clinical trials to demonstrate the similarity of two treatments with a high level of confidence. An important corollary is that obtaining a non-significant p-value when comparing two treatment groups with inadequate numbers of patients does not imply equivalence, since the confidence limits which indicate the range of true treatment differences consistent with the observed data are broad. This point is frequently overlooked in clinical trial design as well as the interpretation of results.

Although many clinical studies in head and neck cancer are planned using a dichotomous response, they may not be analyzed in this way since survival or other types of time-to-failure endpoints often are of primary importance. Sample size estimates are available for this situation if some distributional form for time-to-failure is specified. George and Desu [21] developed sample size requirements for the two-treatment situation where the failure distribution is assumed to be exponential. For determining the number of deaths required in each treatment group, one specifies the Type I error rate (α) and the ratio of median survival times (Δ) that one wishes to detect with power $(1 - \beta)$. Alternatively, one can determine the required duration of the study if the projected rate of patient accrual also is provided. Makuch and Simon [22] have generalized the results of George and Desu to account for the possibility of multiple pairwise comparisons among k treatment groups when $k \geq 2$ treatment groups are under study.

Within the same general framework, Rubinstein, Gail, and Santner [23] have presented several useful tables for planning the size and duration of a clinical trial. Their method allows trial planners to pre-specify several parameters that typically influence the amount of information provided by the complete study. These quantities include the loss to follow-up rate, the accrual rate, the accrual period, and the continuation period. The continuation period is the length of time after accrual has stopped before the analysis is performed. Often this is ignored in planning a study, although varying the length of the continuation period can have a sizable impact on the required size and duration of the study, as indicated by the above authors. To demonstrate, assume the median survival time for patients receiving a standard therapy is one year, and we wish to detect with probability 0.80 an increase in median survival to two years ($\Delta = 2$) for patients receiving an experimental therapy, with $\alpha = 0.05$. Assume the loss to follow-up rate is 0, the yearly accrual rate is 60 patients, and there is no continuation period (i.e., the final analysis is performed immediately upon termination of accrual). Then the estimated total required trial length is 2.26 years. If one were to specify a one year continuation period, while leaving all other design parameters unchanged, the total trial time is 2.56 years. However, because of the one year continuation period, the accrual period would be only $2.56 - 1.0 = 1.56$ years instead of 2.26 years. It follows that fewer patients would be entered on-study in this stituation since accrual is shortened by roughly three-fourths of a year. Thus, the continuation period is an important parameter to consider when designing a study since it can reduce the total number of patients required for the study, while extending the total length of the trial only slightly.

Patient allocation

The most straightforward method for randomly allocating patients involves assigning each patient to one of T treatment groups with probability 1/T. This is referred to as 'pure' randomization. The principle advantages of this approach are simplicity and the complete unpredictability of the next treatment assignment. Peto et al. [24] support the utility of this approach since they contend that any imbalance in prognostic factors can be adjusted for in the analysis of results. But practical considerations argue against this position, unless a trial is quite large or one does not intend to analyze early results while accrual continues. For small clinical trials, Grizzle [25] shows that accounting for stratification at the time of randomization is significantly more efficient than using pure randomization and stratifying at the time of analysis. Also, one can have marked prognostic non-comparability among treatment groups if pure randomization is used. Brown [26] states '... there is much to be gained in persuasiveness or credibility by presentation of data that show the number of patients assigned to the several treatments to be closely balanced with regard to the variables commonly felt to be related to the course of the disease and the response to treatment. No amount of post-stratification and covariance analysis ... will be as convincing as the demonstration that the groups were balanced in the beginning ... '.

Furthermore, if one carries out a two-arm study and a total of 50 patients have been entered, there is a 5% chance of obtaining an 18:32 split in the number of patients per group using purely random assignment. This outcome may prove troublesome to the medical investigator, especially if only 18 patients received the new treatment for which crucial information about efficacy and tolerance is most desired. Although the probability of a split this extreme is small , it is of little consolation to the unfortunate investigator who encounters it. Thus randomized treatment assignment usually is restricted in some way to insure prognostic comparability among the treatment groups, as well as fairly equal numbers of patients in each group.

Perhaps the most commonly used method to achieve comparability is the random permuted blocks design. For this method of stratified randomization, strata are defined so that each stratum comprises a different combination of levels of each factor on which balance is desired. Treatment assignments are independently and randomly generated within each stratum using random permuted blocks. Each random permuted block is composed of $b \cdot T$ random treatment assignments, subject to the constraint that each of the T treatment groups has been assigned to b patients. This process insures protection against unknown time trends in the characteristics of arriving patients. The block length, $b \cdot T$, should not be selected so small that there is a moderate likelihood that an investigator can keep track of treatment assignments and guess the next treatment. Otherwise, the study may be subject to selection bias and defeat one of the primary rationales for randomization. On the other hand, if b is too large, then significant imbalances can arise in the distribution of stratification factors among the treatment groups. Depending on the size of the study and the number of strata, the values of b most widely used in practice lie between 2 and 4 inclusive.

To illustrate this method of patient allocation, assume that two treatment groups (C = control and E = new experimental treatment) are to be compared for patients with advanced (Stage III and IV) resectable head and neck cancer in the larynx or oropharynx. Two important prognostic factors are stage and site (larynx and oropharynx). The total number of strata defined by all combinations of levels of these two factors is $2 \times 2 = 4$. Note that the total number of strata is the product of the number of levels in each factor. Thus the total number of strata increases dramatically with every additional stratification factor. Selecting $b = 2$ implies that, after every four treatment assignments in each stratum-specific block, there must be two 'C's and two 'E's. Every possible ordered treatment assignment per block must be one of the following: CCEE, CECE, CEEC, ECEC, EECC, and ECCE. The overall list of treatment assignments for each stratum is formed by repeatedly and randomly selecting among these six possible ordered treatment assignments. For example, the first 16 treatment assignments for stage III patients with a primary of the larynx might be CECE ECEC EECC CECE. Generally, the randomization list is prepared independently for each stratum. To minimize the potential for bias, the generation of the treatment assignment list should be left to a statistician or some other impartial observer. In addition, the investigator should be kept unaware of the next treatment assignment on the list until the patient is deemed eligible and willing to enter the study, and an informed consent has been obtained.

Although stratification is recommended in most situations, one must also be aware of the dangers of overstratification, i.e., trying to achieve balance on a large number of factors. It is best if the number of stratification factors is limited to those that have an important and independent impact on the primary study endpoint(s). Overstratification can be detrimental in a number of ways. First, sizeable differences can appear in the overall number of patients in each treatment group, leading to a statistically inefficient design. This can occur when many strata have just one or two patients in each of them, and by chance a large majority of the first one or two treatment assignments in each stratum are to the same treatment. Second, overstratification can totally defeat the desired goal of achieving comparability of the treatment groups with regard to the stratification factors [27]. As an example, a sequence of treatment assignments was generated using the permuted block method, with $b = 3$, where Karnofsky performance status (PS) (90 and above versus 80 and below) and N status (0 and 1 versus 2 and 3) are additional factors to the example described previously. In Table 2, the

Table 2. Imbalances of prognostic factors between two treatments in overstratified design

	Stage III				Stage IV			
	PS				PS			
	80 or below		90 or above		80 or below		90 or above	
	N 0+1	N 2+3	N 0+1	N 2+3	N 0+1	N 2+3	N 0+1	N 2+3
Oropharynx	C√	C√	E√	C√	E√	C√	E√	E√
	C√	C√	C√	C√	E	E	C√	C√
	C√	E	C√	E	C	E	E	C
	E	C	C	E	C	C	C	E
	E	E	E	E	E	C	E	E
	E	E	E	C	C	E	C	C
Larynx	C√	C√	E√	E√	E√	E√	E√	E√
	E	C√	E√	C√	E√	C	E√	E√
	C	E	C	E	C	E	C	E√
	E	C	E	C	C	C	E	C
	E	E	C	E	E	C	C	C
	C	E	C	C	C	E	C	C

		C	E
Site:	oropharynx	12	4
	larynx	4	11
Stage:	III	13	4
	IV	3	11
PS:	80 or below	9	4
	90 or above	7	11
N status:	0 or 1	7	9
	2 or 3	9	6
Total, within each teatment		16	15

check marks show the treatment assignments. One can see the distribution of patients in the treatment groups with respect to each factor. Except for N status, and to a lesser extent performance status, distributions of patients are quite unbalanced between the two treatment groups. Although few may consider stopping a study after a total of only 31 patients have been entered, this example is of more than just theoretical interest. For multi-institutional studies, many participating institutions may contribute only a few patients to any particular study. If stratified randomization is performed within each institution, then such imbalances in many institutions could lead to worrisome overall prognostic imbalances for the entire study.

Several methods are available for achieving good balance when there are many stratification factors, or many levels of a given factor such as 'institution'. Zelen [17] has described a method which is particularly suited to multi-institution studies in which randomization is carried out by a central operations office. A randomization list is produced for each prognostic stratum, ignoring institution. To begin the randomization procedure, an investigator contacts the randomization office and reports the required stratification features for a new patient. A tentative treatment assignment is determined by taking the next treatment assignment in the stratum defined by the patient's characteristics. An individual at the operations office then calculates for that institution the difference, DF, between the number of cases on the selected treatment (including the tentative assignment) minus the number of cases for that treatment with the minimum number of cases. If DF is less than some preassigned integer, n, then the tentative assignment is the one given to the investigator. If $DF > n$, the tentative assignment is not given and the next treatment allocation on the randomization list is selected as the tentative assignment. The procedure is repeated until the investigator is provided a treatment assignment. Other more complex procedures to account for large numbers of strata have been described by Efron [28] and Pocock and Simon [27].

Statistical analysis

A brief overview of some of the most frequently encountered statistical methods to evaluate time-to-failure data are provided in order to aid in the interpretation and analysis of such data. Although the term 'failure' will be used to imply death, the methods used to assess survival time apply equally to other well-defined endpoints (e.g. time to first relapse, time to tumor response, or disease-free survival time), provided that they can be accurately and consistently measured. The methods are relatively straightforward and broadly applicable, and can be applied to relatively simple situations. However, many methodological advances continue to occur in this, one of the most active areas of current statistical research. Thus a statistical collaborator is recommended for interim and final analyses of comparative studies in order to ensure that the underlying assumptions of statistical tests have been met and that appropriate inferences are drawn from the data.

The graphical representation of the total survival experience of a group of patients is called a survival curve, and is frequently denoted as $S(t)$. This function represents the probability of surviving at least t time units. To estimate $S(t)$, the time t is calculated for each patient from the start of therapy to either the date of death or the last date of follow-up alive if death was not known to have occurred. This latter date is called the censoring date, and the observation is said to be 'censored' since one is unable to observe the occurrence of the event although a possible change in status may occur with subsequent follow-up. When the event (i.e., death) is observed, then this observation is uncensored. A common method of estimating $S(t)$ for samples of small to moderate size is the product-limit method of Kaplan and Meier [29], which we now describe. Of interest is the interval of time from entry into the trial until death. To calculate the Kaplan-Meier survival estimate for N patients, one needs to record for each patient the time between entry on-study (e.g., date of randomization) and the date of death or if the patient is censored, his most recent follow-up date. Then order the N times in increasing magnitude, i.e., $t_1 \leq t_2 \leq ... \leq t_j \leq ... \leq t_N$. At each ordered time t_i, record the number of deaths d_i at time t_i and the number of patients N_i alive and followed just prior to time t_i. Then the quantity $P_i = (N_i - d_i)/N_i$ estimates the probability of surviving at least to time t_i, given that the patient was alive at time t_{i-1}. The Kaplan-Meier estimate of $S(t_i)$, the probability of survival exceeding time t_i and denoted $\hat{S}(t_i)$, is given by $\hat{S}(t_i) = P_1 \cdot P_2 \cdot ... \cdot P_i$. Once $\hat{S}(1), \hat{S}(2), ...$ have been calculated, a graph is made with time on the horizontal axis and the probability of survival on the vertical axis with values ranging between 0 and 1. Unless $t_1 = 0$, the graph starts at 1 since $\hat{S}(0) = 1$. The coordinates $[t_i, \hat{S}(t_i)]$ are joined by a step function in which the value of $\hat{S}(t_{i-1})$ is drawn horizontally from t_{i-1} to t_i when it drops to $\hat{S}(t_i)$. Note that the step function will only change values at observed death times, not at censoring times.

This procedure is applied to a small subset of survival data from a multi-institutional trial for patients with advanced head and neck squamous carcinoma. The ordered death times (in months) are $1+, 2+, 2+, 3, 3+, 4+,$ $5+, 5+, 7, 9, 10+, 11+, 12, 13, 14, 14+, 15, 18+, 19+$, where censored survival times are denoted by a ' $+$ '. Since $P_i = 1$ whenever no deaths and only censored observations are recorded, every $P_i = 1$ except $P_4 = (16-1)/16$, $P_9 = (11-1)/11$, $P_{10} = (10-1)/10$, $P_{13} = (7-1)/7$, $P_{14} = (6-1)/6$, $P_{15} = (5-1)/5$ and $P_{17} = (3-1)/3$. So the first several steps of the survival function are estimated as $\hat{S}(0) = 1$, $\hat{S}(3) = P(4) = .94$, $\hat{S}(7) = P(4) \cdot P(9) = .85$,

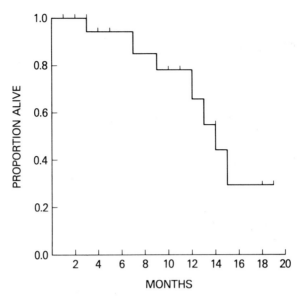

Figure 3. Kaplan-Meier survival curve.

and $\hat{S}(9) = P(4) \cdot P(9) \cdot P(10) = .77$. Similarly, one calculates $\hat{S}(12) = .66$, $\hat{S}(13) = .55$, $\hat{S}(14) = .44$, and $\hat{S}(15) = .29$, where t_{15} is the largest death time. Vertical bars on the graph are made at each censored survival time, as seen in Fig. 3. Whenever survival curves are examined, one should keep in mind that the estimates are not very reliable when relatively few patients are at risk, as may occur at the right-hand side of the curve. For instance, if few patients are at risk for more than a certain time, and after that time none die, then a plateau will appear in the curve. Such a plateau should not be taken as evidence that after a certain time most patients are cured unless there are large numbers of patients at risk at the time of plateau.

The median survival time is defined as the value of t for which $S(t) = 0.50$. The estimated median survival time is often taken to be the time t when $\hat{S}(t) = 0.50$, and is frequently used to report clinical trial results since it is a compact summarization of the survival experience for patients on each therapy. The curve in Fig. 3 does not have a unique point t at which $\hat{S}(t) = 0.50$, but an estimated median can be obtained using linear interpolation. Interpolating between 13 and 14 months, one calculates the estimated median survival time as $13 + (14 - 13) \cdot (.55 - .50)/(.55 - .44) = 13.55$ months. In general, if a neoplasm is completely incurable so that nearly all patients die during the course of a randomized trial, a difference in median survivals for two groups of patients can be reasonably interpreted as indicating superiority of one treatment over another. However, median survival can be misleading if the curves do not drop rapidly through the whole region between 30% and 70% alive. A given curve could form a plateau through this region if no deaths and only censored observations occur. In such a situation, the difference in estimated medians would be imprecise (highly variable) and rather uninformative with regard to any overall difference in survival patterns. For example, a given treatment could cure 49% of a large patient population but still be associated with a median (50%) survival that would not be significantly different from a second treatment that cured no one.

The difference in estimated median survival times is thus not always a suitable measure to characterize differences in survival curves. Furthermore, to compare survival distributions, it is usually inappropriate and inefficient to conduct statistical tests of individual points along the curves [24]. This approach can introduce subjectivity and bias into the analysis if one chooses to make specific comparisons at precisely those points where the largest, or smallest, differences were observed in order to justify an a priori impression regarding comparative treatment efficacy. This practice leads to p-values which cannot be interpreted in the usual way due to the data-dependent nature of the treatment comparisons. Thus, statistical methods which assess the overall survival experience are strongly preferred to the selective comparison of point estimates. Two commonly applied statistical tests of survival curves are Gehan's Generalized Wilcoxon test [30] and the logrank, or Mantel's, test [31]. For simplicity, only the latter test is described here. These statistical tests account for the presence of censored observations, unlike many of the more frequently encountered statistical tests (e.g. t-tests, linear regression) which ignore any distinction between censored and uncensored observations. Survival methods that incorporate censored observations make use of the fact that, for those patients who are lost to follow-up or alive at the time of analysis, their survivals are known only to be at least as great as their last observed values.

To calculate the logrank statistic comparing two treatment groups, a 2×2 table is formed at each death time as depicted in Fig. 4. The quantity a_i is the observed number of deaths at time t_i and b_i is the number of patients alive at time t_i in the experimental treatment group; c_i and d_i are the corresponding quantities in the control group. For each table, one calculates the expected number $E(a_i)$ of deaths in the experimental treatment group as $(a_i + c_i)(a_i + b_i)/N_i$, where $N_i = a_i + b_i + c_i + d_i$. This is the expected number of deaths assuming that no survival difference exists between the two groups. The variance of a_i is

$$V(a_i) = (a_i + c_i)(b_i + d_i)(a_i + b_i)(c_i + d_i)/N_i^2(N_i - 1).$$

The logrank statistic is calculated as

$$(\sum a_i - \sum E(a_i))^2 / \sum V(a_i)$$

Treatment Group	Number of deaths at time t_i	Number of survivors at time t_i	Number of patients at risk just prior to time t_i
Experimental	a_i	b_i	$a_i + b_i$
Control	c_i	d_i	$c_i + d_i$

Figure 4. Distribution of patients at death time t_i, according to treatment and survival status.

where the summation is over all distinct death times.

Survival data are presented by treatment group and T status in Table 3 to demonstrate how the logrank statistic is calculated. The death times, t_i, for the entire population of patients are ordered in increasing magnitude in

Table 3. Calculations for the log-rank test

	Experimental treatment	Control Treatment
T1+T2	11,11+,13+,16,16+,19,21+,	7,8+,9,9+,11+,12,14,15,15+
T3+T4	5,6+,7,9,10,11,11+	3,4,4+,5,6,7,8

	Experimental treatment			Control treatment				
t_i	a_i	b_i		c_i	d_i	N_i	$E(a_i)$	$V(a_i)$
3	0	14		1	15	30	14/30	.2489
4	0	14		1	14	29	14/29	.2497
5	1	13		1	12	27	2·14/27	.4801
6	0	13		1	11	25	13/25	.2496
7	1	11		2	9	23	3·12/23	.6805
8	0	11		1	8	20	11/20	.2475
9	1	10		1	6	18	2·11/18	.4473
10	1	9		0	5	15	10/15	.2222
11	2	7		0	5	14	2·9/14	.4239
12	0	5		1	3	9	5/9	.2469
14	0	4		1	2	7	4/7	.2449
15	0	4		1	1	6	4/6	.2222
16	1	3		0	0	4	4/4	0
19	1	1		0	0	2	2/2	0
Total	8						11.59	3.96

$$x_1^2 = \frac{(8-11.59)^2}{3.964} = 3.25 \text{ on 1 degree of freedom.}$$

the first column. The second column (a_i) and the third column (b_i) describe the number of deaths at each time t_i and the number of survivors at time t_i, respectively, for the experimental treatment patients. The next two columns provide the corresponding information for patients in the control group. The next column, N_i, is the total number of patients from both groups at risk of dying just before time t_i. The last two columns give the expected number of deaths and corresponding variance for the experimental group, using the formulae above. The observed total number of deaths in the experimental treatment group is 8 and the expected number of deaths is 11.59, indicating that fewer deaths were observed in this group than one would have expected if the two treatment groups were equivalent in terms of survival. The variance is 3.964, and one simply calculates the value of the chi-square statistic as $(8 - 11.59)^2/3.964 = 3.25$ on 1 degree of freedom ($p = .08$).

An additional type of analysis frequently discussed in the clinical trial literature is a stratified, or adjusted, analysis. The purpose is to compare all the observations in both treatment groups, adjusting for one or more prognostic factors of interest. A stratified analysis can provide a more powerful test of treatment differences than an unstratified analysis by accounting for factors which represent an important source of variability. This form of analysis is frequently undertaken when there are significant imbalances between two treatment groups in regard to such factors. What is often overlooked is the fact that such adjustment for important variables is worthwhile even if no marked imbalance is present between the treatments. On the other hand, adjustment for unimportant variables can result in a considerable loss of power, and important treatment differences may go undetected. Thus expert statistical advice should be sought before results based on these methods are reported.

Generally speaking, a stratified analysis implies that the patients are first subdivided into smaller and more homogeneous groups called strata. A statistical comparison of treatment effects is made within each stratum separately and then combined over all strata to obtain an overall summary result. To perform a stratified analysis of the data in Table 3, one first notes that T status is an important factor for survival outcome, and thus it is reasonable to adjust for it in the analysis. One performs the same steps as described previously in calculating the adjusted logrank test except that the observed number of deaths, expected number of deaths, and the corresponding variance for the experimental group are calculated within each T class separately. The observed number of deaths is 3 for patients with T1 or T2 primary lesions in the experimental group. The corresponding expected number of deaths and variance is 5.31 and 1.453, respectively. For patients receiving the experimental treatment with T3 or T4 primary lesions, the observed, expected, and variance values are 5, 8.21, and 1.637, respectively.

The overall number of observed deaths in the new treatment group is $3+5 = 8$, as before. However, the corresponding total expected number of deaths is $5.31+8.21 = 13.52$, and the overall variance is $1.453+1.637 = 3.09$. Note that the expected number of total deaths in the experimental treatment group is larger than in the previous unstratified analysis, and the variance in this stratified analysis is smaller. This leads to a highly significant chi-square value on 1 degree of freedom of $(8-13.52)^2/3.09 = 9.86 \, (p < .001)$. Thus the two treatment groups differ very significantly in regard to survival after adjusting for T status, a conclusion that differs from that based on an unstratified analysis. In order to graphically display survival curves which take into account those characteristics adjusted for in the statistical analysis, methods described by Hankey and Myers [32] or Makuch [33] will prove useful.

It is a common misconception that 'stratified' analyses involve comparing the two treatments within each stratum separately, and reporting the p-value for the treatment comparison within each stratum separately. This type of analysis relates more to subgroup analysis and should be distinguished from a stratified procedure, such as that described above, which provides an overall test of comparative treatment efficacy by statistically combining evidence across the baseline strata. Conducting statistical tests within individual patient subgroups can be a hazardous procedure that generally should be avoided without expert statistical guidance. The pitfalls of this and other forms of multiplicity arising in the analysis of clinical trials are discussed further in the next section.

Problems of multiplicities in statistical analysis

Certain features of study design generate multiplicities and create difficulties in applying standard statistical procedures and interpreting the results. First, multiple end-points may be used to evaluate the effect of the therapy on a myriad of symptoms, objective measurements, or laboratory variables. Secondly, the therapeutic effect may be examined in subgroups of the data cross-classified by a variety of patient characteristics, e.g., age, sex, stage of disease, and other baseline factors which may or may not be considered, a priori, to have prognostic value. Thirdly, multiple analyses may be performed on closely-related endpoints (e.g., time to recurrence and survival). Finally, end-point data may be analyzed at frequent intervals throughout the study to detect positive treatment effects as soon as possible, to assure maximum safety and to minimize the impact of possible adverse effects.

The final results of a published study may be the culmination of a series of significance tests at various stages of the study and a detailed exploration of a large data set to substantiate specific claims about a new therapy.

Although it is important to arrive at evidence that is as strong as possible as soon as possible, the investigator must pay a price for the luxury of taking early looks at the data or exploring an unforeseen variety of hypotheses. The more significance tests that are conducted, the greater the possibility of drawing erroneous conclusions unless certain precautions are taken. For example, if two treatment groups are to be compared within only ten sub-groups defined by age, sex and disease stage, there is a 40% chance that at least one of the ten subgroups would turn up a significant treatment difference at the 5% level, even though the treatments had equivalent therapeutic value. This problem is overcome by the choice of a more stringent nominal significance level for each test, so that the overall significance level is maintained at some desired level such as 0.05.

It is often possible, in the design of the study, to avoid multiplicity problems by focusing the trial on a specific class of patients and clearly specifying at most two or three primary end-points in the study protocol. Tukey distinguishes between this type of focused clinical trial and a clinical 'inquiry' in which the goals of therapy and the target population are less well-defined [34]. Results in the latter situation would simply generate new hypotheses to be tested in more well-focused trials by drawing attention to subgroups of patients who appear to benefit from a particular therapy. In a clinical inquiry situation involving subgroup analyses, Tukey recommends a conservative adjustment of significance levels. If there are k subgroups of patients that would have been looked at for treatment differences seriously if results for them appeared interesting, he requires significance at the .05/k level before claiming significance at the .05 level in the subgroups that were indeed looked at. Note that this is an especially strict criterion since, if there are several end-points used to assess improvement, k is the product of the number of plausible end-points multiplied by the number of plausible subgroups. Because of the conservative nature of this adjustment, more focused trials hold greater promise for definitive evidence of treatment efficacy.

An equally serious source of multiplicity arises when the investigator analyzes treatment differences repeatedly as data accumulate. With such inter-

Table 4. Overall probability of achieving a result with a given nominal significance after n repeated tests when there is no difference between the two treatments (expressed as a percentage)

Nominal significance level (%)	Number of repeated significance tests (n)						
	1	2	3	4	5	10	25
1	1	1.8	2.4	2.9	3.3	4.7	7.0
5	5	8.3	10.7	12.6	14.2	19.3	26.6
10	10	16.0	20.2	23.4	26.0	34.2	44.9

im analyses, the probabilities associated with classical fixed sample size significance tests are not appropriate. If an experimenter repeatedly tests accumulating data at constant intervals to test the null hypothesis of no treatment difference at some nominal significance level, say 0.05, the actual probability of obtaining at least one significant difference when the null hypothesis is true increasingly exceeds 0.05 with each additional test. Table 4 shows the probability of achieving a result with a given nominal significance level after n repeated tests on accumulating data when there is no difference in effects of the two treatments [35]. One can see that the probabilities of exceeding critical levels in repeated tests can be substantially above the nominal level even for a modest number of interim looks. For example, the usual 5% significance level (i.e., the probability of falsely rejecting the null hypothesis) for a test performed only once, at the end of the study, increases to 19.3% after 10 repeated examinations of an on-going study. Even if the data were only examined at five approximately equally spaced intervals, probabilities given in this table for n = 5 exceed nominal levels by a multiple of about 3. Thus repeated testing of accumulating data, and stopping the trial when a given nominal significance level is achieved, without taking into account the number of tests performed increases the overall probability of incorrectly rejecting the null hypothesis to levels which may be unacceptable.

Several methods to account for multiple interim looks are available to address whether a trial should be terminated early or continued on to its planned termination. The results from any statistical method which indicate that early stopping is warranted should be taken as one piece of evidence to be integrated with other medical, ethical, and financial aspects of the study before the final decision to terminate is reached. We will describe two useful data-monitoring approaches which have the desirable feature that, if they do not provide evidence that early stopping of patient accrual is warranted, the p-value for the final test is approximately the same as if only a single statistical test were done. Thus the study can be designed as a fixed sample-size trial using the sample size methods described earlier.

The first is a group-sequential method developed by O'Brien and Fleming [36] for the binary outcome situation (e.g., tumor response or no tumor response, alive at three years or dead at three years, etc.). The method presumes that an analysis will be performed a total of N times, with approximately an equal number of patients accrued between each analysis time in each treatment group. One then calculates the usual z-statistic for comparing two proportions, and compares this value to the critical value specified by O'Brien and Fleming to support early stopping. For clinical trials in head and neck cancer, one might reasonably specify that a total of $N = 5$ statistical tests will be performed (four interim analyses and one final analysis) so that the overall probability of falsely rejecting the null hypothesis that the two treatments are equivalent is 0.05. Then one would entertain stopping the trial at the first interim analysis if the value of the z-statistic is 4.56 (p = .00001) or larger. Similar values for the z-statistic (p-value) are 3.23 (p = .0013), 2.63 (p = .0084) and 2.28 (.0025) for the second, third, and fourth interim analysis, respectively. Thus their method does not lead one to recommend stopping the study early unless the evidence is extremely persuasive. If the trial is not stopped early, then the final analysis is performed and a significant treatment difference is claimed if the value of the z-statistic exceeds 2.04 (p = .041). Although the final p-value is slightly less than the overall significance level of 0.05, this should be of little concern since any p-value should be interpreted as a guideline rather than a dogmatic indication of a true treatment difference.

If one wishes to use survival or some other time-to-an-event endpoint to monitor accrual, the approach by Rubinstein and Gail [37] should be useful. Unlike the O'Brien-Fleming procedure, the decision to stop accrual is separated from the formal analysis intended for publication. One should anticipate that several conditions will hold true in a particular clinical trial setting before using this procedure. First, the treatment course should be fairly short and should take place immediately after randomization. Second, once accrual is stopped, the patients already allocated to a particular treatment group should be followed with no change in therapy apart from what was permitted prior to termination. Thus the method is inappropriate if the treatment is administered chronically rather than fixed to a relatively short time period, since there may be a strong temptation to switch all patients to the apparently favorable therapy. Third, one should expect the ratio of death rates between the two groups to remain fairly constant over time. Finally, yearly accrual should be moderately high (50 or more patients) in order for the procedure to lead to possible early termination of the study. Under these conditions, the authors recommend a plan for the sequential monitoring of a trial comparing survival of two treatment groups with power 0.90 to detect a two-fold change in median survival at the two-sided α = 0.05 level. A total of 90 deaths would be required for this case. Then one can monitor the trial annually, or at whatever time intervals one desires, and stop accrual if either of the following conditions are satisfied: (1) the estimated remaining time to death 90, given that accrual is stopped, is estimated to be less than one year, or (2) the value of the logrank statistic is less than -3.84 or greater than 3.84 (this value corresponds to the 0.05 significance level). Once 90 deaths are attained, this monitoring procedure ensures that the final analysis can be undertaken without any statistical adjustment of the p-value while maintaining the overall significance level and power of the trial specified in the design stage. This somewhat surprising result holds true despite the repeated significance tests that were performed to evaluate stopping accrual early.

There are a variety of ways to incorporate data monitoring procedures into the design of a trial to facilitate early stopping. In general, before one considers such trial designs, one should be aware of potential difficulties. First, there is a need for accurate and prompt reporting of all end-point events so that interim data will be correct and ready for up-to-date analysis. Secondly, premature presentation or publication of interim findings may influence participating investigators. If there is little difference between treatments early on, some investigators may lose interest. If there are interesting but nonsignificant differences, some investigators may drop out of the trial; others may continue in an unreliable manner, removing patients prematurely, or perhaps interfering with randomization. It may be wise to have a statistician and a non-participating clinician check interim results, and disclose findings to others only when treatment differences are of sufficient magnitude to merit a discussion to terminate the trial. Thirdly, the end-point used for monitoring the trial may be incorrect, in the sense that important, but unanticipated events would not have a bearing on the statistical rules prescribed *a priori* for terminating the trial. Fourthly, since a clinical trial is a complex scientific experiment, one will have to grapple with possibly inadequate numbers of patients to investigate other hypotheses if the decision is made to stop a trial on the basis of a given criterion. Without adequate attention to these problems, the usefulness of any approach to repeated significance testing or early termination, no matter how carefully planned or technically feasible, will be severely limited.

In summary, multiplicities in the analysis of cancer trials can pose serious problems in the evaluation of new therapies. Proper planning and focused trial design are perhaps the most important measures that can be taken to bypass eventual difficulties in characterizing specific treatment effects. Whenever possible, hypotheses concerning subgroups and multiple end-points for study should be specified before data collection begins, based on reasonable expectations, and limited in number. Likewise, if interim analyses are planned, the end-point should be justifiable and the procedure should be formalized beforehand to account for repeated significance testing.

References

1. Friedman LM, Furberg CD, DeMets DL: Fundamentals of Clinical Trials. London, John Wright, 1981.
2. Proceedings of the Symposium on Designs for Clinical Cancer Research. Cancer Treat Rep. 64:363–538, 1980.
3. Byar DP, Simon RM, Friedewald WT, Schlesselman JJ, DeMets DL, Ellenberg JH, Gail MH, Ware JH: Randomized clinical trials. N Eng J Med 295:74–80, 1976.
4. Gehan EA, Freireich EJ: Non-randomized controls in cancer clinical trials. N Eng J Med 290:198–203, 1974.

5. Byar DP: Necessity and justification of randomized clinical studies. In: Tagnon HJ, Staquet MJ (eds) Controversies in Cancer Treatment. New York, Mason Publishing, 1979, pp 75–82.

6. Shaw LW, Chalmers TC: Ethics in cooperative clinical trials. Ann NY Acad Sciences 169:487–495, 1970.

7. Cox DR: Analysis of Binary Data. New York, Methuen Co., 1970.

8. Cox DR: Regression models and life tables (with discussion). J Royal Stat Soc B 34:187–220, 1972.

9. Farewell VT, D'Angio GJ: A simulated study of historical controls using real data. Biometrics 37:169–176, 1981.

10. Pocock SJ: Randomized clinical trials (letter). Brit Med J 1:1661, 1977.

11. Zelen M: A new design for randomized clinical trials. N Eng J Med 300:1273–1275, 1979.

12. Zelen M: Strategy and alternate randomized designs in cancer clinical trials. Cancer Treat Rep 66:1095–1100, 1982.

13. Fleming TR: Historical controls, data banks, and randomized trials in clinical research: A review. Cancer Treat Rep 66:1101–1106, 1982.

14. Peto R: Clinical trial methodology. Biomedicine 28:24–36, 1978.

15. Schoenfeld D, Gelber R: Designing and analyzing clinical trials which allow institutions to randomize patients to a subset of the treatments under study. Biometrics 35:825–829, 1979.

16. Makuch RW, Simon RM: A note on the design of multi-institution three-treatment studies. Cancer Clin Trials 1:301–303, 1978.

17. Zelen M: The randomization and stratification of patients to clinical trials. J Chron Dis 27:365–375, 1974.

18. Freiman JA, Chalmers TC, Smith H, Jr., et al.: The importance of beta, the type II error and sample size in the design and interpretation of the randomized control trial: Survey of 71 'negative' trials. N Eng J Med 299:690–694, 1978.

19. Casagrande JT, Pike MC, Smith PG: An improved formula for calculating sample sizes for comparing two binomial distributions. Biometrics 34:483–486, 1978.

20. Makuch RW, Simon RM: Sample size requirements for evaluating a conservative therapy. Cancer Treat Rep 62:1037–1040, 1978.

21. George SL, Desu MM: Planning the size and duration of a clinical trial studying the time to some critical event. J Chron Dis 27:15–24, 1974.

22. Makuch RW, Simon RM: Sample size requirements for comparing time-to-failure among k treatment groups. J Chron Dis 35:861–868, 1982.

23. Rubinstein LV, Gail MH, Santner TJ: Planning the duration of a comparative clinical trial with loss to follow-up and a period of continued observation. J Chron Dis 34:469–479, 1981.

24. Peto R, Pike MC, Armitage P, Breslow NE, Cox DR, Howard SV, Mantel N, McPherson K, Peto J, Smith PG: Design and analysis of randomized clinical trials requiring prolonged observation of each patient. Brit J Cancer 34:585–612, 1976 and 35:1–39, 1977.

25. Grizzle JE: A note on stratifying versus complete random assignment in clinical trials. Controlled Clin Trials 3:365–368, 1982.

26. Brown BW, Jr: Statistical controversies in the design of clinical trials — some personal views. Controlled Clin Trials 1:13–27, 1980.

27. Pocock SJ, Simon RM: Sequential treatment assignment with balancing for prognostic factors in the controlled clinical trial. Biometrics 31:103–115, 1975.

28. Efron B: Forcing a sequential experiment to be balanced. Biometrika 58:403–417, 1971.

29. Kaplan EL, Meier P: Nonparametric estimation from incomplete observations. J Am Stat Assn 458–481, 1958.

502

30. Gehan EA: A generalized Wilcoxon test for comparing arbitrarily singly-censored samples. Biometrika 52:203–224, 1965.
31. Mantel N: Evaluation of survival data and two new rank order statistics arising in its consideration. Cancer Chemo Rep 50:163–170, 1966.
32. Hankey BF, Myers MH: Evaluating differences in survival between two groups of patients. J Chron Dis 24:523–531, 1971.
33. Makuch RW: Adjusted survival curve estimation using covariates. J Chron Dis 35:437–443, 1982.
34. Tukey JW: Some thoughts on clinical trials, especially problems of multiplicity. Science 198:679–684, 1977.
35. McPherson K: Statistics: The problem of examining accumulating data more than once. N Eng J Med 290:501–502, 1974.
36. O'Brien PC, Fleming TR: A multiple testing procedure for clinical trials. Biometrics 35:549–556, 1979.
37. Rubinstein LV, Gail MH: Monitoring rules for stopping accrual in comparative survival studies. Controlled Clin Trials 3:325–343, 1982.

Index

508

512